Advances in Face Image Analysis:
Techniques and Technologies

Yu-Jin Zhang
Tsinghua University, Beijing, China

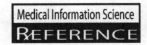

MEDICAL INFORMATION SCIENCE REFERENCE

Hershey · New York

Director of Editorial Content:	Kristin Klinger
Director of Book Publications:	Julia Mosemann
Acquisitions Editor:	Lindsay Johnston
Development Editor:	David DeRicco
Publishing Assistant:	Natalie Pronio
Typesetter:	Casey Conapitski
Production Editor:	Jamie Snavely
Cover Design:	Lisa Tosheff

Published in the United States of America by
Medical Information Science Reference (an imprint of IGI Global)
701 E. Chocolate Avenue
Hershey PA 17033
Tel: 717-533-8845
Fax: 717-533-8661
E-mail: cust@igi-global.com
Web site: http://www.igi-global.com

Library of Congress Cataloging-in-Publication Data

Advances in face image analysis : techniques and technologies / Yu-Jin Zhang, editor.   p. cm.
  Includes bibliographical references and index.
 Summary: "This book reviews and surveys new forward-thinking research and development in face image analysis technologies"--Provided by publisher. ISBN 978-1-61520-991-0 (hardcover) -- ISBN 978-1-61520-992-7 (ebook) 1. Human face recognition (Computer science) I. Zhang, Yu-Jin, 1954-   TA1650.A27 2010
  006.3'7--dc22
                    2009052794

British Cataloguing in Publication Data
A Cataloguing in Publication record for this book is available from the British Library.

Table of Contents

Section 1
Introduction and Background

Chapter 1
Face, Image, and Analysis 1
Yu-Jin Zhang, Tsinghua University, Beijing, China

Chapter 2
Maria De Marsico, Università di Romao "La Sapienza", Italy
Michele Nappi, Università di Salerno, Italy
Daniel Riccio, Università di Salerno, Italy
Sergio Vitulano, Università di Cagliari, Italy

Section 2
Facial Feature Extraction

Chapter 3
Stylianos Asteriadis, Aristotle University of Thessaloniki, Greece
Nikos Nikolaidis, Aristotle University of Thessaloniki, Greece & CERTH, Greece
Ioannis Pitas, Aristotle University of Thessaloniki, Greece & CERTH, Greece

Chapter 4
M. Ashraful Amin, Independent University Bangladesh (IUB), Bangladesh
Hong Yan, City University of Hong Kong, China

Section 5
Facial Expression Classification

Section 6
Invariance Techniques

Detailed Table of Contents

Section 1
Introduction and Background

Chapter 1

    Yu-Jin Zhang, Tsinghua University, Beijing, China

Face image analysis, consisting of automatic investigation of images of (human) faces, is a hot research topic and a fruitful field. This introductory chapter discusses several aspects of the history and scope of face image analysis and provides an outline of research development publications of this domain. More prominently, different modules and some typical techniques for face image analysis are listed, explained, described, or summarized from a general technical point of view. One picture of the advancements and the front of this complex and prominent field is provided. Finally, several challenges and prominent development directions for the future are identified.

Chapter 2

    Maria De Marsico, Università di Romao "La Sapienza", Italy
    Michele Nappi, Università di Salerno, Italy
    Daniel Riccio, Università di Salerno, Italy
    Sergio Vitulano, Università di Cagliari, Italy

In the last decade, many face recognition algorithms based on linear/non-linear methods, neural networks, wavelets, etc. have been proposed. Nevertheless, during Face Recognition Vendor Test 2002 most of them encountered problems outdoors. This lowers their reliability compared to other biometries, and underlines the need for more research. This chapter provides a survey of recent outcomes on the topic, addressing both 2D imagery and 3D models, to provide a starting reference to potential investigators. Tables containing different collections of parameters (such as input size, recognition rate, number of addressed problems) simplify comparisons. Some future directions are finally proposed.

Section 2
Facial Feature Extraction

Chapter 3
Stylianos Asteriadis, Aristotle University of Thessaloniki, Greece
Nikos Nikolaidis, Aristotle University of Thessaloniki, Greece & CERTH, Greece
Ioannis Pitas, Aristotle University of Thessaloniki, Greece & CERTH, Greece

Facial feature localization is an important task in numerous applications of face image analysis that include face recognition and verification, facial expression recognition, driver's alertness estimation, head pose estimation etc. Thus, the area has been a very active research field for many years and a multitude of methods appear in the literature. Depending on the targeted application, the proposed methods have different characteristics and are designed to perform in different setups. Thus, a method of general applicability seems to be away from the current state of the art. This chapter intends to offer an up-to-date literature review of facial feature detection algorithms. A review of the image databases and performance metrics that are used to benchmark these algorithms is also provided.

Chapter 4
M. Ashraful Amin, Independent University Bangladesh (IUB), Bangladesh
Hong Yan, City University of Hong Kong, China

This experimental study determines the characteristics of Gabor and Log-Gabor filters for face recognition. In the experiment, two sixth order data tensor are created; one containing the basic Gabor feature vectors and the other containing the basic Log-Gabor feature vectors. This study reveals the characteristics of the filter orientations for Gabor and Log-Gabor filters for face recognition. These two implementations show that the Gabor filter having orientation zero means oriented at 0 degree with respect to the aligned face has the highest discriminating ability, while Log-Gabor filter with orientation three means 45 degree has the highest discriminating ability. This result is consistent across three different frequencies (scales) used for this experiment. It is also observed that for both the wavelets, filters with low frequency have higher discriminating ability.

Chapter 5
Yuanjia Du, Trident Microsystems Europe B.V., The Netherlands
Ling Shao, The University of Sheffield, UK

In this chapter, the authors present an efficient retrieval technique for human face images based on bag of facial features. A visual vocabulary is built beforehand using an invariant descriptor computed on detected image regions. The vocabulary is refined in two ways to make the retrieval system more efficient. Firstly, the visual vocabulary is minimized by only using facial features selected on face regions which are detected by an accurate face detector. Secondly, three criteria, namely Inverted-Occurrence-Frequency Weights, Average Feature Location Distance and Reliable Nearest-Neighbors, are calculated in advance to make the on-line retrieval procedure more efficient and precise. The proposed system is experimented on the Caltech Human Face Database. The results show that this technique is very effective and efficient on face image retrieval.

Section 3
Feature Dimensionality Reduction

Chapter 6

Sébastien Gadat, Université Paul Sabatier, France

Variable selection for classification is a crucial paradigm in image analysis. Indeed, images are generally described by a large amount of features (pixels, edges ...) although it is difficult to obtain a sufficiently large number of samples to draw reliable inference for classifications using the whole number of features. The authors describe in this chapter some simple and effective features selection methods based on filter strategy. They also provide some more sophisticated methods based on margin criterion or stochastic approximation techniques that achieve great performances of classification with a very small proportion of variables. Most of these "wrapper" methods are dedicated to a special case of classifier, except the Optimal features Weighting algorithm (denoted OFW in the sequel) which is a meta-algorithm and works with any classifier. A large part of this chapter will be dedicated to the description of the description of OFW and hybrid OFW algorithms. The authors illustrate also several other methods on practical examples of face detection problems.

Chapter 7

V. Jadhav Dattatray, Vishwakarma Institute of Technology, India
S. Holambe Raghunath, SGGS Institute of Engineering and Technology, India

Various changes in illumination, expression, viewpoint, and plane rotation present challenges to face recognition. Low dimensional feature representation with enhanced discrimination power is of paramount importance to face recognition system. This chapter presents transform based techniques for extraction of efficient and effective features to solve some of the challenges in face recognition. The techniques are based on the combination of Radon transform, Discrete Cosine Transform (DCT), and Discrete Wavelet Transform (DWT). The property of Radon transform to enhance the low frequency components, which are useful for face recognition, has been exploited to derive the effective facial features. The comparative study of various transform based techniques under different conditions like varying illumination, changing facial expressions, and in-plane rotation is presented in this chapter. The experimental results using FERET, ORL, and Yale databases are also presented in the chapter.

Chapter 8

Le Li, Tsinghua University, Beijing, China
Yu-Jin Zhang, Tsinghua University, Beijing, China

Non-negative matrix factorization (NMF) is a more and more popular method for non-negative dimensionality reduction and feature extraction of non-negative data, especially face images. Currently no NMF algorithm holds not only satisfactory efficiency for dimensionality reduction and feature extraction of face images but also high ease of use. To improve the applicability of NMF, this chapter proposes a new monotonic, fixed-point algorithm called FastNMF by implementing least squares error-based non-negative factorization essentially according to the basic properties of parabola functions. The minimization problem corresponding to an operation in FastNMF can be analytically solved just by this operation, which is far beyond existing NMF algorithms' power, and therefore FastNMF holds much higher efficiency, which is validated by a set of experimental results. For the simplicity of design philosophy, FastNMF is still one of NMF algorithms that are the easiest to use and the most comprehensible. Besides, theoretical analysis and experimental results also show that FastNMF tends to extract facial features with better representation ability than popular multiplicative update-based algorithms.

Section 4
Face Recognition

In this chapter, the authors discuss the problem of face recognition using sparse representation classification (SRC). The SRC classifier has recently emerged as one of the latest paradigm in the context of view-based face recognition. The main aim of the chapter is to provide an insight of the SRC algorithm with thorough discussion of the underlying "Compressive Sensing" theory. Comprehensive experimental evaluation of the approach is conducted on a number of standard databases using exemplary evaluation protocols to provide a comparative index with the benchmark face recognition algorithms. The algorithm is also extended to the problem of video-based face recognition for more realistic applications.

Chapter 10

In this chapter the authors review probabilistic approaches to face recognition and present extended treatment of one particular approach. Here, the face image is decomposed into an additive sum of two parts: a deterministic component, which depends on an underlying representation of identity and a stochastic component which explains the fact that two face images from the same person are not identical. Inferences about matching are made by comparing different probabilistic models rather than comparing distance to an identity template in some projected space. The authors demonstrate that this model comparison is superior to distance comparison. Furthermore, the authors show that performance can be further improved by sampling the feature space and combining models trained using these feature subspaces. Both random sampling with and without replacement significantly improves performance. Finally, the authors illustrate how this probabilistic approach can be adapted for keypoint localization (e.g. finding the eyes, nose and mouth etc.). The authors show that recognition and keypoint localization performance are comparable to using manual labelling.

Chapter 11

    Marios Kyperoundtas, Aristotle University of Thessaloniki, Greece

    Anastasios Tefas, Aristotle University of Thessaloniki, Greece

    Ioannis Pitas, Aristotle University of Thessaloniki, Greece

Large training databases introduce a level of complexity that often degrades the classification performance of face recognition methods. In this chapter, an overview of various approaches that are employed in order to overcome this problem is presented and, in addition, a specific discriminant learning approach that combines dynamic training and partitioning is described in detail. This face recognition methodology employs dynamic training in order to implement a person-specific iterative classification process. This process employs discriminant clustering, where, by making use of an entropy-based measure; the algorithm adapts the coordinates of the discriminant space with respect to the characteristics of the test face. As a result, the training space is dynamically reduced to smaller spaces, where linear separability among the face classes is more likely to be achieved. The process iterates until one final cluster is retained, which consists of a single face class that represents the best match to the test face. The performance of this methodology is evaluated on standard large face databases and results show that the proposed framework gives a good solution to the face recognition problem.

Section 5
Facial Expression Classification

Chapter 12

    Zakia Hammal, Université de Montréal, Canada

This chapter addresses recent advances in computer vision for facial expression classification. The authors present the different processing steps of the problem of automatic facial expression recognition. The authors describe the advances of each stage of the problem and review the future challenges towards the application of such systems to everyday life situations. They also introduce the importance of taking advantage of the human strategy by reviewing advances of research in psychology towards multidisciplinary approach for facial expression classification. Finally the authors describe one contribution which aims at dealing with some of the discussed challenges.

Chapter 13

    Siu-Yeung Cho, Nanyang Technological University, Singapore

    Teik-Toe Teoh, Nanyang Technological University, Singapore

    Yok-Yen Nguwi, Nanyang Technological University, Singapore

This chapter discusses the issues on how advanced feature selection techniques together with good classifiers can play a vital important role of real-time facial expression recognition. Several feature selection methods and classifiers are discussed and their evaluations for real-time facial expression recognition are presented in this chapter. The content of this chapter is a way to open-up a discussion about building a real-time system to read and respond to the emotions of people from facial expressions.

This chapter addresses the recognition of basic facial expressions. It has three main contributions. First, the authors introduce a view- and texture independent schemes that exploits facial action parameters estimated by an appearance-based 3D face tracker. The authors represent the learned facial actions associated with different facial expressions by time series. Two dynamic recognition schemes are proposed: (1) the first is based on conditional predictive models and on an analysis-synthesis scheme, and (2) the second is based on examples allowing straightforward use of machine learning approaches. Second, the authors propose an efficient recognition scheme based on the detection of keyframes in videos. Third, the authors compare the dynamic scheme with a static one based on analyzing individual snapshots and show that in general the former performs better than the latter. The authors provide evaluations of performance using Linear Discriminant Analysis (LDA), Non parametric Discriminant Analysis (NDA), and Support Vector Machines (SVM).

Section 6
Invariance Techniques

Thanks to enormous research efforts, the recognition rates achievable with the state-of-the-art face recognition technology are steadily growing, even though some issues still pose major challenges to the technology. Amongst these challenges, coping with illumination-induced appearance variations is one of the biggest and still not satisfactorily solved. A number of techniques have been proposed in the literature to cope with the impact of illumination ranging from simple image enhancement techniques, such as histogram equalization, to more elaborate methods, such as anisotropic smoothing or the logarithmic total variation model. This chapter presents an overview of the most popular and efficient normalization techniques that try to solve the illumination variation problem at the preprocessing level. It assesses the techniques on the YaleB and XM2VTS databases and explores their strengths and weaknesses from the theoretical and implementation point of view.

While current face recognition algorithms have provided convincing performance on frontal face poses, recognition is far less effective when the pose and illumination conditions vary. Here the authors show how compound image transforms can be used for face recognition in various poses and illumination conditions. The method works by first dividing each image into four equal-sized tiles. Then, image features are extracted from the face images, transforms of the images, and transforms of transforms of the images. Finally, each image feature is assigned with a Fisher score, and test images are classified by using a simple Weighted Nearest Neighbor rule such that the Fisher scores are used as weights. An important feature of this method is that the recognition accuracy improves as the number of subjects in the dataset gets larger.

Perception and recognition of faces presented upright are better than Perception and recognition of faces presented inverted. The difference between upright and inverted orientations is greater in face recognition than in non-face object recognition. This Face-Inversion Effect is explained by the "Configural Processing" hypothesis that inversion disrupts configural information processing and leaves the featural information intact. The present chapter discusses two important findings that cast doubt on this hypothesis: inversion impairs recognition of isolated features (hair & forehead, and eyes), and certain facial configural information is not affected by inversion. The chapter focuses mainly on the latter finding, which reveals a new type of facial configural information, the "Eye-Illusion", which is based on certain geometrical illusions. The chapter proposes that a face is composed of various kinds of configural information that are differently impaired by inversion: from no effect (the Eye-Illusion) to a large effect (the Face-Inversion Effect).

Preface

The analysis of the human face via image (and video) is one of the most interesting and focusing research topics in the last years for the image community. From the analysis (sensing, computing, and perception) of face images, much information can be extracted, such as the sex/gender, age, facial expression, emotion/temper, mentality/mental processes and behavior/psychology, and the health of the person captured. According to this information, many practical tasks can be performed and completed; these include not only person identification or verification (face recognition), but also the estimation and/or determination of person's profession, hobby, name (recovered from memory), etc.

Research on face image analysis has been carried out and is being conducted around various application topics, such as (in alphabetical order) age estimation, biometrics, biomedical instrumentations, emotion assessment, face recognition, facial expression classification, gender determination, human-computer/human-machine interaction, human behavior and emotion study, industrial automation, military service, psychosis judgment, security checking systems, social signal processing, surveillance systems, sport training, tele-medicine service, etc.

To push the deep theoretical study of this important area, to prompt the further development of face analysis techniques, and to guide the people working in image area for applying suitable methods, a comprehensive and detailed volume for the new advancements of face image analysis would be a must, and these are the overall objectives and the main mission of this book. Comprehensive coverage of various branches of face image analysis is provided by more than 30 leading experts from 16 countries and regions around the world.

In addition, new achievements and new challenges often come up together. With the accumulation of research results in face image analysis, the need for a uniform description of this area and a review of recent developments are even increasing. This book tries to set the fundamental knowledge for, and introduce the advancements in recent years in, face image analysis. The principal concern of this book is to provide those in the face image analysis community with a general methodology that allows them to integrate the research results and to apply them in various applications.

The complete coverage of this book is also reflected in the title, "Advances in Face Image Analysis: Techniques and Technologies," where techniques would refer to the different methodologies and models utilized, whereas technologies would refer to the applications and tools applied. This book is intended for scientists and engineers who are engaged in the research and development of face image analysis techniques and who wish to keep their paces with the advances of this field. The objective of this collection is to review and survey new forward-thinking research and development in face image analysis technologies.

Face image analysis is a specialized field of image analysis (that is an important layer of image engineering), though face images have some particularities, the methodologies and techniques presented in this book are ready to be extended to other types of images, and are the foundation of many image analysis applications.

As various face analysis techniques have been widely used in many areas, the audience of such a book should be all persons that study/research in the disciplines such as, image and information processing, computer vision, pattern recognition. Such a book would be suitable for using in specialized courses for graduate students and to be read by researchers in companies of related domains.

The whole book includes 17 chapters and they are organized into six sections. They covers several distinctive research fields in face image analysis and form a solid background for treating feature detection, face recognition, facial expression, etc. They also provide many state-of-the-art advancements and achievements in this field. Some detailed descriptions, respectively for each section and each chapter, are provided in the following.

Section 1 is an "**Introduction and Background**" section, which is for the purpose of providing some historical surroundings information, various achieved results and a brief overview of current research focus of face image analysis, which consists of one opening chapter (Chapter 1) and one surveying chapter (Chapter 2).

Chapter 1 is entitled "*Face, Image, and Analysis*." The 3 terms form a unique composition, face image analysis (FIA). Face image analysis consists of automatic investigation of images of (human) faces, is a hot research topic and a fruitful field. This introductory chapter discusses several aspects of the history and scope of face image analysis and provides an outline of research development publications of this domain. More prominently, different modules and some typical techniques for face image analysis are listed, explained, described, or summarized from a general technical point of view. One picture of the advancements and the front of this complex and prominent field is provided. Finally, several challenges and prominent development directions for the future are identified.

Chapter 2 is entitled "*Face Searching in Large Databases*." With the significant progress of biometric research, increasingly efficient techniques have been developed. Among them, face recognition represents a good solution for local/remote access security even under less controlled conditions. In the last decade, many algorithms based on linear/non-linear methods, neural networks, wavelets, etc. have been proposed. Nevertheless, during Face Recognition Vendor Test 2002 most of them encountered problems outdoors. This lowers the reliability of human face identification compared to other biometrics, and underlines the need for more research. This chapter provides a survey of recent outcomes on the topic, and supply a starting reference to potential investigators. Both 2-D imagery and 3-D models are addressed. Several tables containing different collections of parameters (such as input size, recognition rate, number of addressed problems) make the comparison of different methods without difficulty. Some future directions are finally proposed.

Section 2 is for "**Facial Feature Extraction**", which is a fundamental task in all analysis problems. Once the faces from images are captured, some suitable features should be selected and extracted from these images to represent and describe the face characteristics. These features should represent and/or reflect the particularity of faces in images and provide the base for further treatments. Commonly used features include geometric features, such as distance, angle, curvature, etc; and grey level feature, such as color, texture of faces. Features can also be classified as local ones or holistic ones. This section consists of three chapters (Chapter 3 to Chapter 5) utilizing different techniques.

Chapter 3 is entitled "*A Review of Facial Feature Detection Algorithms.*" Facial feature detection is an important task in numerous applications of face image analysis that include face recognition and verification, facial expression recognition, driver's alertness estimation, head pose estimation etc. Thus, the area has been a very active research field for many years and a multitude of methods appear in the literature. Depending on the targeted application, the proposed methods have different characteristics and are designed to perform in different setups. Thus, a method of general applicability seems to be away from the current state of the art. This chapter intends to offer an up-to-date literature review of facial feature detection algorithms. A review of the image databases and performance metrics that are used to benchmark these algorithms is also provided.

Chapter 4 is entitled "*Gabor and Log-Gabor Wavelet for Face Recognition.*" Gabor wavelet is often applied to extract relevant features from a facial image in practice. This wavelet is constructed using filters of multiple scales and orientations. Based on Gabor's theory of communication, Gabor wavelet and Log-Gabor wavelet are proposed to acquire initial features from 2-D images. Theoretically the main difference between these two wavelets is Log-Gabor wavelet produces DC free filter responses, whereas Gabor filter responses retain DC components. This experimental study determines the characteristics of Gabor and Log-Gabor filters for face recognition. In the experiment, two sixth order data tensor are created; one containing the basic Gabor feature vectors and the other containing the basic Log-Gabor feature vectors. This study reveals the characteristics of the filter orientations for Gabor and Log-Gabor filters for face recognition. These two implementations show that the Gabor filter having orientation zero means oriented at 0 degree with respect to the aligned face has the highest discriminating ability, while Log-Gabor filter with 45 degree of orientation has the highest discriminating ability. This result is consistent across three different frequencies (scales) used for this experiment. It is also observed that for both the wavelets, filters with low frequency have higher discriminating ability.

Chapter 5 is entitled "*Efficient Face Retrieval Based on Bag of Facial Features.*" In this chapter, an efficient retrieval technique for human face images based on bag of facial features is presented. A visual vocabulary is built beforehand using an invariant descriptor computed on detected image regions. The vocabulary is refined in two ways to make the retrieval system more efficient. Firstly, the visual vocabulary is minimized by only using facial features selected on face regions which are detected by an accurate face detector. Secondly, three criteria, namely Inverted-Occurrence-Frequency Weights, Average Feature Location Distance and Reliable Nearest-Neighbors, are calculated in advance to make the on-line retrieval procedure more efficient and precise. The proposed system is experimented on the Caltech Human Face Database. The results show that this technique is very effective and efficient on face image retrieval.

Section 3 is for "**Feature Dimensionality Reduction**". Often a large number of features can be extracted from face images, as human face is a non-rigid natural object and many factors influence the appearance of face in images. The original features extracted correspond to the data in high dimensional space. Directly using these high dimensional data cause not only computational problems but also inaccuracy of analysis results. Therefore, making the reduction of feature dimension, before further treatments is necessary. This section consists of three chapters (Chapter 6 to Chapter 8) describing different methods for this purpose.

Chapter 6 is entitled "*Feature Selection in High Dimension.*" Variable selection for classification is a crucial paradigm in image analysis. Indeed, images are generally described by a large amount of features (pixels, edges …) although it is difficult to obtain a sufficiently large number of samples to draw reliable inference for classifications using the whole number of features. In this chapter, some simple and effective features selection methods based on filter strategy are described. Some more sophisticated methods based on margin criterion or stochastic approximation techniques that achieve great performances of classification with a very small proportion of variables are provided. Most of these "wrapper" methods are dedicated to a special case of classifier, except the Optimal Features Weighting (OFW) algorithm that is a meta-algorithm and works with any classifier. A large part of this chapter will be dedicated to the description of the description of OFW algorithm and hybrid OFW algorithms.

Chapter 7 is entitled *"Transform Based Feature Extraction and Dimensionality Reduction."* Low dimensional feature representation with enhanced discrimination power is of paramount importance to face recognition system. This chapter presents transform based techniques for extraction of efficient and effective features to solve some of the challenges in face recognition. The techniques are based on the combination of Radon transform, Discrete Cosine Transform (DCT), and Discrete Wavelet Transform (DWT). The property of Radon transform to enhance the low frequency components, which are useful for face recognition, has been exploited to derive the effective facial features. The comparative study of various transform based techniques under different conditions like varying illumination, changing facial expressions, and in-plane rotation is presented. The experimental results using FERET, ORL, and Yale databases are also presented.

Chapter 8 is entitled *"FastNMF: Efficient NMF Algorithm for Reducing Feature Dimension."* Non-negative matrix factorization (NMF) is a more and more popular method for non-negative dimensionality reduction and feature extraction of non-negative data, especially face images. Currently, no single NMF algorithm holds not only satisfactory efficiency for dimensionality reduction and feature extraction of face images but also high ease of use. To improve the applicability of NMF, this chapter proposes a new monotonic, fixed-point algorithm called FastNMF by implementing least squares error-based non-negative factorization essentially according to the basic properties of parabola functions. The minimization problem corresponding to an operation in FastNMF can be analytically solved just by this operation, which is far beyond existing NMF algorithms' power. Therefore, FastNMF holds much higher efficiency, which is validated by a set of experimental results. From the point of view of simplicity in design philosophy, FastNMF is also one of NMF algorithms that are the easiest to use and the most comprehensible. Besides, theoretical analysis and experimental results show that FastNMF tends to extract facial features with better representation ability than popular multiplicative update-based algorithms.

Section 4 is for **"Face Recognition"**. Based on the dimensionality reduced features, further treatment would make the recognition of the identity of faces possible. Face recognition is currently the most prominent direction in face image analysis, with both a large numbers of research publications and a various types of application systems, for both verification and identification. This section consists of three chapters (Chapter 9 to Chapter 11) concentrated on employing newly developed theories and tools for face recognition.

Chapter 9 is entitled *"Sparse Representation for View-Based Face Recognition."* In this chapter, the problem of face recognition using sparse representation classification (SRC) is discussed. The SRC classifier has recently emerged as one of the latest paradigm in the context of view-based face recognition. The main aim of the chapter is to provide an insight of the SRC algorithm with thorough discussion of the underlying "Compressive Sensing" theory. Comprehensive experimental evaluation of the approach is conducted on a number of standard databases using exemplary evaluation protocols to provide a comparative index with the benchmark for face recognition algorithms. The algorithm is also extended to the problem of video-based face recognition for more realistic applications.

Chapter 10 is entitled "*Probabilistic Methods for Face Registration and Recognition.*" In this chapter many probabilistic approaches to face recognition are reviewed and the extended treatment of one particular approach is presented. Here, the face image is decomposed into an additive sum of two parts: a deterministic component that depends on an underlying representation of identity and a stochastic component that explains the difference of two face images from the same person. Inferences about matching are made by comparing different probabilistic models rather than comparing distance to an identity template in some projected space. It is demonstrated that this model comparison is superior to distance comparison. Furthermore, its performance can be further improved by sampling the feature space and combining models trained using these feature subspaces. Both random sampling with and without replacement significantly improves performance. Finally, this probabilistic approach can be adapted for keypoint localization. The recognition and keypoint localization performance are comparable to those using manual labelling.

Chapter 11 is entitled "*Discriminant Learning Using Training Space Partitioning.*" Using large training databases often introduces a level of complexity that often degrades the classification performance of face recognition methods. In this chapter, an overview of various approaches that are employed in order to overcome this problem is presented first. In addition, a specific discriminant learning approach that combines dynamic training and partitioning is described in detail. This face recognition methodology employs dynamic training in order to implement a person-specific iterative classification process. This process employs discriminant clustering by making use of an entropy-based measure; the algorithm adapts the coordinates of the discriminant space with respect to the characteristics of the test face. As a result, the training space is dynamically reduced to smaller spaces, where linear separation of the face classes is more likely to be achieved. The process iterates until one final cluster is retained, which consists of a single face class that represents the best match to the test face. The performance of this methodology is evaluated on standard face databases and results show that the proposed framework gives a good solution to the face recognition problem.

Section 5 is for "**Facial Expression Classification**". This task has long time attracted the attention of sociologists and become a focused theme recently in engineering community. Different classes of expression have been defined. The sociologists often classify facial expression into 18 groups, while many computer scientists follow the classification scheme of psychoanalyst to classify facial expression into 6 basic kinds. Another classification scheme combining also the knowledge from anatomy uses 44 action units to describe various facial expressions. This section consists of three chapters (Chapter 12 to Chapter 14) explaining some recent advancements.

Chapter 12 is entitled "*From Face to Facial Expression.*" This chapter addresses recent advances in computer vision for facial expression classification. The different processing steps of the problem of automatic facial expression recognition are presented. The advances of each stage of the problem are described and the future challenges towards the application of such systems to every day life situations are discussed. The importance of taking advantage of the human strategy by reviewing advances of research in psychology towards multidisciplinary approach for facial expression classification is also introduced. Finally, one contribution that aims at dealing with some of the discussed challenges is provided.

Chapter 13 is entitled "*Facial Expression Analysis by Machine Learning.*" Considering a facial expression is formed by contracting or relaxing different facial muscles on human face that results in temporally deformed facial features, some challenges of such system are discussed. For instances, lighting condition is a very difficult problem to constraint and regulate. On the other hand, real-time processing is also a challenging problem since there are so many facial features to be extracted and processed. Often, conventional classifiers are not even effective to handle those features and then produce good classification performance. This chapter discusses the issues on how the advanced feature selection techniques together with good classifiers can play a vital important role of real-time facial expression recognition. Several feature selection methods and classifiers are discussed and their evaluations for real-time facial expression recognition are presented. This chapter opens-up a discussion about building a real-time system to read and respond to the emotions of people from facial expressions.

Chapter 14 is entitled "*Subtle Facial Expression Recognition in Still Images and Videos*." This chapter addresses the recognition of basic facial expressions. It has three main contributions. First, a view- and texture independent schemes that exploits facial action parameters estimated by an appearance-based 3D face tracker is introduced. The learned facial actions associated with different facial expressions by time series are represented. Two dynamic recognition schemes are proposed: one is based on conditional predictive models and on an analysis-synthesis scheme; another is based on examples allowing straightforward use of machine learning approaches. Second, an efficient recognition scheme based on the detection of key-frames in videos is proposed. Third, the dynamic scheme with a static one based on analyzing individual snapshots is compared, the result shows that in general the former performs better than the latter. Evaluations of performance using Linear Discriminant Analysis (LDA), Non parametric Discriminant Analysis (NDA), and Support Vector Machines (SVM) are provided.

Section 6 deals with some "**Invariance Techniques**". Many techniques have been developed for face images obtained under frontal pose and optimal lighting conditions, though their performances attend reasonable high score, the recognition performance severely degrades with pose and lighting variations, as well as expression variations. These variations, for example, could make one's face image more like other person's images than his/her own image. This section consists of three chapters (Chapter 15 to Chapter 17) presenting suitable techniques for cope with these variations for face recognition.

Chapter 15 is entitled "*Photometric Normalization Techniques for Illumination Invariance*." Thanks to the enormous research effort made by different research groups from universities and companies around the world, the recognition rates achievable with the state-of-the-art face recognition technology are steadily growing, even though some issues still pose major challenges to the technology. Amongst these challenges, coping with illumination-induced appearance variations is one of the biggest and still not satisfactorily solved. A number of techniques have been proposed in the literature to cope with the impact of illumination ranging from simple image enhancement techniques, such as histogram equalization, to more elaborate methods, such as anisotropic smoothing or the logarithmic total variation model. This chapter presents an overview of the most popular and efficient normalization techniques that try to solve the illumination variation problem at the preprocessing level. It assesses the techniques on the YaleB and XM2VTS databases and explores their strengths and weaknesses from the theoretical and implementation point of view.

Chapter 16 is entitled "*Pose and Illumination Invariance with Compound Image Transforms*." While current face recognition algorithms have provided convincing performance on frontal face poses, recognition is far less effective when the pose and illumination conditions vary. This chapter shows how compound image transforms can be used for face recognition in various poses and illumination conditions. The method works by first dividing each image into four equal-sized tiles. Then, image features are extracted from the face images, transforms of the images, and transforms of transforms of the images. Finally, each image feature is assigned with a Fisher score, and test images are classified by using a simple Weighted Nearest Neighbor rule such that the Fisher scores are used as weights. Experimental results using the full color FERET dataset show that with no parameter tuning, the accuracy of rank-10 recognition for frontal, quarter-profile, and half-profile images is ~98%, ~94% and ~91%, respectively.

The proposed method also achieves perfect accuracy on several other face recognition datasets such as Yale B, ORL and JAFFE. An important feature of this method is that the recognition accuracy improves as the number of subjects in the dataset gets larger.

Chapter 17 is entitled "*Configural Processing Hypothesis and Face-Inversion Effect*." Perception and recognition of faces presented upright are better than that of faces presented inverted. The difference between upright and inverted orientations is greater in face recognition than in non-face object recognition. This face-inversion effect is explained by the "Configural Processing" hypothesis that inversion disrupts configural information processing and leaves the featural information intact. This chapter discusses two important findings that cast doubt on this hypothesis: inversion impairs recognition of isolated features (hair & forehead, and eyes), and certain facial configural information is not affected by inversion. The chapter focuses mainly on the latter finding, which reveals a new type of facial configural information, the "Eye-Illusion", which is based on certain geometrical illusions. The eye-illusion tended to resist inversion in experimental tasks of both perception and recognition. It resisted inversion also when its magnitude was reduced. Similar results were obtained with "Headlight-Illusion" produced on a car's front, and with "Form-Illusion" produced in geometrical forms. However, the eye-illusion was greater than the headlight-illusion, which in turn was greater than the form-illusion. These findings were explained by the "General Visual-Mechanism" hypothesis in terms of levels of visual information learning. The chapter proposes that a face is composed of various kinds of configural information that are differently impaired by inversion: from no effect (the eye-illusion) to a large effect (the face-inversion effect).

In summary, the *17 chapters* in *6 sections*, a total of *148 figures, 54 tables, 243 equations, 124 key terms and definition*, and the list of more than *800 cited references* of this book offer a comprehensive and vivid image about the recent achievements and current state of face image analysis, and provide a set of general and detailed information on the advances in face image analysis.

Yu-Jin Zhang
Tsinghua University, Beijing, China

Acknowledgment

With great pleasure, the time has come to write this page.

First, sincere thanks should go to the other 32 authors, coming from 16 countries and regions (9 from Asia, 18 from Europe, 2 from North America, and 3 from Oceania). They have made great contributions to this project, such as promptly submitting own chapters with their domain knowledge and research results, as well as carefully reviewing others' chapters for the quality and also the readability and coherence of this book.

IGI Global has provided excellent assistance and guidance along with this project. Special gratitude goes to editors Elizabeth Ardner and Dave DeRicco for their valuable communication and suggestion throughout the development process.

I wish to thank the support made by National Nature Science Foundation of China under grant NNSF-60872084 in providing a comfortable environment for enjoyable scientific works.

Last, but not least, I am indebted to my wife, my daughter and my parents for their encouragement, support, patience, tolerance and understanding during the last two years.

Yu-Jin Zhang
Editor
Tsinghua University, Beijing, China

Section 1
Introduction and Background

Chapter 1
Face, Image, and Analysis

Yu-Jin Zhang
Tsinghua University, Beijing, China

ABSTRACT

Face image analysis, consisting of automatic investigation of images of (human) faces, is a hot research topic and a fruitful field. This introductory chapter discusses several aspects of the history and scope of face image analysis and provides an outline of research development publications of this domain. More prominently, different modules and some typical techniques for face image analysis are listed, explained, described, or summarized from a general technical point of view. One picture of the advancements and the front of this complex and prominent field is provided. Finally, several challenges and prominent development directions for the future are identified.

INTRODUCTION

The face is an important part of human body. Face images can be used to identify a person, to assess people's feeling, to transmit various kinds of information, to communicate with other persons, etc. The information obtained from face images contains abundant meanings, such as the race, gender, age, health, emotion, psychology/ mentation, profession, etc. Therefore, it is not surprise that researches and applications centered on face images is one of the hottest topics in

information science, and even in social science. For example, face recognition stands as the most appealing biometric modality, since it is the natural mode of identification among humans and is very unobtrusive.

After long time intensive research works, together with the progress in electronic equipments and computational devices, some remarkable accomplishments in face image researches have been reported and some real applications have been accomplished. With the accumulation of the research results and application experiences, it is expected that automatic investigation of face images would be possible under various difficult

DOI: 10.4018/978-1-61520-991-0.ch001

conditions in the near future and would allow people to use it in areas such as biometrics, bio-medical applications, human computer interaction, human behavior and emotion study, security and surveillance system, etc.

Various image techniques have been developed to treat different images (and videos, the image sequences) these years. These techniques can be collected into three groups, (i.e., image processing (IP), image analysis (IA), and image understanding (IU)). In a structural sense, IP, IA, and IU build up three interconnected layers of image engineering (IE), a new discipline of information science.

The automatic investigation of face images is based on and evolved from a number of image techniques, such as image segmentation, object detection and object tracking, image classification, image pattern recognition, and image matching etc. According to the above classification of image techniques in image engineering, and the current research and application levels, techniques used to treat face images are mainly under the category of image analysis. Therefore, the automatic investigation of face images is often called face image analysis, though before analysis, many image processing techniques have been served in various pre-processing stages; and after analysis, some image understanding techniques might be used to further interpret the original world.

While human beings are quite good in seeing face images and picking out suitable information for making appropriate decision, the ability of automatic analysis of face images in complex scene by computers is still limited. In other words, face image analysis is a difficult problem for a computer but is relatively straightforward for a human being. This is often explained by the "fact" that the computer is quite suitable for low-level image treatments while the human brain is more preferred for high-level interpretations of scene from images. However, with the theoretical progress and the wide applications of face image analysis in the recent years, this field is undergo-

ing great changes. A general sketch for this field and its advancements will be given in this chapter.

BACKGROUND

In the following, several aspects of the history and scope of face image analysis are discussed, and an outline of research developments and publications is provided.

History and Scope

Face of a person is often the first part perceived by other people. Related researches, especially from psychological and psychophysical point of view, have long been practiced by specialists. Using image analysis techniques to study face images, however, is only considered in recent years with the mature of image techniques. For example, automatic face recognition has been actively studied for over three decades as a means of human identification.

The communication and co-operation between scientists and engineers have put the research and applications in this field forward dramatically. Not only still face images captured in the front, with suitable lighting and without occlusion can be investigate, but also dynamic faces of different ages, different poses, with different lighting conditions, having different expressions can be analyzed.

Getting into 21 century, many techniques have been developed, and more research results have been accumulated. On the other side, the requirements for security, human-machine interaction, etc., are getting more and more attentions. All these greatly contribute to the fast progresses of the field of face image analysis.

Face images consist of large information, and the analysis on these images can provide many cues for various purposes. The scope of face image analysis includes not only face recognition, facial expression classification, but also gender determination, age estimation, emotion assessment, etc.

Developments and Publications

In the last years, face image analysis has experienced significant growth and progress, resulting in a virtual explosion of published information. The progress of research in face image analysis is reflected by the large number of papers published these years. Take "face image analysis" as a key word and search it in the column of "Subject/Title/Abstract" in EI Compendex (http://www.ei.org) on December 2009 provides the results shown in Table 1. The numbers of publication increase in a pace of approximate 6 to 8 times per 10 years.

Face image analysis comprises of a broad area. One of the most concentrated research topics in face image analysis is face recognition in recent years. The number of papers published these years can show an even big figure. Take "face recognition" as key words and search them in the column of "Subject/Title/Abstract" in EI Compendex (http://www.ei.org) on December 2009 gives the results shown in Table 2. The numbers of publication increase even quickly and attend a rate of approaching one order per 10 years in the last period.

A juxtaposition of the data in Table 1 and Table 2 in graphic form is given in Figure 1. The above-mentioned tendency is more directly displayed.

Back to the last 10 years, the progress of theoretical researches and experimental applications in facial image analysis is indexed by the number of papers published these years (Due the delay of recording, the numbers for recent years might not been all accounted yet). Take "facial image analysis" as a key word and search it in the column of "Subject/Title/Abstract" in EI Compendex (http://www.ei.org) with treatment type "Theoretical", as well as "Applications" and "Experimental" provides the results shown in Figure 2. There is a big jump from 2003 to 2004, for both theoretical research and experimental applications.

With the increase of journal and conference publications for researches and applications, a large number of survey papers have been published, such as (Baron, 1981; Ellis, 1986; Bruce, 1990; Samal & Iyengar, 1992; Chellappa, Wilson & Sirohey, 1995; Barrett, 1997; Wayman, 2002; Yang, Kriegman & Ahuja, 2002; Pan et al., 2003; Zhao, Chellappa & Rosenfeld, 2003; Bowyer, Chang & Flynn, 2004; Riaz, Gilgiti & Mirza, 2004; Short, Kittler & Messer, 2004; Bronstein, Bronstein & Kimmel, 2005; Kittler et al., 2005;

Table 1. The numbers of publications with "facial image analysis"

Years	1960–1969	1970–1979	1980–1989	1990–1999	2000–2009	Total
Numbers	2	12	73	867	6371	7325

Table 2. The numbers of publications with "face recognition"

Years	1960–1969	1970–1979	1980–1989	1990–1999	2000–2009	Total
Numbers	10	44	179	1442	13593	15268

Figure 1. The numbers of publications with "face image analysis" and "face recognition"

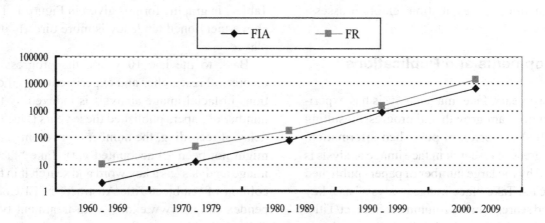

Kong et al., 2005; Tan & Zhang, 2006; Iancu, Corcoran & Costache, 2007; Li & Zhang, 2007; Zou, Kittler & Messer, 2007; Jia & Zhang, 2008; Kruger, Zhang & Xie, 2008; Nikolaos & Feng, 2008; Widanagamaachchi & Dharmaratne, 2008; Yan & Zhang, 2008a; Erik & Trivedi, 2009). A number of specialized books have also been available, such as (Bruce, 1988; Bartlett, 2001; Li & Jain, 2004; Wen & Huang, 2004; Zhou, Chellappa & Zhao, 2006; and Weschler, 2007).

MAIN THRUST

Face image analysis is a complex procedure and should be completed in a number of steps; each of them has specific functions and performs particular tasks. To carry out these tasks and to fulfill these functions, many techniques have been developed. After listing the procedure and modules of face image analysis, two important groups are summarized and their evaluations are discussed below.

Figure 2. The numbers of publications for theoretical researches and experimental applications in face image analysis

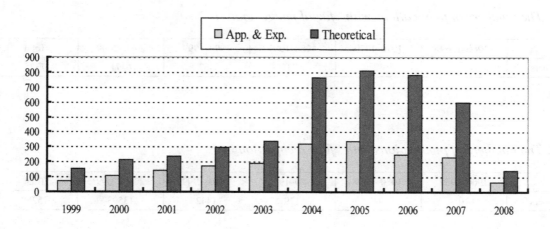

The Modules of Face Image Analysis

The procedure of face image analysis (from input images to output results) consists of several main steps and can be grouped into four modules, as shown in Figure 3.

The functions of these four modules are described shortly as follows:

Face Location: Analyzing faces needs to locate face region from image first, this can include face detection in still image and/or face tracking in video. To determine the position and the extension of faces, often image segmentation techniques are required. This task can be much complicated with the variation of the position and posture of human body in 3-D space, as well as the deviation from the normal lighting conditions.

Feature Extraction: Once the faces from images are captured, to represent and describe the face characteristics, some suitable features should be selected and extracted from these images. These features should represent and/or reflect the particularity of face images. Commonly used features include geometric features, such as distance, angle, curvature, etc; and grey level feature, such as color, texture of faces. Features can also be classified as local ones or holistic ones.

Dimension Reduction: Often a large number of features can be extracted from face images, as a human face is a non-rigid natural object and its image could be obtained under various conditions. The original features extracted correspond to the data in high dimensional space. Directly using these high dimensional data cause not only computational problems but also inaccuracy of

analysis results. Therefore, feature dimensionality reduction is necessary.

Decision Making: Based on the feature-dependent analysis, some decisions about face images can be made toward facial expression classification, face recognition, gender determination, age estimation, etc. Among them, face recognition is currently one of the most popular research topics and can be broadly classified into verification and identification. Verification deals with the validation of identity claims while identification caters for the identifying of unknowns or validation of negative claims.

Subspace Techniques

It is well known that face images are represented by high-dimensional pixel arrays while they are intrinsically belong to a manifold of low dimension. As the dimensionality of face-image data causes a critical issue in the analysis, techniques for reducing this dimensionality have been studied. One of the successful techniques, especially for face recognition is based on subspace methods. First, the value of a pixel in natural images is often highly correlated with the neighborhoods. For example, the surface of a face is typically smooth and has fairly even texture, so the information contained in adjacent pixels have a lot of redundancy. Second, the face is well structured, with the five sense organs arranged in relatively fixed positions. From an image analysis point of view, only interest objects need to be considered. Therefore, the face space is just a subspace of image space. Thus, subspace techniques would be very suitable in this regard.

Figure 3. The procedure and modules of face image analysis

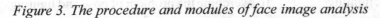
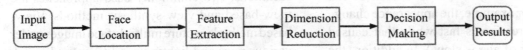

One of the earliest applied subspace techniques is the principal component analysis (PCA) (Kirby & Sirovich, 1990). While PCA minimizes the sample covariance (second-order dependency) of the data, Independent Component Analysis (ICA) minimizes higher order dependencies as well, and the components found by ICA are designed to be non-Gaussian (Bartlett, Movellan & Sejnowski, 2002). More specialized for classification, discriminant techniques have been proposed. One group is based on discriminant analysis. A typical example is linear discriminant analysis (LDA) (Price & Gee, 2005). Another group is based on class-dependence feature analysis CFA (Vijaya et al., 2006).

The above linear analysis methods are suitable for treating fixed and "standard" cases, while for the face images that are captured at different dates with diverse conditions, such as different illuminations, different directions, different expression, etc., which allows any given face to produce a virtually infinite number of different images, some multi-linear and especially non-linear subspace techniques that can identify and parameterize nonlinear subspaces (as well as both active techniques and passive techniques) maybe required (Zou, Kittler & Messer 2007). A list of typical analysis methods in subspace is given in Table 3. See the corresponding references as well as the survey papers and specialized books indicated in the last section for details.

Three-Dimensional Techniques

Faces are non-rigidity and complex 3-D objects in space, though face images captured are generally in 2-D form. The appearance of a face in 2-D images is affected by several factors including identity, age, face pose, facial expression, lighting conditions, occlusion, etc (Their influences can be different. For example, the appearance change caused by expression is fast while that caused by the growing of age is slow.). In addition, the results of face image analysis are also dependent on the size of face in images and the resolution of images. Evaluations on the performance of face recognition, for example, Face Recognition Vendor Test (FRVT) 2002 (Phillips, 2002) have shown that the current state of the art is not sufficient in many applications (Bowyer, Chang & Flynn, 2004).

Modeling and reconstructing 3-D faces are considered to improve the analysis. Many techniques from computer vision can be used for reconstruction, such as shape from shading (SFS), structure from motion (SFM), shape from contour (SFC), and photometric stereo, stereo vision, etc. Some other techniques using structured light, level set theory, etc. To get better results, the above techniques can also be combined with, for example, general human face model, active appearance model (AAM) or 3-D morphable model (3DMM). The models used for modeling 3-D faces can be either directly obtained by using 3-D image acquisition devices or be synthetically generated from 2-D images by using morphing techniques.

Video consists of a sequence of images captured along the time axis, and thus can provide both spatial and temporal information with multiple frames and temporal coherence. These information are also in 3-D space, but different with the above 3-D space. It is possible to improve the performance of face image analysis by taking advantage of the diversity of the information contained in video. However, analyzing faces in video also counts problems caused by the presence of large variations in pose (especially non-frontal poses) and lighting (both in luminosity and direction), as well as poor image resolution. These factors often make the performance of most systems workable in normal situations degraded very quickly, even to be defeated.

To overcome the problem of pose and lighting variations, two commonly used approaches are view-based and view-synthesis methods. View-based methods capture multiple face images under various pose and lighting conditions, and match the probe image with that gallery image which

Table 3. A list of typical analysis methods in subspace

Abbreviation	Full Name	References
2D-LDA	2D Linear Discriminant Analysis	(Li & Yuan, 2005)
2D-PCA	2D Principal Component Analysis	(Yang et al., 2004)
B2D-PCA	Bidirectional 2D-PCA	(Zuo, Zhang & Wang, 2006)
Bayesian	Bayesian	(Moghaddam, Jebara & Pentland, 2000)
CFA	Class-dependence Feature Analysis	(Vijaya et al., 2006)
DLDA	Direct LDA	(Yu & Yang, 2001)
EFM	Enhance Fisher linear discriminant model	(Liu & Wechsler, 2000)
FDA	Fisher Discriminant Analysis	(Kurita & Taguchi, 2005)
FF	Fisher Faces	(Belhumeur, Hespanha & Kriegman, 1997)
FNMF	Fast Non-negative Matrix Factorization	(Li & Zhang, 2009)
GSVD	Generalized Singular Value Decomposition	(Howland & Park, 2004)
ICA	Independent Component Analysis	(Bartlett, Movellan & Sejnowski, 2002)
K2D-PCA	Kernel 2D-PCA	(Wang, Zheng & Hu, 2007)
KFDA	Kernel Fisher Discriminant Analysis	(Mika et al., 1999)
KLDA	Kernel LDA	(Park & Park, 2008)
KPCA	Kernel-based PCA	(Kim, Jung & Kim, 2002)
KTS	Kernel Tensor-Subspace	(Park & Savvides, 2007)
LDA	Linear Discriminant Analysis	(Price & Gee, 2005)
LF	Laplacian Face	(Sundaresan & Chellappa, 2008)
LFA	Local Feature Analysis	(Penev et al., 2004)
LPP	Locality Preserving Projection	(Yu, Teng & Liu, 2006)
NLPCA	Non-Linear PCA	(Kramer, 1991)
NSLDA	Null Space LDA	(Chen et al., 2000)
NMF	Non-negative Matrix Factorization	(Lee & Seung, 1999)
NMSF	Non-negative Matrix Set Factorization	(Li & Zhang, 2007)
NN	Neural Networks	(Micheli-Tzanakou et al., 1995)
OFLD	Optimal LDA	(Yang & Yang, 2001)
PCA	Principal Component Analysis	(Kirby & Sirovic, 1990)
PM	Principal Manifold	(Moghaddam, 2002)
PSA	Probabilistic Subspace Analysis	(Moghaddam, 2002)
SVD	Singular Value Decomposition	(Hong, 1991)
TCF-CFA	Tensor Correlation Filter based CFA	(Yan & Zhang, 2008b)
TPCA	Topological PCA	(Pujol et al., 2001)
UPCA	Unified PCA	(Shan et al. 2008)

has the most similar pose and lighting conditions. View-synthesis methods generate synthetic views from the input probe image that have similar pose and lighting conditions as the gallery images in order to improve the matching performance. The desired views can be synthesized by learning the mapping function between pairs of training images or by combining with some of the above 3-D face models.

Video can be utilized in conjunction with 3-D face models in face image analysis. Using 3-D face models has the advantages of robust against pose and lighting variations. Some studies use reconstructed 3-D models from multiple video frames, and effectively handle the pose and lighting variations observed in medium quality video. Performances on tasks, such as face and facial feature point detection, as well as 3-D reconstruction and 3-D recognition of face images, have been improved a lot.

Face image analyses based on 3-D faces and based on video are both the extensions of 2-D analysis. On the other side, they are both the particular cases of face image analysis based on a set of images. This set of images can be an ordered sequence of frames from a video, or can be an unordered set of photographs; even the temporal information is not available. From this set of images, not only a 3-D face but also its environment could be completely reconstructed.

Finally, one limitation to some existing approaches to 3-D face recognition involves sensitivity to size variation (Bowyer, Chang & Flynn, 2004). Approaches that use a purely curvature-based representation, such as extended Gaussian images, are not able to distinguish between two faces of similar shape but different size. Approaches that use a PCA-type algorithm to can handle size change between faces, but run into problems with change of facial expression between the enrollment image and the image to be recognized.

Benchmark and Database

To evaluate the performance of the techniques for face image analysis, different criteria have been proposed, and new benchmarks have been developed. The design and implementation of a good performance benchmark is a complex process, and some compromising between contrasting goals should be made.

There are five characteristics to be considered by good benchmarks (Huppler, 2009):

1. **Relevant:** A reader of the result believes the benchmark reflects something important.
2. **Repeatable:** There is confidence that the benchmark can be run a second time with the same result.
3. **Fair:** All systems and/or software being compared can participate equally.
4. **Verifiable:** There is confidence that the documented result is real.
5. **Economical:** The test sponsors can afford to run the benchmark.

The first characteristic could be the most important one as without relevance, the benchmark would be worthless. However, the last four items should also be satisfied. Since the tested techniques could be based on different principles and theories, and tested data could be distributed and changed in a non-uniform way, the fairness and repeatability are very critical. The benchmark should be used to fairly evaluate different techniques and to repeatedly measure the performance over the whole range of data that have considered all variations.

In the research of face image analysis, database plays an important role. A number of large databases of face images have been collected and become increasingly popular in the evaluation of techniques for face image analysis. Collecting a high quality database is a resource-intensive task, but the availability of public face databases is important for the advancement of the field. Besides, common databases are necessary to comparatively evaluate algorithms. Some desirable properties for an appropriate evaluation database include (Bowyer, Chang & Flynn, 2004):

1. A large number and demographic variety of people represented.
2. Images of a given person taken at repeated intervals of time.
3. Images of a given person that represent substantial variation in facial expression.
4. High spatial resolution, for example, depth resolution of 0.1 mm or better.
5. Low frequency of sensor-specific artifacts in the data.

Though these five properties are originally declared for 3-D databases for face recognition, they are also valid for 2-D and 3-D databases used for face image analysis. The first three properties are all counts for databases of sufficient size that include carefully controlled variations of these factors. The development of algorithms robust to these variations is critical for real applications. Furthermore, to fully demonstrate the algorithms' performance; their scalability should be considered with the help of such databases.

Recently, as it is relatively easy to collect many images from the Internet and as it is relatively efficient to label them, it has become increasingly popular to evaluate the performance of the techniques for face image analysis on large test sets. However, there is no guarantee that such a set of "found" images accurately captures the range of variation found in the real-world (Pinto, DiCarlo & Cox 2009). A variety of factors conspire to limit the range of variation found in such image sets: (e.g. posing and "framing" of photographs from the web, as photographers typically pose and frame their photos such that a limited range of views are highly over-represented); as well as implicit or explicit selection criteria in choosing and assembling images for the set. Even more, it has shown that an extremely basic recognition system, built on a trivial feature set, was able to

take advantage of low-level regularities in these sets, performing on par with many state-of-the-art systems.

To finish, a question unique to collecting data for facial expression analysis should be pointed out. It is how facial actions are elicited during data collection. To facilitate the collection process, subjects are usually asked to perform the desired actions. However, appearance and timing of these directed facial actions may differ from spontaneously occurring behavior. This problem would be even complicated by the fact that the human face is able to display an astonishing variety of expressions. Recently, some studies for spontaneous facial behavior have been made, for example, see (Zhu et al. 2009).

FUTURE TRENDS

Human analysis of face images are important for recognize a friend or enemy, while automatic analysis of face image continues to be one of the most popular research areas of image engineering, computer vision and machine learning, and is important also for psychological and psychiatric studies. Several challenge and prominent directions can be identified as follows.

Analysis with Sets of Images

To increase the information content for analysis and to tolerate the variations and changes in face images, one could consider using a set of face images as input, instead of using a single face image. In the above mentioned 3-D techniques, either those based on 3-D reconstruction or using a contiguous sequence of frames from a video is working with a set of images. Other techniques working with sets of images include multi-view techniques, taken by individual snapshots from several directions. Compared with video-based techniques, no temporal information is available here in general.

It is a common sense that a large set of images contains more information than every individual image in it: it provides a clue not only on possible appearance on one's face, but also on the typical patterns of variation (Shakhnarovich & Moghaddam, 2004). Technically, just as a set of images known to contain an individual's face allows one to represent that individual by an estimated intrinsic subspace, so the unlabeled input set leads to a subspace estimate that represents the unknown subject. The recognition task can then be formulated in terms of matching the subspaces.

Multi-Modality Analysis

With the progress of various devices for image capturing, multi-sensor information become available and multi-modality analysis of face images turn into consideration. It is not surprise to know that, for example, attempts have been made recently to fuse the visible and infrared modalities to increase the performance of face recognition.

Using multi-modality analysis can provide more comprehensive, accurate, and robust results than that obtained from a single sensor. For example, one problem often encountered with visible light is the variability of lighting conditions. With the thermal infrared images, not only the ability to see in the dark could be improved, but also some facial physiological information (coming from, e.g., vascular network and vessel) could be captured and that inherent information are invariant under light variation (Buddharaju & Pavlidis, 2007). This will certainly increase the ability to extract information and improve decision capability.

Mimic of the Human's Skill

Analyzing the face image and making decision based on the appearance are difficult tasks for a computer but are often easily completed by human beings. What features are taken and what analyses are performed by human beings in the procedure are not clearly described, yet. To mimic the human's skill, one type of techniques is to imitate the behavior of human beings from the bionic point of view, and another type of techniques is to execute a sequence of processes to perform the similar task.

Face image analysis requires making judgment on the similarity among different features and different faces, which is considered a difficult task. One research attempt in this direction is to (A) obtaining reliable facial similarity judgments from human observers, (B) developing 'objective' approaches to similarity to supplement measurements from humans, (C) automatically mapping measured facial features to a space where the natural metric predicts human similarity judgments (Holub, Liu & Perona, 2007). By a learning process, the measured facial features can be mapped to metric spaces in which similar looking faces are near one another. Thus, the subjective judgment of facial similarity has been placed on a solid computational footing.

New Theories and Tools

Image engineering is always supported by new academic advancements and technical developments from various disciplines. Introducing/incorporating suitable theories and tools into face image analysis should be taken into account.

For example, in exploiting the sparsity in face images, the distributed compressive sensing theory has been introduced into analysis (Nagesh & Li, 2009). Considering the different images of the same subject as an ensemble of inter-correlated signals, the training images of a given subject can be represented with sufficient information for good classification by only two feature images: one captures the holistic (common) features of the face, and another captures the different expressions in all training samples. In addition, a new test image of a subject can be fairly well approximated using only the two feature images from the same subject. Thus, the storage space and operational dimensionality could be drastically reduced by keeping only these two feature images or their random measurements. Based on this, an efficient expression-invariant classifier has been designed.

CONCLUSION

Face image analysis is a particular type of image analysis, so it is undergo the similar procedure as general image analysis. It has a long history since it is related to the most important human perception. It was considered simple since it is often completed with no trouble by human beings. It attracts many attentions in research community recently since it is a really challenge problem.

Face image analysis is undergoing a fast evolution. There are two notable directions in this evolution: the transition from linear to general, possibly non-linear and disconnected manifolds; and the introduction of probabilistic and specifically Bayesian methods for dealing with the uncertainty and with similarity.

To guide any serious effort towards solving the problem in face image analysis, one needs to define detailed specifications of what the problem is and what would constitute a solution. Thus, the that incremental progress in research can be precisely quantified and different approaches can be compared through a standard procedure. The development of a robust algorithm for face image analysis, which is capable of functioning in unconstrained, real-world environments, will have far-reaching applications in our modern digital world.

ACKNOWLEDGMENT

This work was supported by the National Nature Science Foundation of China under grant NNSF-60872084.

REFERENCES

Baron, R. (1981). Mechanisms of human facial recognition. *International Journal of Man-Machine Studies*, *15*, 137–178. doi:10.1016/S0020-7373(81)80001-6

Barrett, W. A. (1997). A survey of face recognition algorithms and testing results. *Proc. Asilomar Conference on Signals, Systems & Computers*, *1*, 301-305.

Bartlett, M. S. (2001). *Face Image Analysis by Unsupervised Learning*. Amsterdam: Kluwer Academic Publishers.

Bartlett, M. S., Movellan, J. R., & Sejnowski, T. J. (2002). Face recognition by independent component analysis. *IEEE Trans. NN*, *13*(6), 1450–1464.

Belhumeur, P. N., Hespanha, J. P., & Kriegman, D. J. (1997). Eigenfaces vs. Fisherfaces: Recognition using class specific linear projection. *IEEE Trans. PAMI*, *19*(7), 711–720.

Bowyer, K. W., Chang, K., & Flynn, P. (2004). A survey of approaches to three-dimensional face recognition. *Proc. ICPR*, *1*, 358-361.

Bronstein, A. M., Bronstein, M. M., & Kimmel, R. (2005). Three-dimensional face recognition. *IJCV*, *64*(1), 5–30. doi:10.1007/s11263-005-1085-y

Bruce, V. (1988). *Recognizing Faces*. London: Erlbaum.

Bruce, V. (1990). Perceiving and Recognizing Faces. *Mind & Language*, 342–364. doi:10.1111/j.1468-0017.1990.tb00168.x

Buddharaju, P., & Pavlidis, I. (2009). Physiological Face Recognition Is Coming of Age. *IEEE Trans. PAMI*, *29*(4), 613–626.

Chellappa, R., Wilson, C. L., & Sirohey, S. (1995). Human and machine recognition of faces: A survey. *Proceedings of the IEEE*, *83*(5), 705–741. doi:10.1109/5.381842

Chen, L. F., Liao, H. Y., Ko, M. T., et al. (2000). A new LDA-based face recognition system which can solve the small sample size problem. *PR, 33,* 1713-1726.

Ellis, H. D. (1986). Introduction to aspects of face processing: Ten questions in need of answers. *Aspects of Face Processing,* 3-13.

Erik, M. C., & Trivedi, M. M. (2009). Head pose estimation in computer vision: A survey. *IEEE Trans. PAMI, 31*(4), 607–626.

Holub, A., Liu, Y. H., & Perona, P. (2007). On constructing facial similarity maps. *Proc. CVPR,* 1-8.

Hong, Z. (1991). Algebraic feature extraction of image for recognition. *PR, 24,* 211-219.

Howland, P., & Park, H. (2004). Generalizing discriminant analysis using the generalized singular value decomposition. *IEEE Trans. PAMI, 26*(8), 995–1006.

Huppler, K. (2009). The art of building a good benchmark. *LNCS, 5895,* 18–30.

Iancu, C., Corcoran, P., & Costache, G. (2007). A review of face recognition techniques for in-camera applications. *Proc. International Symposium on Signals, Circuits and Systems, 1,* 1-4.

Jia, H. X., & Zhang, Y. J. (2008). Human detection in static images. *Pattern Recognition Technologies and Applications: Recent Advances,* 227-243.

Kim, K. I., Jung, K., & Kim, H. J. (2002). Face recognition using kernel principal component analysis. *IEEE Signal Processing Letters, 9*(2), 40–42. doi:10.1109/97.991133

Kirby, M., & Sirovich, L. (1990). Application of the Karhunen-Loeve procedure for the characterization of human faces. *IEEE Trans. PAMI, 12,* 103–108.

Kittler, J., Hilton, A., Hamouz, M., et al. (2005). 3D assisted face recognition: A survey of 3D imaging, modeling and recognition approaches. *Proc. CVPR,* 114-120.

Kong, S. G., Heo, J., & Abidi, B. (2005). Recent advances in visual and infrared face recognition -- A review. *Computer Vision and Image Understanding, 97*(1), 103–135. doi:10.1016/j.cviu.2004.04.001

Kramer, M. A. (1991). Nonlinear principal components analysis using auto-associative neural networks. *AIChE Journal. American Institute of Chemical Engineers, 32*(2), 233–243. doi:10.1002/aic.690370209

Kruger, U., Zhang, J. P., & Xie, L. (2008). Developments and applications of nonlinear principal component analysis - A review. *Lecture Notes in Computational Science and Engineering, 58,* 1–43. doi:10.1007/978-3-540-73750-6_1

Kurita, T., & Taguchi, T. (2005). A kernel-based Fisher discriminant analysis for face detection. *IEICE Transactions on Information and Systems, E88*(3), 628–635. doi:10.1093/ietisy/e88-d.3.628

Lee, D. D., & Seung, H. S. (1999). Learning the parts of objects by non-negative matrix factorization. *Nature, 401,* 788–791. doi:10.1038/44565

Li, L., & Zhang, Y. J. (2007). Non-negative matrix-set factorization. *Proc. ICIG,* 564-569.

Li, L., & Zhang, Y. J. (2009). FastNMF: Highly efficient monotonic fixed-point nonnegative matrix factorization algorithm with good applicability. *Journal of Electronic Imaging, 18*(3), 033004. doi:10.1117/1.3184771

Li, M., & Yuan, B. (2005). 2D-LDA: A novel statistical linear discriminant analysis for image matrix. *PRL, 26*(5), 527–532.

Li, S. Z., & Jain, A. K. (2004). *Handbook of Face Recognition.* New York: Springer.

Liu, C. J., & Wechsler, H. (2000). Robust coding schemes for indexing and retrieval from large face databases. *IEEE Trans. IP, 9*(1), 132–137.

Micheli-Tzanakou, E., Uyeda, E., & Ray, R. (1995). Comparison of neural network algorithms for face recognition. *Simulation, 65*(1), 37–51. doi:10.1177/003754979506500105

Mika, G., Ratsch, J., Weston, B., et al. (1999). Fisher discriminant analysis with kernels. *Proc. IWNNSP IX,* 41-48.

Moghaddam, B. (2002). Principal manifolds and probabilistic subspaces for visual recognition. *IEEE Trans. PAMI, 24*(6), 780–788.

Moghaddam, B., Jebara, T., & Pentland, A. (2000). Bayesian face recognition. *PR, 33*(11), 1771-1782.

Nagesh, P., & Li, B. X. (2009). *A Compressive Sensing Approach for Expression-Invariant Face Recognition*. CVPR.

Nikolaos, E., & Feng, D. (2008). Building highly realistic facial modeling and animation: A survey. *The Visual Computer, 24*(1), 13–30.

Pan, Z., Healey, G., & Prasad, M. (2003). Face recognition in hyperspectral images. *IEEE Trans. PAMI, 25,* 1552–1560.

Park, C. H., & Park, H. (2008). A comparison of generalized linear discriminant analysis algorithms. *PR, 41*(3), 1083-1097.

Park, S. W., & Savvides, M. (2007). Individual kernel tensor-subspaces for robust face recognition: A computationally efficient tensor framework without requiring mode factorization. *IEEE Trans. SMC-B, 37*(5), 1156–1166.

Penev, P. S., Ayache, M., & Fruchter, J. (2004). Independent manifold analysis for sub-pixel tracking of local features and face recognition in video sequences. *SPIE, 5404,* 523–533.

Phillips, P. J., Grother, P., Micheals, R., et al. (2002). Face recognition vendor test 2002: Evaluation report. *NIST,* TR-IR 6965. Retrieved from http://www.itl.nist.gov/iad/894.03/face/face.html

Pinto, N., DiCarlo, J. J., & Cox, D. D. (2009). How far can you get with a modern face recognition test set using only simple features? *CVPR,* 2591-2598.

Price, J. R., & Gee, T. F. (2005). Face recognition using direct, weighted linear discriminant analysis and modular subspaces. *PR, 38*(2), 209-219.

Pujol, A., Vitria, J., & Lumbreras, F. (2001). Topological principal component analysis for face encoding and recognition. *PRL, 22*(6-7), 769–776.

Riaz, Z., Gilgiti, A., & Mirza, S. M. (2004). Face recognition: a review and comparison of HMM, PCA, ICA and neural networks. *E-Tech,* 41-46.

Samal, A., & Iyengar, P. A. (1992). Automatic recognition and analysis of human faces and facial expressions: A survey. *PR, 25,* 65-77.

Shakhnarovich, G., & Moghaddam, B. (2004). Face Recognition in Subspaces . In *Handbook of Face Recognition*. Berlin: Springer-Verlag.

Shan, S., et al. (2008). Unified principal component analysis with generalized covariance matrix for face recognition. *Proc. CVPR,* 1-7.

Short, J., Kittler, J., & Messer, K. (2004). Comparison of photometric normalisation algorithms for face verification. *Proc. ICAFGR,* 254-259.

Sundaresan, A., & Chellappa, R. (2008). Model driven segmentation of articulating humans in Laplacian Eigenspace. *IEEE Trans. PAMI, 30*(10), 1771–1785.

Tan, H. C., & Zhang, Y. J. (2006). Automatic facial expression analysis. *Encyclopedia of Human Computer Interaction,* 60-67.

Vijaya, K., Bhagavatula, V. K., & Savvides, M. (2006). Correlation pattern recognition for face recognition. *Proceedings of the IEEE, 94*(11), 1963–1975. doi:10.1109/JPROC.2006.884094

Wang, H. X., Zheng, W. M., & Hu, Z. L. (2007). Local and weighted maximum margin discriminant analysis. *Proc. CVPR*, 1, 1-8.

Wayman, J. L. (2002). Digital signal processing in biometric identification: A review. *Proc. ICIP, 1*, 37-40.

Wen, Z., & Huang, T. S. (2004). *3D Face Processing: Modeling, Analysis and Synthesis*. Amsterdam: Kluwer Academic Publishers.

Weschler, H. (2007). *Reliable Face Recognition Methods: System Design, Implementation and Evaluation*. New York: Springer.

Widanagamaachchi, W. N., & Dharmaratne, A. T. (2008). 3D face reconstruction from 2D images: A survey. *Proc. Digital Image Computing: Techniques and Applications*, 365-371.

Yan, Y., & Zhang, Y. J. (2008a). State-of-the-art on video-based face recognition. *Encyclopedia of Artificial Intelligence*, 1455-1461.

Yan, Y., & Zhang, Y. J. (2008b). Tensor correlation filter based class-dependence feature analysis for face recognition. *Neurocomputing, 71*(16-18), 3534–3543. doi:10.1016/j.neucom.2007.09.013

Yang, J., & Yang, J. Y. (2001). An optimal FLD algorithm for facial feature extraction. *SPIE, 4572*, 438–444.

Yang, J., Zhang, D., Frangi, A. F., et al. (2004). Two-dimensional PCA: A new approach to appearance-based face representation and recognition. *IEEE Trans. PAMI, 26*(1):), 131-137.

Yang, M. H., Kriegman, D. J., & Ahuja, N. (2002). Detecting faces in images: A survey. *IEEE Trans. PAMI, 24*(1), 34–58.

Yu, H., & Yang, J. (2001). A direct LDA algorithm for high-dimensional data with application to face recognition. *PR, 34*(10), 2067-2070.

Yu, W. W., Teng, X. L., & Liu, C. Q. (2006). Face recognition using discriminant locality preserving projections. *Image and Vision Computing, 24*(3), 239–248. doi:10.1016/j.imavis.2005.11.006

Zhao, W., Chellappa, R., & Rosenfeld, A. (2003). Face recognition: A literature survey. *ACM Computing Surveys, 35*, 399–458. doi:10.1145/954339.954342

Zhou, S. K., Chellappa, R., & Zhao, W. (2006). *Unconstrained Face Recognition*. New York: Springer Science + Business Media, Inc.

Zhu, Y. F., Torre, F., Cohn, J. F., et al. (2009). Dynamic cascades with bidirectional bootstrapping for spontaneous facial action unit detection. *Proc. the Third International Conference on Affective Computing and Intelligent Interaction and Workshops*, 1-8.

Zou, X., Kittler, J., & Messer, K. (2007). Illumination invariant face recognition: A survey. *Proc. International Conference on Biometrics: Theory, Applications, and Systems*, 1-8.

Zuo, W., Zhang, D., & Wang, K. (2006). Bidirectional PCA with assembled matrix distance metric for image recognition. *IEEE Trans. SMC-B, 36*, 863–872.

KEY TERMS AND DEFINITIONS

Image Engineering (IE): is a general terms for all image techniques, abroad subject encompassing mathematics, physics, biology, physiology, psychology, electrical engineering, computer science, automation, etc. Its advances are also closely related to the development of telecommunications, biomedical engineering, remote sensing, document processing, industrial applications, etc.

Image Processing (IP): includes primarily the acquisition, representation, compression, enhancement, restoration, and reconstruction of images, etc. Its main concern is the manipulation of an image to produce another (improved) image.

Image Analysis (IA): concerns the extraction of information from an image. In a general sense, it can be said that an image in yields data out. Here, the extracted data can be the measurement results associated with specific image properties or the representative symbols of certain object attributes.

Image Understanding (IU): refers to a body of knowledge used in transforming data extracted by image analysis into certain commonly understood descriptions, and making subsequent decisions and actions according to this interpretation of the images.

Stereo Vision: is a type of techniques for computing depth information based on images captured with two or more cameras. The main idea is to observe a scene from two or more viewpoints and to use the disparity to refer the position, structure and relation of objects in scene.

Photometric Stereo: is an important technique for recovering surface orientation. This technique requires a set of images, which are taken from the same view angles but with different lighting conditions. This technique is easy to implement, but requires the control of the lighting in the application environment.

Shape From Contour (SFC): is a scene recovering technique with only one image. It recovers the surface orientation of objects with the contour information projected on the image.

Shape From Shading (SFS): recovers the shape information of a 3-D scene from a single image. The image shading caused by the object surface illumination in space is used to reconstruct the surface orientation.

Structure From Motion (SFM): recovers the information on the relationship among objects in space and/or the structure of scene by solving the optical flow equations.

Chapter 2
Face Searching in Large Databases

Maria De Marsico
Università di Roma "La Sapienza", Italy

Michele Nappi
Università di Salerno, Italy

Daniel Riccio
Università di Salerno, Italy

Sergio Vitulano
Università di Cagliari, Italy

ABSTRACT

Both government agencies and private companies are investing significant resources to improve local/ remote access security. Badge or password-based procedures have proven to be too vulnerable, while biometric research has significantly grown, mostly due to technological progresses that allow using increasingly efficient techniques, yet at decreasing costs. Suitable devices capture images of user's face, iris, etc., or other biometric elements such as fingerprints or voice. Each biometry calls for specific procedures. Measures from user's data make up the so called biometric key, which is stored in a database (enrolment) or used for recognition (testing). During recognition, a subject's key is matched against those in the database, producing a similarity score for each match. However, some drawbacks exist. For example, iris scanning is very reliable but presently too intrusive, while fingerprints are more socially accepted but not applicable to non-consentient people. On the other hand, face recognition represents a good solution even under less controlled conditions. In the last decade, many algorithms based on linear/non-linear methods, neural networks, wavelets, etc. have been proposed. Nevertheless, during Face Recognition Vendor Test 2002 most of them encountered problems outdoors. This lowers their reliability compared to other biometries, and underlines the need for more research. This chapter provides a survey of recent outcomes on the topic, addressing both 2D imagery and 3D models, to provide a starting reference to potential investigators. Tables containing different collections of parameters (such as input size, recognition rate, number of addressed problems) simplify comparisons. Some future directions are finally proposed.

DOI: 10.4018/978-1-61520-991-0.ch002

INTRODUCTION

Secure access to restricted areas or services, has long since been a major issue. Many agencies are increasingly motivated to improve authentication through bodily or behavioural characteristics, referred to as biometries (Perronnin, 2003). Biometric systems process raw data to extract and store a biometric template. They may implement verification or identification. Verification is a 1:1 match that compares a probe biometric template against a stored one, whose identity is being claimed. Identification implies a 1:N comparison of a query biometric template against all stored templates, to determine its identity. Face recognition is less reliable than, say, fingerprints or iris, yet it seems a good compromise: it requires lighter computation, and produces less psychological discomfort, since people is quite accustomed to be photographed, even if a privacy violation is sometimes asserted (Johnson, 2004). It also has the great advantage of being applicable in places with large concourse of possibly unaware visitors. More recent works exploit 3D face models. Progress of technology also influences related algorithms. The first ones directly worked on clouds of points (after a suitable triangulation), while more recent ones work on a mesh, sometimes considering information from both the 3D shape and the texture.

Despite advances in research, real-world scenarios remain a challenge, because five key factors can significantly affect recognition performances: illumination, pose, expression, time delay, occlusions. This also motivated the generation of several 2D face images databases providing as many variations as possible on their images, to validate the performances of the proposed methods. FERET (Phillips, 2000), CMU-PIE (Sim, 2003), AR Faces (Martinez, 2002), Face Recognition Grand Challenge (FRGC) ver2.0 (Phillips, 2005) represent some of the most popular ones. On the other hand, there are few 3D face models databases, with very little amount of data. The 3D_RMA is an example whose models are represented by clouds of points.

It has long been the only publicly available database, and its quality is rather low. 3D meshes are available today from newer technologies, but in most cases they make up proprietary databases. Table 1 and Table 2 report the most popular 2D and 3D face databases. Their main characteristics are summarized, in particular available distortions: illumination(i), pose(p), expression(e), occlusions(o), time delay(t), indoor/outdoor(i/o).

Neither a common benchmark database is presently used to test existing face recognition algorithms, nor a unique standard evaluation protocol. Performance is typically characterized by Recognition Rate (RR), False Acceptance Rate (FAR) or False Rejection Rate (FRR) under closed-world assumptions. However Sherrah (Sherrah, 2004) recently underlined the importance of minimizing the false alarm rate, which is a more difficult criterion.

In the following, Section II describes recent 2D face recognition research trends, while highlighting achieved results; Section III analyzes what currently prevents a wider commercial adoption of face biometry. It also provides a more general way to evaluate performances for existing face recognition algorithms. A discussion about 3D-based face recognition is presented in Section IV. Finally, Section V closes the chapter with some considerations on state of the art and possible future trends, suggesting multimodality as a good solution to address reliability.

LITERATURE ABOUT AUTOMATIC FACE RECOGNITION

Face Recognition can be considered as a special example of pattern recognition, in particular as a template matching problem. Such problem is hard, as it is intrinsically non linear and must be addressed within a high-dimensional space. The following subsections will summarize the most widely investigated approaches for 2D face recognition. The aim is to present general issues,

Table 1. Most important face databases. The ∗ points out most used databases. Image variations are indicated by: (i) illumination, (p) pose, (e) expression, (o) occlusion, (i/o) indoor/outdoor conditions and (t) time delay.

Name	RGB/ Gray	Image Size	Number of people	Pictures / person	Number of conditions	Available	Web Address
AR Face Database*	RGB	576 × 768	126	26	i, e, o, t	yes	http://rvl1.ecn.purdue.edu/~aleix/ aleix_face_DB.html
Richard's MIT database	RGB	480 × 640	154	6	p, o	yes	
CVL Database	RGB	640 × 480	114	7	p, e	yes	http://www.lrv.fri.uni-lj.si/facedb.html
The Yale Face Database B*	Gray Scale	640 × 480	10	576	p, i	yes	http://cvc.yale.edu/projects/yalefacesB/ yalefacesB.html
The Yale Face Database*	Gray Scale	320 × 243	15	11	i, e	yes	http://cvc.yale.edu/projects/yalefaces/ yalefaces.html
PIE Database*	RGB	640 × 486	68	~ 608	p, i, e	yes	http://www.ri.cmu.edu/projects/project_418.html
The UMIST Face Database	Gray	220 × 220	20	19 to 36	p	yes	http://images.ee.umist.ac.uk/danny/ database.html
Olivetti Att - ORL*	Gray	92 × 112	40	10		yes	http://www.uk.research.att.com/faceda- tabase.html
(JAFFE) Database	Gray	256 × 256	10	7	e	yes	http://www.mis.atr.co.jp/~mlyons/jaffe. html
The Human Scan Database	Gray	384 × 286	23	~66		yes	http://www.humanscan.de/support/ downloads/facedb.php
The University of Oulu Physics- Based Face Database	Gray	428 × 569	125	16	i	Cost $50	http://www.ee.oulu.fi/research/imag/ color/pbfd.html
XM2VTSDB	RGB	576 × 720	295		p	Frontal $153 Side $229.5	http://www.ee.surrey.ac.uk/Research/ VSSP/xm2vtsdb/
FERET*	Gray RGB	256 × 384	1136		p, i, e, t	yes	http://www.itl.nist.gov/iad/humanid/ feret/
FRGC v2.0	Gray RGB	1200×1600			p, i, e, t	yes	http://www.frvt.org/FRGC/

rather than the details of the single prototypes. Ongoing studies are still refining the theoretical background of many of them.

Linear/Non Linear Projection Methods

An efficient dimensional reduction technique is usually searched to project the problem onto a lower-dimensionality space. Eigenfaces (Kirby, 1990) are one of the first approaches in this sense.

An N×N image I is linearized to represent a point in a N^2-dimensional space. Figure 1 shows how a convenient space is found, where comparisons are actually performed. To this aim, Sirovich and Kirby (1990) adopt the PCA (Principal Component Analysis). After linearization the mean vector over all images is calculated, and then subtracted from all the original face vectors. The covariance matrix is computed, to extract a limited number of its eigenvectors corresponding to the great-

Table 2. Most important databases of 3D face models. Image variations are indicated by: (p) pose, (e) expression, (o) occlusion

Name	Type	Data Size	Number of people	3D Models / person	Number of conditions	Texture Image	Available	Web Address
3D RMA	Cloud of points	4000 points	120	3	p	No	Yes	http://www.sic.rma.ac.be/~beumier/DB/3d_rma.html
SAMPL	Range Image	200 x 200	10	33 (for 2 sub.), 1 (for 8 sub.)	p,e	Yes	Yes	http://sampl.eng.ohio-state.edu/~sampl/
Univ. of York 1	Range Image	-	97	10	p,e,o	No	Yes	http://www-users.cs.york.ac.uk/~tomh/3DfaceDatabase.html
Univ. of York 2	Range Image	-	350	15	p,e	No	Yes	http://www-users.cs.york.ac.uk/~tomh/3DfaceDatabase.html
Gavab-DB	Tri-Mesh		61	9	p.e.	No	Yes	http://gavab.escet.urjc.es/recursos_en.html

est eigenvalues. These few eigenvectors, also referred to as eigenfaces, represent a base in a low-dimensionality space. When testing a new image, the corresponding eigenface expansion is computed and compared against the entire database, according to a suitable distance measure (usually the Euclidean distance). As the PCA is only performed for training the system, this method is very fast during testing.

LDA (Linear Discriminant Analysis) (Lu, 2003) has been proposed as a better alternative to PCA, since it expressly provides discrimination among the classes. While PCA deals with the overall input data, no matter what is the underlying structure, LDA mainly aims at finding a base

of vectors able to provide the best discrimination among the classes, i.e. to maximize the between-class differences and minimize the within-class ones.

It is worth noticing that LDA provides better classification performances than PCA only when a wide training set is available, as discussed by Martinèz (Martinèz, 2009). Further studies also strengthen such argument by expressly tackling the classical SSS (Small Sample Size) problem. Some mixed approaches, such as the Fisherfaces (Belhumeur, 1997), preliminary exploit PCA just to reduce the dimensionality of the input space; afterwards, LDA is applied to the resulting space, to perform the actual classification. However,

Figure 1. The general scheme of the Linear/Non-linear methods

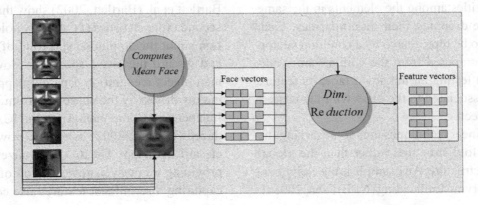

recent works (Yu, 2001) demonstrate that such combination takes to discard discriminant information together with redundant one. Therefore, LDA is often rather applied directly on the input space. In (Dao-Qing, 2007) authors observe that, when the small-sample-size problem is encountered, optimization of the Fisher index does not necessarily take to obtain optimal performances from the system. On the contrary, a two-parameter regularized scheme is proposed, wherein the optimization criterion is based on the posterior error rate. LDA-based techniques also suffer from a scalability problem, which is addressed by incremental methods. For example, the innovation in (Zhao, 2008) with respect to other literature methods consists in extracting a projection matrix in a full space instead of in a subspace.

PCA, LDA and Bayesian analysis are unified under the same framework in (Wang, & Tang, 2004), after modelling face difference with three components: intrinsic difference, transformation difference, and noise. The inherent relationship among different subspace methods is exploited to extract discriminating information. Better recognition performance is achieved than standard subspace methods. Lu et al. (2003) propose an hybrid between D-LDA (Direct LDA) and F-LDA (Fractional LDA), a variant of LDA, in which weighed functions avoid that too close output classes can induce a misclassification of the input. DCV (Discriminant Common Vectors) (Cevikalp, 2005) represents a further development of this approach. Its main idea relies in collecting similarities among the elements in the same class while dropping their dissimilarities. Each class can so be represented by a common vector, which is computed from the within scatter matrix. When testing an unknown face, its feature vector is associated to the class with the nearest common vector.

Other linear techniques aim at preserving the local manifold structure, rather than the global Euclidean structure. An example is the Neighborhood Preserving Embedding (NPE) (Yan, 2005a).

Each data point in the ambient space is represented as a linear combination of its neighbours. Then an optimal embedding is found, preserving the neighborhood structure in the space of reduced dimensionality. The Locality Preserving Projections (LPP) method (Iordanis, 2008) relies on a further linear dimensionality reduction algorithm, preserving the local structure of the image space. In the LPP-based approach in (Yan, 2005b), the manifold structure is modeled by a nearest-neighbor graph of a set of feature images, called Laplacianfaces. As LPP is non-orthogonal, it is difficult to reconstruct the original data. In (Han, 2006) the Orthogonal Locality Preserving Projection (OLPP) method produces orthogonal basis functions that can have more locality preserving power than LPP, and therefore more discriminating power too, since these two characteristics are potentially related.

The above methods, as well as related ones, generally show scarce performance in presence of occlusions or large variations in viewpoints, just due to their linearity. Better results are obtained by a more recent linear approach by Wright et al. (Wright, 2009). It exploits the theory of sparse signal representation. The whole set of training feature vectors from k distinct object classes is used to obtain the sparsest linear representation of a given test sample. This approach allows to use unconventional feature spaces, such as merely down-sampled images, given a sufficiently high number of training samples. Other strategies can make the recognition robust to local alterations. Bartlett et al. (Bartlett, 2002) show that first and second order statistics (PCA) only hold information about the amplitude spectrum of an image, and discard the phase spectrum. However, human object recognition capability appears to be mainly driven by the phase-spectrum. Therefore Independent Component Analysis (ICA) is introduced (Bartlett, 2002) as a more powerful face classification tool. The ICA generalizes PCA, yet providing a better characterization of data, and capturing discriminant features also considering the high-order statistics. Moreover, a non-linear version of ICA has also been investigated (see for example (Gao, 2006)), while in (Haifeng, 2008) ICA is combined with the neighborhood preserving analysis.

As mentioned above, linear subspace analysis methods hardly represent the complex and nonlinear variations of real face images, such as illumination, facial expression and pose variations. For this reason, nonlinear versions of such methods have also been proposed. In (Chalmond, & Girard, 1999) a kind of Non Linear PCA (NLPCA) is introduced. Alternatively, linear and nonlinear techniques are used together. Kernel methods have also been adopted in nonlinear approaches. They first embed data in suitable spaces, and then search for patterns therein.. The key issue is that nonlinear patterns appear as linear in the new space, so that they can be better studied. Kernel-based Nonlinear Discriminant Analysis (KNDA) (QingShan, 2003), combines the nonlinear kernel trick with the Fisher Linear Discriminant Analysis (FLDA) method. This method gives better performances than Kernel-based Principal Component Analysis (KPCA). Kernel machine-based Discriminant Analysis (KDA) (Huang, 2005) can be seen as an enhanced kernel D-LDA method, It is worth mentioning that some authors notice that the difference in performance is often too light to justify the higher computational costs of nonlinear approaches. This is for example the case with PCA and a number of popular nonlinear PCA methods. In (Huang, & Yin, 2009) the authors show that the difference in recognition rate between PCA and computational demanding nonlinear PCA methods is insignificant.

The Neural Networks

Neural classifiers show the advantage of reducing misclassifications among neighbour classes. Basically, a net with a neuron for every pixel in the image is considered. Nevertheless, because of the pattern dimensions (an image is about 112x92

pixels) neural networks are not directly trained with input images, but a dimensionality reduction technique is applied before.

Cottrell and Fleming (1990) introduce a second neural net operating in auto-association mode (Figure 2), which approximates the vector x, representing a face image, by a new vector h with smaller dimensions, which is inputted to the classification net. However, this kind of neural network does not behave better than the Eigenfaces, even in optimal circumstances. Conversely, Self Organizing Maps (SOM) are invariant with respect to minor changes in the image sample, while convolutional networks provide a partial invariance with respect to rotations, translations and scaling. In general, the structure of the network is strongly dependent on its application field. In a quite recent work (Lin, 1997), authors present the Probabilistic Decision Based Neural Network, which is modelled for three different applications (a face detector, an eyes locator and a face recognizer).

As a finale example, the work by Meng et al. (2002) introduces a hybrid approach where PCA extracts the most discriminating features, which are then used as the input of a Radial Basis Function (RBF) neural network. The RBFs perform well for face recognition problems, as they have a compact topology and high learning speed. The authors also face some typical problems: overfitting, overtraining, small sample size, and the singular problem. In general, neural network-based approaches encounter problems when the number of classes increases. Moreover, they are not suitable for recognition tasks with a single model image, because multiple model images per person are necessary for training the system towards "optimal" parameter setting.

Gabor Filters and Wavelets

Gabor filters represent capture important visual spatial features, such as localization, frequency and orientation. Besides being applied to whole

Figure 2. The structure of a neural network based approach

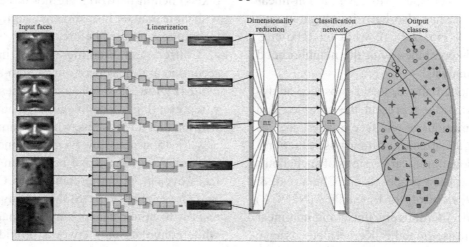

face images, in (Lades, 1993) they are also applied to specific areas of the face, corresponding to nodes of a rigid grid. In each such node, the Gabor coefficients are extracted and combined in jets. The nodes are linked to form a Dynamic Link Architecture (DLA), so that the comparisons among different subjects can rely on a graph matching strategy. Wiskott et al. (1997) go further using DLA and develop an Elastic Bunch Graph Matching (EBGM) method based on Gabor wavelets, to label and recognize human faces. In general, DLA is superior to other face recognition techniques, in terms of rotation invariance; however, the matching process is computationally expensive. F. Perronnin and J.-L. Dugelay (2003) propose a novel probabilistic deformable model

for face mapping, with a similar philosophy to EBGM. It is based on a bi-dimensional extension of the 1D-HMM (Hidden Markov Model). There are two main differences between this method and the original EBGM. First, all the parameters of M are automatically trained, so accounting for the elastic properties of the different parts of the face. Secondly, the model M is shared among all faces, so that little enrolment data is necessary. Liu (2004) proposes a quite different approach (Figure 3). A mother wavelet is defined and forty Gabor filters are derived (five scales and eight orientations). Each filter is convoluted with the input face image, producing forty filtered copies. The resulting Gabor wavelet features are chained to derive an augmented feature vector.

Figure 3. The convolution of Gabor kernels and dimensionality reduction of the filter responses

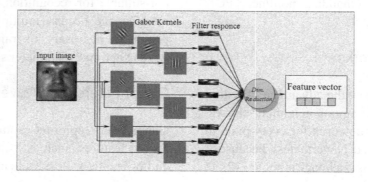

In order to reduce its dimensionality, both PCA and Enhanced Fisher Linear Discriminant Model (EFM) are investigated. The computational cost is dramatically increased by the number of required convolutions. Garcia et al. (2000) propose a faster wavelet-based approach, with a novel method for recognizing frontal views of faces under roughly constant illumination. Such method is based on the analysis of a wavelet packet decomposition of the face images, because very fast implementations of this procedure are available in hardware. An efficient and reliable probabilistic metric, which is derived from the Bhattacharrya distance, is also used to classify the face feature vectors into person classes, so that even very simple statistical features can provide a good basis for face classification.

Fractals and Iterated Function Systems (IFSs)

Fractal based recognition techniques are less computationally expensive than linear, non-linear and NN-based ones. Moreover, no retraining of the system is necessary when new images are added. The Iterated Function Systems (IFS) theory (Riccio, & Nappi, 2003) has been mainly investigated for still image coding, and has been subsequently extended to image indexing, thanks to its ability to describe the image content in a very compact

way (Figure 4). Furthermore, the fractal code of an image is invariant with respect to a wide set of global transformations, such as rotations (multiples of $\pi/2$), contrast scaling and channel shifting, just to cite some of them.

In (Kouzani, 1997) the fractal code of a face image is used for training a neural network, which works as classifier on the face database. Subsequently Tan and Yan propose a different IFS based strategy (Tan, & Yan, 1999), in which the IFS code of the face image is associated as a feature vector and stored in the database. During identification, only one iteration of every IFS code in the database is applied to the test image and the one producing the greater PSNR (Picked Signal to Noise Ratio) is returned. The linear cost of the testing operation represents the actual limit of this technique, when the face database size becomes considerable. The better way to cope with this drawback is to store the information extracted during the coding process, instead. In fact, Komleh et al. investigate on the discriminating power of the IFS parameters (Komleh, 2001). At first they consider contrast, brightness, range/domain match and rotation separately and then combine them together. The combination of IFS parameters provides better recognition rate than testing each one singly.

Figure 4. The feature extraction process of fractal based techniques

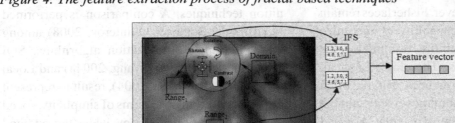

OPEN QUESTIONS IN FACE RECOGNITION

As stated above, Automatic Face Recognition (AFR) can be thought as a very complex object recognition problem, which is very difficult to solve, since the search is done among objects from the same class. Moreover, in most cases, no more than one visible image is available to enrol the subject and train the system, and different difficulties rise under uncontrolled conditions.

Changes in Illumination

Differences in appearance induced by illumination may be greater than differences between individuals. Therefore, many approaches for illumination invariance have been explored. Adini et al. (1997) investigate how changes in illumination can affect performances of some face recognition methods. None of the experimented techniques seems able to solve the problem by itself.

Gao et al. (Gao, & Leung, 2002) define a new approach extending the edge map technique, namely the Line Edge Map: face contours are extracted and combined in segments, which are in turn organized in lines. The Hausdorff distance is also modified in order to manage these new feature vectors. A novel pre-filtering criterion is applied, before performing the real testing operation. This approach outperforms other methods, such as Linear Subspaces or Eigenfaces, presented in (Belhumeur, 1997). However, Fisherfaces remain superior thanks to their capability to maximize the between-person variability, minimizing the within-person differences. Therefore, Li et al. (2004) argue that performances can be often further improved by combining several suitable linear methods. One of the most recent ICA-based methods has been proposed by Kim et al. (2003). The face is split in different regions that overlap on the boundaries. For each class containing all the elements belonging to the same face region, the residual space (the space spanned by the PCA after removing a few leading eigenfaces) is computed and the ICA is applied. The results underline that the PCA components in the residual space are the same found in the normal space, while ICA components are different, so that performances improve. Moreover, splitting the face in several regions simplifies the statistical model of the illumination variations, making the recognition task more robust with respect to them.

Not much has been made on generative methods yet. One of the few such methods has been proposed by Georghiades et al. (2001). The face shape and the albedo are extracted by few subject images, by means of shape from shading. The 3D model is then used to synthesize a wide set of face views in different pose and illumination. The main underlying hypothesis is that, for each fixed pose of the object/face, all its views under different illuminations form a convex cone in the image space. Such convex cone is therefore computed for every subject and pose, and then approximated by means of a low-dimensional linear subspace. In the testing phase the pose of the subject is esteemed, and the identity with the nearest convex cone is assigned, using the Euclidean distance. This method is better than many others in terms of recognition rate. The reverse of the medal is the non-trivial computational cost of the training phase. As for robustness to lighting variations in purely 2D methods, the present trend is to exploit some image normalization technique, rather than devising distortion invariant recognition techniques. A comparison is performed in (Ruiz-del-Solar, & Quinteros, 2008) among many lighting normalization algorithms. SQI (Self Quotient Image) (Wang, 2004a) and Local Binary Pattern (Ahoen, 2004), result to represent the best compromise in terms of simplicity, speed and authentication accuracy when the adopted classifier is of eigen-space based type.

Using some kind of input different from intensity images might overcome the above problems. For example, the infrared imagery deals with subsurface features, and some recent works demonstrate that it can be actually considered as a biometric feature (Chen, 2003). Combining the information from visible and infrared images can improve recognition performances (Socolinsky, & Selinger, 2004). However, a drawback of thermal images is their dependence on the skin temperature. On the other hand, it has been observed that the hyperspectral signature of the face is less dependent on the temperature than the thermal radiance. Different people show a high variability of the hyperspectral properties of the facial tissue, though these are constant for the same person across time and under different illumination. These observations suggest investigating them as a possible biometry (Pan, 2003).

Changes in Pose

It often happens that gallery (stored) face images are caught in quite controlled conditions, in a rather predefined pose, while probes might be caught in a less controlled setting.

Multi-view face recognition directly extends frontal face recognition. Related algorithms require gallery images at every pose. On the other hand, in face recognition across pose we aim at recognizing a face from a quite novel viewpoint. The problem of pose changes has been addressed by extending linear subspace approaches. For example, (Okada, 2002) addresses large 3D pose variations by means of parametric linear subspace models. The authors investigate two different linear models, namely the Linear Principal Components MAPing (LPCMAP) model: and the Parametric Piecewise Linear Subspace (PPLS) model. The experimental results, though with a relatively small number of subjects, show that the recognition system is robust against large 3D head pose variations covering 50 degree rotations along each axis. Gross et al. (2002) propose to use the light-field to achieve a greater robustness and stability to pose variation. The light-field is a 5D function of position (3D) and orientation (2D), which specifies the radiance of light in free space. Any image of the object corresponds to a curve in the light-field. The input face images are therefore vectorized in light-field vectors, next used for training and testing the system. Generative methods have also been proposed for pose variations. In (Zhang, 2008), starting from one frontal and one in profile image, both 3D shape and texture information are recovered. Such novel 3D virtual face model subsequently allows generating face images in completely arbitrary poses. In (Xiujuan, 2007) the frontal image of a face in non frontal pose is reconstructed from a single image, in order to avoid the computationally expensive process of 3D model generation. The underlying assumption is that there exist a linear mapping between subregions (patches) of non frontal and frontal images.

Occlusion

Local approaches represent one possible approach to better recognize partially occluded objects. In general, these techniques divide the face into different parts and then use a voting space to find the best match. However, a voting technique can easily misclassify a test image, since it does not take into account how good a local match is. Martinez (Martinez, & Kak, 2001) adopts a probabilistic approach to address this problem. Each face image is divided into k different local parts, each modelled by a Gaussian distribution, which accounts for the localization error problem. Performed experiments demonstrate that the suppression of 1/6 of the face does not decrease accuracy, while even for those cases where 1/3 of the face is occluded, the identification results are very close to those obtained without occlusions. Worse results are obtained when the eye area is occluded rather than the mouth area. The probabilistic approach proposed by Martinez only identifies a partially occluded face, while the method by Kurita et al. (2003) also reconstructs the occluded part of the face and detects the occluded regions in the input image, by means of an auto-associative neural network. The network is first trained on the non-occluded images in normal conditions. During testing the original face can be reconstructed by replacing occluded regions with the recalled pixels. As a further example, Sahbi and Boujemaa (2002) propose a method, to deal with both occlusions and illumination changes, based on salient feature extraction in challenging conditions. These features are used in a matching process using the dynamic space warping. Such process aligns each feature in the query image, if possible, with its corresponding feature in the gallery set. Even in (Kazuhiro, 2008) the main idea is to exploit a local feature extraction process. In the specific case at hand, local SVM kernels are combined by local Gaussian summation kernel. The difference in recognition accuracy between global kernel SVMs and local kernel ones significantly grows with the size of the occluded region, till to reach a factor of 6. The method in (Hyun, 2008) differs from others since the proposed algorithm locates occluded regions first, in order to exclude them from the actual recognition phase. The obtained accuracy performances are about double than those obtained by a global method, e.g. PCA.

Age

A non-negligible time lapse between the training and testing images may introduce critical variations in the face appearance, therefore reducing recognition performances. Some addressing strategies require to periodically upgrade the gallery or to retrain the system. This solution is quite impractical and only applies to those systems granting some services, which frequently perform the authentication task. Alternatively, the age of the subject could be simulated. Several related techniques are given in literature, though none has been investigated in the face recognition framework: Coordinate Transformations, Facial Composites, Exaggeration of 3D Distinctive Characteristics. Lanitis et al. (2002) propose a method based on age functions. Every image in the face database

is described by a set of parameters b, and for each subject the best age function is drawn depending on his/her b. The main advantage of this approach is that different subject-based age functions allow taking into account external factors which contribute to age variations. Notice that the number of database subjects is very small, emphasizing the absence of a standard FERET-like database, which systematically models the age variations.

Final Remarks on 2D Face Recognition Testing

Methods presented in previous sections have both advantages and drawbacks. Stating which one is the best is very difficult, and strongly depends on the working requirements. Moreover, most of the above approaches have been tested on different datasets, so that it is sometimes hard to effectively compare them. One way to make a more general evaluation is to pick a wider set of significant parameters, rather than considering the recognition rate only. As shown in Table 3, the parameter set may include several aspects that need to be taken into account during testing. Examples are the number of databases and their characteristics, probe and gallery sets dimension, input size and so on. Table 3 summarizes the characteristics of a number of methods.

3D FACE RECOGNITION

In a recent work, Xu et al. (Xu, 2004) demonstrated that depth maps a more robust face representation, less affected by illumination changes, than intensity images, since a 3D model, either range data or polygonal mesh, retains a complete information about the face geometry. In a 3D face model, facial features are represented by local and global curvatures that can be considered as the real signature which identifies persons.

Two main face models are commonly used in 3D applications, namely 2.5D and 3D images (see

Table 3. A summary of characteristics of 2D face recognition methods

Method		Databases	Recognition Rate	EXPR	ILL	POSE	OCCL	AGE
Authors	Name							
(Martinez, 2002)	PCA	AR-Faces	70%		no	no	no	no
(Martinez, 2002)	LDA	AR-Faces	88%		no	no	no	no
(Belhumeur, 1997)	Fisherfaces	YALE	99.6%	yes	yes	no	no	no
(Yu, & Yang, 2001)	Direct LDA	ORL	90.8%	yes	yes	yes	no	no
(Lu, 2003)	DF-LDA	ORL UMIST	96% 98%		yes no	no no	no no	no no
(Dao-Qing, 2007)	RDA	ORL YALE FERET	85% 78% 82%	yes	yes	no	no	no
(Zhao, & Pong, 2008)	ILDA	FERET CMU-PIE	96% 88%	yes	yes	yes	no	yes
(Cevikalp, 2005)	DCV	Yale AR-Faces	97.33% 99.35%		yes	no	no	no
(Bartlett, 2002)	ICA	FERET	89%	yes	no	no	no	no
(Haifeng, 2008)	ICA-NPA	FERET CAS-PEAL	93% 85%	yes	yes	no	no	no
(Lin, 1997)	PDBNN	SCR FERET ORL	100% 99% 96	yes yes yes	yes yes yes	yes no yes	no no no	no no no
(Meng, 2002)	RBF	ORL PropertyDB	98.1% 100%	yes		yes	no	no
(Perronnin, 2003)	HMM	FERET	97%	yes	no	no	no	no
(Lades, 1993)	DLA	PropertyDB	90.3%	yes		yes	no	no
(Liu, 2004)	Gabor EFM	FERET ORL	99% 100%	yes yes	no no	no yes	no no	no no
(Wiskott, 1997)	EGM	FERET PropertyDB	80% 90%	yes yes		yes yes	no no	no no
(Garcia, 2000)	WPA	MIT FERET	80.5% 89%	yes	yes		no	no
(Kouzani, 1997)	IFS	PropertyDB	100%	no	no	no	no	no
(Tan, & Yan, 1999)	IFS	ORL	95%				no	no
(Komleh, 2001)	IFS	MIT	90%			yes	no	no
(Chen, 2003)	Th-Infrared	PropertyDB	98%	yes	yes	no	no	no
Socolinsky, & Selinger, 2004)	Thermal	PropertyDB	93%	yes	yes	no	no	no
(Pan, 2003)	Hyperspectral	PropertyDB	92%	no	yes	no	no	no
Open Question Methods								
(Gao, & Leung, 2002)	LEM	Bern AR-Faces Yale	72.09% 86.03% 85.45%	yes	yes yes yes	yes no no	no no no	no no no
(Kim, 2003)	ICA	Subset of AR Faces, Yale, ORL, Bern and FERET	98%		yes	yes	no	no
(Li, 2004)	Linear Methods LDA/GSVD LDA/QR	CMU_PIE/Pose27	100% 99.53%	no	yes	no	no	no
(Li, 2004)	Linear Methods LDA/GSVD LDA/QR	YaleB/Pose00	99% 98.03%		yes	no	no	no
(Zhang, 2008)	AA-LBP	CMU-PIE	93%	yes	yes	yes	no	no
(Xiujuan, 2007)	LLR	CMU-PIE	94%	no	no	yes	no	no
(Georghiades, 2001)	Cones Gen.	Yale B	97%	no	yes	yes	no	no
(Okada, 2002)	LinearSubspaces	ATR-Database	98.7%	no	no	yes	no	no
(Gross, 2002)	Eigen Lights	CMU-PIE	36%	no	yes	yes	no	no

continued on following page

Table 3. continued

Method		Databases	Recognition Rate	EXPR	ILL	POSE	OCCL	AGE
Authors	Name							
(Martinez, & Kak, 2001)	Martinez	AR-Faces	65%	no	no	no	yes	no
(Kazuhiro, 2008)	SVM-GSK	ORL AR-Faces	90% 80%	yes	yes	no	yes	nl
(Hyun, 2008)	S-LNMF	AR-Faces	87%	yes	yes	no	yes	no
(Kurita, 2003)	NeuralNetworks	AR-Faces	79%	no	no	no	yes	no
(Sahbi, & Boujemaa, 2002)	DSW	ORL AR Faces					yes	
(Lanitis, 2002)	Age Functions	PropertyDB	71%	yes	yes	no	no	yes

Figure 5. (a) 2D image, (b) 2.5 image and (c) 3D image (© [2004] IEEE)

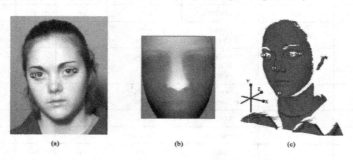

Figure 5). A 2.5D image (range image) consists of a two-dimensional representation of a 3D point set (x,y,z), where each pixel in the X-Y plane stores the depth value z, like in a grey-scale image. 2.5D images depend on the external appearance as well as environmental conditions. Taking several scans from different viewpoints allows building a whole 3D head model. On the contrary, 3D images are a global representation of the whole head, and the facial surface is further related to the internal anatomical structure. A further difference between 2.5D and 3D images is that the latter are not affected by self-occlusions of the face, when the pose is not full-frontal.

The simplest 3D face representation is a 3D polygonal mesh, consisting of a list of points (vertices) connected by edges (polygons). Among the many ways to build a 3D mesh, the most popular ones are combining several 2.5D images, properly tuning a 3D morphable model, or exploit-

ing a 3D acquisition system (3D scanner). However, aligning a 3D polygonal mesh within an absolute reference frame is generally computationally expensive, and existing methods are not always convergent. In addition, the assertion that 3D data acquisition (laser and structured light scanners) is light independent is not completely true; 3D sensors could be affected by a strong light source or by reflective surfaces, so it can be reasonably asserted that different light sources might generate quite different 3D data sets.

Not so many papers have been published at present about 3D face recognition. Many criteria can be adopted to compare existing 3D face algorithms, by taking into account the type of problems they address, such as mesh alignment, morphing, etc., or their intrinsic properties. Indeed, some approaches perform very well only on faces with neutral expression, while some others try also to deal with expression changes. Sometimes, the distance between the target and the camera can affect the size of the facial surface, as well as its height, depth, etc. Therefore, approaches exploiting a curvature based representation cannot distinguish between two faces with similar shape, but different size. Some methods try to overcome this problem by point-to-point comparison or by volume approximation. However, the lack of an appropriate standard dataset containing a large number and variety of people, and of image variations, is one of the great limitations to empirical experimentation for existing algorithms. In general, 3D face recognition systems are tested on proprietary databases, with few models and with a limited number of variations per model.

Methods in this section have been grouped in three main categories: 2D image-based, 3D image-based and multimodal systems. The first category includes methods which are still based on comparisons among 2D intensity images, yet supported by some 3D data and procedure that increase the system robustness. The second class groups approaches based on 3D facial representations, like range images or meshes. Finally, the third category includes methods combining 2D image and 3D image information.

2D-Based Class

The underlying idea is to use a 3D generic face model to improve robustness of 2D methods with respect to pose, illumination and facial expression variations. An example of this approach is given by Blanz et al. (Blanz, & Vetter, 2003). They propose to automatically synthesize a number of facial variations by using a morphable model (see Figure 6). The resulting images are used to augment the given training set, containing only a single frontal 2D image for each subject. Hu et al. (2004) show that linear methods such as PCA and LDA can be further extended to cope with changes in pose and illumination by using a Nearest Neighbour approach. Their results show that

Figure 6. Face reconstruction from a single image (© [2003] IEEE)

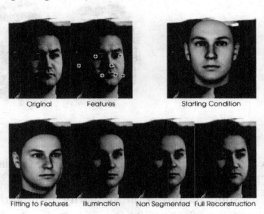

using virtual faces for particular poses increase the recognition rate.

3D-Based Class

The first problem to address is how to obtain a correct alignment between two face surfaces. One possible approach exploits an acquisition system based on a morphable model, which is pre-aligned within a given reference frame. The work by Ansari (2003) presents an example of this kind of methods.

The Iterative Closest Point (ICP) algorithm (Besl, & McKay, 1992) is an alternative approach to alignment. It could be used to reduce misalignment during the registration phase as well as to approximate the volume difference between two surfaces. However, it leads to convergence problems when the initial misalignment of the data sets is too large; it is possible to address this limitation with a coarse pre-alignment. An ICP-based approach is given by Cook et al. (2004). They use ICP only to establish the correspondence between 3D surfaces, in order to cope with the non-rigid nature of faces. Once the registration is completed, faces are compared by using the statistical Gaussian Mixture Model (GMM), and the distribution of the errors is then parameter-

Figure 7. Examples of 3D mesh segmentation based on local curvature (© [2004] Moreno A. B.)

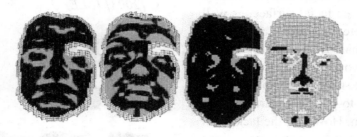

ized. Irfanoglu et al. (2004) exploit a quite similar ICP-based approach.

Despite its power in similarity estimation between two faces, ICP has a serious drawback, since it treats the 3D shape of the face as a rigid object, so that it is unable to handle changes in expression. In (Medioni, & Waupotitsch, 2003), authors propose an ICP-based approach, that first aligns two face surfaces and calculates a map of differences between them; afterwards, statistic measures are applied in order to obtain a compact description of this map. A different use of the ICP algorithm is to approximate the surface difference between two faces (see for example (Lu, 2004)).

A further interesting aspect concerns the analysis of the 3D facial surface in order to extrapolate information about the shape. Some approaches are based on a curvature-based segmentation, which detects a set of fiducial regions (see Figure 7). In 1991, Gordon (1991) presents a method based on the idea that some facial descriptors, such as the shape of forehead, jaw line, eye corner cavities and cheeks, remain generally similar although they are taken by different range images for the same subject. Chua *et al.* (2000) report similar observations. It is worth noticing that this is not completely true when detection errors or changes in expression occur. Another interesting segmentation approach based on Gaussian curvature has been proposed by Moreno et al. (2003).

Creating mathematical models to represent local curvatures is the leading idea behind a further kind of approach to the analysis of facial shape. A 3D surface can be effectively repre-sented in a compact fashion, using few character-izing features descriptors. In addition, a local curvature-based representation better copes with the non-rigid nature of face due to facial expres-sions. In fact, even though expressions change the facial surface globally, local curvature rela-tions are preserved. Unfortunately, such repre-sentations are not able to handle information about the size of face, thus not allowing to distinguish two similar faces but with different sizes. Tanaka et al. (1998) propose an approach along this line.

In 3D face recognition PCA is applied to data treated as a cloud of points rather than a surface. Moreover, new axes that best summarize the vari-ance across the vertices are determined. Thus, the PCA is able to work with different facial poses producing a descriptive model of the facial shape. This approach has been extended by Hesher et al. (2002). The method applies the PCA directly to range images, while the Euclidean distance is used to measure similarities among the resulting feature vectors. Further investigations on PCA in the 3D setting have been carried out by Heseltine et al. (Heseltine, 2004a; Heseltine, 2004b).

2D and 3D-Based Class

Multimodal approaches combine information coming from 2D images as well as 3D models of faces. Chang (2004) underlines four important conclusions: (1) 2D and 3D individually have similar recognition performance, (2) Combining 2D and 3D results by a simple weighting scheme outperforms either 2D or 3D alone, (3) Combining

Figure 8. PCA-based recognition experiments performed using 2D and 3D Eigenfaces

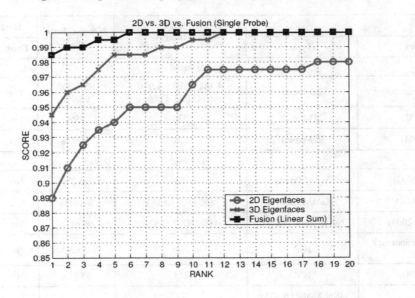

Figure 9. Facial surface representation: (a) texture mapping on the facial surface (b) and on the canonical form; (c) the resulting flattened texture and (d) the canonical image (© [2003] Bronstein A.)

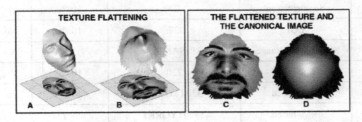

Figure 10. Colour mapping of residual 3D distance (a) from two different subjects and (b) from the same subject (© [2004] IEEE)

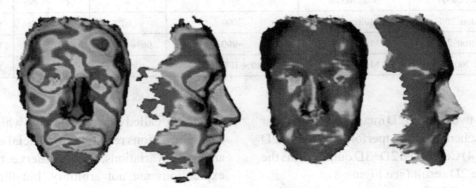

Table 4. The main information about the experimental results of most of the discussed 3D methods

Method		No. Images	Recogn. Rate %	Database Characteristics			
Authors	Type			Expr.	Ill.	Pose	Occl
2D based							
(Blanz, & Vetter, 2003)	2D-based	4,488 (PIE) + 1,940 (FERET)	95% and 95,9%	Yes	Yes	Yes	No
(Lu, 2003)	2D-based	220	85%	Yes	Yes	Yes	No
(Hu, 2004)	2D-based	41.368	< 95%	Yes	Yes	Yes	No
3D based							
(Ansari, 2003)	Set of Points	52	96.2%	No	No	No	No
(Cook, 2004)	GMM (ICP)	360 (3D_RMA)	97,33%	Yes	No	Yes	No
(Irfanoglu, 2004)	Set of Points (ICP)	90 (3D_RMA)	96,66%	Yes	No	Yes	No
(Medioni, & Waupotitsch, 2003)	ICP	700	98%	No	No	Yes	No
(Lu, 2004)	ICP	113	95.5%	Yes	Yes	Yes	No
(Gordon, 1991)	Local Shape Descriptors	24	100%	No	No	No	No
(Moreno, 2003)	Local Shape Descriptors	420 (GavabDB)	78%	Yes	Yes	Yes	No
(Chua, 2000)	Segmentation	24	100%	Yes	No	No	No
(Tanaka, 1998)	EGI	37	100%	No	No	No	No
(Wang, 2004b)	Sphere-Spin-Images	31 (SAMPL)	91,68%	No	No	Yes	No
(Hesher, 2002)	PCA-based	220	100%	Yes	No	No	No
(Heseltine, 2004a)	PCA-based	330 (YORK)	<87,3%	Yes	No	Yes	No
(Heseltine, 2004b)	PCA-based	1770 (YORK)	<88,7%	Yes	No	Yes	No
(Iordanis, 2008)	3D	2500 (BU-3DFE)	86%	Yes	No	No	No
Multimodal							
(Chang, 2004)	Multimodal	-	98.8%	Yes	Yes	Yes	No
(Bronstein, 2003)	Multimodal	-	-	Yes	No	Yes	No
(Tsalakanidou, 2003)	Multimodal	3000	91,67%	Yes	Yes	Yes	Yes
(Papatheodorou, 2004)	Multimodal	~900	66%-100%	Yes	Yes	Yes	No
(Ajmal, 2007)	Multimodal	4950 (FRGC)	99%	Yes	No	No	No

results from two or more 2D images using a similar weighting scheme also outperforms a single 2D image, and (4) Combined 2D+3D outperforms the multi-image 2D result (see Figure 8).

(Bronstein, 2003) presents a method based on a bending invariant canonical representation

(Figure 9), called canonical image, which models the deformations resulting from facial expression and pose variations. They observe that facial expressions are not arbitrary, but they can be modelled by using isometric transformations. The canonical image stores these geometric invariants.

The 2D face image is mapped onto the canonical image shape by flattening the texture coordinates onto the canonical surface.

As a further example of "hybrid" systems, Tsalakanidou (2003) presents an Hidden Markov Model (HMM) approach to integrate depth data and intensity image. Papatheodorou and Ruecker (2004) propose a 4D registration method based on Iterative Closest Point (ICP), with the addition of textural information. Measurement of facial similarity involves a 4D Euclidean distance (colour mapped as shown in Figure 10) between four dimensional points, characterized by the three spatial coordinates plus the texel intensity information. In case of frontal pose, results show that the use of both texture and shape improves performances, depending on pose and expression. In (Ajmal, 2007) the authors present an hybrid 2D-3D classification algorithm, based on Scale-Invariant Feature Transform (SIFT). SIFTs, when applied to the 2D face projection, allow to discard most models, in a first database filtering step; during a second phase, only candidate models are compared through a local match.

All 3D based methods introduced so far are summarized in Table 4, together with a small set of parameters, that can be considered meaningful for a more complete and accurate evaluation of discussed approaches.

DISCUSSION AND REMARKS

The approaches discussed herein address only part of existing open questions. The current state of the art makes it clear that none of the existing techniques is able to cope by itself with all possible distortions that a face can undergo. A serious obstacle to an overall comparison of different proposals is the lack of a wide standard face database, modelling a real world scenario in terms of differences in gender and ethnic group as well as expression, illumination, pose, etc.

In Section II many strategies have been analyzed, showing that almost all methods claim satisfactory recognition rates, but only when tested on standard databases or some parts of them. Subsection II-A highlights that linear/non-linear approaches overcome other methods when illumination changes occur. However, this class of methods is noticeably affected by changes in pose, and they perform worse when both variations are present. Similarly, methods that cope with variations in pose and illumination, such as Line Edge Map (Gao, & Leung, 2002) suffer from the presence of occlusions and age variations.

Similarly, 3D image analysis has the potential to increase the recognition performances of the 2D face recognition with respect to pose, illumination and expression variations, but there are many challenging problems to be still addressed, such as alignment of meshes or sensitiveness of the acquisition process. Another important issue for face recognition is the detection of occlusive objects, like glasses and hair. At present, no 3D face recognition method addresses occlusions. Finally, a smart integration between the texture image and facial surface is necessary. Most 2D+3D approaches work on 2D and 3D data separately, with possible overlap of the same information taken from two differences sources, and merge final results together. In particular, combining 2D and 3D approaches leads to results that overcome both 2D and 3D, in terms of recognition rate. Nevertheless, this kind of systems inherit common problems of 3D processing, particularly concerning the acquisition process.

The above discussion suggests that only a proper combination of more current methods in a single face multibiometric system can be robust enough to be applied in a real-world scenario.

REFERENCES

Adini, Y., Moses, Y., & Ullman, S. (1997). Face recognition: The problem of compensating for changes in illumination direction. *IEEE Transactions on Pattern Analysis and Machine Intelligence, 19*(7), 721–732. doi:10.1109/34.598229

Ahonen, T., Hadid, A., & Pietikainen, M. (2004). Face recognition with local binary patterns. In N. Sebe, M. S. Lew & T. S. Huang (Eds.), *The Eighth European Conference on Computer Vision* (ECCV 2004) (pp. 469–481).

Ajmal, S., Mian, M. B., & Robyn, O. (2007). An Efficient Multimodal 2D-3D Hybrid Approach to Automatic Face Recognition. *IEEE Transactions on Pattern Analysis and Machine Intelligence, 29*(11), 1927–1943. doi:10.1109/TPAMI.2007.1105

Ansari, A., & Abdel-Mottaleb, M. (2003). 3-D face modeling using two views and a generic face model with application to 3-D face recognition. In *Proc. IEEE Conf. on Advanced Video and Signal Based Surveillance*, Miami, FL, USA, July (pp. 37–44).

Barrett, W. A. (1997). A survey of face recognition algorithms and testing results. In *Conference Record of the Thirty-First Asilomar Conference on Signals, Systems & Computers* (pp. 301–305).

Bartlett, M., Stewart, M., Javier, R., & Sejnowski, T. J. (2002). Face recognition by independent component analysis. *IEEE Transactions on Neural Networks, 13*(6), 1450–1464. doi:10.1109/TNN.2002.804287

Belhumeur, Peter N., Hespanha, J. P., Kriegman, David. (1997). Eigenfaces vs. fisherfaces: Using class specific linear projection. *IEEE Transactions on Pattern Analysis and Machine Intelligence, 19*(7), 711–720. doi:10.1109/34.598228

Besl, P. J., & McKay, N. D. (1992). A method for registration of 3-d shapes. *IEEE Transactions on Pattern Analysis and Machine Intelligence, 14*(2), 239–256. doi:10.1109/34.121791

Blanz, V., & Vetter, T. (2003). Face recognition based on fitting a 3D morphable model. *IEEE Transactions on Pattern Analysis and Machine Intelligence, 25*(9), 1063–1074. doi:10.1109/TPAMI.2003.1227983

Bronstein, A., Bronstein, M., & Kimmel, R. (2003). Expression-invariant 3D face recognition. Proc. Audio & Video-based Biometric Person Authentication (AVBPA). In *Lecture Notes in Computer Science*, Vol. 2688. Springer, pp. 62–69.

Cevikalp, H., Neamtu, M., Wilkes, M., & Barkana, A. (2005). Discriminative common vectors for face recognition. *IEEE Transactions on Pattern Analysis and Machine Intelligence, 27*(1), 4–13. doi:10.1109/TPAMI.2005.9

Chalmond, B., & Girard, S. C. (1999). Nonlinear modeling of scattered multivariate data and its application to shape change. *IEEE Transactions on Pattern Analysis and Machine Intelligence, 5*(21), 422–432. doi:10.1109/34.765654

Chang, K., Bowyer, K., Flynn, P. (2004). An evaluation of multi-modal 2D + 3D face biometrics. *IEEE Trans. Pattern Anal. Machine Intell.* (PAMI 2004).

Chen, X., Flynn, P. J., & Bowyer, K. W. (2003). PCA-based face recognition in infrared imagery: Baseline and comparative studies. In *IEEE Internat. Workshop on Analysis and Modeling of Faces and Gestures* (pp. 127–134).

Chua, C. S., Han, F., & Ho, Y. K. (2000). 3D human face recognition using point signature. In *IEEE Internat. Conf. on Automatic Face and Gesture Recognition (FG 2000)*, France, March, pp. 233–238.

Cook, J., Chandran, V., Sridharan, S., & Fookes, C. (2004). Face recognition from 3D data using iterative closest point algorithm and Gaussian mixture models. In *Internat. Symposium on 3D Data Processing, Visualization and Transmission (3DPVT 2004)*, Thessaloniki, Greece, 6–9 September.

Cottrell, G. W., & Fleming, M. (1990). Face Recognition using unsupervised feature extraction. In *International Neural Networks Conference* (pp. 322-325).

Dao-Qing, D., & Pong, C. Y. (2007). Face Recognition by Regularized Discriminant Analysis. *IEEE Transactions on Systems, Man and Cybernatics – Part B, 37*(4), 1080-1085.

Gao, P., Woo, W. L., & Dlay, S. S. (2006). Nonlinear independent component analysis using series reversion and Weierstrass network. In *Vision Image and Signal Processing* (pp. 115-131).

Gao, Y., & Leung, M. K. H. (2002). Face recognition using line edge map. *IEEE Transactions on Pattern Analysis and Machine Intelligence, 24*(6), 764–779. doi:10.1109/TPAMI.2002.1008383

Garcia, C., Zikos, G., & Tziritas, G. (2000). Wavelet packet analysis for face recognition. *Image and Vision Computing, 18*, 289–297. doi:10.1016/S0262-8856(99)00056-6

Georghiades, A. S., Belhumeur, P. N., & Kriegman, D. J. (2001). From few to many: Illumination cone models for face recognition under variable lighting and pose. *IEEE Transactions on Pattern Analysis and Machine Intelligence, 23*(6), 643–660. doi:10.1109/34.927464

Gordon, G. (1991). Face recognition based on depth maps and surface curvature . In *Geometric Methods in Computer Vision* (pp. 1–12). SPIE.

Gross, R., Matthews, I., & Baker, S. (2002). Eigen light-fields and face recognition across pose. In *IEEE Internat. Conf. on Automatic Face and Gesture Recognition*, May (pp. 1–7).

Haifeng, H. (2008). ICA-based neighborhood preserving analysis for face recognition . *Computer Vision and Image Understanding, 3*(112), 286–295.

Han, J., Cai, D., He, X., & Zhang, H.-J. (2006). Orthogonal laplacianfaces for face recognition. *IEEE Transactions on Image Processing, 15*, 3608–3614. doi:10.1109/TIP.2006.881945

Heseltine, T., Pears, N., & Austin, J. 2004a. Three-dimensional face recognition: An eigensurface approach. In *Internat. Conf. on Image Processing (ICIP 2004)*, October, Singapore.

Heseltine, T., Pears, N., & Austin, J. (2004b). Three-dimensional face recognition: A fischersurface approach. *Image Analysis and Recognition: Internat. Conf. (ICIAR 2004)*, Porto, Portugal (pp. 684–691).

Hesher, C., Srivastava, A., & Erlebacher, G. (2002). Principal component analysis of range images for facial recognition. *Internat. Conf. on Imaging Science, Systems and Technology (CISST 2002)*.

Hu, Y. X., Jiang, D. L., Yan, S. C., & Zhang, H. J. (2004). Automatic 3D Reconstruction for Face Recognition. In *IEEE International Conf. on Automatic Face and Gesture Recognition (FGR 2004)*, Seoul . *Korea & World Affairs*, (May): 843–850.

Huang, J., Chen, W.-S., Yuen, P. C., & Dai, D.-Q. (2005). Kernel machine-based one-parameter regularized Fisher discriminant method for face recognition. *IEEE Trans. Syst. Man Cybern. B, 35*(4), 659–669. doi:10.1109/TSMCB.2005.844596

Huang, W., & Yin, H. (2009). *Comparison of PCA and Nonlinear PCA for Face Recognition*. Signal Processing, Pattern Recognition and Applications.

Hyun, J. O., Kyoung, M. L., & Sang, U. L. (2008). Occlusion invariant face recognition using selective local non-negative matrix factorization basis images. In *Image and Vision Computing* (pp. 1515–1523).

Iordanis, M., Sotiris, M., & Michael, G. S. (2008). Bilinear Models for 3-D Face and Facial Expression Recognition. *IEEE Transactions on Information Forensics and Security*, 3(3), 498–511. doi:10.1109/TIFS.2008.924598

Irfanoglu, M. O., Gokberk, B., & Akarun, L. (2004). 3D shape-based face recognition using automatically registered facial surfaces. In *Internat. Conf. on Pattern Recognition (ICPR2004)*, Cambridge (pp. 183–186).

Johnson, M. L. (2004). Biometrics and the threat to civil liberties. *Computer*, 37(4), 90–92. doi:10.1109/MC.2004.1297317

Kazuhiro, H. (2008). Robust face recognition under partial occlusion based on support vector machine with local Gaussian summation kernel. *Image and Vision Computing*, 26, 1490–1498. doi:10.1016/j.imavis.2008.04.008

Kim, T.-K., Kim, H., Hwang, W., Kee, S.-C., & Kittler, J. (2003). Independent component analysis in a facial local residue space. In *IEEE Computer Society Conference on Computer Vision and Pattern Recognition* (Vol. 1, pp. 579–586).

Kirby, M., & Sirovich, L. (1990). Application of the Karhunen-Loeve procedure for the characterization of human faces. *IEEE Transactions on Pattern Analysis and Machine Intelligence*, 12(1), 103–108. doi:10.1109/34.41390

Komleh, E. H., Chandran, V., & Sridharan, S. (2001). Face recognition using fractal codes. In *International Conference on Image Processing* (pp. 58–61).

Kouzani, A. Z., He, F., & Sammut, K. (1997). Fractal face representation and recognition. In *IEEE Internat. Conf. on Systems, Man, and Cybernetics* (pp. 1609–1613).

Kurita, T., Pic, M., & Takahashi, T. (2003). Recognition and detection of occluded faces by a neural network classifier with recursive data reconstruction. In *IEEE Conf. on Advanced Video and Signal Based Surveillance*, July (pp. 53–58).

Lades, M., Vorbruggen, J. C., Buhmann, J., Lange, J., van der Malsburg, C., Wurtz, R. P., & Konen, W. (1993, March). Distortion invariant object recognition in the dynamic link architecture. *IEEE Transactions on Computers*, 42, 300–311. doi:10.1109/12.210173

Lanitis, A., Taylor, J. C., & Timothy, F. C. (2002). Toward automatic simulation of aging effects on face images. *IEEE Transactions on Pattern Analysis and Machine Intelligence*, 24(4), 442–455. doi:10.1109/34.993553

Li, Q., Ye, J., & Kambhamettu, C. (2004). Linear projection methods in face recognition under unconstrained illuminations: A comparative study. In *IEEE Computer Society Conf. on Computer Vision and Pattern Recognition (CVPR04)*.

Lin, S.-H., Kung, S.-Y., & Lin, L.-J. (1997). Face recognition/detection by probabilistic decision-based neural network. *IEEE Transactions on Neural Networks*, 8(1), 114–132. doi:10.1109/72.554196

Liu, C. (2004). Gabor-based kernel PCA with fractional power polynomial models for face recognition. *IEEE Transactions on Pattern Analysis and Machine Intelligence*, 26(5), 572–581. doi:10.1109/TPAMI.2004.1273927

Lu, J., Plataniotis, Kostantinos, N., & Venetsanopoulos, A. N. (2003). Face Recognition Using LDA-Based Algorithms. *IEEE Transactions on Neural Networks*, 14(1), 195–200. doi:10.1109/TNN.2002.806647

Lu, X., Colbry, D., & Jain, A. K. (2004). Three-dimensional model based face recognition. In *Internat. Conf. on Pattern Recognition (ICPR2004)*, Cambridge (pp. 362–366).

Martinez, A. M. (2002). Recognizing imprecisely localized, partially occluded, and expression variant faces from a single sample per class. *IEEE Transactions on Pattern Analysis and Machine Intelligence*, *24*(6), 748–763. doi:10.1109/TPAMI.2002.1008382

Martinez, A. M., & Kak, A. C. (2001). PCA versus LDA. *IEEE Transactions on Pattern Analysis and Machine Intelligence*, *23*(2), 228–233. doi:10.1109/34.908974

Medioni, G., & Waupotitsch, R. (2003). Face recognition and modeling in 3D. In *IEEE Internat. Workshop on Analysis and Modeling of Faces and Gesture Recognition (AMFG'03)*, Nice, France, October (pp. 232–233).

Meng, J. E., Shiqian, W., Juwei, L., & Hock, L. T. (2002). Face recognition with radial basis function (RBF) neural networks. *IEEE Transactions on Neural Networks*, *13*(3), 697–710. doi:10.1109/TNN.2002.1000134

Moreno, A. B., Sanchez, A., Velez, J. F., & Diaz, F. J. (2003). Face recognition using 3D surface-extracted descriptors. In *Irish Machine Vision and Image, (IMVIP'03)*, September.

Okada, K., & von der Malsburg, C. (2002). Pose-invariant face recognition with parametric linear subspaces. In *IEEE Internat. Conf. on Automatic Face and Gesture Recognition*, May (pp. 64–69).

Pan, Z., Healey, G., Prasad, M., & Tromberg, B. (2003). Face recognition in hyperspectral images. *IEEE Transactions on Pattern Analysis and Machine Intelligence*, *25*(12), 1552–1560. doi:10.1109/TPAMI.2003.1251148

Papatheodorou, T., & Rueckert, D. (2004). Evaluation of automatic 4D face recognition using surface and texture registration. In *IEEE Internat. Conf. on Automatic Face and Gesture Recognition* Seoul . *Korea & World Affairs*, (May): 321–326.

Perronnin, F., & Dugelay, J.-L. (2003). An introduction to biometrics and face recognition. In *IMAGE'2003: Learning, Understanding, Information Retrieval, Medical* (pp. 1-20).

Phillips, J. P., Moon, H., Rizvi, A. S., & Rauss, P. J. (2000). The FERET evaluation methodology for face-recognition algorithms. *IEEE Transactions on Pattern Analysis and Machine Intelligence*, *22*(10), 1090–1104. doi:10.1109/34.879790

Phillips, P. J., Flynn, P. J., Scruggs, T., Bowyer, K. W., Chang, J., Hoffman, K., et al. (2005). Overview of the Face Recognition Grand Challenge. In *IEEE Conf. Computer Vision and Pattern Recognition (CVPR)* (pp. 947-954).

Qing Shan, L., Rui, H., Han Qing, L., & Song De, M. (2003). Kernel-based nonlinear discriminant analysis for face recognition. *Journal of Computer Science and Technology*, *18*(6), 788–795. doi:10.1007/BF02945468

Riccio, D., & Nappi, M. (2003 September). Defering range/domain comparisons in fractal image compression. In *Internat. Conf. on Image Analysis and Processing* (Vol. 1, pp. 412–417).

Ruiz-del-Solar, J., & Quinteros, J. (2008). Illumination compensation and normalization in eigenspace-based face recognition: A comparative study of different pre-processing approaches. In *Pattern Recognition Letters* (pp. 1966–1979).

Sahbi, H., & Boujemaa, N. (2002). Robust Face Recognition Using Dynamic Space Warping. In *Biometric Authentication, International ECCV 2002 Workshop Copenhagen* (pp. 121–132).

Sherrah, J. (2004 May). False alarm rate: A critical performance measure for face recognition. In *Sixth IEEE Internat. Conf. on Automatic Face and Gesture Recognition*, (pp. 189–194).

Sim, T., Baker, S., & Bsat, M. (2003). The CMU pose, illumination, and expression database. *IEEE Transactions on Pattern Analysis and Machine Intelligence*, 25(12), 1615–1618. doi:10.1109/TPAMI.2003.1251154

Socolinsky, D. A., & Selinger, A. (2004). Thermal face recognition over time. In *Internat. Conf. on Pattern Recognition (ICPR04)*.

Tan, T., & Yan, H. (1999). Face recognition by fractal transformations. In *IEEE Internat. Conf. on Acoustics, Speech, and Signal Processing (ICASSP'99)* (pp. 3537–3540).

Tanaka, H. T., Ikeda, M., & Chiaki, H. (1998). Curvature-based face surface recognition using spherical correlation – principal directions for curved object recognition. In *Internat. Conf. on Face & Gesture Recognition (FG'98)*, Nara, Japan, April (pp. 372–377).

Tsalakanidou, F., Tzovaras, D., & Strintzis, M. G. (2003). Use of depth and colour Eigenfaces for face recognition. *Pattern Recognition Letters*, 24(9-10), 1427–1435. doi:10.1016/S0167-8655(02)00383-5

Wang, H., Li, S., & Wang, Y. (2004). Face recognition under varying lighting conditions using self quotient image. In *International Conference on Face and Gesture Recognition* (pp. 819–824).

Wang, Y., Pan, G., & Wu, Z. (2004 June). Sphere-spin-image: A viewpoint-invariant surface representation for 3D face recognition. In *Internat. Conf. on Computational Science (ICCS'04)* (LNCS 3037, pp. 427–434).

Wiskott, L., Fellous, J. M., Kruger, N., & von der Malsburg, C. (1997). Face recognition by elastic bunch graph matching. *IEEE Transactions on Pattern Analysis and Machine Intelligence*, 19(July), 775–779. doi:10.1109/34.598235

Wright, J., Yang, A. Y., Ganesh, A., Sastry, S. S., & Ma, Y. (2009). Robust Face Recognition via Sparse Representation. *IEEE Transactions on Pattern Analysis and Machine Intelligence*, 2(31), 210–227. doi:10.1109/TPAMI.2008.79

Xiaogang, W., & Xiaoou, T. (2004). A unified framework for subspace face recognition. *IEEE Transactions on Pattern Analysis and Machine Intelligence*, 26(9), 1222–1228. doi:10.1109/TPAMI.2004.57

Xiujuan, C., Shiguang, S., Xilin, C., & Wen, G. (2007). Locally Linear Regression for Pose-Invariant Face Recognition. *IEEE Transactions on Image Processing*, 7(16), 1716–1725. doi:10.1109/TIP.2007.899195

Xu, C., Wang, Y., Tan, T., & Quan, L. (2004). Depth vs. intensity: Which is more important for face recognition? *Internat. Conf. on Pattern Recognition (ICPR 2004)* (Vol. 4, pp. 342–345).

Yan, S., He, X., Cai, D., & Zhang, H.-J. (2005). Neighborhood preserving embedding. In *IEEE International Conference on Computer Vision* (pp. 1208–1213).

Yan, S., Hu, Y., Niyogi, P., He, X., Cai, D., & Zhang, H.-J. (2005). Face recognition using laplacianfaces. *IEEE Transactions on Pattern Analysis and Machine Intelligence*, 27, 328–340. doi:10.1109/TPAMI.2005.55

Yu, H., & Yang, J. (2001, October). A direct LDA algorithm for high-dimensional data with application to face recognition. *Pattern Recognition*, 34, 2067–2070. doi:10.1016/S0031-3203(00)00162-X

Zhang, X., Gao, Y., & Leung, M. K. H. (2008). Recognizing Rotated Faces From Frontal and Side Views: An Approach Toward Effective Use of Mugshot Databases. *IEEE Transactions on Information Forensics and Security, 3*(4), 1966–1979. doi:10.1109/TIFS.2008.2004286

Zhao, H., & Pong, C., Y. (2008). Incremental Linear Discriminant Analysis for Face Recognition, *IEEE Transactions on Systems, Man and Cybernetics – Part B, 38*(1), 210-221.

KEY TERMS AND DEFINITIONS

Biometric Systems: They allow the recognition of individual physical or behavioural features (e.g. face, fingerprint, iris, etc.) and work in two operation modes, namely verification and identification. Verification entails a one-to-one comparison, to check if the person is who he/she claims to be. Identification corresponds to a one-to-many comparison to find out who the person is, as in dangerous or missing people identification.

Face Recognition: It can be intended as a special case of pattern recognition, where both intra-class and inter-class variations are bound to the specific features of the object to be recognized. Like in the general case, illumination, pose and occlusions are issue to be addressed, but in this case also expression variations and time lapse must be considered.

Dimensional Reduction Technique: In many cases the adopted object (face) recognition technique entails the use of an high number of features, each possibly defined by more measures. This takes to the need of exploring a vector space of very high dimensionality, with a consequent overwhelming computational complexity. For this reason, many researchers aim at finding efficient and effective dimensionality reduction techniques in order to operate in a more manageable vector space, which has to maintain original patterns and distribution of vectors.

Neural Classifiers: Artificial neural networks are relatively crude electronic networks of *neurons* inspired to the neural structure of the brain. They process items one at a time, and *learn* by comparing their classification of the item with the known true classification of the item. The errors from the initial classification of the first record is fed back into the network, and used to modify the networks algorithm the second time around, and so on for many iterations.

Gabor Filters: A powerful tool to process and code images. A Gabor filter is a linear filter whose impulse response is defined by a harmonic function multiplied by a Gaussian function. They are exploited together with wavelets, thanks to their ability to capture relevant visual characteristics such as spatial localization, spatial frequency and orientation.

Partitioned Iterated Function Systems: A fractal-based approach for image coding and indexing. In the basic mechanism for fractal image coding is as follows, the original image is partitioned into a set of non-overlapping square regions called ranges. From the same image, another set of square regions is selected. These regions, called domains, are larger in size and may overlap. Typically, there are many more domains than there are ranges. The aim of fractal coding is to approximate every range by an affine transformed version of a suitable domain.

3D Morphable Model: A technique to derive a 3D object model from a single 2D shot. Given a single photograph of a face, its 3D shape is estimated by approximating its orientation in space and the illumination conditions in the scene. Starting from a rough estimate of size, orientation and illumination, the algorithm optimizes these parameters along with the face's internal shape and surface colour to find the best match to the input image. The face model extracted from the image can be rotated and manipulated in 3D.

3D Face Recognition: A way to overcome limitation of 2D face recognition by relying on a 3D face model. Actually, a 3D model provides more geometrical information on the shape of the face and is unaffected by illumination and pose variations. The development of 3D acquisition systems and then the 3D capturing process are becoming cheaper and faster too. This definitely makes the 3D approach more and more applicable to real situations out of the laboratories.

Iterative Closest Point: An algorithm to minimize the difference between two clouds of points. ICP is often employed to reconstruct 3D surfaces from different scans, to robots self localization and achieve optimal path planning. The algorithm iteratively revises the transformation (translation, rotation) needed to minimize the distance between the points of two raw scans.

Multimodal (Biometric) Approaches: Multimodal biometric systems are those which concurrently exploit more than one physiological or behavioral trait for enrollment, verification, or identification. They provide an effective alternative to unimodal architectures, as flaws of an individual system can be compensated by the availability of a higher number of cooperating biometries. They can be classified by distinguishing *truly multi-modal* systems, where the same biometry is processed through different input modalities, *multi-biometric* systems, where more biometries are jointly used, and *multi-expert* systems, where different classifiers for the same biometry are fused together.

Section 2
Facial Feature Extraction

Chapter 3
A Review of Facial Feature Detection Algorithms

Stylianos Asteriadis
Aristotle University of Thessaloniki, Greece

Nikos Nikolaidis
Aristotle University of Thessaloniki, Greece & CERTH, Greece

Ioannis Pitas
Aristotle University of Thessaloniki, Greece & CERTH, Greece

ABSTRACT

Facial feature localization is an important task in numerous applications of face image analysis that include face recognition and verification, facial expression recognition, driver's alertness estimation, head pose estimation etc. Thus, the area has been a very active research field for many years and a multitude of methods appear in the literature. Depending on the targeted application, the proposed methods have different characteristics and are designed to perform in different setups. Thus, a method of general applicability seems to be away from the current state of the art. This chapter intends to offer an up-to-date literature review of facial feature detection algorithms. A review of the image databases and performance metrics that are used to benchmark these algorithms is also provided.

INTRODUCTION

Face image processing and analysis is a research field that deals with the extraction and analysis of information related to human faces from sources such as still images, video and 3D data. This research area, which one can position within the general field of computer vision, has attracted the interest of a significant part of the research community during the last years. Face image analysis deals with a variety of problems that include face detection and tracking, face recognition and verification, facial expression and emotion recognition, facial features detection and tracking, eye gaze tracking, virtual face synthesis and animation, etc.

Facial feature (or landmark) detection in images and videos deals with estimating the position of prominent features of a human face. The detected features are, in most cases, the eyes, the eyebrows, the nose and the mouth. The result of the detection can be either a list of characteristic points on those features, namely the eye corners,

DOI: 10.4018/978-1-61520-991-0.ch003

the center of the iris, the corners or the center of the eyebrows, the nose tip, the nostrils, the corners or the center of the mouth, or the corresponding image region defined either by its bounding box or, more accurately, by its contour (e.g. lips contour). A considerable amount of work has been published recently in this area. The increasing interest for facial feature detection methods is due to their wide range of applications within the field of face image analysis. For example, face recognition and verification methods (Lam & Yan, 1998; Karungaru, Fukumi, & Akamatsu, 2004; Campadelli & Lanzarotti, 2004) used in security or access control applications frequently involve a pre-processing step of facial features localization. The detected features can be subsequently used for the registration of the test image with the images in the face database or for the actual face recognition/verification task. Furthermore, the strong need for man-machine interaction paradigms has created a high interest for facial expression recognition, head pose and eye gaze estimation and facial feature tracking techniques (Bhuiyan, Ampornaramveth, Muto, & Ueno, 2003; Yilmaz & Shah, 2002). Such techniques often include a facial feature detection step in order to perform image registration, initialize the tracking of facial features, etc. Also, applications such as drivers' attention assessment (Smith, Shah, & Vitoria Lobo, 2003) or visual speech understanding require the detection of fiducial points on faces, whereas face detection techniques sometimes involve a facial feature detection step in order to verify that the candidate region is indeed a face.

Depending on the approach, facial feature detection methods utilize facial geometry, luminance, edge, color and shape information. In their vast majority, the published methods involve a face detection step and seek for facial features only within the detected face region. These methods give more robust results than the second category of methods that do not involve face detection and search for facial features over the entire image. In the first group of approaches, no scaling problems exist, as these are solved at the face detection step. On the contrary, methods that belong to the second category must make an initial estimation of the expected dimensions of the sought facial features. As a consequence, their use is limited to applications where the distance between the camera and the face is approximately known. Such applications include driver's attention determination (Smith et al., 2003), face recognition in controlled image acquisition setups, etc.

In terms of the approach used, facial feature detection techniques can be roughly categorized into model/template matching techniques and feature based techniques. Model matching techniques try to identify image areas whose characteristics match those of a model of the facial feature to be detected (e.g. an eye or mouth model). The models/ templates involved in such techniques might refer to image intensity, edges, color distribution, etc. Despite being usually time consuming, template-matching techniques tend to provide better results than other methods. On the other hand, feature based techniques try to detect facial features by taking advantage of the facial feature properties, e.g. the fact that some facial features (e.g. the eyes or the mouth) are darker (Bhuiyan et al., 2003; Shih & Chuang, 2004; Perlibakas, 2003; Lai, Yuen, Chen, Lao, & Kawade, 2001) or have different color distribution than the rest of the face (Smith et al., 2003), or that facial feature areas exhibit a large concentration of edges. It should be noted, however, that the classification of the various methods to one of these two categories is rather difficult, since many methods involve elements from both categories or the characteristics of the method make this distinction not very obvious.

Both template and feature based techniques often involve geometric constraints derived from the facial geometry. Such constraints provide an efficient way to verify detection results or suppress falsely identified features. Another common characteristic of many methods that search for multiple facial features is that eyes (which are usually the most prominent feature) are detected first and their position is used, along with rules stemming from facial geometry, to initialize the search of the other features.

In this chapter, a review of facial feature detection techniques published during the last years will be provided. Due to the large volume of published work, the review is a non-exhaustive one and does not cover face detection/tracking. Furthermore, it focuses on facial feature detection on images acquired from visible light cameras, and, thus, it does not include facial feature tracking techniques since these form a different category of methods or eye detection techniques (e.g. eye or eye gaze tracking techniques) that incorporate active illumination from infrared sources, as these require special setups and are of no general applicability.

TEST DATABASES AND EVALUATION CRITERIA

Various test databases are used for the performance evaluation of facial feature detection algorithms. The BioID (*The BioID face database,* n.d.) is one of the most widely used databases. It contains 1521 grayscale, frontal facial images of dimensions 384×286 pixels, acquired under various lighting conditions in front of a complex background. The database contains tilted and rotated faces, subjects that wear eye-glasses and, in a few cases, subjects that have their eyes shut or pose various expressions. Thus, it is considered (Zhou & Geng, 2004) as one of the most challenging databases for the facial feature detection task. Examples of images from the BioID database are shown in Figure 1. The database contains ground-truth information for 20 facial feature points, namely the eye centers and corners, eyebrow corners, nostrils and nose tip, mouth corners and upper and lower points of the lips, chin and temples. Another dataset that is quite challenging is the one constructed for the Face Recognition Grand Challenge (FRGC) (P. J. Phillips et al., 2005). The dataset contains a training set ("large

still training set") that consists of 12,776 color images from 222 subjects obtained in controlled and uncontrolled conditions. The validation set contains images from 466 subjects collected in 4,007 subject sessions. The database contains also a second training set ("3D training set") that contains 3D scans, and controlled and uncontrolled still images from 943 subject. The images dimensions are either 1704×2272 or 1200×1600 pixels. The dataset includes ground truth data for eyes, nose and mouth center. Most other databases are much simpler and include head-and-shoulder images with uniform background that are taken under controlled lighting conditions. The XM2VTS database (Messer, Matas, Kittler, Luettin, & Maitre, 1999) is a popular example. The database includes 2360 color images of dimensions 720×576 pixels and contains ground-truth information for eye centers and corners, nostrils and mouth corners. The database of the University of Bern consists of 450 grayscale images with size 512×342 pixels. The AR database (Martinez & Benavente, 1998) consists of more than 4000 color images of dimensions 768×576 pixels depicting 126 persons. The images were acquired under various illumination conditions. Both AR and Bern databases contain head-shoulders images that were acquired over a uniform background. The FERET database (P. Phillips, Wechsler, Huang, & Rauss, 1998) consists of 14051 grayscale images of individuals, taken in front of a non-complex background. The size of the images is 256×384 pixels. The YALE face database (Belhumeur, Hespanha, & Kriegman, 1997) consists of 165 grayscale facial images of faces, depicting 11 persons. The people in the database pose various expressions and the dimensions of the images are 320×243 pixels. Ground truth is provided for the eye centers and the middle of the upper lip. The database used in (Kanade, Cohn, & Tian, 2000) consists of 1917 video sequences of 182 subjects taking variable poses and expressions. The videos were taken under relatively controlled light conditions and

Figure 1. Example images from the BioID database (The BioID face database, n.d.)

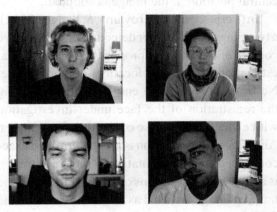

the color quality is very good. The frame sizes are 640×480 pixels.

A number of objective criteria are used for evaluating the performance of facial feature detection algorithms on the databases described above. These criteria require ground truth information regarding the actual position of the facial features and consider a detection to be correct when the position of the found feature is sufficiently close to its actual position, the proximity being defined by means of various distance metrics and appropriate thresholds. The number of correct detections over the number of test images are then used to evaluate the correct detection ratio. A performance criterion proposed in (Jesorsky, Kirchberg, & Frischholz, 2001) for the eye center detection task and subsequently used by many authors is the following:

$$d_{eye} = \frac{\max(d_l, d_r)}{s} < T_{eye} \qquad (1)$$

In the previous formula, d_l and d_r are the distances between the ground truth positions of the left and right eye centers and the corresponding eye centers found by the algorithm. The criterion is normalized by the distance s between the two ground truth eye centers (inter-ocular distance)

and, thus, unlike other similar criteria used in the literature, it is scale independent. Correct detection is declared when deye is smaller than a threshold T_{eye} and the correct detection rate is evaluated over all available test images. Thus, this performance index results in a compact, single-figure performance indicator. Obviously, the value of T_{eye} should be chosen according to the accuracy requirements of the application, a smaller threshold implying a stricter criterion. Common threshold values are T_{eye}=0.25 and T_{eye}=0.1. Plots of correct detection rates versus the value of Teye are also used to provide a more complete view of the algorithm's performance. A variation of the formula in (1) was used in (Cristinacce, Cootes, & Scott, 2004) for the performance evaluation of methods searching for *n* features:

$$m_e = \frac{1}{ns}\sum_{i=1}^{n}d_i < T \qquad (2)$$

where d_i is the distance between the ground truth of *i*-th feature point and the detected one, s is the ground-truth inter-ocular distance, and n is the number of feature points. Cootes *et al* in (Cootes, Edwards, & Taylor, 1998) used the mean absolute error of the detected feature points with respect to the ground-truth ones, normalized by the face width.

The above criteria are used to measure the performance of methods that search for specific points (eye centers, mouth corners, nostrils, etc.). No specific criteria have been proposed for the evaluation of methods that try to detect entire regions of facial features (e.g. eye regions). In such cases, a correct region detection is usually declared when the found region contains the feature being searched.

METHODS INVOLVING FACE DETECTION

Model/Template Matching Techniques

In (Jesorsky et al., 2001), a two stage technique for eye center localization is proposed. The technique utilizes the modified Hausdorff distance $H(A,B)$ introduced in (Dubuisson & Jain, 1994) between the set of edge points A found on the image and a set of points B of an edge model of the face. To detect the position of the face, an area of interest with predetermined width/height ratio is defined for the test image and is scaled to fixed dimensions. The Sobel edge intensity image is extracted from the area of interest and local thresholding, applied so as to equally distribute the resulting binary edge pixels on the image, is performed. Then, the face position on the binary edge image A is found as the best match with the face edge model B. This is accomplished by finding the parameters p of a geometric transform $T_p()$ such as a combination of rotation, translation and scaling, which results in the minimum Hausdorff distance between the edge image A and the transformed model $T_p(B)$

$$\hat{p} = \arg \min_p H(A, T_p(B)) \tag{3}$$

Subsequently, a more detailed face model is used on the face area found in the previous step, in order to detect face characteristics. The procedure is the same as before and the transformation T_p of the previous step, together with the $T_{p'}$, resulting from this refinement step are used to locate the eye positions. Finally, a Multi-Layer Perceptron (MLP), trained with pupil images is used for finding the exact pupil locations. The method was tested on the BioID and XM2VTS databases and, for T_{eye}=0.25 in (1), the correct detection rates were 91.8% and 98.4% respectively. A drawback of this method is that, for the coarse face localization,

the rather unrealistic hypothesis that faces lie in a central position in the image is adopted.

In (Feris, Gemmell, Toyama, & Kruger, 2002), a two-stage approach for detecting mouth and eye corners and nostrils is proposed. After an initial estimation of the face location, Gabor Wavelet Networks (GWNs) are employed for achieving the registration of the face under investigation with a face in a database of training face images. An affine transformation is also determined to account for different orientations. Once registration is achieved, the positions of facial features on the training image are used as initial estimates of the face features on the test image. A second level of GWNs, trained for each one of the 8 feature regions (mouth corners, nostrils and eye corners), is used for deriving refined estimates for the facial features of interest. The method was tested on the Yale and FERET databases and the criterion used for declaring a correct detection was that detected features should be no more than 3 pixels away from the corresponding ground truth points. The performance was evaluated independently for each feature and the biggest correct detection rate was obtained for the eye corners (95.5%), while the worst results were obtained for the mouth corners (87.5%).

In (Cristinacce et al., 2004), a multi-stage approach is used to locate 17 features on and around the mouth and eyes. First, the face is detected using the boosted cascaded classifier algorithm by Viola and Jones (Viola & Jones, 2001), (Viola & Jones, 2004). For the detection of the facial features, a boosted cascade detector was trained for each feature using manually labelled examples. These examples were subsequently sampled 5 times with small random rotations and scale changes to provide a total of 5275 training patches for each feature. During detection, the search region within the face bounding box for each feature is defined and the location within this region, which provides the best score of the corresponding feature detector, is declared as the position of this feature. Results are improved using a novel shape constraint, the Pairwise Reinforcement of Feature Responses (PRFR). According to this approach, a pairwise distribution is defined as the distribution of the true location of feature *i* given the location found by feature detector *j* in the reference frame defined by the whole face region. Thus, $17^2=289$ histograms $H_{ij}(x_i-x_j)$ are evaluated for all possible pairs of locations x_j found by feature detector *j* and true feature locations x_i in order to approximate the pairwise distribution $P_{ij}(x_i|x_j)$. The computation of the histograms is done on a set of training images by recording the true position of every feature and the positions found by the various feature detectors. Using these histograms and a number of possible feature positions helps to improve feature detection. More specifically, instead of finding the single most probable image location for the *j*-th feature, a list of the *k* most probable image locations q_{jt} $(t=1,...,k)$ for this feature is generated by using the corresponding feature detector. In order to estimate the location $\hat{x}_i$ of feature i, the sum of all probabilities $P_{ij}(x_i|q_{jt})$ for all q_{jt} is found. The estimated feature location $\hat{x}_i$ maximizes the quantity:

$$\hat{x}_i = \arg\max_{x_i}\sum_{j=1}^{n}\sum_{t=1}^{k}P_{ij}(x_i \mid q_{jt}) \qquad (4)$$

A refinement of this method can be obtained by employing a variation of the Active Appearance Model (AAM) algorithm (Cootes et al., 1998) that uses four values as model parameters for each pixel, namely the normalized gradients in the *x* and *y* directions and its "edgeness" and "cornerness". The method was tested on the BioID and XM2VTS databases using the evaluation criterion in (2). For $T=0.1$ on the BioID database, the method achieves 96% correct detection rates for all 17 features. When only eye detection is considered, correct detection rates are 96% on

the BioID database and 93% on the XM2VTS, using the criterion (1) with $T_{eye}=0.1$.

In (Reinders, Koch, & Gerbrands, 1996), a three-layer neural network, trained as a classifier using backpropagation is utilized to detect small eye subregions, namely patches around the eye corners and the two eyelids. These patches are searched for within search regions around the eye which are set manually or found by an eye region detection algorithm. In order to handle variable illumination, as well as scale and shape variations, the feature vectors used as input to the neural network comprised of local orientation information, namely magnitude and orientation of intensity gradient. To improve detection, the results of the neural network, i.e. the candidate eye corner and eyelid positions, are post-processed using a-priori knowledge about the geometrical structure of the eye. The method was tested on persons of different poses and expressions. A feature point (corner, eyelid position) was declared to be successfully detected if its *x* and *y* coordinates were no more than 2 pixels away from the manually labelled ones. The correct detection rates were 96% on average for all the detected feature points.

In (Asteriadis, Nikolaidis, Hajdu, & Pitas, 2006), eyes and eye centers are detected inside face areas found by the algorithm described in (Viola & Jones, 2001). The Canny edge detector is applied on the output of the face detector and, for each pixel, the vector that points to the closest edge pixel is calculated. The magnitude (length) and the slope (angle) of each vector are assigned to the corresponding pixel. Thus, instead of the intensity values of each pixel, the proposed algorithm uses the produced vector length and angle maps (Figure 2). These maps encode the geometry of the face and are quite robust to variable lighting conditions. PCA is subsequently applied on a set of training eye images to derive eigenvectors for these maps. In order to detect the eye regions on an image, the length and angle maps of candidate regions are evaluated and are projected on the subspaces spanned by the eigenvectors found during training. The similarity of the candidate regions in the new feature spaces with the features derived for a pair of prototype eye models is used to declare eye presence. Subsequently, after a light reflection removal step, eye centers are found by detecting inside the eye regions dark small areas containing strong edges. The method was tested on the XM2VTS and the BioID databases and the correct detection rates were 98% and 98.8% respectively, for T_{eye}=0.25 in (1). An improved variant of this method that also deals with mouth corner detection is presented in (Asteriadis, Nikolaidis, & Pitas, 2009).

A four step technique is employed in (Vukadinovec & Pantic, 2005), for the detection of 19 facial points on images depicting faces in neutral expression. The facial points that are searched are the eye upper and lower points and corners, the eyebrow and nose corners, the mouth upper and lower points and corners, as well as the chin. The face is first detected based on a real-time face detection method (Fasel, Fortenberry, & Movel-

lan, 2005). After the face is detected, each feature is searched for in a region of interest (ROI). In order to define these ROIs, iris and mouth center detection take place. In more detail, the left and right iris are searched for within the upper left and right face regions respectively. The position of an iris in its ROI is decided based on the horizontal and vertical intensity histograms. The peak of these histograms shall give the horizontal and vertical position of the iris, respectively. The positions of the irises help to estimate a ROI for detecting the medial point of the mouth. The vertical position of this point is found by applying a procedure similar to the one used for the iris detection on thresholded edge images. The horizontal position coincides with the horizontal position of the midpoint of the line segment joining the eyes (after aligning the face image horizontally). The positions of the irises and the mouth middle point are used for defining 20 ROIs for the facial feature extraction step. For the detection of the facial points in their corresponding ROIs, feature patch templates are used. These are centered around the point of interest and were obtained by applying a bank of Gabor filters on the grayscale values of each patch. Such patch templates were learnt using a representative set of positive and negative examples and Gentleboost classification was further used for deciding whether a point corresponds to the point of interest in the corresponding ROI. The method was trained and tested on the Cohn Kanade database (Kanade et al., 2000). Successful detection was declared when the detected characteristic was less than 10% of the inter-ocular distance away from the corresponding, manually annotated point. An average successful detection of 93% for all feature points was achieved. However, the authors note that success is not guaranteed in case of face images with size much different than the ones of the test database.

Figure 2. Elements used in the eye detection method presented in (Asteriadis et al., 2006): (a) Face image, (b) edge map, (c) vector slopes, (d) vector lengths

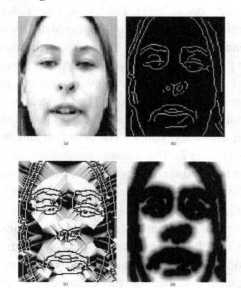

Feature Based Methods

In (Yilmaz & Shah, 2002), a method for detecting eyes, eyebrows and the mouth for facial pose recovery is proposed. Initially, the facial area is detected and the probability distribution of chromatic information of eyes and eyebrows is subsequently used to locate candidate positions for these facial features. This is done by comparing distributions of candidate face areas with distributions extracted by averaging training data. Sobel edge detection is then used to locate the mouth, since a large number of edges exist at the mouth area. This is done using an appropriate confidence function which is minimized in areas of large edge concentration. The areas scanned in order to detect the mouth are specified relatively to the positions of eyes and eyebrows found at the previous step.

In (Bhuiyan et al., 2003), eyes, eyebrows, nose and mouth regions are detected, following the detection of the face. Face detection is done using skin color segmentation in the YIQ color space. Empirically set thresholds are used to segment the Y and I components and detect skin-like regions. The largest skin-colored connected component is labelled as the face area. A genetic algorithm that operates on the luminance of the detected face area and involves a template face image is subsequently employed to improve face localization. Subsequently, histogram equalization and noise filtering are employed. The features of interest are detected using the fact that they are usually darker than other face parts (cheeks, forehead, etc.). Thus, the image is thresholded and a binary image where the features of interest correspond to white areas is extracted. Morphological operations are subsequently used to remove small holes and the resulting binary map is used to tag the facial features. Each one of the six features is assigned a unique tag, depending on its location on the face area. The method works well in cases where the assumption that features of interest are darker than the rest of the face holds, but might fail when applied on subjects with beard or eyeglasses with thick dark frames.

In (Perlibakas, 2003), eye and mouth regions are searched for inside face-defining ellipses and contours. A sequence of bottom hat morphological operations, followed by thresholding, are used to detect dark regions in the face area. The candidate regions are tested to verify whether they correspond to eye or lip regions by taking into account a number of heuristic rules (Han, Liao, Yu, & Chen, 2000; Chan & Lewis, 1999), that involve the expected face size, the maximum and minimum dimensions and aspect ratios of eyes and lips. Subsequently, all possible pairs of eyes are identified and, those that conform to certain rules regarding their size, shape and mean luminance are considered as candidate eye pairs. Eyes and mouth triplets that are far from the center of the face ellipse are removed. Also, triplets where the orientation of the line that connects the two eyes differs significantly from that of the ellipse minor axis, are removed. The method was tested on 600 images from the FERET, BioID and PICS (Stirling Psychology Department, n.d.) databases, with a success rate of 71.2%.

In (Gourier, Hall, & Crowley, 2004), eyes, nose, mouth and chin are detected following the detection of skin-colored elliptic facial regions. The face images found are normalized in dimension and the intensity is used to locate facial features. The first and second order derivatives of a 2D Gaussian function along the two dimensions (G_x, G_y, G_{xx}, G_{xy}, G_{yy}) are convolved with the image, resulting in a five-dimensional vector in each pixel. A set of training images is used to obtain such Gaussian derivatives which are clustered using the K-means algorithm. The clusters obtained are exploited in order to distinguish between hair, salient facial features (eyes, nose, mouth, chin) and other skin areas. Further geometrical analysis regarding the size and the shape of the detected connected regions is used to decide whether a connected region of pixels belonging to a particular cluster belongs to the corresponding feature or not.

In (Shih & Chuang, 2004), the bounding boxes of the eyes, nose and mouth are searched for. Two empirically selected thresholds are applied on the edge map of an image for the extraction of the head and face boundaries. Projections along the *x*- and *y*- directions are subsequently applied on the binary edge image of the face region (see the description of (Zhou & Geng, 2004) for more details) in order to find the limits of the four bounding boxes of the eyes, nose and mouth. In cases where the above procedure results in facial features that are very close to each other, a geometric model is used in order to detect the facial features. This model describes the relations between distances of various facial features (e.g. nostrils to mouth vertical distance or distance between the mouth corners) and the inter-ocular distance *D* (Figure 3). In particularly difficult situations involving poor illumination and shadows, another approach is proposed. According to this approach, the eyes are detected first using Gabor filters, as follows. A training database of facial images is convolved with a bank of Gabor filters (Fasel, Smith, Bartlett, & Movellan, 2002; Hjelmaas, 2000). The test image is also convolved with such filters and a pixel is declared to belong to a fiducial point if its Euclidean distance from the closest output in the training database is smaller than an empirical threshold. Subsequently, the other features are localized by using the geometrical model described above. This technique provides a complete methodology to detect head/face boundaries and facial features and seems to perform well even in

Figure 3. Geometric face model used in (Shih & Chuang, 2004)

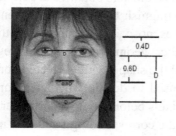

difficult cases. However, no results were reported in cases of subjects wearing eyeglasses.

In (Zhou & Geng, 2004) the authors introduce the Generalized Projection Functions (*GPF*) and use them to locate the eye centers in a face area found using the algorithm proposed in (Wu & Zhou, 2003). The Generalized Projection Functions are a linear combination of the Integral Projection Functions (*IPF*) and the Variance Projection Functions (*VPF*). The horizontal mean Integral Projection Function and Variance Projection Function of an image *I(x,y)* along the interval $[x_1, x_2]$ are defined as follows:

$$IPF_h(y) = \frac{1}{x_2 - x_1} \sum_{x=x_1}^{x_2} I(x, y) \tag{5}$$

$$VPF_h(y) = \frac{1}{x_2 - x_1} \sum_{x=x_1}^{x_2} [I(x_i, y) - IPF_h(y)]^2 \tag{6}$$

The corresponding vertical functions are defined in a similar manner. In general, the values of projection functions (*PF*) change rapidly when object boundaries (edges) are encountered. For example, a strong vertical boundary can be declared to exist at *x* if $\vartheta PF_v(x)/\vartheta x > T$. The GPF along the horizontal direction is defined as follows:

$$GPF_h(y) = (1 - \alpha) \cdot IPF_h(y) + \alpha \cdot VPF_h(y) \tag{7}$$

where $0 \leq a \leq 1$.

The approximate positions of eye areas were found using the algorithm proposed in (Wu & Zhou, 2003). Subsequently, GPFs were used to accurately locate the bounding box of the eye by finding maxima of the derivatives of the horizontal/vertical *GPFs* (Figure 4).

The eye center were then found by taking the center of the bounding box. The method was

Figure 4. GPF derivatives (Zhou & Geng, 2004) in an image area depicting an eye

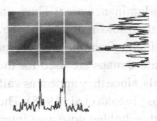

tested on the BioID, JAFFE (*The JAFFE database*, n.d.) and NJUFace face databases. The best results for all three databases were achieved by using *GPFs* with α=0.6. More specifically, by setting T_{eye} <0.25 in (1) for successful detection, the correct detection rates were 94.81% on the BioID, 97.18% on JAFFE and 95.82% on NJUFace.

A technique for eye, mouth and nose region detection is presented in (Lai et al., 2001). The method uses skin and lip color information to define candidate face regions, whereas accurate face detection is performed using spline wavelets. The face region is converted into a binary image using the average of the Integral Optical Density (*IOD*) (Castleman, 1979) as a threshold. The average of *IOD* is defined as:

$$IOD = \frac{\iint_D Y_k(x,y)dxdy}{\iint_D dxdy} \qquad (8)$$

where $Y_k(x,y)$ denotes a binary image generated by applying threshold k on the greyscale image. More specifically, the threshold k is selected so that the average of *IOD* obtains a value in the experimentally selected interval [0.14,0.20]. The authors claim that the above thresholding procedure results in a binary image where eyes, nose and mouth are clearly defined. The bounding boxes of the features of interest are subsequently extracted by applying projections on the binary image (see the description of (Zhou & Geng, 2004) for more details on projections). Subsequently, the *IOD*

thresholding technique is applied separately within each bounding box in order to obtain more accurate feature localization. The algorithm achieved a correct detection rate of 86% on low resolution images from the Omron database, captured under various illumination conditions and backgrounds.

In (Lam & Yan, 1998), mouth, nose, eyes and eyebrows are detected and subsequently used for face recognition. Active contours are used to extract the face boundary. Corner detection using the approach described in (Xie, Sudhakar, & Zhuang, 1993) follows and corner regions with specific characteristics are classified as corners belonging to the eye or mouth corners class. More specifically, the following parameters of the detected corners are evaluated:

• the curvature, i.e. the acute angle between the lines that define the corner;
• the orientation of the line that bisects the angle between the two corner lines;
• the difference between the grey level averages in the two regions defined by the corner lines.

If the corner parameters fall within empirically selected value ranges, then the corner is declared as an eye/mouth corner. An approach based on deformable templates and snakes is then used to extract the shape of the eyes and mouth, starting from the detected corners. Using the location of the eye corners, nose and eyebrows centers are detected. The horizontal position of the eyebrow center is defined by the line that is perpendicular to the midpoint of the line segment that connects the two eye centers, whereas its vertical position is found by evaluating local minima of the vertical integral projection function. The vertical position of the nose center is defined by the symmetry axis of the face, whereas its horizontal position is defined by taking the minima of vertical integral projections.

In (Gargesha & Panchanathan, 2002), a hybrid technique involving a combination of methods for the detection of eyes, nose and lips in frontal facial images is presented. The technique used for eye detection combines luminance and chrominance information with curvature analysis and uses PCA or Radon transform for refining the results. First, an initial estimate of the eyes position is obtained as follows: Two maps, based on the chrominance and luminance components in the YC_bC_r color space, are created using the methodology proposed in (Hsu, Abdel-Mottaleb, & Jain, 2001). The luminance map is extracted by applying morphological dilations and erosions on the Y component. The two maps are subsequently combined with the multiplication operation and segmented by an empirical threshold. In this way, a binary image is calculated. The curvature map (Tanaka, Ikeda, & Chiaki, 1998) of the face intensity surface is also derived. Eyes correspond to concave regions on this map. The extracted map is binarized. The two binary maps are combined with the *AND* operator to provide an image where eyes, as well as other regions of the face are highlighted. Subsequently, PCA is applied on this binary image in order to achieve accurate localization of the eyes. More specifically, pairs of highlighted regions of the binary image that satisfy certain geometric constraints are projected onto the "eye space", created through PCA from a set of training eye images. The within and from eye space distances are used to declare eye existence in a way similar to the face detection technique in (Menser & Muller, 1999). Another variant, based on the Radon transform is also presented. The Radon transform can be used to distinguish symmetric highlighted regions in the binary image from non-symmetric regions. The Radon transform of a symmetric image is very similar to the Radon transform of a version of this image that is inverted with respect to the horizontal and vertical axis, a property that does not hold for non-symmetric images (Figure 5).

This property is used to identify candidate eye regions, since their shape is usually ellipsoid and, thus, symmetric. Additional geometric constraints are used to declare the existence of a pair of eyes.

Nose tip detection within a search region is based on the observation that the area around the nose tip is a low luminance area. Thus, an empirical luminance threshold is found for the extraction of a binary image from the nose region. Furthermore, curvature maps are used for the detection of the nostrils, since they appear as valley regions in such maps (Tanaka et al., 1998). The combination of the thresholded nose area image with the curvature map of the same area gives a binary image with the tip of the nose highlighted. The position of the nose along with chrominance information (utilized in a way similar to (Hsu et al., 2001)) is then used to define the search region for the lip corner detection. Lip corners within this search region are found by taking the vertical projection $P_r(x)$ of the output of a horizontal edge detector and searching for positions where $P_r(x)$ exceeds a threshold. The vertical position of the lip corners is determined by the position of the

Figure 5. (a) Non-symmetric image, (b) eye-like symmetric image, (c) radon transform of non-symmetric image, (d) radon transform of symmetric image, (e) radon transform of mirrored and inverted non-symmetric image, (f) radon transform of mirrored and inverted symmetric image

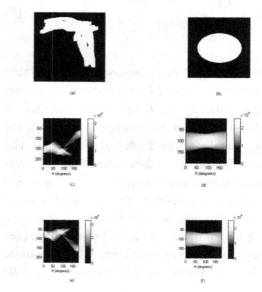

darkest pixels on the columns that correspond to the horizontal positions of the corners. The basic drawback of the proposed method is that, in the case of Radon transform, symmetrical non-eye regions might be erroneously identified as eyes. Furthermore, nose and lip detection depend highly on the successful localization of features at previous steps, whereas non-uniform illumination conditions and the existence of a moustache or beard might mislead the algorithm.

The iris detection algorithm, proposed in (Kawaguchi & Rizon, 2003), utilizes a Sobel edge detector on head-and-shoulder images with simple background to detect the face. For iris detection, the valley image of the face is found by subtracting the morphological closing of the image from the original image. Subsequently, a threshold is defined as the largest T value satisfying the following inequality:

$$\frac{1}{N} \sum_{i=T}^{\text{MAX}} h(i) \geq 0.1 \qquad (9)$$

where MAX denotes the maximum grayscale value of the valley image, N the number of pixels in the face area and $h(i)$ the valley image histogram. Initial guesses are localized as valley points, i.e. points whose luminance in the valley image is greater than the calculated threshold. Candidate iris locations are then detected based on a cost function that takes into account the extent to which the valley region is circular (by using the Hough transform), the separability between the iris and the surrounding area, and the luminance of the grayscale image at this region. A pair of candidate iris regions is indeed a pair of irises if the correlation between the two regions is sufficiently high. The method was tested on two databases: The database of the University of Bern and the AR database. Correct detection rates were 95.3% and 96.8% respectively, failing to detect eyes in cases where people were slightly leaning ahead.

In (Ioannou, Karidakis, Kollias, & Karpouzis, 2007), the upper, lower, rightmost and leftmost parts of eye, eyebrow and mouth masks, as well as the nostrils are detected. For the initialization of the algorithm, eye areas are searched for using a feed-forward back propagation Neural Network. The network input consists of a 13-dimensional vector that includes the Y, C_r and C_b values of each pixel, as well as the 10 most important DCT coefficients of the 8×8 area around each pixel. The output of the neural network is a mask indicating eye/non-eye pixels with boundaries that do not strictly coincide with the eye boundaries. Edges above the detected eye masks are used to define masks for eyebrow detection. Nostrils are also detected based on the fact that their luminance is low in comparison to other parts of the face. The relative position of the detected regions with respect to the eyes is used for false alarms removal.

More accurate eye detection is achieved by the combination of four eye masks. The first mask is created by applying an adaptive low-luminance threshold on the initially detected eye mask. The center of the mask provided by the neural-network is fairly close to the eyes center. Thus, considering the closest horizontal edges of such points, a new mask limited by the eyelids is found. For the creation of the third mask, a region-growing technique is employed. By iteratively thresholding the grayscale image with its 3×3 standard deviation map, regions of high complexity, such as the eye area, are extracted. Finally, by thresholding the eye area, the darkest regions are extracted and used for the creation of a fourth mask.

For the creation of the mouth mask, three intermediate masks have to be found. The first one is extracted similarly to the NN-based eye mask. For the extraction of the second mask, the horizontal morphological gradient is calculated and the longest component that is not too close to the nostrils is defined as the mouth mask. As for third mask, the low luminance of the mouth corners is taken into account. Simple thresholding and connected components labeling provides with two possibilities: Either a connected closed-mouth area, or more components of an open mouth, separated by the teeth. In the first case, the mouth mask is automatically extracted while, in the second, the components that obey to certain rules regarding their position are selected. The convex hull of the result is further combined with horizontal edge maps to achieve upper and lower lip detection.

Prior to mask fusion for each characteristic, a confidence value, based on its position, is attributed to each mask. Rather than selecting the mask with the highest confidence value, the mask fusion technique combines results extracted from all masks, favoring the ones with the highest scores. The method was tested on the ERMIS (IST-2000-29319, n.d.) database, but no performance results were reported, as it was, actually, a preprocessing step to facial expression recognition.

In (Nguyen, Perez, & Torre Frade, 2008) linear regression prediction is used to coarsely localize the eyes in faces detected using the Viola-Jones face detector (Viola & Jones, 2004). Subsequently, Support Vector Machines (SVM) is employed for finding the location of the iris centers. SVMs operate on the pixels in the candidate eye areas. Instead of utilizing all pixels in these areas in a uniform way, weights, obtained through training, are imposed on the pixel intensities. The authors consider SVM parameter learning and feature (pixel) weighting in a common optimization framework, to achieve similar results with non-weighted SVM but at a lower computational cost. Results are reported for the FERET (P. Phillips et al., 1998) database. Visual inspection of these results shows that, for a threshold value of $T = 0.05$ in (1) the correct detection rate is approximately 88%.

In (Ding & Martinez, 2008), the authors utilize the Viola-Jones face detector (Viola & Jones, 2004) in video sequences and apply a Gaussian model on the position and the scale of each detection at every frame in order to refine results and reduce false positives. To detect the eye centers, they utilize classifiers that are trained to classify image

patches (obtained by moving a search window) to two main classes, namely regions corresponding to eye centers and regions in the area surrounding the eyes. The authors use a subclass training approach (Zhu & Martinez, 2006) that separates each class into subclasses through the application of a K-means algorithm. Training involves a large number of examples from the two classes namely patches depicting eye centers and neighboring areas. The same approach is used (after training with appropriate examples) for the detection of eye and mouth corners and the nose region. Color and luminance properties of each facial feature are used to extract characteristic points on them. Eyebrows are detected as non-skin color areas above the (already detected) eyes. A Gaussian defined in the HSV color space is used to model skin color for this purpose. The nose contour is extracted by first projecting the image gradient in the (already detected) nose area on the x and y axes which leads to a tighter estimate (bounding box) for the nose. The outer gradient curve of this bounding box is taken to be the nose edge. Nostrils are also detected within this bounding box as local intensity minima. In a similar manner, the mouth contour is extracted by using saturation, hue and gradient information. Finally, the chin contour is detected as a set of edge pixels forming an ellipsoid shape.

METHODS THAT DO NOT INVOLVE FACE DETECTION

Model/Template Matching Techniques

In (Smith et al., 2003), a system to evaluate drivers' attention that involves facial feature detection as the first step is proposed. The method uses histogram-like structures called color predicates (Kjeldsen & Kender, 1996) that model the color distribution for each of the areas of interest. These color predicates are evaluated using a set of training facial images where the areas of interest are manually selected. Lip color predicates are initially used to detect the lips on the face. Subsequently, skin color predicates are used to detect the skin area. Since eyes are not skin-colored, they are detected as holes in the upper part of the skin area. The proposed feature detection method was found to perform well. However, the reported good performance stems mainly from the fact that, in this application, the position of the camera with respect to the driver's face is fixed and, thus, the size and approximate position of the facial features on the image can be assumed to be known.

Feature Based Methods

In (Wu & Zhou, 2003), eye-related patches are found and further used as a cue for detecting faces in images. First, small image patches that are darker than most of their neighbors are found. To do this, each pixel intensity is compared to the average intensity of eight patches around it (Figure 6). If a pixel is found to be darker than most of its surrounding neighborhoods, it is marked as eye-related pixel. A concentration of eye-related pixels forms an eye-related patch. The eye-related patches whose dimensions exceed significantly the hypothesized width or height of the eye are excluded. Furthermore, if many pixels in the neighborhood of a pixel that is not marked as eye-related belong to eye-related regions, the pixel is marked as eye-related. Those of the new eye-related patches that are much larger or smaller than the expected dimensions, or whose height to width ratio is too big, are excluded. If two eye-related patches satisfy the following constraints:

$$1.5w_e < d_{ij} < 2.5w_e \qquad (10)$$

$$|x_i - x_j| < h_e \qquad (11)$$

where

Figure 6. *The 8 neighborhoods of a pixel used in the method presented in (Wu & Zhou, 2003)*

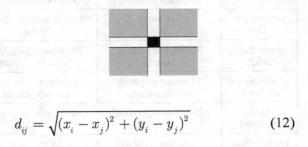

$$d_{ij} = \sqrt{(x_i - x_j)^2 + (y_i - y_j)^2} \qquad (12)$$

while (x_i, y_i) and (x_j, y_j) are the centroids of the two segments, w_e and h_e the expected width and height of the eye, and d_{ij} the distance between the centroids of the two patches, then these segments are declared as eyes and a face is detected.

The method was tested on part of the FERET database, and on the BioID database. The evaluation criterion used was the same as that of (1) with a correct detection threshold T_{eye}=0.25. The detection rates were 98.75% on the FERET database and 98.6% on the BioID. One drawback of the method is that it makes prior assumptions about the size of the eyes and, thus, it can be used only when faces are of known approximate dimensions.

In (D'Orazio, Leo, Cicirelli, & Distante, 2004), the Hough transform is used for the detection of the iris of the eye on the edge map of the image. After one of the two eyes is found, the second eye is searched within the limits of two predetermined zones left and right of the found eye. The two regions are then compared pixel by pixel and if their difference is less than a predefined threshold they are denoted as an eye pair. Faces used in the test database utilized in the paper were of known size and search regions were adjusted accordingly.

In (Ohmoto, Ueda, & Ohno, 2008), the authors detect ten facial features in order to compute head pose and eye gaze. Their final aim is to detect temporal periods when a person is lying. For face tracking, the authors use the method proposed in (Kawato & Tetsutani, 2004), where eyes are localized in the frame, based on blink detection. Eyes positions are used to provide an initial position

Table 1. Summary of reviewed methods

Method	Detected Features	Main Characteristics	Pros	Cons
(Jesorsky et al., 2001)	Eye pupils	Model searching, Hausdorff distance	Scale-independent	Hypothesis that faces lie in the center of the image
(Feris et al., 2002)	Mouth, eye corners, nostrils	Model matching, Gabor wavelet networks	Does not require an "external" face detector	Depends on training data
(Cristinacce et al., 2004)	17 feature points on mouth and eyes	Model matching, boosted cascade detection	Good results, scale independent	Sensitive to face alignment during training
(Reinders et al., 1996)	Eye corners, eyelids	Model searching, neural networks	Can handle various head poses	Sensitive to eye region initialization
(Asteriadis et al., 2006), (Asteriadis et al., 2009)	Eye centers, eye and mouth corners	Model searching, edge information, distance vector fields	Robustness to various lighting conditions and scale parameters	Sensitive to face detector choice
(Vukadinovec & Pantic, 2005)	19 facial points	Model based, intensity information and Gabor filters	Good results for strict criteria	Success not guaranteed when testing and training data differ in scale
(Yilmaz & Shah, 2002)	Eyes, eyebrows, mouth	Chromatic and edge information, chromatic probability distributions and Sobel filters	Head pose independent	High dependence on chrominance values
(Bhuiyan et al., 2003)	Eyes, eyebrows, nose, mouth	Luminance information, morphological operations	Scale independent	Highly depends on luminance values and might not work in case of glasses-beard
(Perlibakas, 2003)	Eyes, lips	Luminance information, morphological operations, facial geometry	Scale independent	Low success rates
(Gourier et al., 2004)	Eyes, nose and mouth regions	Luminance, Gaussian of derivatives of training images	Scale independent	Sensitive to facial geometry considerations
(Shih & Chuang, 2004)	Eyes, nose and mouth regions	Projections of edge maps	Can handle different poses	Sensitive to pre-determined thresholds
(Zhou & Geng, 2004)	Eye centers	Projections of grayscale values	Insensitive to lighting variations	Highly depends on predetermining coarse eye regions
(Lai et al., 2001)	Eyes, nose and mouth regions	Thresholding of grayscale face images	Can handle low resolution images	Sensitive to facial shadows, beard, glasses
(Lam & Yan, 1998)	Eye and mouth contours, nose and eyebrow specific points	Corner detection, grayscale values projections, snakes	Small head rotations can be handled	Needs high resolution images so that facial patches maintain certain properties
(Gargesha & Panchanathan, 2002)	Eyes, nose and lip regions	Color transformations and curvature map followed by PCA or Radon transform	Scale variations are handled	Detection of certain features depends on successful localization of other features
(Kawaguchi & Rizon, 2003)	Irises	Morphological closing, geometrical facial properties	Face rotations can be handled	Requires simple background
(Ioannou et al., 2007)	Eye, eyebrows, mouth corners and nostrils	Luminance and edge information, neural networks	Confidence values are attributed to each feature detector	Face needs to be well aligned
(Nguyen et al., 2008)	Irises	Luminance, support vector machines	High success rates	Requires good initial alignment of face region

continued on following page

Table 1. continued

Method	Detected Features	Main Characteristics	Pros	Cons
(Ding & Martinez, 2008)	Eye centers and corners, mouth corners and contour, eyebrows, nostrils, nose contour	Color transformations and projections, k-means clustering of image patches	Handles large appearance variability	Requires good scale adjustment of the search regions
(Wu & Zhou, 2003)	Eye regions	Luminance information, areas of high contrast and geometrical constraints	Good success rates	Requires prior knowledge or assumptions regarding features size
(D'Orazio et al., 2004)	Eye centers	Edge map, Hough transform	Good success rates	Head rotations cannot be tackled
(Smith et al., 2003)	Lips and eyes areas	Trained color predicates	Good success rates	Knowledge of face size is implied
(Ohmoto et al., 2008)	Eye centers and corners, nostrils, mouth centers	Grayscale values projection, edge map	Handles head rotation to some extent	Infrared lighting is necessary for detecting pupils

estimate for the face and subsequently the rest of the features (eye corners, pupil centers, nostrils, mouth corners) are detected. Eye corners are detected using the edge map of the eyes area, and pupil centers are extracted from the projections of grayscale values of the eyes area (see the description of (Zhou & Geng, 2004) for additional details). Nostrils and mouth corners are found as points in the darkest regions of predefined areas.

CONCLUSION AND FUTURE TRENDS

A review of some facial feature detection methods published during the last years was attempted in this chapter. A concise view of all reviewed methods that includes the detected features, the main characteristics of each method, its advantages and disadvantages is provided in Table 1. The spectrum of reviewed works provides a fairly representative sample of the ideas behind facial feature detection and reveals the multitude of approaches that have been used so far. Despite the very good results obtained by the majority of the methods when applied on one of the test image databases or in controlled environments, the problem of facial feature detection on images obtained in uncon-

strained environments under difficult or varying lighting conditions is still far from being solved. Things are getting worse due to the fact that most methods rely on face detection whose performance in complex and unconstrained environments has largely improved in the last years but is still far from perfect. In conclusion, facial feature detection is still an open research issue, which is expected to attract considerable attention in the years to come. No particular approach seems to prevail and thus one can safely assume that diversity will continue to be a major characteristic of this research area in the near future. However, one can safely bet that the main research target from now on will be (or at least, should be) robustness and satisfactory performance in real world conditions. As face detection is starting slowly to enter a commercialization phase (e.g. in digital cameras), the same should be expected, sooner or later, for facial feature detection. Utilization of a series of novel fundamental tools such as powerful classifiers approaches) or robust key point detectors and descriptors is expected to help in advancing the current state of the art. In addition, advances in capturing devices make *3D* facial data (point clouds, meshes) readily available and direct scientists towards finding ways to take advantage of such data in order to obtain improved face analysis results. Thus, techniques for facial features detection in such data emerge (Dibeklioglu, Salah, & Akarun, 2008; Xu, Tan, Wang, & Quan, 2006) and this topic is expected to attract the interest of the corresponding community in the near future.

ACKNOWLEDGMENT

The research leading to these results has received funding from the European Community's Seventh Framework Programme (FP7/2007-2013) under Grant Agreement 211471 (i3DPost).

REFERENCES

Asteriadis, S., Nikolaidis, N., Hajdu, A., & Pitas, I. (2006). A novel eye detection algorithm utilizing edge-related geometrical information. In *14th European Signal Processing Conference (EUSIPCO)*.

Asteriadis, S., Nikolaidis, N., & Pitas, I. (2009). Facial feature detection using distance vector fields. *Pattern Recognition, 42*(7), 1388–1398. doi:10.1016/j.patcog.2009.01.009

Belhumeur, P. N., Hespanha, J. P., & Kriegman, D. J. (1997). Eigenfaces vs Fisherfaces: Recognition using class specific linear projection. *IEEE Transactions on Pattern Analysis and Machine Intelligence, 19*(7), 711–720. doi:10.1109/34.598228

Bhuiyan, M. A., Ampornaramveth, V., Muto, S., & Ueno, H. (2003). Face detection and facial feature localization for human-machine interface. *National Institute of Informatics Journal, 5*, 25–39.

Campadelli, S. P., & Lanzarotti, R. (2004). An efficient method to detect facial fiducial points for face recognition. In *17th International Conference on Pattern Recognition* (Vol. 1, pp. 532-525).

Castleman, K. R. (1979). *Digital image processing*. Englewood Cliffs, NJ: Prentice Hall.

Chan, S. C. Y., & Lewis, P. H. (1999). A pre-filter enabling fast frontal face detection. In *3rd International Conference on Visual Information and Information Systems* (pp. 777-784)

Cootes, T. F., Edwards, G. J., & Taylor, C. (1998). Active appearance models. In *5th European Conference on Computer Vision* (Vol. 2, pp. 484-498).

Cristinacce, D., Cootes, T., & Scott, I. (2004). A multi-stage approach to facial feature detection. In *15th British Machine Vision Conference* (pp. 231-240).

D'Orazio, T., Leo, M., Cicirelli, G., & Distante, A. (2004). An algorithm for real time eye detection in face images. In *17th International Conference on Pattern Recognition* (Vol. 3, pp. 278-281).

Dibeklioglu, H., Salah, A. A., & Akarun, L. (2008). 3D facial landmarking under expression, pose, and occlusion variations. In *IEEE Second International Conference on Biometrics: Theory, Applications and Systems*.

Ding, L., & Martinez, A. M. (2008). Precise detailed detection of faces and facial features. In *IEEE Conference on Computer Vision and Pattern Recognition* (CVPR) (pp. 1-7).

Dubuisson, M. P., & Jain, A. K. (1994). A modified Hausdorff distance for object matching. In *12th International Conference on Pattern Recognition* (pp. 566-568).

Fasel, I. R., Fortenberry, B., & Movellan, J. R. (2005). Gboost: A generative framework for boosting with applications to realtime eye coding. *Computer Vision and Image Understanding, 98*(1), 182–210. doi:10.1016/j.cviu.2004.07.014

Fasel, I. R., Smith, E. C., Bartlett, M. S., & Movellan, J. R. (2002). A comparison of Gabor filter methods for automatic detection of facial landmarks. In *IEEE International Conference on Automatic Face and Gesture Recognition* (pp. 231-235).

Feris, R. S., Gemmell, J., Toyama, K., & Kruger, V. (2002). Hierarchical wavelet networks for facial feature localization. In *5th International Conference on Automatic Face and Gesture Recognition* (pp. 125-130).

Gargesha, M., & Panchanathan, S. (2002). A hybrid technique for facial feature point detection. In *5th IEEE Southwest Symposium on Image Analysis and Interpretation* (pp. 134-138).

Gourier, N., Hall, D., & Crowley, J. L. (2004). Facial features detection robust to pose, illumination and identity. In *International Conference on Systems Man and Cybernetics* (pp. 617-622).

Han, C. C., Liao, H. Y. M., Yu, G. J., & Chen, L. H. (2000). Fast face detection via morphology- based pre-processing. *Pattern Recognition, 33,* 1701–1712. doi:10.1016/S0031-3203(99)00141-7

Hjelmaas, E. (2000). Feature-based face recognition. In *Norwegian Image Processing and Pattern Recognition Conference.*

Hsu, R. L., Abdel-Mottaleb, M., & Jain, A. K. (2001). Face detection in color images. In *IEEE International Conference on Image Processing* (Vol. 1, pp. 1046-1049).

Ioannou, S., Karidakis, G., Kollias, S., & Karpouzis, K. (2007). Robust feature detection for facial expression recognition. *EURASIP Journal On Image and Video Processing, 2007.* IST-2000-29319. (n.d.). *ERMIS, Emotionally Rich Man-machine Intelligent System.* Retrieved from http://www.image.ntua.gr/ermis

Jesorsky, O., Kirchberg, K. J., & Frischholz, R. W. (2001). Robust face detection using the Hausdorff distance. In *3rd International Conference on Audio and Video-based Biometric Person Authentication* (pp. 90-95).

Kanade, T., Cohn, J., & Tian, Y.-L. (2000). Comprehensive database for facial expression analysis. In *International Conference on Automatic Face and Gesture Recognition* (pp. 46- 53).

Karungaru, S., Fukumi, M., & Akamatsu, N. (2004). Face recognition using genetic algorithm based template matching. In *IEEE International Symposium on Communications and Information Technology* (pp. 1252-1257).

Kawaguchi, T., & Rizon, M. (2003). Iris detection using intensity and edge information. *Pattern Recognition, 36*(2), 549–562. doi:10.1016/S0031-3203(02)00066-3

Kawato, S., & Tetsutani, N. (2004). Detection and tracking of eyes for gaze-camera control. *Image and Vision Computing, 22*(12), 1031–1038. doi:10.1016/j.imavis.2004.03.013

Kjeldsen, R., & Kender, J. (1996). Finding skin in color images. In *2nd International Conference on Automatic Face and Gesture Recognition* (pp. 312-317).

Lai, J., Yuen, P. C., Chen, W., Lao, S., & Kawade, M. (2001). Robust facial feature point detection under nonlinear illuminations. In *2nd International Workshop on Recognition, Analysis and Tracking of Faces and Gestures in Real-Time Systems* (pp. 168-174).

Lam, K., & Yan, H. (1998). An analytic-to-holistic approach for face recognition based on a single frontal view. *IEEE Transactions on Pattern Analysis and Machine Intelligence, 20*(7), 673–686. doi:10.1109/34.689299

Martinez, A. M., & Benavente, R. (1998). The AR face database (Tech. Rep. No. 24). *CVC.*

Menser, B., & Muller, F. (1999). Face detection in color images using principal components analysis. In *7th International Conference on Image Processing and Its Applications* (Vol. 2, p. 620-624).

Messer, K., Matas, J., Kittler, J., Luettin, J., & Maitre, G. (1999). XM2VTSDB: The extended M2VTS database. In *2nd International Conference on Audio and Video-based Biometric Person Authentication* (pp. 72-77).

Nguyen, M. H., Perez, J., & de la Torre Frade, F. (2008). Facial feature detection with optimal pixel reduction SVMs. In *8th IEEE International Conference on Automatic Face and Gesture Recognition.*

Ohmoto, Y., Ueda, K., & Ohno, T. (2008). Real-time system for measuring gaze direction and facial features: towards automatic discrimination of lies using diverse nonverbal information. *AI & Society, 23*(2), 187–200. doi:10.1007/s00146-007-0138-x

Perlibakas, V. (2003). Automatical detection of face features and exact face contour. *Pattern Recognition Letters, 24*(16), 2977–2985. doi:10.1016/S0167-8655(03)00158-2

Phillips, P., Wechsler, H., Huang, J., & Rauss, P. (1998). The FERET database and evaluation procedure for face-recognition algorithms. *Image and Vision Computing, 16*(5), 295–306. doi:10.1016/S0262-8856(97)00070-X

Phillips, P. J., Flynn, P. J., Scruggs, T., Bowyer, K. W., Chang, J., & Hoffman, K. (2005). Overview of the face recognition grand challenge . In *IEEE Computer Vision and Pattern Recognition conference* (*Vol. 1*, pp. 947–954). CVPR.

Reinders, M. J. T., Koch, R. W. C., & Gerbrands, J. J. (1996). Locating facial features in image sequences using neural networks. In *2nd International Conference on Automatic Face and Gesture Recognition* (pp. 230-235).

Shih, F. Y., & Chuang, C.-F. (2004). Automatic extraction of head and face boundaries and facial features. *Information Sciences Informatics and Computer Science: An International Journal, 158*(1), 117–130.

Smith, P., Shah, M., & da Vitoria Lobo, N. (2003). Determining driver visual attention with one camera. *IEEE Transactions on Intelligent Transportation Systems, 4*(4), 205–218. doi:10.1109/TITS.2003.821342

Stirling Psychology Department. U. of. (n.d.). *Psychological Image Collection at Stirling (PICS image database).* http://pics.psych.stir.ac.uk/.

Tanaka, H. T., Ikeda, M., & Chiaki, H. (1998). Curvature-based face surface recognition using spherical correlation principal directions for curved object recognition. In *3rd IEEE International Conference on Automatic Face and Gesture Recognition* (pp. 372-377).

The BioID face database. (n.d.). Retrieved from http://www.bioid.com/downloads/facedb /face-database.html

The JAFFE database. (n.d.). Retrieved from http://www.mis.atr.co.jp/ mlyons/jaffe.html

Viola, P., & Jones, M. (2001). Rapid object detection using a boosted cascade of simple features . In *IEEE Computer Vision and Pattern Recognition* (*Vol. 1*, pp. 511–518). CVPR.

Viola, P., & Jones, M. (2004). Robust real-time face detection. *International Journal of Computer Vision, 57*(2), 137–154. doi:10.1023/B:VISI.0000013087.49260.fb

Vukadinovec, D., & Pantic, M. (2005). Fully automatic facial feature point detection using Gabor feature based boosted classifiers. In *International Conference on Systems Man and Cybernetics.*

Wu, J., & Zhou, Z.-H. (2003). Efficient face candidates selector for face detection. *Pattern Recognition*, *36*(5), 1175–1186. doi:10.1016/S0031-3203(02)00165-6

Xie, X., Sudhakar, R., & Zhuang, H. (1993). Corner detection by a cost minimization approach. *Pattern Recognition*, *26*, 1235–1243. doi:10.1016/0031-3203(93)90208-E

Xu, C., Tan, T., Wang, Y., & Quan, L. (2006). Combining local features for robust nose location in 3D facial data. *Pattern Recognition Letters*, *27*(13), 1487–1494. doi:10.1016/j.patrec.2006.02.015

Yilmaz, A., & Shah, M. A. (2002). Automatic feature detection and pose recovery for faces. *In Asian Conference on Computer Vision* (pp. 23-25).

Zhou, Z. H., & Geng, X. (2004). Projection functions for eye detection. *Pattern Recognition*, *37*(5), 1049–1056. doi:10.1016/j.patcog.2003.09.006

Zhu, M., & Martinez, A. (2006). Subclass discriminant analysis. *IEEE Transactions on Pattern Analysis and Machine Intelligence*, *28*(8), 1274–1286. doi:10.1109/TPAMI.2006.172

KEY TERMS AND DEFINITIONS

Facial Features Detection: Localization of characteristic points or areas of interest (e.g. eyes or eye centers) on the face.

3D Facial Features Detection: Localization of characteristic facial points on 3D (e.g. mesh or point cloud) facial data.

Face Detection: Localization of the face (e.g. through a bounding box) on an image or video frame.

Radon Transform: An integral transform whose inverse is usually used in tomographic reconstruct (e.g. in CT scans). Essentially, it computes the projection along a line of a specific direction.

Integral Projection Function (or Projection): The set of the sums of pixel values along consecutive image lines (or columns)

Gabor Filters: linear filters with impulse response defined by a Gaussian function multiplied with a harmonic. They are used in object detection and object pose estimation, as they give different responses for different directionalities.

Chapter 4
Gabor and Log–Gabor Wavelet for Face Recognition

M. Ashraful Amin
Independent University Bangladesh (IUB), Bangladesh

Hong Yan
City University of Hong Kong, China

ABSTRACT

In practice Gabor wavelet is often applied to extract relevant features from a facial image. This wavelet is constructed using filters of multiple scales and orientations. Based on Gabor's theory of communication, two methods are proposed to acquire initial features from 2D images that are Gabor wavelet and Log-Gabor wavelet. Theoretically the main difference between these two wavelets is Log-Gabor wavelet produces DC free filter responses, whereas Gabor filter responses retain DC components. This experimental study determines the characteristics of Gabor and Log-Gabor filters for face recognition. In the experiment, two sixth order data tensor are created; one containing the basic Gabor feature vectors and the other containing the basic Log-Gabor feature vectors. This study reveals the characteristics of the filter orientations for Gabor and Log-Gabor filters for face recognition. These two implementations show that the Gabor filter having orientation zero means oriented at 0 degree with respect to the aligned face has the highest discriminating ability, while Log-Gabor filter with orientation three means 45 degree has the highest discriminating ability. This result is consistent across three different frequencies (scales) used for this experiment. It is also observed that for both the wavelets, filters with low frequency have higher discriminating ability.

DOI: 10.4018/978-1-61520-991-0.ch004

INTRODUCTION

Face recognition research is important for both psychology and information science. How do we humans recognize faces and how faces are represented or encoded in our brain, are both long debated issues. Some of the theories of face recognition characteristics have been implemented in computer-based face recognition system. Following is a brief summary of the common approaches to face recognition.

An appearance based holistic approach to face recognition was introduced by Kirby & Sirovich (1990), and Turk & Pentland (1991) by representing facial images as eigenfaces. Subsequently, the concept of Fisher-Faces was introduced (Belhumeur et al., 1997; Etemad & Chellappa, 1997; Zhao et al., 1998). Liu & Wechsler (2001) introduced an enhanced Fisher classifier method for face coding and recognition. It relied on an enhanced Fisher Linear Discriminant model that used integrated shape and texture features (Liu & Wechsler, 2001). In a recent work, Vasilescu & Terzopoulos (2002) proposed a different type of facial representation named Tensor-Face.

In the actual practice of face detection, the image size can be quite small and Zhao et al. (1999) demonstrated that the image size could be very small for holistic face recognition. For example, a Linear Discriminant Analysis (LDA) system used 12×11 image for face recognition. Lin et al.'s (1997) Probabilistic Decision-Based Neural Network (PDBNN) system used 14×10, while neuropsychological research has shown that for human perception a minimum image of 18×24 is acceptable. Moreover, Zhao et al. (1999) insisted that there exists a universal face subspace of fixed dimension. For holistic recognition this means that the image size does not matter as long as it is larger than the subspace dimension. Zhao et al. also showed that smaller images perform slightly better perhaps due to the improvement of signal-to-noise ratio with the decrease in image size. More studies on the size of image and filter size were discussed in a recent paper by Zhang et al. (2006).

Lin et al. (1997) used a PDBNN method to create fully automatic face detection and recognition system. Shan et al. (2003) presented a method for lighting, expression and viewpoint independent face recognition by improving the eigenfaces method (Turk & Pentland, 1991). Bartlett et al. (2002) presented an in-depth analysis of the Independent Component Analysis (ICA) and its strength over the eigenface approach for face recognition. A comparative study on the effect of image compression techniques on the PCA, LDA and ICA was performed by Delac et al. (2007). Different ICA (Cao et al., 2004), two-dimensional (2D) PCA (Pang et al., 2008), and marginal fisher analysis-based face recognition approaches are also available in recently published works (Xu et al., 2005). Yan & Zhang (2008a, 2008b) proposed a method for face recognition based on correlation filter based class-dependence feature analysis.

Lades et al. (1993) applied Gabor wavelet for face recognition, using the Dynamic Link Architecture (DLA) framework. At first the DLA computes the Gabor jets and then it performs a flexible template comparison between the resulting image decompositions, applying graph-matching methods. In a later work Wiskott et al. (1997) expanded the DLA and developed a Gabor wavelet-based elastic bunch graph matching method that was used to recognize human faces. Lyons et al. (1999, 2000) proposed a two-class categorization of gender, race, and facial expression from facial image based on the 2D Gabor wavelet representation and the labeled elastic graph matching. Donato et al. (1999) have compared a method based on Gabor representation with other techniques, finding that the former provided better performance. In a series of work, Liu combined Gabor features with enhanced Fisher linear discriminant methods (Liu, 2002), kernel PCA with fractional power polynomial models on the Gabor features

(Liu, 2004) and, Liu & Wechsler (2003) applied Gabor+PCA+ICA method for face recognition. Gabor representation of face (Liu, 2002; Liu, 2004; Liu & Wechsler, 2003; Lyons et al., 1999; Lyons et al., 2000; Wiskott, 1997), facial expression (Amin et al., 2005; Dailey et al. 2002), and gait (Tao et at., 2007) have shown good performance in classification and identification. Among other feature extraction and subspace projection method includes local binary pattern (LBP) texture features (Ahonen at al., 2006), effective part-based local representation method named locally salient ICA (LS-ICA) (Kim et al., 2005), and appearance based face recognition method called the Laplacianface approach (He et al., 2005).

There are two implementations of Gabor wavelet in vision science that are adopted from Gabor's theory of communication (Gabor, 1946). One was proposed by Daugman (1985) in 1985, and the other one is Log-Gabor implementation proposed by Field (1987) in 1987. In this paper the results for applying Gabor and Log-Gabor filter to extract the initial features for face recognition are investigated. This experiment constructs 24 different filters for each of the Gabor and Log-Gabor wavelet. For both the wavelets, filters are created at eight orientations $\{0, \pi/8, \pi/4, 3\pi/8, \pi/2, 5\pi/8, 3\pi/4, 7\pi/8\}$ for three scales (frequencies). Two major observations are (1) the recognition accuracy for the Gabor filter is maximum at orientation zero ($0°$) and for Log-Gabor filter at orientation three ($45°$) for a given frequency, if the orientation is considered with respect to the aligned face, (2) lower the frequency of a filter at a given orientation, higher the recognition accuracy.

The system is built based on the following hypothesis: If a set of subjects are represented as, $s=\{s_1, s_2, \ldots\}$ then the set of images portrayed by the ith subject at the jth pose (or expression) is represented as, $e_{i,j}=\{e_{i,j,1}, e_{i,j,2}, \ldots\}$ in the image space. In this context, after applying Gabor or Log-Gabor filters on each of the images of $e_{i,j}$,

will produce $G_{i,j}=\{G_{i,j,1}, G_{i,j,2}, \ldots\}$ as $e_{i,j,k} \xrightarrow{Gabor/Log-Gabor} G_{i,j,k}$. Application of PCA on each of the Gabor or Log-Gabor feature vectors of $G_{i,j}$ will produce $P_{i,j} = \{P_{i,j,1}, P_{i,j,2}, \ldots\}$ as $G_{i,j,k} \xrightarrow{PCA} P_{i,j,k}$. Then classifiers (PNN) can be trained with a sub-set of $\{(P_{i,j,k})\}$ to learn the class information. This means that after applying Gabor-PCA or Log-Gabor-PCA transformation of an image ($e_{i,j,k}$), classifiers can still be used on the lower dimensional representation ($P_{i,j,k}$) of the image ($e_{i,j,k}$) to identify the person (i) in that image. More precisely, it is possible for a classifier to associate the facial image ($e_{i,j,k}$) in a lower dimensional (Gabor-PCA or, Log-Gabor-PCA) representation ($P_{i,j,k}$) with the person (i) in the image.

FACE RECOGNITION SYSTEM AND EXPERIMENTAL SETUP

A typical facial recognition system will have four major generic components that are (1) facial image acquisition, (2) facial image pre-processing, (3) facial feature extraction, and (4) face recognition. These steps are briefly discussed in the following sections.

Facial Data Acquisition

Different background and lighting will influence the performance of face or any type of object recognition and tracking system (Huanga et al., 2008). Images from 30 subjects are collected in a daily life environment for the experiment. Three image sequences for three different poses and one image sequence for different expressions are taken. Each sequence contains 100 frames. Here in Figure 1 we provide some of the frames of a subject's four sequences. (This data can be downloaded from www.spl.it.cityu.edu.hk/~amin/face.html.

Figure 1. An example of raw images for a subject's 4 different poses and expressions

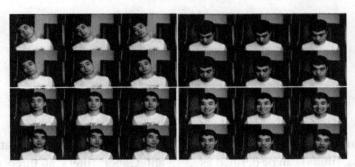

Facial Data Preprocessing

Two main issues of image processing will strongly affect the performance of the system are the brightness distribution across a facial image and the facial geometric correspondence. To ensure the above-mentioned criteria in facial images, an affine transformation (rotation, scaling and translation) is used to normalize the face geometry and invariant intensity for all the actors. The normalization is achieved by identification of three landmark points: the center of the top lip and the center of both the eyes as shown in Figure 2. Similar method is also adopted by Bartlett et al. (2002), Buhmann et al. (1990), Liu & Wechsler (2001) and Zhang (2006).

In the proposed method a gray level raw image of size 640×480 is cropped into a 240×292 facial region image where the centers of left and right eyes are positioned at (56,88) and (148,88), and

the center of the top lip is positioned at (102,224) (Figure 2).

Facial Feature Extraction

The Gabor Wavelet

Gabor wavelet was introduced to image analysis due to their biological relevance and computational properties (Daugman, 1980; Daugman, 1985; Daugman, 1988; Jones & Palmer, 1987; Marcelja, 1980). In face recognition, Gabor filters as feature generator are widely used (Donato et al., 1999; Lades et al., 1993; Liu, 2002; Liu, 2004; Liu, & Wechsler, 2003; Lyons et al., 1999; Lyons et al., 2000; Wiskott et al. 1997). The Gabor wavelet, whose kernels are similar to the 2D receptive field profiles of the mammalian cortical simple cells, exhibit desirable characteristics of spatial locality and orientation selectivity, and are optimally

Figure 2. Affine transformation to normalize facial geometry and intensity

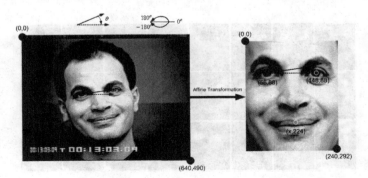

Figure 3. The magnitude of the Gabor kernels at three different scales (v={0,1,2})

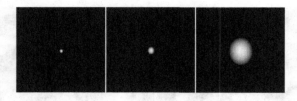

localized in the space and frequency domains. The Gabor wavelet (kernels, filters) can be defined as follows (Daugman, 1988; Lades et al., 1993; Liu, 2002; Marcelja, 1980):

$$\psi_{\mu,\nu}(z) = \frac{\left\|k_{\mu,\nu}\right\|^2}{\sigma^2} e^{-\frac{\left\|k_{\mu,\nu}\right\|^2 \|z\|^2}{2\sigma^2}} \left[e^{ik_{\mu,\nu}z} - e^{-\frac{\sigma^2}{2}} \right] \quad (1)$$

Where μ and v define the orientation and scale of the Gabor kernel $z = (x, y)$, $\|\bullet\|$ denotes the Euclidean norm operator, and wave vector $k_{\mu,\nu}$ is defined as follows:

$$k_{\mu,\nu} = k_{\nu} e^{i\varphi_{\mu}} \quad (2)$$

where $\varphi_{\mu} = \mu\pi/8$ and $k_{\nu} = k_{max}/f^{\nu}$. Here, k_{max} is the maximum frequency, and f is the spacing factor between kernels in the frequency domain. In Figure 3 magnitude of Gabor kernels at 3 different scales can be seen.

For our experiment, a lattice of phase-invariant Gabor filters at three scales $v=\{0,1,2\}$ in Equation (1), and eight orientations $\mu=\{0,1,2...,7\}$ in Equation (1) are applied on each preprocessed facial image. The Gabor filter/kernel representation of a facial image is obtained by convolving the Gabor filters/kernels with the facial image. So, from a single facial image 24 Gabor responses are recorded. Figure 4 presents 24 Gabor magnitude representation of the normalized facial image of Figure 2.

Here it may be noted that the dimension of the preprocessed image is 240×292 and the scale size is relative to this image size. According to Bachmann (1991) and Buhmann et al. (1990), as an image feature detector, the Gabor filters exhibits "some" invariance to background, translation, distortion, and size. However, if the change in background, translation, distortion, or size is too large then this invariance property of the Gabor wavelet may not hold, so in this sense the filter scale and image size is related.

Figure 4. The magnitude of Gabor representation at eight orientations $\mu = \{0, 1, 2, ..., 7\}$ and three scales $v = \{0, 1, 2\}$

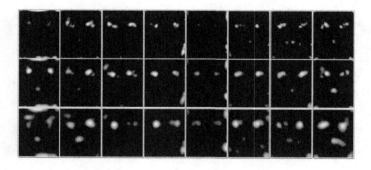

The Log-Gabor Wavelet

According to Field (1987) the implementation of Equation (1) will have the problem of the tails of the two Gaussians crossing over the DC for lower frequency Gabors. He proposed Log-Gabor function which will always yield a spectrum that approaches zero amplitude toward the DC component, regardless of central frequency of the function or phase angle used in the inverse Fourier transform. In the Fourier domain, the real part of the Log-Gabor filter can be expressed as:

$$LG(r,\theta) = \exp\left\{-\left(\frac{\left(\log\left(\frac{R(r_i,\theta_j)}{f}\right)\right)^2}{2\log(\frac{\sigma_1}{f})^2}\right)\right\}\exp\left\{-\left(\frac{\Phi(r_i,\theta_j)^2}{2\sigma_2^2}\right)\right\}$$

(3)

In the equation, r_i and θ_j represent any given point in the polar coordinates, R represents a given radius vector (the spatial frequency dimension or the spread of the filter), f is the center spatial frequency of the Log-Gaussian function, σ_1 is the spatial frequency bandwidth of the Log-Gaussian, Φ represents a given theta 'arc vector' (the orientation dimension), and σ_2 is the orientation bandwidth of the Gaussian function.

Hansen & Hess (2006) represent this procedure with the illustration of Figure 5. The image on the left in Figure 5 is the 2D polar coordinate reference map depicting the cardinal axes of the polar coordinate system, where the radius r is spatial frequency axis, and the theta θ "arc" is orientation

axis. The second image from the left is the radial Log-Gaussian filter component, and third is the Gaussian θ component. The combination of the radial Log-Gaussian and θ Gaussian components generates the Log-Gabor filter as shown in the first image after the equality sign in Figure 5. Finally in Figure 5, an example of this filter in the spatial domain that has been assigned an even-symmetric local absolute phase angle is provided showing the real component of the filter generated.

In Figure 6 the magnitude of three Log-Gabor filters used in the experiment are provided. Here note the difference in magnitude at the center of the filters acquired from Log-Gabor wavelet in Figure 6 with the filters acquired using Gabor wavelet as shown in Figure 3. For the Log-Gabor wavelet the response at the center of a filter is minimum and for the Gabor filter it is maximum.

In Figure 7 the magnitude representation of the Log-Gabor of the same image of Figure 2 are depicted. Here also notice the differences with the intensity images of Figure 4. Particularly, the difference is more visible for the low frequency filter responses which are provided at the last row of the Figure 4 and Figure 7.

The Gabor or Log-Gabor Feature Representation

The result of a Gabor or Log-Gabor transformation can be seen as a 4th order tensor $T(u,v,l,m)$ (Figure 4 and Figure 7) which is a 8×3×29×35 tensor, where $l=\{1,2,...,29\}$ and $m=\{1,2,...,35\}$ are the indexes along the sub-sample points of the width and height of the image respectively (8 pixel sub-sampling is used as shown in Figure

Figure 5. An illustration of the different stages of the Log-Gabor filter creation

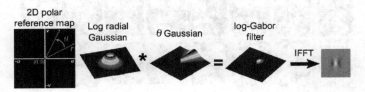

Figure 6. The magnitude of the Log-Gabor kernels at three different scales

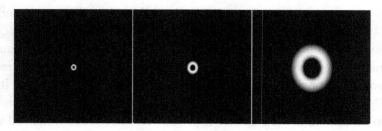

8), and u = {1,2,…8}, v={1,2,3}, are the indexes along the orientation and scale of the Gabor (or Log-Gabor) filter response.

Here, the entries of the 4th order tensor are complex numbers and the magnitude part of this 4th order tensor is defined as the Gabor or Log-Gabor face. In Gabor or Log-Gabor facial representation, there are 24 components for a single facial image, and each one is the magnitude part of the output which is obtained by convolving a facial image with 24 filters or kernels. For our experiment we have s={1,2,…,30}subjects, p={1,2,…4} poses per subject and each pose has e={1,2,…,100} facial images. Applying Gabor or Log-Gabor filters on each image, data tensor $DG(s,p,e,u,v,l,m)$ from Gabor and $DLG(s,p,e,u,v,l,m)$Log-Gabor filter responses are created. A pictorial representation for the tensor DG is provided in Figure 9. Similar representation for the tensor DLG is also possible.

For better illustration, the Gabor filter responses are presented in image form. In reality,

the output of a Gabor function using the convolution $\left| I(x,y) * \psi_{\mu,\nu}(x,y) \right|$ will return a basic Gabor feature vector for the μth orientation at ν^{th} scale, which in this case is a vector of size $n = l * m = 29 * 35 = 1015$. This means, the practical representation of the whole data set is in-fact a 6th order tensor $DG(s,p,e,u,v,n)$ which is a 30×4×100×8×3×1015tensor. Hence, during implementation if we want to refer to the response of the kernel $\psi_{\mu,\nu}(x,y)$ for the ith person's j^{th} pose's k^{th} image in the tensor, we can write $DG(i,j,k,\mu+1,v+1,:)$. For rest of the paper we follow this notation to refer to an element in the tensor. Here, the response for a kernel is considered as a single component even though it is a 1015 element vector and for each facial image, 24 different components (feature vectors) exist in the tensor. The Log-Gabor data tensor DLG is also a 6th order tensor and accessed using similar process.

Figure 7. The magnitude of Log-Gabor representation at eight orientations and three scales

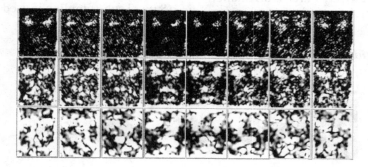

Figure 8. Sub-sampling of the image to acquire Gabor filter responses

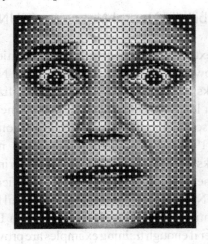

Principle Component Analysis (PCA)

Principle Component Analysis (PCA) is a simple statistical method to reduce the dimensionality while minimizing mean squared reconstruction error (Turk & Pentland, 1991). It is commonly applied to reduce the dimension of Gabor features. Assume that X is a data matrix containing M Gabor feature vector of a given scale and orientation as the column vectors, first the mean column vector Ξ, for the Gabor feature vectors of X is calculated. Then the mean is subtracted from each of the Gabor feature vectors and kept in the matrix A. Finally, the covariance matrix can be calculated as:

$$\Im = \frac{1}{M} AA^T \qquad (4)$$

Here the matrix AA^T of size 1015×1015 needs to be constructed to calculate the covariance matrix $\Im$, however, it is too large for the memory constrains. Rather, the method described in Turk & Pentland (1991) is employed to construct the covariance matrix $\Im$ replacing AA^T with A^TA. The original data X of α-dimensional space is projected as data Y_ε to a subspace spanned by ε principal eigenvectors for the top ε eigenvalues of the covariance matrix $\Im$. If Ω_ε contains top ε principal eigenvectors of the covariance matrix $\Im$, then,

$$Y_\varepsilon = \Omega_\varepsilon^T A \qquad (5)$$

For two important reasons the covariance matrix is not created from the whole data set. First, even if we follow the method proposed in Turk & Pentland (1991), matrix A^TA of size 12000×12000 (total number of Gabor feature vectors is 30×4×100) is needed which is even larger than AA^T (1015×1015) in size. Thus, we chose 10 subjects to construct $\Im$. Moreover, $\Im$ is not created from all the Gabor feature vectors of those 10 subjects. Rather, from the tensor DG 400 feature vectors as $DG(i,j,k,$u,v$:)$ are selected for an orientation and scale, where $i=\{1,2,\ldots,10\}$, $j=\{1,2,..,4\}$ and $k=\{1,11,..,91\}$. This makes it

Figure 9. The 7th order data tensor's pictorial view

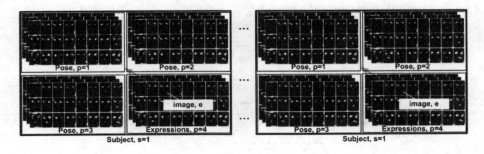

possible to create a manageable sized covariance matrix following Turk & Pentland (1991), since, $A^T A$ is of size 400×400. All the data of *DG* are projected on the top 50 principle components of the covariance matrix and the projected tensor $PG(s,p,e,u,v,r)$ is acquired. Here, *PG* is a 30×4×100×8×3×50 tensor with $r=\{1,2,...,50\}$ representing the features associated with the top 50 principle components. The top 50 principle components are chosen because the sum of the top 50 eigenvalues of the covariance matrix is more than 90% of the sum of all the eigenvectors.

Secondly, the covariance matrix is not created from the whole data set, because, for a face recognition system it is not possible to recalculate the covariance matrix each time a new subject is added to the database, if a system is built based on a covariance matrix ($\Im$) that is created from all the example data in hand then it means each time new images for a subject is added to the database, $\Im$ needs to be recalculated. Hence, the classification accuracy such systems provide may not be as credible as a system that creates $\Im$ from small number of subjects than the actual number it intends to identify. The method proposed here does not have this problem as images from one third of the subjects are applied in the $\Im$ calculation. This method is followed for each orientations and scales, which means that the PCA process is run 24 times. In a similar way *PLG* is constructed from the tensor *DLG*.

Classification

Probabilistic Neural Networks (PNN)

The next task is to perform classification of these lower dimensional feature vectors. Neural networks are excellent in greater generalization through learning hence neural learning methods have also been applied to face recognition (Lin et al., 1997). We applied probabilistic neural networks (PNN) for classification of 'principle component features' for person identification. The PNN learns rapidly than the traditional back-propagation, guarantees to converge to a Bayes classifier if enough training examples are provided, enables faster incremental training, and is robust to noisy examples (Specht, 1990).

In Figure 10, *R* is the number of elements (features) in the input vector, and *Q* is the total number of training pairs, including input and output. This is also the number of neurons in layer 1 (radial basis layer), and *WI* and b_1 are the weight matrix and bias vector of the redial basis layer. *K* is the number of classes of input data, and the number of neurons in layer 2 (competitive layer), and *LW* is the weight matrix of the competitive layer.

A subset of feature vectors are selected from tensor *PG* for an orientation and scale as PG(i,j,k,u,v:) where $i=\{1,2,...,30\}$, $j=\{1,2,...,4\}$ and $k=\{1,5,...,97\}$ to train the PNN, this means for each subject's each pose, 25 projected feature vectors are selected as training dataset, and rest of the feature vectors are kept apart for testing. In this experiment $R=\{1,2,...,50\}$, $Q=30\times4\times25$

Figure 10. A typical probabilistic neural network

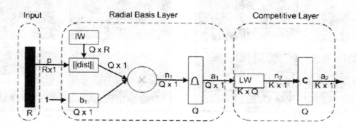

and *K*=30, and the value of *R* changes as we test the classification accuracy of different number of features.

In the training phase *IW=X^T*, *X* is the training pattern matrix of size *R×Q* containing *Q* training patterns as column vectors and, *LW=T* where *T* is the training class matrix of size *K×Q* containing *Q* training class information as column vectors. The entries to the matrix *T* are Boolean and if the *i^{th}* pattern (column) in *X* belongs to the class *k* then the *k^{th}* entry of the *i^{th}* column in matrix *T* is set to 1 and rest of the entries of that column is set to 0.

In the testing phase, when a test input vector is presented, the ‖*dist*‖ box (Figure 10) produces a vector whose elements indicate how close the input is to the vectors of the training set. These elements are multiplied element by element by the bias, and passed as the argument *n* to the radial basis transfer function of Equation (6) (please refer to Figure 10 for visualization of this process).

$$a_1(i) = e^{-n_1(i)^2} \qquad (6)$$

An input vector close to a training vector is represented by a number close to 1 in the output vector a_1. In the second layer, the multiplication $T * a_1$ sums the elements of a_1 due to each of the *K* input classes. Finally, the second-layer uses a comparative transfer function and produces a 1

corresponding to the largest element of n_2, and 0 elsewhere. It illustrates that the network has classified the test input vector into a specific one of the *K* classes because that class had the maximum probability of being correct as it is most similar with an example of that class. This method is followed for each orientation and scale. So, 24 PNNs are created for each length $((1),(1,2),…,(1,2,…,50))$ of feature vectors, hence 24×50 PNNs are created for this experiment. The classification accuracies of the PNNs on the test data is provided in the next section. Similar process is followed for training and testing of face recognition performance of the Log-Gabor feature vectors of the tensor *PLG*.

RESULTS OF THE EXPERIMENT AND DISCUSSION

In the experiment, classification accuracies for the same training and test set for each of the 24 filter responses is acquired for both the Gabor-PCA and Log-Gabor-PCA representations. The results are provided in Figures 11 to 16. Discriminating ability for a given orientation and scale can be logically determined from the classification accuracies acquired for the features produced by that specific filter. In Figure 11, the recognition accuracies for the smallest frequency filter are provided for all

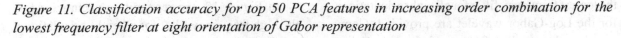

Figure 11. Classification accuracy for top 50 PCA features in increasing order combination for the lowest frequency filter at eight orientation of Gabor representation

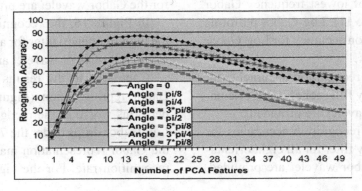

Figure 12. Classification accuracy for top 50 PCA features in increasing order combination for the lowest frequency filter at eight orientation of Log-Gabor representation

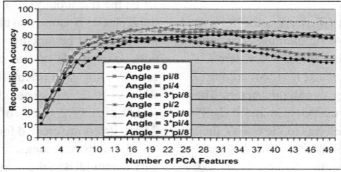

Figure 13. Classification accuracy for top 50 PCA features in increasing order combination for the medium frequency filter at eight orientation of Gabor representation

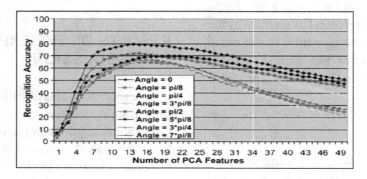

eight orientations for the Gabor wavelet. Here note that, each time the number of features is increased by one starting with the feature corresponding to the topmost principle component.

In Figure 12, the recognition accuracies for the lowest frequency filter for all eight orientations for the Log-Gabor wavelet are provided. Compared to the results of lowest frequency Gabor representation (Figure 11), Log-Gabor performs better as the recognition accuracy for Log-Gabor crosses the 90% mark.

In Figure 13, the recognition accuracies for the medium frequency filter for all eight orientations for the Gabor wavelet are provided.

In Figure 14, the recognition accuracies for the medium frequency filter for all eight orientations for the Log-Gabor wavelet are provided.

Compared to the results of Figure 13, Log-Gabor performs better in Figure 14. As the number of feature increases the recognition accuracy for Gabor decreases gradually, however for the Log-Gabor it decreases drastically.

In Figure 15, the recognition accuracies for the high frequency filter for all eight orientations for the Gabor wavelet are provided.

In Figure 16, the recognition accuracies for the high frequency filter for all eight orientations for the Log-Gabor wavelet are provided.

Compared to the results of high frequency Gabor representation (Figure 15), Log-Gabor performs worse as the recognition accuracy for Log-Gabor drops under the 70% mark, whereas, the Gabor representation maintains a near 80% recognition rate. For the high frequency filters

Figure 14. Classification accuracy for top 50 PCA features in increasing order combination for the medium frequency filter at eight orientation of Log-Gabor representation

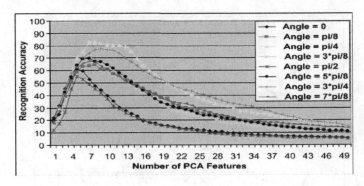

Figure 15. Classification accuracy for top 50 PCA features in increasing order combination for the high frequency filter at eight orientation of Gabor representation

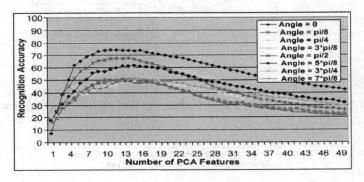

Figure 16. Classification accuracy for top 50 PCA features in increasing order combination for the high frequency filter at eight orientation of Log-Gabor representation

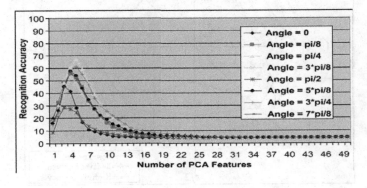

Figure 17. Rader Plot of best accuracies for Gabor wavelet at different frequencies for the in-house database

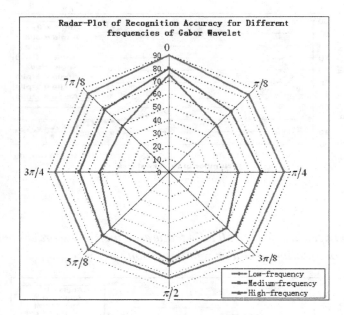

Figure 18. Rader Plot of best accuracies for Log-Gabor wavelet at different frequencies for the in-house database

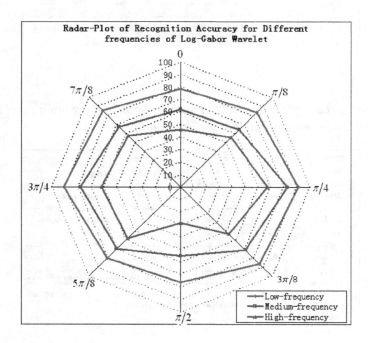

the recognition rate for the Gabor representation decreases slowly while for the Log-Gabor representation this rate is very dramatic and is at the peak for 3 to 5 features and then dives to almost zero (Figure 16).

In Figure 17 and Figure 18 the radar-plots for the best classification accuracy at eight orientations for three different frequencies is provided for Gabor and Log-Gabor wavelet consecutively. Eight axes represent eight orientations and three colors represent three different frequencies.

In this experiment we observed that the recognition accuracy for a lower frequency filter is higher than high frequency filter for both Gabor and Log-Gabor wavelet. This can be seen in Figure 17 and Figure 18 as the line representing the recognition accuracies for comparatively higher frequencies is totally encapsulated by the lines representing comparatively lower frequencies. This means for a given filter orientation the recognition accuracy is **Low-frequency > Medium-frequency > High-frequency**. That is, from the figures red-circle is inside blue circle, and blue-circle is inside green-circle for both Gabor and Log-Gabor wavelets.

Furthermore, the maximum recognition accuracy is acquired for the 0 orientation for the Gabor filters representation of each frequency (Figure 17), whereas for the Log-Gabor implementation the maximum recognition accuracy is shown by the $\pi/4$ filter (Figure 18). The second highest recognition accuracy for Gabor wavelet is acquired for the orientation $0+\pi/2=\pi/2$. The second highest recognition accuracy for Log-Gabor wavelet also follows this trend of adding $\pi/2$ with the best filter's orientation which is the filter with orientation $\pi/4+\pi/2=3\pi/4$.

Results and Observations for Different Databases

Above results are acquired for in-house database. To verify the consistency of the characteristics found from the empirical experiments from the testing on the in-house database, the same procedure is followed for two publicly available benchmark databases namely the ORL database and CMU facial expression database.

In Figure 19 and Figure 20 best recognition accuracies for eight orientations for each of the

Figure 19. Rader Plot of best accuracies for Gabor wavelet at different frequencies for the ORL Database

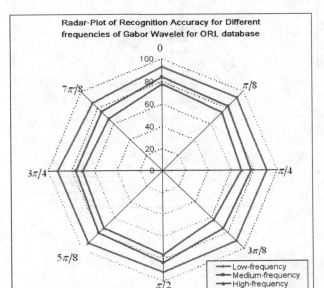

Figure 20. Rader Plot of best accuracies for Log-Gabor wavelet at different frequencies for the ORL Database

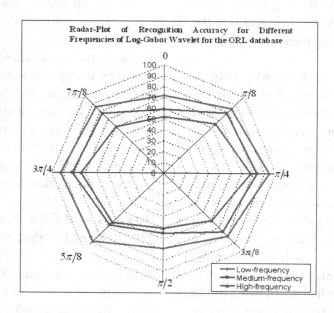

Figure 21. Rader Plot of best accuracies for Gabor wavelet at different frequencies for the CMU Database

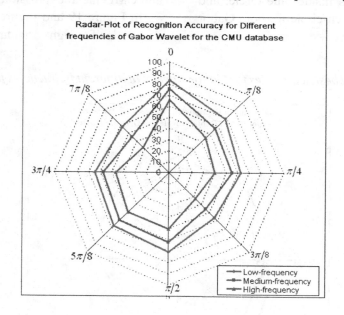

Figure 22. Rader Plot of best accuracies for Log-Gabor wavelet at different frequencies for the CMU Database

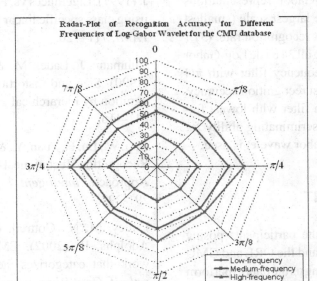

three frequencies are provided as radar plots. Here notice that the accuracy is not the same as the in-house database however, the characteristics are similar. For this database for both Gabor and Log-Gabor representation, a lower frequency representation has higher recognition rate hence have higher discriminating ability. Also the maximum recognition accuracy is acquired for the 0 orientation for the Gabor filters representation for each frequency (Figure 19), whereas for the Log-Gabor implementation the maximum recognition accuracy is shown by the $\pi/4$ filter (Figure 20). Similar results are observed for the CMU database and these are provided in Figure 21 and Figure 22.

FUTURE TRENDS AND CONCLUSION

The Gabor filter based method has been used in biometric application for many years. In this work we investigated the characteristics of two different implementations adopted based on Gabor's (1946) theory of communication. To determine the characteristics of each of the filters acquired from Gabor and Log-Gabor wavelets, three different scales (frequencies) and eight different orientations are considered. The discriminating ability of these 24 filters is determined from their classification accuracy from a face recognition problem.

The experiment reveals the following characteristics of the Gabor representations: (1) among 8 basic Gabor representations for a given scale (frequency) filter the $0°$ orientation has the highest recognition rate, (2) among 3 basic Gabor representations for a given orientation filter the largest scale (smallest frequency) has the highest recognition rate. (3) 1 and 2 concludes that among all 24 basic Gabor representations lowest frequency filter with $0°$ orientation have the highest recognition accuracy. Hence, the $0°$ orientation filter with lowest frequency has the highest discriminating ability for face recognition if Gabor wavelet is used.

The characteristics of the Log-Gabor representations are as follows: (1) among 8 basic Log-Gabor representations for a given scale (frequency), the

$\pi/4$ orientation has the highest recognition rate, (2) among 3 basic Log-Gabor representations for a given orientation the largest scale (smallest frequency) has the highest recognition rate. (3) 1 and 2 concludes that among all 24 basic Log-Gabor representations lowest frequency filter with $\pi/4$ orientation have the highest recognition accuracy. Hence, the $\pi/4$ orientation filter with lowest frequency has the highest discriminating ability for face recognition if Log-Gabor wavelet is used.

ACKNOWLEDGMENT

We would like to thank the participants posing for the in-house database, and the ORL and CMU facial databases for providing us the data to perform verification.

This work was supported by a grant from the City University of Hong Kong (Project No. 9610034).

REFERENCES

Ahonen, T., Hadid, A., & Pietikainen, M. (2006). *Face description with local binary patterns: Application to face recognition* (pp. 2037–2041). IEEE Trans. on PAMI.

Amin, M. A., Afzulpurkar, N. V., Dailey, M. N., Esichaikul, V., & Batanov, D. N. (2005). Fuzzy-C-Mean Determines the Principle Component Pairs to Estimate the Degree of Emotion from Facial Expressions. *FSKD*, 484-493.

Bachmann, T. (1991). Identification of spatially quantized tachistoscopic images of faces: How many pixels does it take to carry identity? *European Journal of Cognitive Psychology*, 87–103.

Bartlett, M. S., Movellan, J. R., & Sejnowski, T. J. (2002). Face recognition by independent component analysis. *IEEE Transactions on Neural Networks*, 1450–1464. doi:10.1109/TNN.2002.804287

Belhumeur, P. N., Hespanha, J. P., & Kriegman, D. J. (1997). Eigenfaces vs. Fisherfaces: Recognition using class specific linear projection. *IEEE Trans. PAMI*, 711–720.

Buhmann, J., Lades, M., & von der Malsburg, C. (1990). Size and distortion invariant object recognition by hierarchical graph matching. *IJCNN*, 411-416.

Cao, W., Lu, F., Yuan, Y., & Wang, S. (2004). Face Recognition Technique Based on Modular ICA Approach. *Intelligent Information Processing*, 291-297.

Dailey, M. N., Cottrell, G. W., Padgett, C., & Adolphs, R. (2002). EMPATH: A neural network that categorizes facial expressions. *Journal of Cognitive Neuroscience*, 1158–1173. doi:10.1162/089892902760807177

Daugman, J. G. (1980). Two-Dimensional Spectral Analysis of Cortical Receptive Field Profiles. *Vision Research*, 847–856. doi:10.1016/0042-6989(80)90065-6

Daugman, J. G. (1985). Uncertainty Relation for Resolution in Space, Spatial Frequency, and Orientation Optimized by Two-Dimensional Cortical Filters. *Journal of the Optical Society of America*, 1160–1169.

Daugman, J. G. (1988). Complete Discrete 2D Gabor Transforms by Neural Networks for Image Analysis and Compression. *IEEE Trans. PAMI.*, 1169-1179.

Delac, K., Grgic, M., & Grgic, S. (2007). Image Compression Effects in Face Recognition Systems. In Delac, K., & Grgic, M. (Eds.), *Face Recognition* (pp. 75–92).

Donato, G., Bartlett, M. S., Hager, J. C., Ekman, P., & Sejnowski, T. J. (1999). Classifying Facial Actions. *IEEE Trans. PAMI*, 974-989.

Etemad, K., & Chellappa, R. (1997). Discriminant analysis for recognition of human face images. *Journal of the Optical Society of America*, 1724–1733.

Field, D. J. (1987). Relations between the statistics of natural images and the response properties of cortical cells. *Journal of the Optical Society of America*, 2379–2394.

Gabor, D. (1946). Theory of communication. *Journal of Institute of Electronic Engineers*, 429-457.

Hansen, B. C., & Hess, R. F. (2006). The role of spatial phase in texture segmentation and contour integration. *Journal of Vision (Charlottesville, Va.)*, 595–615.

He, X., Yan, S., Hu, Y., Niyogi, P., & Zhang, H. (2005). Face recognition using Laplacianfaces. *IEEE Trans. on PAMI*, 328–340.

Huanga, K., Wanga, L., Tana, T., & Maybank, S. (2008). A real-time object detecting and tracking system for outdoor night surveillance. *Pattern Recognition*, 432–444. doi:10.1016/j.patcog.2007.05.017

Jones, J., & Palmer, L. (1987). An Evaluation of the Two-Dimensional Gabor Filter Model of Simple Receptive Fields in Cat Striate Cortex. *Journal of Neurophysiology*, 1233–1258.

Kim, J., Choi, J., Yi, J., & Turk, M. (2005). Effective representation using ICA for face recognition robust to local distortion and partial occlusion. *IEEE Trans. on PAMI*, 1977–1981.

Kirby, M., & Sirovich, L. (1990). Application of the Karhunen-Loeve Procedure for the Characterization of Human Faces. *IEEE Trans. PAMI*, 103-108.

Lades, M., Vorbruggen, J. C., Buhmann, J., Lange, J., Von Der Malsburg, C., Wurtz, R. P., & Konen, W. (1993). Distortion Invariant Object Recognition in the Dynamic Link Architecture. *IEEE Transactions on Computers*, 300–311. doi:10.1109/12.210173

Lin, S. H., Kung, S. Y., & Lin, L. J. (1997). Face recognition/detection by probabilistic decision based neural network. *IEEE Transactions on Neural Networks*, 114–132.

Liu, C. (2002). Gabor Feature Based Classification Using the Enhanced Fisher Linear Discriminant Model for Face Recognition. *IEEE Transactions on Image Processing*, 467–476.

Liu, C. (2004). Gabor-Based Kernel PCA with Fractional Power Polynomial Models for Face Recognition. *IEEE Trans. PAMI*, 572-581.

Liu, C., & Wechsler, H. (2001). A shape- and texture-based enhanced fisher classifier for face recognition. *IEEE Transactions on Image Processing*, 598–608.

Liu, C., & Wechsler, H. (2003). Independent Component Analysis of Gabor Features for Face Recognition. *IEEE Transactions on Neural Networks*, 919–928.

Lyons, M. J., Budynek, J., & Akamatsu, S. (1999). Automatic Classification of Single Facial Images. *IEEE Trans. PAMI*, 1357-1362.

Lyons, M. J., Budynek, J., Plante, A., & Akamatsu, S. (2000). Classifying Facial Attributes Using a 2-D Gabor Wavelet Representation and Discriminant Analysis. *FG*, 202-207.

Marcelja, S. (1980). Mathematical Description of the Responses of Simple Cortical Cells. *Journal of the Optical Society of America*, 1297–1300. doi:10.1364/JOSA.70.001297

Pang, Y., Tao, D., Yuan, Y., & Li, X. (2008). Binary Two-Dimensional PCA. *IEEE Trans. on Systems, Man, and Cybernetics, Part B*, 1176-1180.

Samal, A., & Iyengar, P. (1992). Automatic recognition and analysis of human faces and facial expressions: A survey. *Pattern Recognition*, 65–77. doi:10.1016/0031-3203(92)90007-6

Shan, S., Gao W., & Zhao, D. (2003). Face Identification Based On Face-Specific Subspace. *International Journal of Image and System Technology*, 23-32.

Specht, D. F. (1990). Probabilistic Neural Networks. *Neural Networks*, 109–118. doi:10.1016/0893-6080(90)90049-Q

Tao, D., Li, X., Wu., X., & Maybank, S. J. (2007). General Tensor Discriminant Analysis and Gabor Features for Gait Recognition. *IEEE Trans. PAMI*, 1700-1715.

Turk, M., & Pentland, A. (1991). Eigenfaces for Recognition. *Journal of Cognitive Neuroscience*, 71–86. doi:10.1162/jocn.1991.3.1.71

Vasilescu, M. A. O., & Terzopoulos, D. (2002). Multilinear Analysis of Image Ensembles: TensorFace. *ECCV*, 447-46.

Wiskott, L., Fellous, J.-M., & Von Der Malsburg, C. (1997). Face recognition by elastic bunch graph matching. *IEEE Trans. PAMI*, 775–779.

Xu, D., Tao, D., Li, X., & Yan, S. (2007). Face Recognition - a Generalized Marginal Fisher Analysis Approach. *International Journal of Image and Graphics*, 583–591. doi:10.1142/S0219467807002817

Yan, Y., & Zhang, Y.-J. (2008a). Tensor Correlation Filter Based Class-dependence Feature Analysis for Face Recognition. *Neurocomputing*, 3434–3438. doi:10.1016/j.neucom.2007.11.006

Yan, Y., & Zhang, Y.-J. (2008b). 1D Correlation Filter Based Class-Dependence Feature Analysis for Face Recognition. *Pattern Recognition*, 3834–3841. doi:10.1016/j.patcog.2008.05.028

Yang, M. H., Kriegman, D., & Ahuja, N. (2002). Detecting Faces in Images: A Survey. *IEEE Trans. PAMI*, 34-58.

Zhang, B., Shan, S., Chen, X., & Gao, W. (2006). Histogram of Gabor Phase Patterns (HGPP), A Novel Object Representation Approach for Face Recognition. *IEEE Transactions on Image Processing*, 57–68.

Zhao, W., Chellappa, R., & Krishnaswamy, A. (1998). Discriminant analysis of principal components for face recognition. *FG*, 336–341.

Zhao, W., Chellappa, R., & Phillips, P. J. (1999). *Subspace linear discriminant analysis for face recognition. Technical report, CAR-TR-914*. MD: Center for Automation Research, University of Maryland.

Zhao, W., Chellappa, R., Phillips, P. J., & Rosenfeld, A. (2003). Face Recognition: A Literature Survey. *ACM Computing Surveys*, 399–458. doi:10.1145/954339.954342

KEY TERMS AND DEFINITIONS

Face Recognition: This topic covers the scientific study of recognizing faces by human and machine.

Human Biometrics: This topic studies the measurement of different distinctive characteristics of human from human physiology (face, fingerprint, etc) and behavior (talking, gait, etc) to differentiae individuals from each other.

Filter: A filter is the process that is designed to examine an input or output image request for certain qualifying criteria and then process or forward it accordingly. In other words, a filter lets pass-through the relevant information by filtering out the undesirable information from an image.

Wavelets: A wavelet is a mathematical function that can be applied on an image to acquire relevant information from different frequency and orientation viewpoint.

Gabor Wavelet: Gabor is a special type of wavelet that has a function similar to the one that Dennis Gabor proposed in 1946 to characterize telecommunication signals.

Log-Gabor Wavelet: Log-Gabor wavelet is a modified version of the Gabor wavelet that provides responses free from any DC component.

Tensor Representation: A tensor is a generalized form of matrix. Matrix is two-dimensional arrays where as it can be seen as a multidimensional array. Gabor wavelet responses are acquired from different frequency and orientation filters and collection of all the filter responses for all the instances is put into a tensor and this is called tensor representation or more precisely Gabor tensor representation.

Chapter 5
Efficient Face Retrieval Based on Bag of Facial Features

Yuanjia Du
Trident Microsystems Europe B.V., The Netherlands

Ling Shao
The University of Sheffield, UK

ABSTRACT

In this chapter, the authors present an efficient retrieval technique for human face images based on bag of facial features. A visual vocabulary is built beforehand using an invariant descriptor computed on detected image regions. The vocabulary is refined in two ways to make the retrieval system more efficient. Firstly, the visual vocabulary is minimized by only using facial features selected on face regions which are detected by an accurate face detector. Secondly, three criteria, namely Inverted-Occurrence-Frequency Weights, Average Feature Location Distance and Reliable Nearest-Neighbors, are calculated in advance to make the on-line retrieval procedure more efficient and precise. The proposed system is experimented on the Caltech Human Face Database. The results show that this technique is very effective and efficient on face image retrieval.

INTRODUCTION

The last decade has witnessed great interest in research on content-based image retrieval. This has paved the way for a large number of new techniques and systems, and a growing interest in associated fields to support such systems. Likewise, digital imagery has expanded its horizon in many directions, resulting in an explosion in the volume of image data required to be organized. As a result, image retrieval techniques are becoming increasingly important in multimedia information systems (Datta, et al. 2005).

Early image retrieval techniques focused on the retrieval of entire images (Smeulders, et al. 2000). Given a query image, the goal was to retrieve entire scenes or it was assumed that images contain a single object occupying most of the image. Background clutter or partial occlusions were not explicitly handled. Intra-class variations, camera viewpoint or illumination variations were usually not explicitly modeled. Later, some ap-

DOI: 10.4018/978-1-61520-991-0.ch005

proaches tried to extract 'objects' from images by segmenting them into regions with coherent image properties like color or texture, however, such systems enjoyed only limited successes since the segments and description of segments are crude (Sivic, 2006).

Recently, Local Invariant Regions based retrieval has emerged as a cutting edge methodology in specific object retrieval. The first influential image retrieval algorithm using local invariant regions was introduced by Schmid and Mohr (Schmid & Moger, 1997). The local regions that are invariant to rotation, translation and scaling are detected around Harris corner points (Harris & Stephens, 1988). Differential greyvalue invariants are used to characterize the detected invariant regions in a multi-scale way to ensure invariance under similarity transformations and scale changes. Semi-local constraints and a voting algorithm are then applied to reduce the number of mis-matches. Van Gool et al. (2001) described a method for finding occurrences of the same object or scene in a database using local invariant regions. Both geometry-based and intensity-based regions are employed. The geometry-based regions are extracted by first selecting Harris corner points as 'anchor points' then finding nearby edges detected by Canny's detector (Canny, 1986) to construct invariant parallelograms. The intensity-based regions are defined around local extrema in intensities. The intensity function along rays emanating from a local extremum is evaluated. An invariant region is constructed by linking those points on the rays where the intensity function reaches extrema. Color moment invariants introduced in (Mindru, et al. 1998) are adopted as region descriptor for characterizing the extracted regions. A voting process is carried out by comparing the descriptor vectors of the query and test images to select the most relevant images to the query. False positives are further rejected using geometric and photometric constraints. An image retrieval technique based on matching of

distinguished regions is presented in (Obdrzalek & Matas, 2002). The distinguished regions are the Maximally Stable Extremal Regions introduced in (Matas, et al., 2002). An extremal region is a connected area of pixels that are all brighter or darker than the pixels on the boundary of the region. Local invariant frames are then established on the detected regions by studying the properties of the covariance matrix and the bi-tangent points. Correspondences between local frames are evaluated by directly comparing the normalized image intensities. Matching between query and database images are then done based on the number and quality of established correspondences.

The limitation of the above cited methods is that region description and matching are conducted during retrieval, which makes fast indexing unfeasible. Sivic et al. (2004) proposed a search engine like algorithm for objects in video materials which enables all shots containing the same object as the query to be retrieved efficiently. Regions are first detected by the Harris affine detector and maximally stable extremal region detector (Matas, et al., 2002). Each region is then represented by a 128 dimensional invariant vector using SIFT descriptor (Lowe, 2004). Vector quantization is applied on the invariant descriptors so that the technology of text retrieval can be employed. Sivic and Zisserman (2003) further developed a method for obtaining the principal objects, characters and scenes in a video by measuring the reoccurrence of spatial configurations of viewpoint invariant features. James Philbin et al. (2007) developed a similar system which used SIFT features and adopte the technology of text retrieval architecture to retrieve specific buildings in a large (1M+) image database.

Inspired by Sivic's work (Sivic et al., 2004 & Sivic et al., 2003), we propose a new technique to refine visual vocabulary and construct configuration relations between visual words. The proposed technique shows better results than existing techniques in near-frontal human face image retrieval. We have two major contributions in this paper:

- Inverted-Occurrence-Frequency Weights (IOFW) and Average Feature Location Distance (AFLD) are introduced to refine visual vocabulary by giving different weights to different visual words. The weights are determined by occurrence distribution of vectored features which are hard assigned to a visual word.
- Reliable Nearest-Neighbors (RNN) is proposed to construct connections between each visual word. Therefore, a visual words distribution based model is built for each specific human face.

In the following section, we first briefly review invariant region detectors and descriptors; Section 3 illustrates how we build and refine the visual vocabulary, followed by Section 4 in which experimental results are shown and compared with other techniques. Finally, we conclude this paper in Section 5.

DETECTORS AND DESCRIPTORS

Detecting and matching specific face features across different images is the main operation for our work. This operation typically involves three distinct steps. Firstly, a 'feature detector' identifies a set of image locations presenting rich visual information and whose spatial configuration is well defined. The spatial extent or 'scale' of the feature may also be identified in this first step, as well as the local shape near the detected location. The second step is 'description': a vector characterizing local visual appearance is computed from the image near the nominal location of the feature. 'Matching' is the third step: a given feature is associated with one or more features in other images.

A number of feature detectors (Harris & Stephens, 1988 & Matas et al, 2002 & Beaudet, 1978 & Kadir et al., 2004 & Mikolajczyk & Schmid, 2004), feature descriptors (Lowe, 2004 & Freeman & Adelson, 1991 & Belongie et al., 2002 & Ke & Sukthankar, 2004) and feature matchers (Schmid & Moger, 1997 & Lowe, 2004 & Carneiro & Jepson, 2004 & Moreels & Perona, 2004) have been proposed in the literature. They can be variously combined or concatenated to produce different systems. Typical region detectors include *Harris Detector, Hessian Detector, Affine Invariant Harris/Hessian Detector, Difference of Gaussian filters, Kadir-Brady Detector* and *MSER Detector. SIFT, PCA-SIFT, Steerable filters, Differential Invariants* and *Shape context* are some state-of-the-art region descriptors. In (Moreels & Perona, 2005), the authors evaluated some state-of-the-art region detectors and descriptors. Their results showed that Hessian-Affine combined with SIFT is the most robust to viewpoint changes; Harris-Affine combined with SIFT and Hessian-affine combined with shape context are the most reliable for illumination variations and scaling, respectively, followed by Hessian-Affine combined with SIFT, which is slightly worse.

SIFT (Lowe, 2004) is popular in general object recognition as well as for other machine vision applications. One of the interesting features of the SIFT approach is its capability to capture the main gray-level features of an object's view by means of local patterns extracted from a scale-space decomposition of the image. Bicego et al. (2006) investigated the application of the SIFT approach in the context of face authentication and confirmed its applicability. Despite the wide applicability and potential of SIFT, the research which applies SIFT to face retrieval and recognition is rarely studied due to the challenges of face images, e.g. different facial expressions.

In this paper, we use Hessian-Affine detector combined SIFT for region detection and description due to their outstanding performance in (Moreels & Perona, 2005). In the matching stage, dot products are used to calculate distance between feature vectors. Matches are confirmed only when the ratio of vector angles between the nearest neighbor and the second nearest is less than a threshold.

BUILDING AND REFINING FACIAL VOCABULARY

Face Detection and Crop

Face detection and crop is a required first step in our face recognition system, as it can effectively exclude background cluttering from facial visual vocabulary. Additionally, the visual vocabulary will be much smaller since only interest points across face regions are detected and described. Figure 1 shows some match results before face detection and crop. A number of points in the background are detected and further used for matching, resulting in a lot of false matches.

The algorithm we use for face detection was proposed by Nilsson et al. (2007). They used local Successive Mean Quantization Transform features (SMQT) for illumination and sensor

insensitive operation in face detection, and a split up Sparse Network of Windows (SNoW) is used to speed up the original classifier. Figure 2 illustrates the match results after face detection. Compared with results in Figure 1, the mismatches caused by background cluttering are eliminated. An alternative technique for face detection is *Viola & Jones* face detector, which is used in (Sivic et al., 2005).

Building Vocabulary

After face detection, Hessian-affine region detector is used to detect affine invariant regions across face areas and then the SIFT descriptor is adopted to describe the regions into 128- dimensional vectors. The objective in this sub-section is to quantize the descriptor vectors into clusters which will be the visual 'words' for retrieval. In order to evaluate the capability of the system on retrieving images not used for vocabulary building, our vocabulary is constructed from half of the images in the dataset, and the other half is used for querying. The vector quantization is carried out by K-means clustering. Euclidean distance is used as the distance function for K-means clustering.

Figure 1. The first row shows 3 images which share similar background. The second row illustrates the detected invariant regions. Many regions on the background are detected which are not useful for face retrieval. The third and fourth rows show the results of matching. Many mismatches occur because of background cluttering.

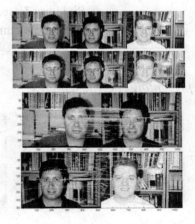

Figure 2. The first row contains face regions of images in Figure 1. The second row gives the match results. The mismatches caused by background cluttering are eliminated.

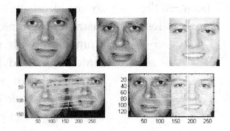

The distance between two descriptor vectors x_1, x_2, is then calculated as follows:

$$d(x_1, x_2) = \sqrt{(x_1 - x_2)^T (x_1 - x_2)} \qquad (1)$$

The centroid of each cluster represents one visual word. Each centroid is the mean of the descriptor vectors in that cluster. Note that, no prior knowledge is used for building the vocabulary, i.e. we do not know which face images belong to which persons during vocabulary building. With this characteristic, our algorithm can be easily extended to video retrieval in which prior knowledge about face ownership is difficult to obtain. Our vocabulary building mechanism is also different to the training procedures in face recognition, where prior knowledge about the face images is intensively studied. After the vocabulary has been built, all the descriptor vectors and additional information are saved for further use.

Defining Vocabulary

In the initial visual vocabulary, some words are rather specific, e.g. eyes from the same person (Figure 3), others are generic, e.g. parts of the cheeks from different persons (Figure 4). In this sub-section, our objective is to refine the visual vocabulary by assigning certain weights to visual words and descriptor vectors according to their properties. Generally, based on Inverted-Occurrence-Frequency-Weights (IOFW) and Average Feature Location Distance (AFLD), more specific words should obtain larger weights; and each descriptor vector ought to have a weight based on information of its Reliable Nearest Neighbors (RNN). All the weights are automatically calculated and saved in the vocabulary and "info-matrix" for fast indexing during retrieval.

IOFW Combined with AFLD

Sivic and Zisserman (2003) used a Term Frequency Inverse Document Frequency (TF-IDF) scheme

Figure 3. One of the visual words representing specific features

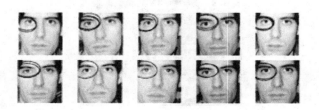

Figure 4. One of the visual words representing generic features

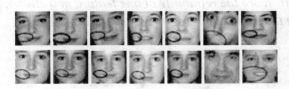

to score the relevance of an image to the query. Inspired by that, we propose IOFW combined with AFLD as follows:

$$w_i = \ln \frac{N}{N_i \times AD_i} \qquad (2)$$

where N is the number of images in the database, and N_i is the number of images in the database with at least one feature in cluster i, AD_i is the average spatial distance between every two features in cluster i. For a specific cluster I, if lots of images in the database have features in it, cluster I probably contains only generic features like Figure 4, then its weight should be small. As we use face detection, all corresponding specific features appear approximately in the same spatial locations on the detected face areas. Therefore, AD_i can be used to distinguish whether or not the features in cluster I are from images of the same person. The combination of IOFW and AFLD can

avoid clusters containing only few features that are spread across images to gain a large weight. However, when there exist significantly scaling and viewpoint changes in the face images, AFLD should be omitted. Since the face images in our experiments are all taken from the front with similar sizes, AFLD is useful for vocabulary refinement.

RNN

Text retrieval techniques rank documents based on the criterion whether the query words appear close together in the retrieved texts (measured by word order). This analogy is relevant for querying objects by an image, where matched covariant regions in a retrieved image in the database should have a similar spatial layout to that of the corresponding regions in the query image (Sivic, 2006 & Schmid & Moger, 1997 & Schaffalitzky & Zisserman, 2002). Sivic and Zisserman implemented this idea (2003). In the indexing stage, they first retrieve images using TF-IDF alone, and

Figure 5. Illustration of spatial consistency voting (Sivic, 2006). To verify a pair of matching regions (A, B), a circular search area is defined by the k (=5 in this example) spatial nearest neighbors in both images. Each match which lies within the search areas in both images casts a vote in support of match (A, B). In this example three supporting matches are found. Matches with no support are rejected.

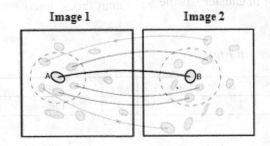

Figure 6. Illustration of refinement of vocabulary using RNN. Circular regions that have the same color belong to the same cluster. To score the reliability of one feature in a cluster, its K (=5 in this example) spatial nearest neighbors in that image (circles in gray area) are used.

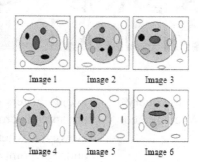

then re-rank them based on a measure of spatial consistency (Figure 5). In this paper, we further develop Sivic and Zisserman's idea to use spatial consistency to rank features in each cluster.

Figure 6 shows an example of RNN scoring. The red circles represent features for which we want to score the reliability, while the other circles are the red circle's nearest neighbors. If features in red belong to the same Cluster *j*, the normalized RNN reliability score of the *i*th feature in Cluster *j* is defined as:

$$w_{i,j}^{RNN} = \frac{\sum_{k=1}^{K} NN_{k,j}^{p}}{K \times ND_j} \qquad (3)$$

where K is the number of nearest neighbor regions used (i.e. K=5 in Figure 6), *p* indicates which cluster feature *i*'s *k*th nearest neighbor belongs to, is the occurrence frequency of Cluster *p* in feature *i*'s *k*th nearest neighbor in Cluster *j*. is the

number of features in Cluster *j*. In the example of Figure 6, there are 6 features in Cluster *j*, and 8 different clusters (circles in other colors) appear as 5 nearest neighbors of features (red circle) in Cluster *j*. Their occurrences are shown in Table 1.

In the final retrieval stage, ranking of images in the database is first arranged according to the descriptor vector distances between regions on the query image and visual words in the vocabulary; after that, images are re-ranked using Equation (2), then spatial consistency information as in Equation (3) is applied to further re-rank images. The ranked Images in the database are then output as final results.

EXPERIMENTS

To evaluate our system, we use the Caltech Human Face database from (Li et al., 2004), which contains 435 images representing 27 sets of human faces. Each set contains a number of face

Table 1. Occurrences of clusters in Figure 6

Yellow	6	Bright Green	6	Blue	5	Black	4
Dark Green	3	Brown	3	Turquoise	2	Pink	1

Table 2. Number of images for each person in the database (N) and number of images used to build visual vocabulary (Nv)

Set	1	2	3	4	5	6	7	8	9	10	11	12	13	14
N	21	20	5	22	21	23	20	5	19	5	5	5	20	19
Nv	11	10	2	11	11	11	10	3	10	3	2	3	10	10
Set	15	16	17	18	19	20	21	22	23	24	25	26	27	28
N	25	22	5	19	20	20	19	20	22	5	20	18	5	
Nv	13	11	2	9	10	10	10	10	11	3	10	9	2	

images of a particular person taken at different backgrounds with different facial expressions and lighting conditions. Half of the database is used to build visual vocabulary (depicted in Table 2). In total, 500 visual words representing 14406 features are created for the visual vocabulary. 15 query images are randomly selected from the database for experiments (Figure 7).

We also test our system on the movie *Groundhog Day*. Instead of retrieving single images, the system is designed to retrieve shots that contain the same actor/actress as the query does. The movie contains 145342 frames in 817 shots, in which 129 shots contain faces.

Evaluation Methods

To evaluate the accuracy of the proposed face retrieval algorithm, we use Average Precision (AP) computed as the area under the *Precision-Recall* curve. *Precision* is the number of retrieved positive images relative to the total number of images retrieved; *Recall* is the number of retrieved positive images relative to the total number of positives in the database.

$$precision = \frac{TP}{TP + FP} \qquad (4)$$

$$recall = \frac{TP}{TP + TN} \qquad (5)$$

where TP, TN, and FP stand for true positive, true negative and false positive, respectively.

Retrieval Performance

In this subsection, we discuss some quantitative results of our method and compare it with results of techniques that use all features to build a vocabulary as Sivic and Zisserman did (2003).

Figure 7. 15 query images used for experiments

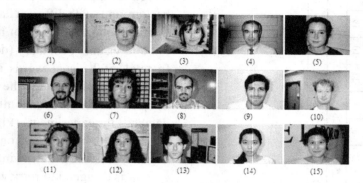

Figure 8. Sample of results returned by the systems. (a) is results returned by the proposed system while (b) results from the system using only the spatial consistency criterion, (c) results of the bag-of-features method alone. The ranking of images in all sets is lowered from left to right. Note that, although (c) shows more relevant images than (b), its precision is lower.

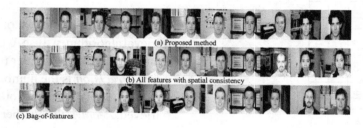

Figure 9. Comparison of results with significant background cluttering. (a) is the results returned by the proposed system while (b) results from the systems using only the spatial consistency criterion and (c) results of the bag-of-features method alone. Note that, the images in (b) and (c) have a similar background pattern (window or window-like).

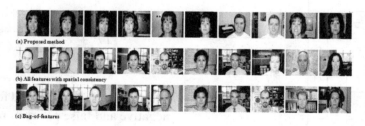

Figure 8 shows an example of results for query (2), which is one of the images we used for building the visual vocabulary. We can see that the proposed system can retrieve more images that are relevant to the query and the precision is higher than other systems. Another example is shown in Figure 9 for query (7), which is not used during vocabulary building. The results show the robustness and scalability of our algorithm for retrieving face images that are not used for building the visual vocabulary. The results show that our system outperforms the system without

Table 3. The TP, TN (FP) and Recall results of 15 query images using facial features and all features

Query	TP		TN(FP)		Recall	
	All features	Facial features	All features	Facial features	All features	Facial features
1	8	9	3	2	72.73%	81.82%
2	6	9	5	2	54.55%	81.82%
3	8	10	3	1	72.73%	90.91%
4	10	10	1	1	90.91%	90.91%
5	9	9	1	1	90.00%	90.00%
6	8	10	2	0	80.00%	100.00%
7	0	8	10	2	0.00%	80.00%
8	10	10	0	0	100.00%	100.00%
9	12	12	1	1	92.31%	92.31%
10	9	5	2	6	81.82%	45.45%
11	9	9	1	1	90.00%	90.00%
12	10	9	0	1	100.00%	90.00%
13	10	10	1	1	90.91%	90.91%
14	7	9	3	1	70.00%	90.00%
15	7	6	2	3	77.78%	66.67%
Total	123/158 (77.85%)	135/158 (85.44%)	35/3112 (1.06%)	23/3112 (0.74%)	77.85%	85.44%

Figure 10. The results when using a query image (in red rectangle) with partial occlusion

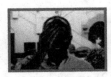 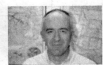

face detection significantly. The method without face detection is hugely under-performing due to the mis-matches on the informative background which contains many features.

Table 3 shows the results of our face retrieval system on the 15 query images. For each query, we retrieve the same number of ranked images as that is used during vocabulary building. For example, we retrieve 11 images for query 1 since 11 face images of the same person as in query 1 are used during vocabulary building. In that case, FP=TN, and *precision=recall*. From the table we see that most of the images containing the same human faces as the query images are retrieved correctly; and the false positives are extremely

low. Comparing our system with the one which uses all features across the image to build visual vocabulary, the overall true positive rate increases from 79.11% to 85.44%, and the overall false positive rate goes down from 1.06% to 0.74%. Some query images have lower positive rates (Query 10 and Query 15) than others because lighting conditions change a lot and there is shortage of distinctive features on those face images. As we use reliable neighbors to refine the vocabulary, people who have distinctive features on their faces (like Query 6 and Query 8) are more likely to be retrieved by the system.

When the face region in the query image is partially occluded or suffers from modest lighting

Figure 11. Illustration of two images in very different lighting conditions: (a) two images that are taken under different lighting conditions; (b) after face detection; (c) matches between images. All the matched regions found are wrong.

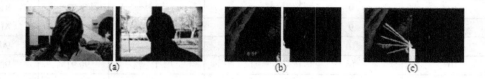

Figure 12. Precision (y-axis): Recall (x-axis) curves for 15 queries images. From top-left to bottom-right, the figures refer to query images from (1) to (15). Note that, all the curves are drawn based on top 20 output results, therefore, not all the Recall curves converge to one.

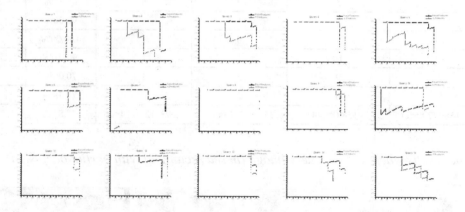

changes (Figure 10), the results of the proposed system are still acceptable. However, when the lighting conditions of the query image and the candidate images in the database are extremely different, the system would fail (Figure 11). Therefore, pre-processing may be required to our system in this aspect. Robustness to large illumination changes will be our main task for our future work.

Figure 12 shows the Precision-Recall curves of 15 query images in Figure 7. We can see that AP of the proposed system is higher than that of the system with no face detection in all the cases except for Queries (10) and (12). Note that, our system has relatively low performance on Query (10) as shown in Table 3 and Figure 12. We think the reason comes from the fact that most of the distinctive features of Query (12) are on hair regions, which do not contribute to the retrieval system after face cropping in our proposed method.

CONCLUSION AND FUTURE WORK

As not specifically designed to work on deformable objects, SIFT features are regarded to be biased towards textured regions (Sivic & Zisserman, 2003). Accordingly, research using bag-of-SIFT-features on face retrieval is rarely published or further studied. In this paper, we have demonstrated that SIFT features could nevertheless be used for efficient face retrieval. A visual vocabulary consisting of facial features only has been built for fast indexing. Three criteria, Inverted Occurrence Frequency Weights, Average Feature Location Distance and Reliable Nearest-Neighbors, are utilized to refine the vocabulary based on the properties of face images. The performance evaluation shows a great improvement of the proposed system over algorithms using the bag-of-features method and with spatial consistency re-ranking only. 8% or more improvement of retrieval rates has been achieved.

The advantages of the proposed face retrieval algorithm include: efficient indexing, since the visual vocabulary is built beforehand; small vocabulary size, because of face detection; high retrieval accuracy for the reason of vocabulary refinement techniques.

As no particular illumination normalization is used in the current work, our system may fail to handle face images with extreme lighting conditions. Also, large viewpoint variations are not covered. Therefore, our future work will be mainly focused on problems of lighting and viewpoint changes.

REFERENCES

Beaudet, P. R. (1978). Rotationally Invariant Image Operators. *IJCPR*, 579-583.

Belongie, S., Malik, J., & Puzicha, J. (2002). *Shape Matching and Object Recognition Using Shape Contexts*. Pattern Analysis and Machine Intelligence PAMI.

Bertero, M., Poggio, T., & Torre, V. (1988). Ill-posed problems in early vision. In *Proceedings of the IEEE*, 869–889.

Bicego, M., Lagorio, A., Grosso, E., & Tistarelli, M. (2006). On the Use of SIFT Features for Face Authentication. In *Conference on Computer Vision and Pattern Recognition Workshop*.

Bigun, J. (1997). Retinal vision applied to facial features detection and face authentication. *Pattern Recognition Letters*, *23*, 463–475.

Canny, J. (1986). A Computational Approach to Edge Detection. *IEEE Transactions on Pattern Analysis and Machine Intelligence*, *8*, 679–714. doi:10.1109/TPAMI.1986.4767851

Carneiro, G., & Jepson, A. D. (2004). *Flexible Spatial Models for Grouping Local Image Features*. Computer Vision and Pattern Recognition.

Datta, R., Li, J., & Wang, Z. (2005). Content-based image retrieval: approaches and trends of the new age. In *Proceedings of the 7th ACM SIGMM international workshop on Multimedia information retrieval* (pp. 253 - 262).

Ferrari, V., Tuytelaars, T., & Van Gool, L. (2001). Real-time affine region tracking and coplanar grouping. In *Conference on Computer Vision and Pattern Recognition* (pp. 226-233).

Freeman, W., & Adelson, E. (1991). The design and use of steerable filters. *Pattern Analysis and Machine Intelligence*, *13*, 891–906. doi:10.1109/34.93808

Harris, C., & Stephens, M. (1988). A combined corner and edge detector. In *Proceedings of the 4th Alvey Vision Conference* (pp. 147-151).

Kadir, T., Zisserman, A., & Brady, M. (2004). An Affine Invariant Salient Region Detector. In *Conference of European Computer Vision* (pp. 228-241).

Ke, Y., & Sukthankar, R. (2004). *PCA-SIFT: A More Distinctive Representation for Local Image Descriptors*. Computer Vision and Pattern Recognition.

Li, F., Fergus, R., & Perona, P. (2004). Learning generative visual models from few training examples: an incremental Bayesian approach tested on 101 object categories. *Computer Vision and Pattern Recognition Workshop on Generative-Model Based Vision*. Retrieved from http://www.vision.caltech.edu/Image_Datasets/Caltech101/Caltech101.html

Lowe, D. G. (2004). Distinctive Image Features from Scale-Invariant Keypoints. *International Journal of Computer Vision, 60*, 91–110. doi:10.1023/B:VISI.0000029664.99615.94

Matas, J., Chum, O., Urba, M., & Pajdla, T. (2002). Robust wide baseline stereo from maximally stable extremal regions. In *Proceedings of British Machine Vision Conference* (pp. 384-396).

Mikolajczyk, M., & Schmid, C. (2004). Scale & Affine Invariant Interest Point Detectors. *International Journal of Computer Vision, 60*, 63–86. doi:10.1023/B:VISI.0000027790.02288.f2

Mind ru, F., Moons, T., & Van Gool, L. (1998). Color-Based Moment Invariants For Viewpoint And Illumination Independent Recognition Of Planar Color Patterns. In *International Conference on Advances in Pattern Recognition* (pp. 113–122).

Moreels, P., & Perona, P. (2004). *Common-Frame Model for Object Recognition*. NIPS.

Moreels, P., & Perona, P. (2005). Evaluation of features detectors and descriptors based on 3D objects. In *IEEE International Conference on Computer Vision* (Vol. 1, pp. 800- 807).

Nilsson, M., Nordberg, J., & Claesson, I. (2007). Face Detection using Local SMQT Features and Split up Snow Classifier. In *IEEE International Conference on Acoustics, Speech and Signal Processing* (Vol. 2, pp. 589-592).

Obdrzalek, S., & Matas, J. (2002). Object recognition using local affine frames on distinguished regions. In *Proceedings of British Machine Vision Conference*.

Philbin, J., Chum, O., Isard, M., Sivic, J., & Zisserman, A. (2007). Object retrieval with large vocabularies and fast spatial matching. In *Proceedings of Computer Vision and Pattern Recognition*.

Schaffalitzky, F., & Zisserman, A. (2002). Automated scene matching in movies. In *Proceedings of the International Conference on Image and Video Retrieval* (pp. 186-197).

Schmid, C., & Moger, R. (1997). Local Grayvalue Invariants for Image Retrieval. *IEEE Transactions on Pattern Analysis and Machine Intelligence, 19*, 530–535. doi:10.1109/34.589215

Shakhnarovich, G., & Moghaddam, B. (2004). *Handbook of Face Recognition*. Berlin: Springer Verlag.

Sivic, J. (2006). *Efficient visual search of images and videos*. Ph.D. Thesis, University of Oxford, Oxford, UK.

Sivic, J., Everingham, M., & Zisserman, A. (2005). Person spotting: video shot retrieval for face sets. In *International Conference on Image and Video Retrieval*.

Sivic, J., Schaffalitzky, F., & Zisserman, A. (2004). Efficient Object Retrieval from Videos. In *Proceedings of the 12th European Signal Processing Conference*.

Sivic, J., & Zisserman, A. (2003). Video Google: A Text Retrieval Approach to Object Matching in Videos. In *Proceedings of the International Conference on Computer Vision*.

Smeulders, M., Santini, S., Gupta, A., & Jain, R. (2000). Content-based image retrieval at the end of early years. *IEEE Transactions on Pattern Analysis and Machine Intelligence, 22*, 1349–1380. doi:10.1109/34.895972

Wiskott, L., Fellous, J., Kruger, N., & Von der Malsburg, C. (1997). Face recognition by elastic bunch graph matching. *IEEE Transactions on Pattern Analysis and Machine Intelligence, 19,* 775–779. doi:10.1109/34.598235

Zhang, G., Huang, X., Li, S., Wang, Y., & Wu, X. (2004). Boosting local binary pattern (lbp)-based face recognition . In *SINOBIOMETRICS*. Berlin: Springer Verlag.

KEY TERMS AND DEFINITIONS

Image Retrieval: An image retrieval system is a computer system for browsing, searching and retrieving images from a large database of digital images.

Face Detection: Face detection is a computer technology that determines the locations and sizes of human faces in arbitrary (digital) images.

SIFT Features: Scale-invariant feature transform (or SIFT) is an algorithm in computer vision to detect and describe local features in images. The algorithm was published by David Lowe in 1999.

Feature Clustering: Cluster analysis or clustering is the assignment of a set of observations into subsets (called clusters) so that observations in the same cluster are similar in some sense. Clustering is a method of unsupervised learning, and a common technique for statistical data analysis used in many fields, including machine learning, data mining, pattern recognition, image analysis and bioinformatics.

ROC Curve: In signal detection theory, a receiver operating characteristic (ROC), or simply ROC curve, is a graphical plot of the sensitivity vs. (1−specificity) for a binary classifier system as its discrimination threshold is varied. The ROC can also be represented equivalently by plotting the fraction of true positives (TPR = true positive rate) vs. the fraction of false positives (FPR = false positive rate). Also known as a Relative Operating Characteristic curve, because it is a comparison of two operating characteristics (TPR & FPR) as the criterion changes.

Recall Rate: Recall is the fraction of the documents that are relevant to the query that are successfully retrieved. In binary classification, recall is called sensitivity. So it can be looked at as the probability that a relevant document is retrieved by the query. It is trivial to achieve recall of 100% by returning all documents in response to any query. Therefore recall alone is not enough but one needs to measure the number of non-relevant documents also, for example by computing the precision.

Precision Rate: Precision is the fraction of the documents retrieved that are relevant to the user's information need. In binary classification, precision is analogous to positive predictive value. Precision takes all retrieved documents into account. It can also be evaluated at a given cut-off rank, considering only the topmost results returned by the system. This measure is called precision at n or P at n.

Section 3
Feature Dimensionality Reduction

Chapter 6
Feature Selection in High Dimension

Sébastien Gadat
Université Paul Sabatier, France

ABSTRACT

Variable selection for classification is a crucial paradigm in image analysis. Indeed, images are generally described by a large amount of features (pixels, edges ...) although it is difficult to obtain a sufficiently large number of samples to draw reliable inference for classifications using the whole number of features. The authors describe in this chapter some simple and effective features selection methods based on filter strategy. They also provide some more sophisticated methods based on margin criterion or stochastic approximation techniques that achieve great performances of classification with a very small proportion of variables. Most of these "wrapper" methods are dedicated to a special case of classifier, except the Optimal features Weighting algorithm (denoted OFW in the sequel) which is a meta-algorithm and works with any classifier. A large part of this chapter will be dedicated to the description of the description of OFW and hybrid OFW algorithms. The authors illustrate also several other methods on practical examples of face detection problems.

INTRODUCTION

High dimensional data Most of nowadays encountered examples of face analysis tasks involve high-dimensional input variables. To detect faces in an image, we usually consider the set of all possible gray-level pixels of the image as informative features. In this case, features are considered as

"low level" features contrary to more sophisticated "high level features" built from linear or non linear combination of the gray-level pixels such as linear filters, edges (mostly coming from some thresholding step), Fourier and Wavelet coefficients, principal components ...

In the case of high level features, the number of variables may thus become very large and can even exceed the number of images. Imagine for instance one thousand samples of images described

DOI: 10.4018/978-1-61520-991-0.ch006

by 60×85 pixels, signals are thus defined by 5100 low-level features and the number of samples become rapidly too small to describe efficiently the data. Consequently, algorithms involving face detection tasks must generally solve some large dimensional problems while a large amount of variables may not be so good to reach accuracy and robustness properties as we will see in the next paragraph.

In this chapter, we focus on the problem of selecting features associated to the detection of "faces" (versus "non-faces") when images are described by high-dimensional signals.

A statistical remark and the curse of dimensionality Let us first discuss in further details why abundance of variables can significantly harm classification in the context of face detection. From a statistical point of view, it is important to remove some irrelevant variables which act as artificial noise in data, especially in the case of images, and limit accuracy of detection tasks.

Moreover, in high dimensional spaces, we face the curse of dimensionality and it is generally impossible to draw some reliable conclusions from databases built with little number of examples regarding some large number of features. This phenomenon has been first pointed by Bellman (1961). Let us describe briefly this statistical property which can be summarized as the exponential growth of hyper-volume as a function of dimensionality. Consider for instance the learning task of face detection. The signal is denoted I while the presence of a face in the signal is Y ($Y = 1$ when a face is present and $Y = 0$ otherwise). A good statistical prediction of Y given I corresponds to a good knowledge of the joint law Y|X. If we called the dimension of the space E_d where I lives, the problem is equivalent to find a correct interpolation of this joint law given a Learning Set of size N when the samples are drawn in the space E_d. As d increases, the number of samples N necessary to build a design of fixed precision increases exponentially. For instance, N = 100 uniformly-spaced sample points suffice to sample a unit interval of dimension one with no more than 0.01 distance between points although an equivalent sampling of a 10-dimensional (d = 10) unit hypercube with a lattice spacing of 0.01 between adjacent points would require N = 10^{20} sample points. Thus, it will be exponentially hardest to approximate the joint law Y|X when d is increasing.

In addition, let us remind the classical Bias/ Variance trade-off (see (Geman, Bienenstock, and Doursat, 1992). If one want to predict Y with a function f applied to signal I using observations in a Learning Set D, the square loss decomposition for the prediction f(X) is given as

$$E_D\left[f(X) - Y\right]^2 = \underbrace{\left[E_D f(X) - Y\right]^2}_{\text{Bias}} + \underbrace{E_D\left[f(X) - E_D f(X)\right]^2}_{\text{Variance}}.$$

(1)

In the former decomposition, the bias is typically a non increasing function of the dimension d while the variance term may drastically increase with d. It is thus necessary to follow a Bias/Variance trade-off to find a good prediction f and a good complexity d. One of the goals of the selection of features is to reduce this phenomenon by restricting the set of features to the "good" ones.

At last, we can notice some efficiency issues, since the speed of many classification algorithms is largely improved when the complexity of the data is reduced. For instance, the complexity of the q-nearest neighbour algorithm varies proportionally with the number of variables. In some cases, the application of classification algorithms like Support Vector Machines described in Vapnik (1998) or q-nearest neighbours on the full features space is not possible or realistic due to the time needed to apply the decision rule.

Knowledge interest from an intellectual point of view, it looks motivating to find the useful features from a large set of variables as this knowledge may be used to improve some pre-processing task. For instance, in the field of bio-informatics and micro-array (Guyon, Weston, Barnhill, and

Vapnik, 2002), it is even more important to locate responsible genes of some pathology than to obtain the best performance of classification of the micro-array.

In the framework of face analysis, variable selection can be applied to detect some areas where are located useful variables. Then, one may think to improve some classification or detection procedures by feeding to classical algorithms good set of variables. Moreover, some image analysis algorithms require placing some landmarks on "mean" faces. Thus, using some selection of features makes also possible to detect the good characteristic points of the shape and thus good location for landmarks.

All these simple remarks show that there exists some strong evidence of the interest of reducing the dimension of the input signal I to infer some reliable conclusions for the response Y.

BACKGROUND AND RELATED WORK

Statistical Considerations

Let us define a precise statistical background for the problem of variable selection. Several i.i.d. realizations of images I are observed in a Learning Set which contains n samples $(I_1,...,I_n)$. Each sample I_i is described by p attributes (e.g. features, variables) which are denoted as $(X^1,...,X^p)$ whereas some labels $(Y_1,...,Y_n)$ are given with the observed signals. The whole dataset D is thus given by $\left\{(I_1,Y_1),...,(I_n,Y_n)\right\}$ and obviously the joint law Y|I is unknown.

We aim to find an optimal subset of the initial features that optimizes the classification task given the dataset D.

For this, we formally call A any classification algorithm which can be used on the Learning Set D with any subset of variables $(X^j)_{j\in w},\, w \subset \left\{1,...p\right\}$. If we call $\subset$ the signal reduced to features in w,

an optimal features selection method would theoretically yield the optimal subset w* which minimizes

$$P(A_D(I^{w^*}) \neq Y). \tag{2}$$

Numerical problems First, one may think of measuring the predictive ability of each feature, in spite of considering interaction between variables. This may not be a good idea in the case of features which are highly correlated and consequently redundant. It may not be relevant too in the case of variables which look poorly effective one by one but could be much more efficient when they are aggregated with some other variables. Consequently, it seems important to look at collaborative selection and explore subsets of variables.

Following the classification task of predicting Y (faces) when I (images) are observed, the main goal is to find a subspace $F \subset E_d$ where the joint law Y|X is easiest to describe than the law in the space E_d. Even if there would exist some empirical criterion to measure the efficiency of the description Y|X, select the optimal F for this criterion will generally be possible only after a whole exploration of subsets of E_d. To optimize any criterion on subspaces, the exhaustive search of optimal subset in E_d requires testing 2^d subsets. Such numerical optimization is un-tractable: for instance, using a face database of 30×30 images and looking for an optimal subset that optimizes an empirical classification error computed in 1 ms would require more than 10^{250} centuries of computation!

Each algorithm of variables selection repeats some iterations: each iteration is referred to one computation for the method. In the sequel, we will look for algorithms of features selection which have a very low number of computation in view of the number of subsets of features. We will then refer to low computational cost methods. For the next detailed algorithms in this section, we will provide this computational cost.

Algorithm 1 General scheme of filter methods

for k = 1 to p **do**
Select variable X^k.
Compute an individual criterion on X^k based on the Learning Set D.
end for
Rank them by decreasing discriminative power according to the criterion computed.

Filtering versus Wrapping There are two main families of features selection for classification in high dimensional space: filters and wrappers methods.

Let us first describe the general scheme of filter methods. Most of filter methods work by measuring individual performances of each variable and sort them by decreasing order. Then, one has to select among them a small number of useful variables according to the former performance. Consequently, filter methods have a very low computation cost since only p (the number of variables) iterations are needed to rank them. The general scheme of filter methods for a set of p variables is as follow.

Moreover, filter methods are robust against over fitting since they do not use any unstable exploration subset technique and generally have a very low variance. However, these methods suffer from theoretical justification about the optimality of the subset ω^* since most of them do not link individual performance of each variable with the classification algorithm A. At last, most of filter methods do not take into account the interactions between variables although it seems important to feed A with no redundant variables.

The second class of features selection algorithms is wrapper methods. In order to obtain a sparse selection of features, these methods measure the efficiency of subsets of variables. They also use different heuristics to penalize the number of features used, or some stochastic search among subsets of variables. These methods consider thus some interactions between variables and can select no redundant features. Moreover, they are theoretically justified and based on a cost functional optimization. But they are prone to over fit the data and are numerically more costly than filter methods. The general scheme of wrapper methods for a set of p variables and a classifier A is as follow.

Finally, the number of computation of filter methods is generally set to p although the computational cost of wrapper methods is k_{max} which is not easily theoretically tractable. Hopefully, this number k_{max} is generally small (but sometimes higher than p) for practical experiments which make wrapper methods competitive. Further considerations are referred to by Guyon and Eliseef (2003) or Blum and Langley (1997).

Assessing numerical performances of features selection methods We measure the performance of the methods using the evolution of the misclassification error rate with the number of selected features. Measuring classification error rate of any pattern detection algorithm A when both train and test set are available is easy. But when only

---

Algorithm 2 General scheme of wrapper methods

Define k_{max} the maximum number of iteration.
for k = 1 to k_{max} **do**
Select a subset of variables w_k.
Compute a criterion based on the Learning Set D, w_k and the classifier A.
Update the set of variables (it may be deletion, addition, weights,...).
end for
Rank variables using decreasing power (it may be deletion, addition, weights,...).

---

one data set D is available, it is not completely obvious and Stone (1974) solved the problem by using some cross-validation technique. In our work, we will avoid these considerations since we will use a learning and test set.

Flexibility of the methods The last important point is the ability of each method to be ran with several classifiers A. Indeed, there does not exist a better classifier A to detect "faces" vs. "non-faces" and it is important to be able to use a features selection method with several different A. It is always possible using filter methods as these methods do not use the classifier A to build the good subset of features, but it is generally impossible with wrapper methods since each one is dedicated to a special case of classifier as pointed in the general scheme above (most of them are concerned with the SVM classifier, see Guyon and Eliseef (2003) for instance).

Filter Methods

For sake of completeness, we recall in this paragraph a list of classical and effective filter methods of features selection for classification. We will illustrate most of these methods on the experimental section.

Fisher Scoring and Signal to Noise (S2N) ratio. As pointed in the last paragraph, each filter method is associated to ranking criterion. The Fisher score ranking can be computed even in the case of multi-class detection problem. Assume each Y_i to belong to $\{1, ..., c\}$ where c is the number of classes and define n_i the number of samples of the Learning Set in class i. Let μ_i^j and $\left\{\sigma_i^j\right\}^2$ the mean and variance of the variable X^j in the class i while μ^j and $\left\{\sigma^j\right\}^2$ are mean and variance of variable X^j in the whole Learning Set. We then denote

$$F_j = \frac{\sum_{i=1}^{c} n_i (\mu_i^j - \mu^j)^2}{\sum_{i=1}^{c} n_i \left\{\sigma_i^j\right\}^2}. \tag{3}$$

Fisher score corresponds to the ratio of between-class variance divided by the within-class variance. This criterion is very popular and numerically simple to compute. In the two-class case (Y is equal to 0 or 1), F_j is simply reduced to

$$F_j = \frac{\left(\mu_0^j - \mu_1^j\right)^2}{n_0 / n \left\{\sigma_0^j\right\}^2 + n_1 / n \left\{\sigma_1^j\right\}^2}. \tag{4}$$

The Fisher score corresponds indeed to the variance comparison test used by statisticians. The S2N filter method is largely inspired from the last Fisher score and can be applied in the two-class case. The S2N is computed for each variable as

$$S2Nj = \frac{|\mu_0^j - \mu_1^j|}{\sigma_0^j + \sigma_1^j}. \tag{5}$$

The T-test ranking is based on the comparison of two samples using a Student statistic.

Relief and weighted features selection algorithms Relief is a variable selection method introduced in Kira and Rendell (1992) and is very effective for assessing variable performance. It belongs to the large class of methods which are trying to maximize margins between each class for each feature. The algorithm defines iteratively a weight over the p features during T iterations. The principle of the method is to quantify the importance of the variables in the weights distribution. Useful features will have large positive weights although bad features will obtain small negative weights. Initial weights w are set to 0 and the several steps are as follow. In the sequel, we denote s^j the amplitude of each variable j.

Algorithm 3 Relief features Selection (Kira and Rendell, 1992)

for t = 1 to T do
Select following a uniform law one sample (I_n, Y_n) among D.
Call the nearest hit (resp. miss) in the same (resp. opposite) class $NH(I_n)$ (resp. $NM(I_n)$).
for j = 1 to p do

$$w^i = w^j + \frac{\left|I_n^j - NM(I_n)^j\right|}{T_{S^j}} - \frac{\left|I_n^j - NH(I_n)^j\right|}{T_{S^j}} \quad \text{end for}$$

end for

Sun (2007) has shown the link between the original iterative Relief algorithm and an optimal margin condition. Define $\rho_n(w)$ as:

$$\rho_n(w) = \sum_{j=1}^{p} w_j \left(\frac{\left|I_n^j - NM(I_n)^j\right|}{S^j} - \frac{\left|I_n^j - NH(I_n)^j\right|}{S^j} \right), \tag{6}$$

then the optimal weight w solves the optimization problem:

$$w^* = \arg_{w\|w\|_2 = 1, w \geq 0} \max \sum_{n=1}^{N} \rho_n(w). \tag{7}$$

Relief is robust and Kononenko (1994) extended to the multi-class case but it has no mechanism to eliminate redundant features.

In this chapter, we will omit some classical approaches such as Principal Component Analysis (PCA) (some details can be found in the book of Jolliffe (2002)) or Independent Component Analysis (see Jutten and Herault (1991) for instance) since these approaches does not provide some selection of variables among the initial set of features. Indeed, these approaches are dimensionality reduction technique and provide some new representations of the images using some linear transformation of the initial set of features but new variables are linear combinations of all the original variables. To avoid this important

disadvantage, Zhou, Hastie, and Tibshirani (2006) used some sparse criterion. It yields the Sparse Principal Component Analysis based ℓ^1 penalty.

Wrapper Methods

In the recent years, some more sophisticated wrapper approaches have been developed for features selection. Most of them are based on some margin criterion to measure the accuracy of subsets of features.

Sparse representations and features selection We start this paragraph with a short description of some classical considerations related to sparse solutions of some constrained optimization problems. This method is dedicated to features selection with some SVM classification algorithm. Let us briefly describe first the algorithm of SVM (Vapnik, 1998). The SVM procedure aims to solve the following problem:

$$\min_{w,b} \left\{ \|w\|_2^2 + C \sum_{i-1}^{n} \xi_i \; |Y_i(wI_i + b) \geq 1 - \xi_i, \xi_i \geq 0 \right\} \tag{8}$$

where $w \in \mathbb{R}^p$ is the normal vector of the SVM, b is the intercept (additional constant) of the model, and ξ_i are margin parameters to ensure solvability of the optimization problem. The classification algorithm then produces the rule based on

$$\text{sign}(wI + b) \in \{+1; -1\}. \tag{9}$$

This problem is solved using the Karush-Kuhn-Tucker conditions for constrained optimization problems. Indeed, this optimization does not yield some variable selection algorithm. But large improvements can be done considering some other norm on the vector w as pointed by Elisseef, Weston, and Schölkopf (2003). Some ideal optimization problem would be

$$\min_{w,b} \left\{ \|w\|_0 + C \sum_{i=1}^{n} \xi_i \mid Y_i(wI_i + b) \geq 1 - \xi_i, \xi_i \geq 0 \right\}, \tag{10}$$

where $|w|_0$ denotes the number of components of w which does not vanish. The idea is to find a linear separation which has an important number of vanishing w and well separates the two classes due to the minimisation of the $\sum \xi_i$. The function of the (ξ_i) is to enable an imperfect separation on the Learning Set (when $\xi_i > 1$) in view to obtain some more vanishing w. This last optimization step would produce some sparse representation of w (lots of w_i are 0). This produces a features selection algorithm since only variable X^j such that $w_j \neq 0$ are used for prediction. Unfortunately, Amaldi and Kann (1998) have shown that solving some l_0 type problems is NP-Hard and a statistical approximation idea is to replace $|w|_0$ by $|w|_p^p$ where the parameter $p \to 0$. A very special case of this idea is used in the Lasso approach for linear models (Tibshirani, 1996) and more recently by Candes and Tao (2005) with the Dantzig selector.

Finally, Elisseef, Weston and Schölkopf(2003) proposed to solve the following optimization problem:

$$\min_{w} \left\{ \|w\|_p^p \mid Y_i(wI_i + b) \geq 1, \|w\|_0 \leq r \right\} \tag{11}$$

for $p = 1$. This approach appears to be competitive with some state of the art results on several databases. We will illustrate this method in the experimental section, and will refer to this method as L0-SVM. Note also that Wright, Yang, Ganesh, Shankar Sastry and Ma (2009) have used the ℓ^1 penalty to yield sparse selection on face image analysis.

Recursive features Elimination Guyon, Weston, Barnhill and Vapnik (2002) introduced the RFE as a new algorithm of variables selection dedicated to the optimization of a features subset for the SVM classification. The RFE method hierarchically constructs a sequence of subsets $F_k \subset F_{k-1} \subset ... \subset F_1 = \{X^1, ..., X^p\}$. Each iteration k of the algorithm produces elimination following a backward elimination scheme. Using Elisseef, Weston and Schölkopf (2003) notation for the dual variables $(\alpha_i)_i$ of the SVM optimization problem, one can show that

$$W^2(\alpha) = \sum_{i,j} \alpha_i \alpha_j Y_i Y_j K(I_i, I_j) \tag{12}$$

where K is the kernel used for the SVM. Moreover, $W^2(\alpha)$ is a measure of predictive ability of each SVM and is inversely proportional to the margin of the separation in the Learning Set. Thus, $W^2(\alpha)$ is small when the margin of the SVM is large and its prediction reliable.

If we denote $W^2(\alpha)_j$ the vector given by dual variables α while features X^j is removed from the Learning Set. If we denote q the number of variables to select, the RFE algorithm can be summarized as follow:

Note that when the kernel used in the SVM is linear, this algorithm is equivalent to remove the smallest corresponding value of $|w_i|$ in the original SVM optimization problem.

Indeed, all these methods try to optimize the generalization ability of any classification algorithm while maximizing the margin between the two classes of the Learning Set.

Algorithm 4 Recursive features Elimination [GE03]

$F_1 = \{X^1, \dots X^p\}$
$R = p$
While $r > q$ do
Compute the optimal SVM with features of F_{p-r+1} and $W^2(\alpha)$.
Compute for each remaining features X^j the accuracy index $W^2_{-j}(\alpha)$
Remove the remaining features X^j with smallest value $W^2(\alpha) - W^2_{-j}(\alpha)$.
$r = r-1$
end while

Features selection using Random Forest. The Random Forest (RF) algorithm of Breiman (2001) is an improvement of the classical Classification and Regression Tree (CART) method introduced by Breiman, Friedman, Stone and Olshen (1984) and belongs to the class of aggregation methods. Older ideas of Amit and Geman (1997) and Ho (1998) have inspired the RF randomization on variables. Its aim is to generate lots of elementary un-pruned trees of classification using a randomization step on variables. More precisely, each tree is built using a uniform random sampling step: for each node of each tree, randomly choose m (around $\sqrt{p}$) variables on which to base the decision at that node and compute the best split.

Some features selection algorithm can be added at the end of the RF algorithm. One natural criterion on the usefulness of variables for the classification is then the number of time each features has been used in the Random Forest.

Iterative algorithms Some feature selection method based on the Boosting idea of Friedman, Hastie, and Tibshirani (2000) has been developed based in the work of Xiao, Li, Tian and Tang (2006). The Boosting recursively builds some weak classifiers which are aggregate to obtain the final decision rule. The main idea is to compute successively some classifiers dedicated to learn some hard situations using some weighting techniques among the samples of the dataset. This approach yields some robust classification based on few classifiers (selected features) which has been built for the aggregation.

Other methods based on the Genetic Algorithm idea have been developed recently. These algorithms are based on some stochastic evolutions of a population of features. This is for instance the case of the works of Sun and Lijun (2007), van Dijck, van Hulle, and Wevers (2004) or Gadat (2008).

STOCHASTIC ALGORITHM FOR WEIGHTING VARIABLES (OFW)

In this section, we present a recent wrapper algorithm derived from the works of Gadat and Younes (2007) and Gadat (2008).

Optimal Features Weighting

Notations: OFW is an optimization algorithm which minimizes a classification error rate. For this, let us note any classification algorithm A, which can be run given any database D and any subset of features $w \subset \{1, \dots, p\}$. It provides different classifiers A_w for each choice w and OFW is dedicated to the optimization of the subset used to feed A. We will denote e the error rate $e(w) = P(A_w(X) \neq Y)$. To estimate this last error, we will use the following strategy: extract uniformly with replacement two subsets T_1 and T_2 in D and define $e(w, T_1, T_2) = P_{T_2}(A_{w, T_1}(X) \neq Y)$. This last expression denotes the empirical error on T_2 of the classifier learnt with features w and samples T_1, e is then estimated as:

$$e(w) \simeq E_{T1, T2}[\hat{e}(w, T_1, T_2)] := q(w). \tag{13}$$

Cost Functional: To select a group of relevant variables, one can think first about a hard selection method:

$$q(w^*) = \arg\min_{w \subset F} q(w).$$ (14)

Unfortunately, as pointed by Amaldi and Kann (1998), this is numerically un-tractable and we will address a soft selection procedure. Consider P a probability distribution over the features space $F = (X^1, ..., X^p)$ as in Relief. Any w of size q will be sampled with respect to $P^{\otimes q}$. Our goal is to minimize ε defined as

$$\varepsilon(P) = E_{w \sim P^{\otimes q}} \big[q(w) \big]$$ (15)

with respect to the selection parameter P. If P* is optimal, it is likely to find useful variables when $P^*(X^j)$ is large. Thus, the idea is similar to the RELIEF one: give important weights for useful features and very small positive weights for the bad ones.

Constrained optimization: We provide here a stochastic algorithm that minimizes (15). Denote S_F the simplex of probability measures on F.

$$S_F := \left\{ P \mid \left[\sum_{j=1}^{p} P\left(X^j\right) = 1 \atop \forall j \in \{1...p\} P(X^j) \geq 0 \right] \right\}$$ (16)

and the affine projection on S_F is not reduced to the Euclidian projection on the supporting hyperplane of the simplex. We refer to the paper of Gadat and Younes (2007) for the computation of this projection. Denote π_{S_F} the standard projection on the hyper-plane. A natural idea is to use:

$$\frac{dP_t}{dt} = -\pi_{S_F}\left(\nabla\varepsilon(P_t)\right)$$ (17)

and a discretized version of (17) is

$$P_{n+1} = P_n - \alpha_n \pi_{H_F}\left(\nabla\varepsilon(P_n)\right).$$ (18)

This equation can be implemented provided $P_n \in S_F$ but the positivism constraints of equations (16) are not guaranteed by (18). To impose positivism constraints, we use a constrained process

$$\frac{dP_t}{dt} = -\pi_{S_F}\left(\nabla\varepsilon(P_t)\right) = -\pi_{H_F}\left(\nabla\varepsilon(P_t)\right) + dZ_t$$ (19)

In view of (19), dZ_t is a stochastic process which accounts for the jumps appearing when a re-projection is needed on S_F. In other words, $d|Z|_t$ is positive if and only if P_t hits the boundary ∂S_F of our simplex.

Stochastic optimization within the Robbins-Monro case: Denote $C(w,X^j)$ the number of occurrences of X^j in w:

$$C(w, X^j) = |\{i \in \{1,...k\} \mid w_i = X^j\}|.$$ (20)

Proposition 1. If P is any point of S_F, then

$$\forall X^j \in F \quad \nabla_P \varepsilon\left(X^j\right) = \sum_{w \in F^k} \frac{C(w, X^j) P^{\otimes k}(w)}{P\left(X^j\right)} q(w).$$ (21)

This computation is also un-tractable as it is necessary to cover all subsets $w \in F^k$. We next design a stochastic algorithm which simulates an approximation of (19). Duflo (1996) and Benaïm (2000) stated that stochastic approximations can be seen as noisy discretization of deterministic ODE's. They are expressed under the form

$$X_{n+1} = X_n + \varepsilon_n F(X_n, \xi_{n+1}) + \alpha_n^2 \eta_n \qquad (22)$$

where X_n is the current state of the process, ξ_{n+1} a random perturbation, and η_n a secondary error term. If the distribution of ξ_{n+1} only depends on the current value of X_n (Robbins-Monro case), then one defines an average drift $X \rightarrow G(X)$ by

$$dX_t = G(X_t) \qquad (23)$$

and the Equation (22) can be shown to evolve similarly to the ODE $dX_t = G(X_t)$. From proposition 1, we remark that

$$\nabla_P \varepsilon(X^j) = E_{w \sim P^{\otimes k}} \left[\frac{C(w, X^j) q(w)}{P(X^j)} \right]. \qquad (23)$$

Then, given any step n, it is natural to define the approximation term of the gradient descent (19) by:

$$d_n = \pi_{H_F} \left(\frac{C(w_n, \cdot) \hat{e}(w_n, T_1^n, T_2^n)}{P_n(\cdot)} \right) \qquad (24)$$

where w_n is a random variable extracted from F with law $P_n^{\otimes k}$ and T_1, T_2 are independently sampled into the Learning Set D. Following the definition of d_n and the generic notations introduced in equation (22), we obtain

$$E_{\xi_{n+1}} \left[F(X_n, \xi_{n+1}) \right] = E_{w_n, T_1^n, T_2^n} \left[d_n(\omega_n, T_1^n, T_2^n) \right]$$
$$= E_{w_n, T_1^n, T_2^n} \left[\pi_{H_F} \left(\frac{C(w_n, \cdot) \hat{e}(w_n, T_1^n, T_2^n)}{P_n(\cdot)} \right) \right]$$
$$= E_{w_n} \left[\pi_{H_F} \left(\frac{C(w_n, \cdot) E_{T_1^n, T_2^n} \left[\hat{e}(w_n, T_1^n, T_2^n) \right]}{P_n(\cdot)} \right) \right]$$
$$= E_{w_n} \left[\pi_{H_F} \left(\frac{C(w_n, \cdot) q(w_n)}{P_n(\cdot)} \right) \right]$$
$$= E_{w_n} \left[F(P_n, w_n) \right] = \pi_{H_F} \left(\nabla \varepsilon(P_n) \right).$$
$$(25)$$

Thus, the mean effect of (25) is equivalent to (22) and the final algorithm follows the iterative scheme:

Convergence of OFW

Theorem 1 stands for the convergence of the algorithm.

Theorem 1. Let α_n chosen such that $\sum \alpha_n = \infty$ and $\sum \alpha_n^2 < \infty$, then (P_n) *converges to a trajectory given by equation* (19).

In our simulation, we will use a Harmonic-like sequence $\alpha_n = C_1 / (C_2 + n)$ with a suitable choice of C_1 and C_2 ($C_1 = C_2 = 1000$ in order to have a very slow decreasing sequence α_n). Theorem 1 ensures the convergence of the OFW stochastic algorithm towards the differential flow (19). Thus this differential flow and OFW both converge to arg min ε.

Comments on the original OFW algorithm

Convergence speed of OFW As described precisely in Theorem 2.2.12 of Duflo (1996), denoting P^* the limit of P_n, OFW satisfies in the usual cases (when the energy ε does not have any degenerated minimum on P^*) the following convergence

---

Algorithm 5 Optimal features Weighting algorithm [GY07]

$F = \{X^1, \ldots X^p\}$

$n = 0$ and $P_0 = U_F$ (uniform law over F).

while $\left\| P_{n-\lfloor n/\mu \rfloor} - P_n \right\| > \varepsilon$ **do**

Extract w_n from F^* with respect to P_n^k.

Extract T_1^n and T_2^n of size T with uniform independent samples over D.

Compute $\hat{e}(w_n, T_1^n, T_2^n)$ and the drift vector d_n given by equation (25).

Define

$$P_{n+1} = \pi_{S_F} \left[P_n - \alpha_n d_n \right] \text{ end while}$$

$$\sqrt{n} \left(P_n - P^* \right) \to N(0, \sum{}^2). \qquad (26)$$

The classical convergence rate $n^{1/2}$ may be optimistic in some rare cases depending on the energy ε in the neighbourhood of P^*, and this rate can fall to $\sqrt{\log n / n}$ or even n^τ with $\tau < 1/2$. Duflo (1996) provides further details about the different rate of convergence. The OFW algorithm is much faster than an exhaustive search between subsets and slower than a classical filter selection approach. It takes for instance around 30 minutes of learning on a standard 2 Ghz PC with a data-set of several hundred images described by 2000 gray-level pixels.

Advantages From a theoretical point of view, OFW is satisfying since it really solves a minimization problem related to the problem of variable selection.

Moreover, OFW considers interactions between features since each $P(X^j)$ is based on the ability of X^j to predict efficiently Y with other features among F.

At last, OFW is not dedicated to a special case of classification algorithm such as SVM or CART for instance. It may be applied to several A and this flexibility characteristic is useful. Indeed, there does not exist a better classifier A among all classification algorithms, thus it is of major importance to be able to optimize the features selection depending on the classifier A which performs the best on a given database. Lê Cao, Gonçalves, Gadat, and Besse (2007) successfully applied OFW in Bio-Informatics with CART. To the best of our knowledge, this is not the case for other methods of features selection.

Some theoretical and practical issues concerning OFW can be studied. Statistically, there does not exist mathematical clue about the amount of over-fitting with OFW. More precisely, recall that $e(w) = P(A_w(I) \neq Y)$ and denote P^0 the Oracle distribution which minimizes the energy

$$\varepsilon^{\circ}(P) = E_w \left[\varepsilon(w) \right]. \qquad (27)$$

OFW yields P^* and solves the optimization problem

$$\varepsilon^D(P) = E_w \left[q(w) \right], \qquad (28)$$

where $q(w) = P_D(A_w(I) \neq Y)$ (the probability of error using A_w and samples D). To derive the statistical stability of OFW, it is important to control the deviation $| P^* - P^0 |$ as the number of samples in D increases.

Another clue would be to study the convergence rate and to implement some stochastic schemes to improve the speed of OFW. This may be done using classical averaging method on stochastic algorithms as pointed in Duflo (1996) or with a modification of the original O.D.E. considering the approach of Cabot, Engler and Gadat (2009).

From a practical point of view, one can think about an integration of a hybrid process to compose features all along the learning process.

Hybrid OFW for Binary Features

We present here a dynamical model for a population of features which is an improvement of OFW. From a pre-processed initialization of a set of variables, a stochastic algorithm recursively builds and improves the set of variable. This algorithm simulates again a Markov chain which estimates a probability distribution P on the set of features. The features are structured as binary trees and we show that such forests are a good way to represent the evolution of the features set.

Tree Structure of Features for Hybrid OFW and Cost Functional

Tree structured features. Let F_0 be the initial set of features constructed from the original set of variables $\{X_1, ..., X_p\}$ which are binary valued. F_t will be the set of features at time t. For several reasons given in next paragraphs, we will structure features following a structure of binary trees. For an elementary features X^j, we associate the elementary tree (and keep the same notation X^j):

$$X^j := X^j.$$
$$\diagup \diagdown$$
$$\varnothing \quad \varnothing$$

Now, a tree features A follow the recursive structure of binary tree: each node contains a composition of elementary features, and terminal nodes (leaves) are elementary features of F_0. Moreover, each non-terminal node in A must be the concatenation of its descendants so that one can easily infer how any tree has been formed. The root of A, denoted r(A), is the upper node of A. Tree features A, B are aggregated with the construction rule "::"

$$\mathcal{A} :: \mathcal{B} = \quad r(\mathcal{A}) \cup r(\mathcal{B}).$$
$$\diagup \diagdown$$
$$\mathcal{A} \quad \mathcal{B}$$

The computation of any tree A with upper node $r(A) = \left\{ X^{i_1}, ..., X^{i_q} \right\}$ on I will be

$$A(I) = X^{i_1}(I) \times ... \times X^{i_q}(I). \tag{29}$$

Remark 1. As the computation $r(I)$ does not use the tree structure, one may wonder why we use this complicated tree representation. Indeed, it will be useful in our evolutionary algorithm to modify F_t with this tree representation and not with a simple structure of list. For instance, consider T the aggregation of two trees:

$$T = \{X^1; X^2; X^3\}$$
$$\diagup \diagdown$$
$$\{X^1; X^2\} \quad \{X^3\}$$

Without any tree structure, it is impossible to decide whether if $\{X^1, X^2, X^3\}$ as been created with the aggregation of $\{X^1, X^2\}$ and X^3 or $\{X^1, X^3\}$ and $X^2 X^2$ or $\{X^2, X^3\}$ and X^1. Using our representation, it is easy to recover the hierarchical process used to build T. This will have a theoretical importance in the sequel.

Global energy Following the initial OFW, we weight each tree A of any forest F with a probability P. This enables us to define the energy cost ε_{err}:

$$\varepsilon_{err}\left(P,F\right) = E_w\left[q\left(w\right)\right]. \qquad (30)$$

Define $I(A.l, A.r)$ as the empirical mutual information function between the sons of A. The structural functional over any forest F is given by:

$$\varepsilon_{struct}\left(F\right) = \underbrace{\sum_{A\in F}|A|}_{\varepsilon_s^1(F)} + \underbrace{\sum_{A\in F} I(A.l, A.r)}_{\varepsilon_s^2(F)}. \qquad (31)$$

First term limits the size of the following the Rissanen (1983) principle although the second term favours the concatenation of correlated trees as in the work of Fleuret and Geman (2001). Our goal is to minimize $\varepsilon_s(F) + \varepsilon_{err}(F) = \varepsilon$ over the space of forests and probability on forests. We will denote (P_t, F_t) the continuous process associated to our hybrid algorithm. Note that for any time t ≥ 0, P_t is a probability over trees in F_t.

Exploring Forests with Reversible Jumps

Operations on trees We describe first the transitions to be applied to F_t. Forests evolve following three simple rules: aggregating two trees, cutting or reviving one tree. These transitions are precisely described in the paper of Gadat (2008). For instance, the following aggregation is an acceptable transition:

$$X^1X^2 \; :: \; X^1X^3 = X^1X^2X^3 \; :=A.$$

$$
\underbrace{X^1 \quad X^2}_{A1} \quad \underbrace{X^1 \quad X^3}_{Ar} \quad X^1X^2 \quad X^1X^3
$$

$$X^1 \quad X^2 X^1 \quad X^3$$

Note that we can reform left and right sons (A.r and A.l) from A cutting his main node. It is manifest that without this tree structure, from the equivalent composition

$$\underbrace{X^1X^2}_{B.l} \; :: \; \underbrace{X^1X^3}_{B.r} = X^1X^2X^3 := B$$

We could not obtain antecedents of B. This remark shows the usefulness of trees for the weak reversibility of the whole process.

Jump process: The jump process corresponds to the modifications performed at time t on F_t. It enables the dynamical system to explore the space of features according to Metropolis-Hastings strategy. The time differences between jumps are assumed to be mutually independent, and independent from the rest of the process. Jumps occur as a Poisson process (inter-jump times are i.i.d. exponential). Coupled with a constrained stochastic differential equation on P_t, this allows the inference algorithm to visit the set of possible states and is suitable regarding the discrete nature of the problem. At jump times, the transitions $F_t \rightarrow F_{t+dt}$ will correspond to the operations described above. Each of these rules will be designed using an accept/reject scheme as follows. Denote (P_t,F_t) the current state.

1   Choose one operation randomly among birth, aggregate or cut and trees to apply the chosen operation.
2   The way we propose our transitions from (P,F) define a probability among all the reachable state which is denote $Q((P,F),.)$.

Accept the transition according to the probability:

$$Q\left[\binom{P}{F};\binom{\tilde{P}}{\tilde{F}}\right] = \min\left(1; \frac{Q_0\left[(P,F);(\tilde{P},\tilde{F})\right]}{Q_0\left[(\tilde{P},\tilde{F});(P,F)\right]} e^{\varepsilon}\left(\tilde{P},\tilde{F}\right) - \varepsilon\left(P,F\right)\right).$$

(32)

Gadat (2008) has provided the precise settings for distribution Q_0 and evolution (P_t,F_t) to (P_{t+dt},F_{t+dt}). The important fact for the jump process is its ergodic nature described by the following proposition.

Proposition 2. (Reversibility of the jumps) The dynamic of (P_t,F_t) induced by operations on forests is reversible.

It is important here to underline why the building process of (P_t,F_t) must be reversible.

- From its stochastic nature, the process may be mistaken for an iteration because of the Metropolis-Hastings strategy. We may need to cancel each decision easily.

- Furthermore, the acceptation rate computation (32) involves the ratio $Q_0(x, y)/Q_0(y, x)$. If the features are not structured as tree, one cannot compute equation (32) since from any set of variables x, the unique pair of its antecedents is unknown.

Coupled Stochastic Process

Between two jumping times s_j, s_{j+1}, F_t is constant and P_t evolves following a constrained diffusion with a drift given by

$$Q\left[\binom{P}{F};\binom{\tilde{P}}{\tilde{F}}\right] = \min\left(1; \frac{Q_0\left[(P,F);(\tilde{P},\tilde{F})\right]}{Q_0\left[(\tilde{P},\tilde{F});(P,F)\right]} e^{\varepsilon}\left(\tilde{P},\tilde{F}\right) - \varepsilon\left(P,F\right)\right).$$

. This evolution is just a noisy equation based on equation (19):

$$\nabla \varepsilon_{err}$$

(33)

In (32), W_t is a Brownian motion and σ_t is a covariance matrix used to project W_t in $_t dP_t = -\nabla \varepsilon_{err}\left(P_t\right) dt + \sigma_{F_t} dW_t + dZ_t$. At last dZ_t is the projection term described in equation (19). The exact construction of solutions to equations (33) relies on each Skorokhod Map defined for each simplex explored by P_t. Further details can be found in the papers of Gadat (2008), Dupuis and Ishii (1991) or Dupuis and Ramanan (1999). We can then ensure the global existence and uniqueness of the coupled process. Denote Φ the stationary solution of the reflected jump diffusion based on (couples equations (32) and (33)), we have:

Theorem 2. (Stationary solution Φ) Let (Ω, T, Q) a probability space with an increasing filtration $(T_t)_t$, let $(W_t)_{t \geq 0}$ a standard Brownian motion and $(N_t)_{t \geq 0}$ a Poisson jump process, adapted and independent. There exists a unique stationary solution called $\Phi = (P,F)$ of:

$$H_{F_t}$$

(34)

Stochastic Approximation and Hybrid OFW

The computation of

$$d\binom{P_t}{F_t} = -\binom{\nabla^{F_t}\varepsilon(P_t)dt + \sum^{F_t} dW_t + dZ_t}{0} + \int_{F,P} Q\left[\binom{P_t}{F_t};\binom{P}{F}\right] N\left(d\binom{P}{F};dt\right).$$

$_t$ is still un-tractable. However, it is yet possible to design a stochastic algorithm which approximates the behaviour of solution given by Theorem 2. We provide a pseudo-code which describes the hybrid-OFW. Jumps are distributed with a Poisson process $P(\lambda)$. Recall here that the conversion between iterations n and time t is given by

$$\nabla \varepsilon_{err}$$

(35)

Algorithm 6 Hybrid Optimal features Weighting algorithm [Gad08]

F_0 is defined using initial elementary trees built with $\{X^1,...X^p\}$.

n=0 and $P_0 = t_n = \sum_{i=0}^{n} \alpha_i$.

Define $S_O=0$ the initialization of the jumping times.

for $j=1 ...\infty$ **do**

Define S_j as the first time of jump after S_{j-1} using $S_j - S_{j-1} \sim exp(\lambda)$.

while $t_n \leq S_j$ **do**

Extract w_n from U_{F_O} with respect to $F_{l_n}^k$.

Extract P_n^k and T_1^n of size T with uniform independent samples over D.

Compute $\hat{e}(w_n, T_2^n, T_1^n)$ and the drift vector d_n given by equation (25).

Compute a Gaussian increment on T_2^n denoted S_{F_n}.

Define

$d\xi_n$ $n{\rightarrow}n+1$

end while

Modify $P_{n+1} = \pi_{S_{F_{l_n}}} \left[P_n - \alpha_n d_n + \sqrt{\alpha_n} d\xi_n \right]$ and P_n according the transition described in equation (32).

end for

Gadat (2008) has provided a proof assuming $\sum \alpha_i = \infty$ and $\sum \alpha_i^2 < \infty$.

EXPERIMENTS AND CONCLUSION

Dataset Description and Objectives

We have designed two sequences of experiments for the problem of selecting variables for the detection of "face" versus "non-face".

- We use first the AT&T ORL (Olivetti) database composed of 400 samples of 92 × 112 faces with 256 grey levels per pixel. Our features are the Sobel vertical and horizontal edge detectors, this yields a dimension of 20608. As no test set is available, we split the data in two parts. We use for non faces samples of images of the same size taken on the Web. Some samples extracted from the database are shown in Figure 1.

- We use also the MIT-CBCL database that contains face images of 19 × 19 pixels. These images are described with the binary edge detectors of Fleuret and Geman (2001). We then obtain 1926 binary features defined by their orientation, vagueness and position. The database provides both learning and test set, each one described with face and non face images. Some samples extracted from the database are shown in Figure 2.

The datasets are summarized in the Table 1.

We use a linear SVM (polynomial with degree 1) and a shrinkage parameter tuned using a cross validation step. At last, we compare the performance of filter methods (Fisher and Relief) and wrapper methods (OFW, RFE, L0-SVM, RF) on the two databases. As hybrid OFW requires a large time of computation, we only use it on the MIT-CBCL database since there are fewer variables than in the AT&T database.

Figure 1. Samples of images taken from the ORL database

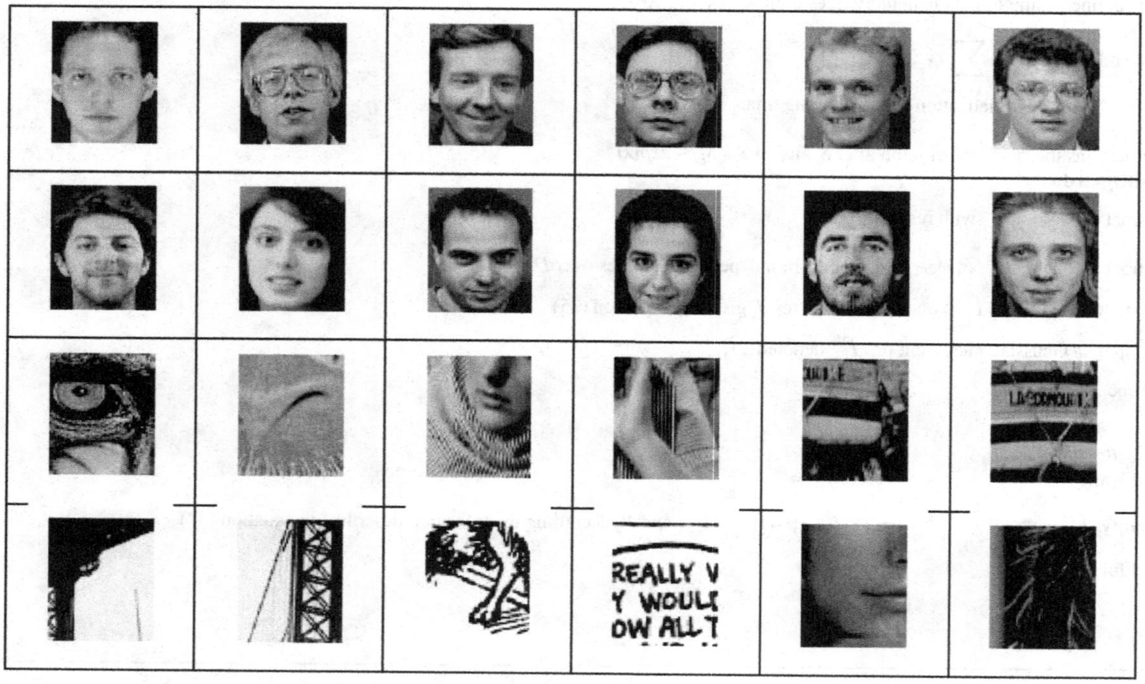

Our objective is to describe the results of several algorithms of features selection according to the misclassification error rate with respect to the number of features selected. We are also interested in the features selected by the several algorithms.

For the two datasets, the experimental protocol is to use each time the whole Learning Set and to select for each integer n from 1 to 1000 (5000 for the ORL database) the n most important features. Then, we compute with these n variables the associated classifier A on the Learning Set and at

last the misclassification error rate of the classifier A on the test set.

Misclassification Error Rate for ORL and MIT-CBCL Databases

No selection Without any selection, A is excellent on the ORL database since the misclassification rate is under 1% but this performance is obtained with almost 20000 features. On the MIT-CBCL database, without any selection, A performs well as it makes only 2.3% error using 1926 features.

Table 1. General description of the experimental setup

Dataset	AT&T ORL (Olivetti)	MIT-CBCL
Dimension of Images	92 x 112	19 x 19
Number of Features	20608	1926
Nature of Features	Sobel Filters	Binary edges (0/1)
Number of Images (Learning Set)	200 faces / 200 non-faces	2429 faces / 4548 non-faces
Number of Images (Test Set)	200 faces / 200 non-faces	472 faces / 23573 non-faces

Figure 2. Samples of images taken from the MIT database

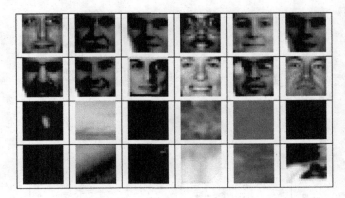

The Figures 3 and 4 show the evolution of the classification error rate with respect to the number of features for some of the algorithms previously described in the paragraphs above for the ORL and MIT-CBCL database.

Performance of filter and wrapper methods On the ORL dataset, the Fisher score obtains average results comparing to those of RFE (for instance less than 10% error rate for 500 variables) as pointed by the Figure 2 whereas the Relief method performs bad. On the MIT-CBCL dataset, the Fisher rule performs poorly (10% of misclassification when wrapper methods obtain less than 5% of misclassification), the Relief method is here much better (results corresponding to average results of wrapper methods).

Wrapper methods perform better here and results provided by RFE, L0-SVM, Random Forests or OFW are similar on the MIT database. On the ORL database, RFE looks better than other methods except for the first hundred features selected.

- A first concluding remark is that wrapper methods, even if they are numerically more costly than the filter methods, get better results of classification. This is explained here by the fact that wrapper methods optimise some theoretical criterion based on

Figure 3. Efficiency of several features extractions methods for the ORL database

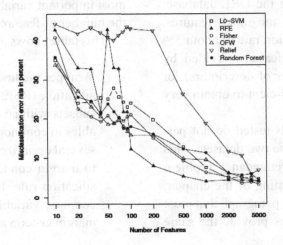

Figure 4. Efficiency of several features extractions methods for the MIT-CBCL database

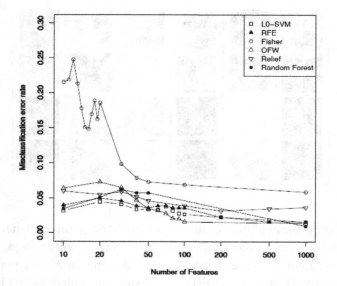

some classification error rate on these datasets and avoid the over fitting phenomenon here. Among the wrapper methods, it is hard to exhibit a "top" method since most of them obtain similar results. This will be explained in the next paragraph regarding the selected subsets of variables.

- Regarding now the evolution of the misclassification error rate with the number of selected features, we remark that the efficiency of wrapper methods is stationary after 100 variables on the MIT database, and after 1000 features on the ORL database: it is useless to select too much features. Moreover, a compression rate of about 5% (number of selected features divided by the initial total number of descriptors) for the two datasets is sufficient to obtain very good detection results.

- The two filter methods tested do not perform very well on these two datasets. This is mainly due to the redundancy problem exhibited in the beginning of the chapter. We will see in the next paragraph that most of the selected features provide the same information to the classifier A. This redundancy may be due to the dataset itself, or to the nature of the features handled (Edges indicator), it would require further investigations to analyse the relation between edges and statistical redundancy but it is far beyond the scope of this chapter.

Comparison of Selected Subsets and Localization of Features

Among the 100 first selected features (thus the 100 most important variables), we display in Table 2 the number of features shared by each methods.

This table shows at last two important points:

- Wrapper methods based on the SVM classification (RFE, OFW, L0) aims to select subsets with an important number of variables in common. This fact is related to the several optimized criteria which are related to margin conditions of some SVM classification rule. It is thus quite logical that common variables are chosen even if the margin criteria are not exactly the same.

Table 2. Number of selected features shared by the several used methods over 100 most important variables

MIT-CBCL database ORL database	OFW+SVM	RFE	L0-SVM	RF	Fisher	Relief
OFW+SVM	#	55	45	10	12	8
RFE	65	#	40	18	20	10
L0-SVM	46	52	#	23	22	12
RF	17	18	11	#	48	15
Fisher	3	6	8	65	#	38
Relief	3	6	7	12	32	#

- Random Forest and the Fisher selection share an important number of selected variables. CART searches in the features space the best variable and the best split to divide each node. The Table 2 shows that most variables chosen by CART have an important Fisher score. This common number is equal to 65 for the ORL database and it explains why the Fisher rule is not so bad in this case.

At last, the representation of the ten most useful features for the six methods on the MIT-CBCL database shows that informative features are selected with several different algorithms. These features are located in meaningful positions, as shown in Figures 5 and 6 such as eyes, nose and mouth contours. We can observe also that the simplest Fisher method mostly select redundant information (correlated features) since for instance the ten most important selected features are located on 4 typical positions whereas the other algorithms spread more the selected features. This

fact explains here why the misclassification rate is not so good with a very small number of features (less than 20 variables).

Performance of Hybrid OFW

The main interest of Hybrid OFW is that it produces some features aggregation. We thus display the 15 useful aggregated (or not) variables learnt after a long run of Hybrid OFW (it lasts about two hours when standard OFW or RFE take few minutes of computation). The first important point is that composed features are built and used by the stochastic process as shown in Figure 7. For instance, the fifteenth aggregation is formed by six elementary edges. Note also that the most weighted composed features use some correlated elementary features, despite the addition of the term F_{t_n}.

Concerning now the misclassification error rate, building composed features clearly improves the discrimination as we obtain a very accurate

Figure 5. Representation of the main edge detectors after learning with Fisher (left), Relief(center) and L0-SVM (right) methods for the MIT-CBCL database.

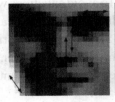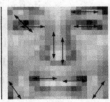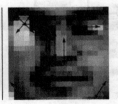

Figure 6. Representation of the main edge detectors after learning with OFW (left), RFE (center) and RF (right) for the MIT-CBCL database

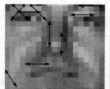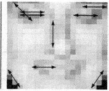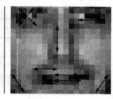

misclassification rate of 1.2% for 100 selected features. This can be explained by the good discrimination of non-faces as the test set is formed of 20% faces, 80% non-faces. Thus, the misclassification rate is largely improved. We can see here that the aggregation technique is powerful for the discrimination of "non-face" signals.

Finally, the main disadvantage of the hybrid OFW is its large computational cost owing to the large number of generation of complex features.

CONCLUSION

As pointed above, selecting relevant features for classification in a large set of variables is not obvious. Existing methods can be splitted in filter or

Figure 7. Representation of the main aggregation of edges detectors selected by Hybrid OFW process for the MIT-CBCL database

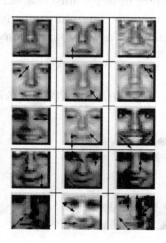

wrapper algorithms. Filter ones are fast, and do not over fit but are not generally as accurate as wrapper ones which tend to over fit. Contrary to filter methods, wrapper methods are generally based on theoretical justifications about margins of classifiers. About these theoretical motivations, OFW and hybrid OFW are very special case since they directly aim to minimize a misclassification rate.

Concerning the accuracy of each method, we show that wrapper methods based on margin conditions behave well for the detection of faces and are generally better then filter ones. However, it does not seem exist a best method among them as pointed in the paragraphs above. Indeed, the main conclusion of the experimental sections is that performances and features selected by algorithm mainly depends on the nature of the optimization problem solved by the methods: wrapper methods based on SVM share a lots of variables in common, it is also the case for Fisher and Random Forest selection which have both a large amount of features in common in the datasets MIT and ORL.

From a practical and intellectual point of view, the experimental section show that in the case of face detection, some characteristic areas of images in the neighbourhood of eyes, noses and mouths are relevant for classification.

At last, OFW and hybrid OFW perform well but the computational time of hybrid OFW curbs its use. To avoid situations with too many variables for the hybrid OFW, one can use a pre-processing step of S2N filtering described above with a low F-test threshold. Moreover, as there is no a better classifier A, it is important that a features selection method can be applied to any classifier. In this connection, OFW has the great advantage to be applied to any A, and permits to be adapted to various situations.

Finally, a challenging question is to understand the number of variables that can be selected without any over fitting regarding the number of samples in the database. For this, it is necessary to properly define and control the variance of the features selection algorithm, which is at the moment an open question.

REFERENCES

Amaldi, E., & Kann, V. (1998). On the approximability of minimizing non zero variables or unsatisfied relations in linear systems. *Theoretical Computer Science, 209*, 237–260. doi:10.1016/S0304-3975(97)00115-1

Amit, Y., & Geman, D. (1997). Shape quantization and recognition with randomized trees. *Neural Computation, 9*, 1545–1588. doi:10.1162/neco.1997.9.7.1545

Bellman, R. (1961). *Adaptive control processes: A guided tour*. Princeton, NJ: Princeton University Press.

Benaïm, M. (2000). Convergence with probability one of stochastic approximation algorithms whose average is cooperative. *Nonlinearity, 13*(3), 601–616. doi:10.1088/0951-7715/13/3/305

Blum, A., & Langley, P. (1997). Selection of relevant features and examples in machine learning. *Artificial Intelligence, 97*(1-2), 245–271. doi:10.1016/S0004-3702(97)00063-5

Breiman, L. (2001). Random forests. *Machine Learning, 45*(1), 5–32. doi:10.1023/A:1010933404324

Breiman, L., Friedman, J., Stone, C., & Olshen, R. (1984). *Classification and regression tree*. San Francisco: Wadsworth International.

Cabot, A., Engler, H., & Gadat, S. (2009). On the long time behaviour of second order differential equations with asymptotically small dissipation. In *Transactions of the American Mathematical Society*.

Candès, E., & Tao, T. (2005). The dantzig selector: statistical estimation when p is much larger than n. *Annals of Statistics, 35*, 2313–2351. doi:10.1214/009053606000001523

Duflo, M. (1996). *Algorithms stochastiques*. Berlin: Springer-Verlag.

Dupuis, P., & Ishii, H. (1991). On Lipschitz continuity of the solution mapping to the Skorokhod problem, with applications. *Stochastics and Stochastics Reports, 35*(1), 31–62.

Dupuis, P., & Ramanan, K. (1999). Convex duality and the Skorokhod problem (Part I & II). *Probability Theory and Related Fields, 115*(2), 153–236. doi:10.1007/s004400050269

Elisseeff, A., Weston, J., & Schölkopf, B. (2003). Use of the zero-norm with linear models and kernel methods. *Journal of Machine Learning Research, 3*, 1439–1461. doi:10.1162/153244303322753751

Fleuret, F., & Geman, D. (2001). Coarse-to-fine face detection. *International Journal of Computer Vision, 41*, 85–107. doi:10.1023/A:1011113216584

Friedman, J., Hastie, T., & Tibshirani, R. (2000). Additive logistic regression: a statistical view of boosting. *Annals of Statistics, 28*, 337–374. doi:10.1214/aos/1016218223

Gadat, S. (2008). Jump diffusion over feature space for object recognition. *SIAM Journal on Control and Optimization, 47*(2), 904–935. doi:10.1137/060656759

Gadat, S., & Younes, L. (2007). A stochastic algorithm for feature selection in pattern recognition. *Journal of Machine Learning Research, 8*, 509–547.

Geman, S., Bienenstock, E., & Doursat, R. (1992). Neural networks and the bias/variance dilemma. *Neural Computation, 4*, 1–58. doi:10.1162/neco.1992.4.1.1

Guyon, I., & Elisseeff, A. (2003). An introduction to variable and feature selection. *Journal of Machine Learning Research, 3*, 1157–1182. doi:10.1162/153244303322753616

Guyon, I., Weston, J., Barnhill, S., & Vapnik, V. (2002). Gene selection for cancer classification using support vector machines. *Machine Learning, 46*(1-3), 389–422. doi:10.1023/A:1012487302797

Ho, T. K. (1998). The random subspace method for constructing decision forests. *IEEE Transactions on Pattern Analysis and Machine Intelligence, 20*(8), 832–844. doi:10.1109/34.709601

Jolliffe, I. T. (2002). *Principal component analysis.* New York: Springer.

Jutten, C., & Herault, J. (1991). Blind separation of sources, part i: An adaptive algorithm based on neuromimetic architecture. *Signal Processing, 24*(1), 1–10. doi:10.1016/0165-1684(91)90079-X

Kira, K., & Rendell, L. A. (1992). A practical approach to feature selection. In *Proceedings of 9th International Conference on Machine Learning* (pp. 249–256).

Kononenko, I. (1994). Estimating attributes: Analysis and extensions of relief. In *Proceedings of European Conference on Machine Learning* (pp. 171–182).

Lê Cao, K. A., Gonçalves, O., Besse, P., & Gadat, S. (2007). Selection of biologically relevant genes with a wrapper stochastic algorithm. *Statistical Applications in Genetics and Molecular Biology, 6*(1). doi:10.2202/1544-6115.1312

Rissanen, J. (1983). A universal prior for integers and estimation by minimum description length. *Annals of Statistics, 11*(2), 416–431. doi:10.1214/aos/1176346150

Stone, M. (1974). Cross-validatory choice and assessment of statistical predictions. *Journal of the Royal Statistical Society. Series B. Methodological, 36*, 111–147.

Sun, Y. (2007). Iterative relief for feature weighting: Algorithms, theories, and applications. *IEEE Transactions on Pattern Analysis and Machine Intelligence, 29*, 1035–1051. doi:10.1109/TPAMI.2007.1093

Sun, Y., & Lijun, Y. (2007). A genetic algorithm based feature selection approach for 3d face recognition. *Biometrics Symposium in 3D Imaging for Safety and Security, Springer - Computational Imaging and Vision, 35*, 95–118.

Tibshirani, R. (1996). Regression shrinkage and selection via the lasso. *Journal of the Royal Statistical Society. Series B. Methodological, 58*, 267–288.

van Dijck, G., van Hulle, M., & Wevers, M. (2004). Genetic algorithm for feature subset selection with exploitation of feature correlations from continuous wavelet transform: a real-case application. *International Journal of Computational Intelligence, 1*, 1–12.

Vapnik, V. (1998). *Statistical learning theory. Adaptive and Learning Systems for Signal Processing, Communications, and Control.* New York: John Wiley & Sons Inc.

Wright, J., Yang, A., Ganesh, A. Y., Shankar Sastry, S., & Ma, Y. (2009). Robust face recognition via sparse representation. *IEEE Transactions on Pattern Analysis and Machine Intelligence, 31*(2), 210–227. doi:10.1109/TPAMI.2008.79

Xiao, R., Li, W., Tian, Y., & Tang, X. (2006). Joint boosting feature selection for robust face recognition. In *Proceedings of the IEEE Conference on Computer Vision and Pattern Recognition (CVPR 06)* (pp. 1415–1422).

Yang, J., & Li, Y. (2006). Orthogonal relief algorithm for feature selection. *Lecture Notes in Computer Science*, *4113*, 227–234. doi:10.1007/11816157_22

Zou, H., Hastie, T., & Tibshirani, R. (2006). Sparse principal component analysis. *Journal of Computational and Graphical Statistics*, *15*, 262–286. doi:10.1198/106186006X113430

KEY TERMS AND DEFINITIONS

Features Selection Methods: General reference to algorithms in Computer Science field. These algorithms are developed for the selection of a small group of variables among a large set of features that describe a signal.

High Dimensional Data: Special framework in machine learning in which the signal is described in a database $D=(I1,...\ In)$ by a very large number of features p. In this framework, this number p is generally not negligible comparing to the number of samples n.

Filter Methods: Reference to very simple features selection algorithms. These methods have a low computational cost but do not provide some very accurate results.

Wrapper Methods: Reference to a second kind of features selection algorithms. These methods are much more complicated and more costly comparing to filter ones but are generally more accurate.

Stochastic Algorithm: Reference to a field of numerical probability research. This field is related to statistical optimization methods. Some very famous methods such as Genetic Algorithms, Simulated Annealing or Robbins Monro methods belong to this large class of Stochastic Algorithms.

OFW: Optimal Feature Weighting is a wrapper method of feature selection which uses a Stochastic approximation algorithm to solve a minimization problem dedicated to classification.

Hybrid OFW: Hybrid Optimal Feature Weighting is an improvement of the original OFW. It is also a wrapper method of feature selection and it uses a Genetic Algorithm like technique to modify the set of features and solve some minimization problem.

Chapter 7
Transform Based Feature Extraction and Dimensionality Reduction Techniques

V. Jadhav Dattatray
Vishwakarma Institute of Technology, India

S. Holambe Raghunath
SGGS Institute of Engineering and Technology, India.

ABSTRACT

Various changes in illumination, expression, viewpoint, and plane rotation present challenges to face recognition. Low dimensional feature representation with enhanced discrimination power is of paramount importance to face recognition system. This chapter presents transform based techniques for extraction of efficient and effective features to solve some of the challenges in face recognition. The techniques are based on the combination of Radon transform, Discrete Cosine Transform (DCT), and Discrete Wavelet Transform (DWT). The property of Radon transform to enhance the low frequency components, which are useful for face recognition, has been exploited to derive the effective facial features. The comparative study of various transform based techniques under different conditions like varying illumination, changing facial expressions, and in-plane rotation is presented in this chapter. The experimental results using FERET, ORL, and Yale databases are also presented in the chapter.

INTRODUCTION

The face recognition process in human is a high-level visual task. Although human can detect and identify faces in a scene with varying conditions without much effort, building an automated system that accomplishes such task is very challenging. The challenges are even more profound when one considers the wide variations in imaging condi-tions. There are inter, and intra subject variations associated with face images. Inter subject variations are limited due to the physical similarity among individuals. Intra subject variations are extensive because of head position (rotation), presence or absence of structural components (beards, glasses, etc.), facial expression, illumination conditions, age, and occlusion by other objects or peoples. These variations are challenges in face recognition.

DOI: 10.4018/978-1-61520-991-0.ch007

Face recognition is one-to-many matching process. It compares a specific face image (the probe) against all of the images in a face database (the gallery). The probe image is identified by determining the image in the gallery that most closely resembles the probe image.

Machine recognition of human faces from still and video images is active research area spanning several disciplines such as image processing, pattern recognition, computer vision etc. Given a still or video image of a scene using a stored database of faces, available information such as race, age, and gender may be used in narrowing the search. The solution of the problem involves segmentation of faces from cluttered scenes, extraction of features from the face region, matching, and identification. Psychophysicists and neuroscientist have been concerned with issues such as, uniqueness of faces, whether face recognition is done holistically or by local feature analysis, and use of facial expression for face recognition. Low dimensional feature representation with enhanced discrimination power is an important requirement of face recognition system. Extracting the effective and efficient features is a great challenge in face recognition (Chellappa 1995).

This chapter presents the different transform based techniques for feature extraction. The various analyses performed on these features to further reduce the dimensionality are discussed in this chapter. This chapter also presents two different techniques for feature extraction, which are computationally efficient and robust to zero mean white noise. These techniques attempt to exploit the capabilities of Radon transform (to enhance low frequency components), discrete cosine transform (DCT), and discrete wavelet transform (DWT) to derive effective and efficient face features. The effectiveness of these transform-based approaches is demonstrated in terms of both absolute performance and comparative performance.

BACKGROUND AND RELATED WORK

Feature selection for face representation is one of central issues to face recognition systems. Appearance based approaches, which generally operate directly on images or appearances of face objects, process the images as two-dimensional holistic patterns. Principle component analysis (PCA) and linear discriminant analysis (LDA) are widely used subspace analyses for data reduction and feature extraction in appearance-based approaches. Most of the appearance based feature extraction techniques can be classified into following types.

- Algorithms based on principal component analysis (PCA)
- Algorithms based on nonlinear PCA
- Algorithms based on linear discriminant analysis
- Algorithms based on nonlinear discriminant analysis

Algorithms Based on Principal Component Analysis

Projecting images into eigenspace is a standard procedure for many appearance based object recognition algorithms. Eigenspace is calculated by identifying the eigenvectors of the covariance matrix derived from a set of training images. The eigenvectors corresponding to non-zero eigenvalues of the covariance matrix form an orthonormal basis that reflects the image. Mathew Turk and Alex Pentland presented a well-known classical approach to the detection and identification of human faces using eigenspace called as principal component analysis (PCA).

PCA is a classical method that has been widely used for human face representation and recognition. The major idea of PCA is to decompose a data space into a linear combination of small collection of bases, which are pair wise orthogonal and capture the directions of maximum variance in the training set. Suppose there is a set of N dimensional training samples x_i, $i=1,2,...,M$. The ensemble covariance matrix C of the training set is given as

$$C = \sum_{i=1}^{M} (x_i - m)(x_i - m)^T \qquad (1)$$

where m is the mean of all samples.

The PCA leads to solve the following eigenvector problem:

$$\lambda V = CV \qquad (2)$$

Where V are the eigenvectors of C and λ are the corresponding eigenvalues. These eigenvectors are ranked in a descending order according to the magnitudes of their eigenvalues that represent the variance of face distribution on eigenfaces. The eigenvector associated with the largest eigenvalue is the eigenvector that finds the greatest variance in the images. There are at most *M-1* eigenfaces with non-zero eigenvalues. These eigenvectors are commonly called eigenfaces. These eigenfaces with large eigenvalues represent the global, rough structure of the training images, while the eigenfaces with small eigenvalues are mainly determined by the local, detail components. Therefore, after projecting onto the eigenspace, the dimension of the input is reduced while the main components are maintained. When testing images have variations caused by local deformation, such as different facial expression, PCA can alleviate this effect (Turk 1999).

This approach is also known as Karhunen-Loeve (KL) transform or expansion. The magnitude and phase spectra of Fourier-Mellin transform and the Analytical Fourier-Mellin transform are jointly processed to derive the facial features. PCA is incorporated on these features to simplify feature data for recognition and discrimination (Yu 2006). DCT has been used to derive the compact facial features to reduce the memory requirement. PCA and LDA are implemented on these features (Chen 2005).

Algorithms Based on Nonlinear PCA (Kernel PCA)

The representation in PCA is based on the second order statistic of the image set and does not address higher order statistical dependencies such as the relationship among three or more pixels. With the Cover's theorem, nonlinearly separable patterns in an input space will become linearly separable with high probability if the input space is transformed nonlinearly into a high dimensional feature space. Face recognition is a highly complex and nonlinear problem because there exists so many image variations. These variations would give nonlinear distribution of face images of an individual. The kernel trick is demonstrated to be able to efficiently represent complicated nonlinear relations of the input data. The kernel trick first maps the input data into an implicit feature space with a nonlinear mapping, and then the data are analyzed in this high dimensional space. The kernel trick has been combined with PCA and developed Kernel Principal Component Analysis (KPCA). KPCA computes the higher order statistics and is able to extract nonlinear features. It is found superior compared with conventional PCA (Hsuan 200), (Belhumeur 1997), (B. Scholof 1998).

Three classes of widely used kernel functions are as follows.

1. Polynomial kernels:

$$k(x,y) = (x.y)^d \qquad (3)$$

Where d is the degree of polynomial.

2. Gaussian or Radial Basis Function kernel:

$$k(x,y) = \exp(\frac{\left\| x - y \right\|^2}{2\sigma^2}) \qquad (4)$$

3. Sigmoid kernels

$$k(x,y) = \tanh(k(x.y) + v) \qquad (5)$$

where $\sigma>0, k>0,$ and $v<0$.

Gabor wavelets with five scales and eight orientations have been used to derive desirable facial features characterized by spatial frequency, spatial locality, and orientation selectivity to cope with the variations due to illumination, and facial expression changes (Liu 2004). The KPCA is then extended to include fractional power polynomial model on Gabor features for enhanced face recognition performance. Gabor based KPCA with doubly nonlinear mapping for face recognition is presented in (Xie 2006). The nonlinear mapping performed in the original feature space not only considers the statistical property of the input features but also adopts the eigenmask to emphasize the important facial feature points. The conventional KPCA is performed on this mapped data.

Algorithms Based on Linear Discriminant Analysis Methods

LDA determines a set of projection vectors (W) maximizing the between-class scatter matrix S_b while minimizing the within-class scatter matrix S_w in the projective feature space.

The within class matrix in the feature space is given as

$$S_w = \sum_{i=1}^{L} \sum_{x_k \in x_i} (x_k - m_i)(x_k - m_i)^{\mathrm{T}} \qquad (6)$$

The between class matrix is given as

$$S_B = \sum_{i=1}^{L} N(m_i - m)(m_i - m)^{\mathrm{T}} \qquad (7)$$

Where m_i is the mean of ith class and m is the overall mean. Subspace is computed from the following equation.

$$S_B V = \lambda S_w V \qquad (8)$$

LDA group images of the same class and separates images of different classes. The rank of S_w is at most $M\text{-}L$. However, in face recognition, usually there are only a few samples for each class and $M\text{-}L$ is far smaller than the face vector length N. So S_w may become singular and it is difficult to compute S_w^{-1}. To avoid this, face data is first projected to a PCA subspace spanned by the largest $M\text{-}L$ eigenfaces. LDA is then performed in the $M\text{-}L$ dimensional subspace, such that S_w is nonsingular.

LDA implemented on the Gabor wavelet features enhances the discrimination information called as Gabor Fisher Classifier (GFC) (Liu 2003). Fourier transform (Jing 2005) and fractional Fourier transform (Jing 2006) have been used to derive the facial frequency features. LDA is performed on these features to enhance the discrimination capability. Wavelet transform is used to extract the low dimensional features called as wavelet faces. LDA is implemented on these features to enhance discrimination power in presence of wide facial expression variations (Jen 2002).

Algorithms Based on Nonlinear Discriminant Analysis

Linear methods such as LDA (Liu 2003), (Quing 2002) could not provide sufficient discrimination information to handle the face recognition problems. To overcome this limitation, kernel approach is proposed. The Kernel Fisher Discriminant Analysis (KFDA), which is a combination of kernel trick with Fisher linear discriminant analysis (FLDA), is introduced to represent facial features for face recognition (Mtiller 2001). The

KFD method uses nonlinear mapping between the input space and the feature space. Let $w_1, w_2, \ldots, w_L$ denote the L number of classes and $N_1, N_2, \ldots, N_L$ denote the number of samples in the class respectively. Let $X = [\bar{x}_1, \bar{x}_2, \ldots \bar{x}_M]$ be the features of the training samples and ϕ be a nonlinear mapping between the input space and the feature space. Let D represent the data matrix in the feature space:

$$D = [\phi(\bar{x}_1)\phi(\bar{x}_2)\ldots\phi(\bar{x}_M)], \qquad (9)$$

Where M is the total number of training samples $(N_1 + N_2 + \ldots N_L)$. A kernel matrix K by means of the dot product in the feature space is defined as:

$$\mathbf{K} = \mathbf{D}^T\mathbf{D} \qquad (10)$$

where $K_{ij} = (\phi(X_i).(\phi(X_j)) i, j = 1, 2, \ldots, M$.

The within class matrix in the feature space is given as

$$S_w = \frac{1}{M}\mathbf{D}\mathbf{D}^T \qquad (11)$$

The between class matrix is given as

$$S_B = \sum_{i=1}^{L} N(m_i - m)(m_i - m)^T = \frac{1}{M}\mathbf{D}\mathbf{W}\mathbf{D}^T \qquad (12)$$

Where m_i is the mean of ith class and m is the overall mean. $W \in R^{M \times M}$ is a block diagonal matrix. $W = diag[W_1, W_2, \ldots, W_L]$, where $W_j \in R^{Nj \times Nj}$ is an $N_j \times N_j$ matrix with all elements equal to $1/N_j, j = 1, 2, \ldots, L$.

A good criterion for class separability should convert these scatter matrices to a number, which becomes large when the between class scatter is large or the within class scatter is small. The KFD projection matrix consists of the eigenvectors V corresponding to the largest eigenvalues λ of

$$S_B V = \lambda S_w V \qquad (13)$$

However, the scatter matrices reside in the high dimensional feature space and are difficult to evaluate. In practice, the kernel matrix K is computed by means of a kernel function rather than by explicitly implementing the nonlinear mapping ϕ. It takes advantage of the Mercer equivalence condition and is feasible because the dot products in the high dimensional feature space are replaced by a kernel function in the input space while computational complexity is related to the number of training examples rather than the dimension of the feature space (Liu, 2006). Kernel matrix K is computed by using kernel function

$$K(x, y) = (x.y)^d \qquad (14)$$

where d is the degree of polynomial. To evaluate this difficulty, S_B and S_w are replaced by the kernel matrix given as

$$KWK\alpha = \lambda KK\alpha \qquad (15)$$

The generalized eigenvalue problem of Equation (15) can be converted into an ordinary eigenvalue problem

$$(KK + \varepsilon I)^{-1}(KWK)\alpha = \lambda\alpha \qquad (16)$$

where ε is a small positive regularization number and $\mathbf{I}$ an $M \times M$ identity matrix. The vector α is normalized so that KFD basis vector V has unit norm.

New kernel function called the cosine kernel has been suggested in (Qingshan 2004) to increase the discrimination capabilities of the original polynomial kernel function. Computational complexity of KFDA has been reduced by using a geometry based feature vector selection scheme. A variant of the nearest feature line classifier is employed to further enhance the recognition performance as it can produce virtual samples to make up for the shortage of training samples. In (Jadhav 2008) Gabor wavelets with five scales and eight orientations whereas in (Jadhav 2007) two level decomposition using discrete wavelet transform were used to derive facial features. The fractional power polynomial kernel maps the input data into an implicit feature space with a nonlinear mapping. Being linear in the feature space, but nonlinear in the input space, kernel is capable of deriving low dimensional features that incorporate higher order statistic. LDA is applied to kernel mapped multiresolution feature data.

All above mentioned subspace algorithms require to be retrained if any new image is added in the database. Two different techniques for feature extraction, which are computationally efficient, and robust to zero mean white noise and having data independent bases have been presented in the following sections.

RADON AND DISCRETE COSINE TRANSFORMS BASED APPROACH

Various changes in illumination, expression, viewpoint, and plane rotation present challenges to face recognition. Dimensionality reduction is essential for extracting effective features and reducing computational complexity in the classification stage. When the training database becomes large, the training time, and the memory requirement increase significantly. Systems based on PCA or LDA require to be retrained when new classes are added to obtain optimal projection results. Therefore, reduction in computational complexity is highly desirable. Discrete Cosine Transform (DCT) has been used for dimensionality reduction in face recognition (Hafed 2001) (Pan 2000). The characteristics of human visual model, features extracted using DCT, and PCA has been used for face recognition (Ramasubramanian 1989).

The combined feature Fisher classifier, which combines holistic and local features for face recognition is presented in (Zhou 2005). In this approach an image is divided into smaller sub-images and the DCT of whole face image and some sub-images is computed to extract holistic and local facial features. DCT based holistic and local features are combined to form image feature vector. LDA is implemented on these feature vectors to enhance the discrimination capability. Local appearance based scheme for face recognition, which uses block based DCT is presented in (Eknel 2006). In this approach, a detected and normalized face image is divided into blocks of 8 X 8 pixels. DCT of each block is computed and its coefficients are ordered using zigzag scanning. The DCT coefficients are concatenated to construct the image feature vector. The face recognition system based on pseudo 2-D Hidden Markov Model, which is implemented on DCT based features, is presented in (Eickeler 2000).

In order to recognize faces, number of features may be required. The Radon transform, which converts rotation into translation, is effective in detection algorithm (Magli 1999). DCT is effective in dimensionality and memory requirement reduction. So to improve the performance, Radon transform and DCT have been combined. This section presents Radon transform and DCT based framework for face recognition called as RDCT. The technique is invariant to in-plane rotation and illumination variations and robust to zero mean white noise. It has data independent bases. The technique computes Radon projections in different orientations and captures the directional features of the face images. The DCT applied on Radon projections provides enhanced directional frequency features of the facial images. For classification, the nearest neighbor classifier has been used.

Radon Transform

The Radon transform of a two dimensional function $f(x,y)$ is defined as

$$R(r,\theta) = \mathsf{R}[f(x,y)] = \int\limits_{-\infty}^{\infty} \int\limits_{-\infty}^{\infty} f(x,y)\delta(r - x\cos\theta - y\sin\theta)\,dxdy$$

$$(17)$$

where, r is the distance of a line from the origin and $\theta \in [0,\pi]$ is the angle between the distance vector and X- axis as shown in Figure 1 (Magli 1999), ((Jafari 2005) (A.Kadyrov 2001). The symbol $\mathcal{R}$ denotes Radon transform operator.

A rotation of $f(x,y)$ by an angle ϕ leads to translation of $R(r,\theta)$ in the variable θ byϕ, i.e.

$$\mathsf{R}\{f(x\cos\phi + y\sin\phi, -x\cos\phi + y\sin\phi)\} = R(r,\theta+\phi)$$

$$(18)$$

The proposed technique uses Radon transform to convert the rotation into translation and then applies translation invariant DCT to extract the rotation (in-plane) invariant features. In addition, due to its excellent energy compaction property, the use of DCT in the proposed approach also helps in reduction of feature vector dimension.

Another advantage of using Radon transform, in the proposed approach, is robustness to zero mean white noise. Let us consider that the noise corrupted image $f(x,y)$ is observed as

$$\hat{f}(x,y) = f(x,y) + \eta(x,y) \qquad (19)$$

where, $\eta(x,y)$ is zero mean white noise. The Radon transform of $\hat{f}(x,y)$ is

$$\mathsf{R}\,[\hat{f}(x,y)] = \mathsf{R}\,[f(x,y)] + \mathsf{R}\,[\eta(x,y)] \qquad (20)$$

Since the Radon transform is line integrals of the image, for the continuous case, the Radon transform of white noise is constant for all of the points and directions and is equal to the mean value of the noise (if integrated over infinite axis), which is assumed to be zero (Jafari 2005), (Xuan 2007) (S. Srisuk 2003). In our case, the signal

(digital image) is discontinuous and composed of a finite number of pixels. Hence, $\mathcal{R}[\eta(x,y)]$ in equation (6) does not become zero. However, in this case, Radon transform improves signal-to-noise ratio as below.

$$SNR_{\text{proj}} = SNR_{\text{image}} + 1.7N\,SNR_{\text{image}} \qquad (21)$$

where, SNR_{image} and SNR_{proj} indicate signal-to-noise ratio of the image and its Radon projection respectively. In practice, N which is radius in pixels, is sufficiently large and hence SNR_{proj} is much higher than SNR_{image} This property of Radon transform makes the proposed algorithm robust to zero mean white noise (Jafari 2005).

Discrete Cosine Transform

DCT is a well-known signal analysis tool used in compression due to its compact representation capability. It has an excellent energy compaction property for highly correlated data. This helps in reduction of feature vector dimension.

Let $f(x,y)$ is represented as discrete image $f(m,n)$ of size $M \times N$. The 2-D DCT of an image $f(m,n)$ is given as

$$B_{pq} = \alpha_p \alpha_q \sum_{m=0}^{M-1} \sum_{n=0}^{N-1} f(m,n) \cos\frac{\pi(2m+1)p}{2M} \cos\frac{\pi(2n+1)q}{2N}$$

$$(22)$$

$$\alpha_p = \begin{cases} 1/\sqrt{M} & p=0 \\ \sqrt{2/M} & 1 \le p \le M-1 \end{cases} \qquad \alpha_q = \begin{cases} 1/\sqrt{N} & q=0 \\ \sqrt{2/N} & 1 \le q \le N-1 \end{cases}$$

Figure 1. Radon transform of the image

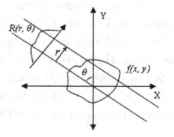

Where M and N denote the size of row and column of $f(m,n)$ respectively (Chen 2005).

Radon Transform and DCT Based Feature Extraction Algorithm (RDCT)

Facial features are the directional low frequency components. Earlier studies show that information in low frequency band plays a dominant role in face recognition (Chen 2005). In this RDCT approach, the global Radon projections for the limited number of orientations are computed to transform an image into Radon space. The line integral of an image during the computation of the Radon transform acts like a low-pass filter. This amplifies low frequency components in the face images. Radon space image for angle 0 to 179^0 is shown in Figure 2. The 2-D DCT is used to derive the facial frequency features from the Radon space. Figure 3 (a) shows DCT of Radon projection at 45^0 and Figure 3 (b) shows the significant coefficients. Significant coefficients of DCT (25% coefficients derived experimentally) in different orientations are concatenated to form the facial feature vector. Such vectors for all the training as well as test images are computed. Because of selection of significant coefficients in the limited directions, the technique is useful in dimensionality reduction. The images are classified using the nearest neighbor classifier (Jadhav 2008). The RDCT algorithm works as follows.

1. Normalize the training images.
2. Find the optimum number of projections.
3. Transform the image into Radon space $R(r,\theta)$ using optimum number of global Radon projections.
4. Compute DCT of Radon space.
5. Select the significant coefficients (25% coefficients) of DCT as feature. Concatenate the significant coefficients to form the feature vector.
6. Find the feature vectors for all the training images. These represent the reference feature

vectors for training images and are stored in the database.

RADON AND WAVELET TRANSFORM BASED APPROACH

Wavelet based representation has many advantages. According to psycho-visual research, there are strong evidences that the human visual system processes images in a multi-scale way. Converging evidences in neurophysiology and psychology are in consistent with the notion that the human visual system analyses image at several spatial resolution scales (Zhang 2004). An appropriate wavelet transform can result in robust representation with respect to illumination and expression changes and is capable of capturing substantial facial features, keeping computational complexity low.

This section presents Radon and Discrete Wavelet transform based framework for face recognition denoted as RDWT. The technique computes Radon projections in different orientations and captures the global directional features of the face images. Further, the wavelet transform applied on Radon space provides the directional multiresolution features of the facial images. For classification, the nearest neighbor classifier has

Figure 2. (a) shows the original images while (b) shows the respective Radon transforms for angle of 0° to 179°

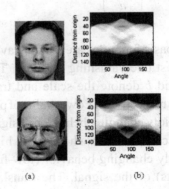

Figure 3. (a) Plot of Discrete Cosime Transform of Radon projection at an angle of 45°, (b) Significant coefficients

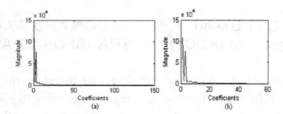

been used. This algorithm is invariant to facial expression and illumination variations.

Multiresolution Features

Wavelet Transform (WT) has the nice features of space frequency localization and multiresolution. The main reasons for WT's popularity lie in its complete theoretical framework, the great flexibility in choosing the bases and the low computational complexity.

Let $L^2(R)$ denote the vector space of a measurable, square integrable, one dimensional signal. Wavelet transform of $f(t) \in L^2(R)$ is defined as

$$(W_a f)(b) = \int f(t) \phi_{a,b}(t) dt \qquad (23)$$

where the wavelet basis function $\phi_{a,b}(t) \in L^2(R)$ can be expressed as

$$\phi_{a,b}(t) = a^{-\frac{1}{2}} \phi \left(\frac{t-b}{a} \right) \qquad (24)$$

These basis functions are called wavelets and have at least one vanishing moment. The arguments a and b denote the scale and translation parameters respectively. Lower value of parameter a gives rapidly changing behavior of signal (high frequency components) whereas; its high value gives slowly changing behavior (low frequency components) of the signal. The translation parameter b determines the localization of $\phi_{a,b}(t)$ in time. The wavelet basis functions in equation

(10) are dilated (scaled) and translated versions of mother wavelet $\phi(t)$ (Mallat 1989). 2-D WT of images can be similarly defined by implementing the one dimensional WT for each dimension (row and column) separately. Figure 4 illustrates the decomposition of an image using Discrete Wavelet Transform (DWT) into four sub-images via the high-pass and low-pass filter. H and L represent the high-pass and low-pass filter, respectively, and $\downarrow 2$ denotes the sub-sampling by 2.

In this approach Radon space image is decomposed using Daubechies wavelet DB3 (because of its symmetry, compact support, and the use of overlapping windows to reflect all changes between pixel intensities). Low frequency sub-image (LL), which possesses high energy, is selected for further decomposition. This component represents the basic figure of an image and is the most informative sub-image gearing with the highest discrimination power.

Radon Transform and DWT Based Feature Extraction Algorithm (RDWT)

In this algorithm, the facial features are the directional multiresolution information of the face images. The features are captured by using DWT of the global Radon projections of an image in different orientations. The optimum number of projections transforms the image into Radon space. In this transformation low frequency components useful in recognition are boosted.

Two level decomposition of Radon space using Daubechies wavelet has been carried out to derive the multiresolution features. The rows of

Figure 4. Multire solution approach used for image decomposition

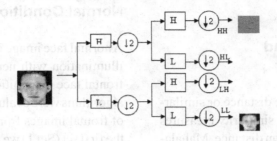

LL part are concatenated to form image feature vector. The feature vectors of training images are stored in the database as reference (Jadhav 2009). The RDWT algorithm works as follows.

1. Normalize the training images.
2. Find the optimum number of projections.
3. Transform the image into Radon space $R(r,\theta)$ using optimum number of global Radon projections.
4. Obtain two levels DWT of Radon space.
5. Concatenate the rows of LL part of decomposed Radon space. This represents the feature vector.
6. Find the feature vectors for all the training images. These represent the reference feature vectors for the training images and are stored in the database.

EXPERIMENTAL RESULTS

In this section, we evaluate the performance of PCA, LDA, KPCA, KLDA, RDCT and RDWT algorithms using three databases: (1) Face Recognition Technology (FERET), (2) an Olivetti Research Laboratory (ORL), and (3) Yale. In the first part of this section, we have briefly described the databases, the characteristics of the images and the normalization procedure. This is followed by the experiments carried out.

Databases and Normalization Procedure

The FERET database, which has become the de facto standard for evaluating the face recognition technologies, consists of more than 13,000 facial images corresponding to more than 1500 subjects. The diversity of the FERET database is across gender, ethnicity, and age. Since images are acquired during different photo sessions, the illumination conditions, facial expressions, and the size of the faces have been varied. The data set used in our experiments consists of 2500 gray frontal FERET face images (normal, varying illumination and varying facial expressions) corresponding to 300 subjects. The images are of size 256 X 384 with 8-bit resolution. The normalization process detects the center of the eyes and crops the image to the size of 128 X 128 (Phillips 2000). The normalized images (from FERET database) used in following experiments are shown in Figure 5.

The ORL face database is composed of 400 images with ten different images for each of the 40 distinct subjects. The variations of the images are across pose, size, time, and facial expression. All the images were taken against a dark homogeneous background with the subjects in an upright, frontal position, with tolerance for some tilting, and rotation of up to about 20⁰. The spatial resolution is of 92 X 112, while gray level resolution is 8-bit. There are 165 images in Yale database, which is of 15 different subjects with 11 images per subject. The images vary in facial expressions, and lighting conditions (ORL and Yale face database).

Distance Measures and Classification Rule

To classify the images, some distance or similarity measure is used. Popular similarity measures include L1 distance, Euclidean distance, Mahalanobis distance and cosine similarity measure. We have used Euclidean distance measure to classify the images. Let X_i represents the reference feature vectors in the database and Y represents the feature vector of test image.

$$\mathbf{X}_i = [x_{1i}...x_{Ni}]^{\mathrm{T}} \tag{25}$$

$$\mathbf{Y} = [y_i \cdots y_N]^{\mathrm{T}} \tag{26}$$

The Euclidean distance used to classify the image is given as

$$D_i = \sqrt{(x_{1i} - y_1)^2 + ...(x_{Ni} - y_N)^2} \qquad i = 1, 2, ...M. \tag{27}$$

Let

$$D = \min(D_i) \tag{28}$$

The test image belongs to class J if $\mathbf{D}=\mathbf{D}_J$. Recognition rate is defined as follows:

$$\mathrm{Re\,cognition\ \ Rate} = \frac{\mathrm{Number\ \ of\ \ correct\ \ matches}}{\mathrm{Total\ \ number\ \ of\ \ test\ \ images}} 100\% \tag{29}$$

To evaluate the performance of the algorithms following experiments were carried out.

Recognition under Normal Conditions

A normal face image is of frontal view under even illumination with neutral facial expression. For frontal face recognition, the performances of the algorithms were evaluated using two different sets of frontal images from grey FERET database. In the first set (Set 1) we used two images per subject in gallery (training set) as well as probe (testing set). In the second set (Set 2), three and four images per subject were used in gallery and probe respectively. In each set, the images in gallery and probe are not overlapping.

The performance of RDCT and RDWT algorithms were evaluated using different number of Radon projections. Recognition rate remains almost unaffected for any variation in number of projections above 60. The results are presented in Table 1. When high frequency sub-image in the decomposition was included in the feature vector along with low frequency sub-image, the recognition rate is slightly improved. This result is represented as RDWT-(H). This improvement is because of extraction of high frequency detail in the facial image by high frequency component in the decomposition process.

The performances of the RDCT and RDWT algorithms are better than the other approaches.

Figure 5. Original and normalized images from the FERET database

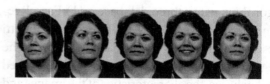

(a) Original imagers

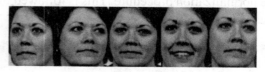

(b) Normalized images

Table 1. Recognition rate of algorithms for normal conditions

Algorithm	% Recognition Rate			
	FERET		ORL	Yale
	Set 1	Set 2		
PCA	87	88	88	88.7
LDA	88.5	90.3	90.5	92
KPCA	87.1	88.6	89.5	90
KLDA	89.3	92	91.5	95
DCT	89	91.5	87.4	92.6
RDCT	96.9	97.8	97.3	98.5
DWT	84.6	87.2	83	90.5
RDWT	97.75	98.5	97.5	98.8
RDWT-H	98.2	98.9	98.2	99

This is due to boosting of low frequency components, which contribute significantly in the recognition process during the computation of Radon projections apart from removal of redundant information in wavelet decomposition and reduced number of Radon projections.

Recognition under Different Illumination Conditions

The effect of illumination variation on face recognition was investigated using FERET, and Yale databases. Two images per subject that have variations in illumination have been selected for testing and two normal images per subject were used for training. To remove the effect of illumi-

nation variations, the DC component of LL sub-images, and DCT (which corresponds to average illumination) was removed before all the rows were concatenated to form the feature vector. The results of these experiments are given in Table 2.

The performance of RDCT, and RDWT algorithms is almost unaffected by illumination variations because of the removal of DC value corresponding to average illumination. The performance of approaches like PCA, LDA is significantly affected because PCA represents faces with their principal components. However, the variations between the images of the same face due to illumination are larger than image variations due to change in face identity.

Table 2. Recognition rate of algorithms under different illumination conditions

Algorithm	% Recognition Rate	
	FERET	Yale
PCA	54	62.2
LDA	76.2	79.8
KPCA	58	64
KLDA	77.4	78.9
RDCT	95.5	96.3
RDWT	97.8	94.5

Table 3. Face recognition results for different facial expressions on different databases

Algorithm	% Recognition Rate		
	FERET	**ORL**	**Yale**
PCA	85	87.4	88.3
LDA	78	75.3	65
KPCA	86.2	82	87
KLDA	90	89	92.4
RDCT	89.6	88.2	89.4
RDWT	97.7	98	97.6
RDWT (H)	88.2	86.4	89.9

Recognition under Facial Expression Variations

Experiments based on the face images with different facial expressions were conducted to assess the robustness of the approach to variations in facial expressions. In this experiment two frontal normal images per subject were used for training. The images having facial expression variations from FERET, ORL, and Yale databases were used for testing. The recognition rate for different databases is given in Table 3. The performance of RDCT algorithm has been affected compared with other approaches. This is because of formation of facial expressions from the local distortions of the facial feature points, which have affected the corresponding local texture and shape properties and have been detected by DCT. Radon projections, which act as low-pass filter (Integration) followed by wavelet decomposition in which LL sub-image is selected, make RDWT algorithm invariant to facial expressions. However, inclusion of high frequency component in feature vector affects the performance of this approach.

Robustness of Algorithms Against Zero Mean White Noise

The robustness of the algorithms to zero mean white noise was tested using one of the combinations of training and testing images of ORL database. Zero mean white noise with variance dependent on the required signal-to-noise ratio (SNR-15, 10 and 7 dB) was added in the test images. No noise was added in the training images. Figure 6 (a) shows an original image while (b), (c), (d) show the images with signal to noise level of 15 dB, 10 dB, and 7 dB respectively. Table 4 shows the effect of noise of different level on the performances of algorithms. These results show that the RDCT and RDWT algorithms have significantly higher robustness to zero mean white noise. Since, the SNR improves significantly in Radon space, RDCT and RDWT algorithms are robust to zero mean white noise.

FUTURE TRENDS AND CONCLUSION

In this chapter, transform based techniques for feature extraction has been reviewed and the sub-

Figure 6. (a) Typical image from CRL database and (b), (c), and (d) are the images corrupted with zero mean white noise with signal to nosie ration of 15dB, 10dB, and 7dB respectively

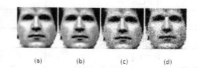

Table 4. Effect of zero mean white noise on the performance of algorithms

Algorithm	SNR			
	No Noise	15 dB	10 dB	7 dB
PCA	88	74.2	62.0	54.5
LDA	90.5	71	65.4	59.6
KPCA	89.5	78.2	67.0	61.2
KLDA	92	79.2	71	68
RDCT	96.2	96	95.2	93.3
RDWT	97.5	97	95	93.5

space analyses performed on these features for face recognition have been discussed. Requirements of high recognition accuracy, high computational efficiency and invariance to changes in scale, facial expression variations, illumination conditions and plane rotation are the challenges in face recognition. Recognition in presence of noise is also the great challenge in face recognition.

RDCT algorithm uses DCT, which has compact data representation property, to extract the features from the Radon space. The algorithm is invariant to in-plane rotation and illumination variations. This algorithm is computationally efficient and has achieved high recognition accuracy. However, the performance of this algorithm is slightly affected by facial expression variations.

In RDWT algorithm, Daubechies wavelet is used to extract the multiresolution features from the Radon space. This computationally efficient algorithm has high recognition accuracy. It is invariant to facial expression and illumination variations. However, it is not invariant to in-plane rotation.

Above mentioned Radon transform based algorithms are not required to be retrained if any new image is included in the database. These algorithms are very robust to zero mean white noise because of the improvement of signal to noise ratio in Radon space. These algorithms can also be implemented using single image per person.

Based on the work presented in the chapter the directions for future research work could be to develop the algorithm for automatic normalization of faces, to develop the computationally efficient algorithm, which will be invariant to variations in scale, rotation, illumination, facial expressions, and robust to noise. Development of the real time system and its hardware realization is also important. Development of multimodal biometric system is also the emerging trend in biometrics.

ACKNOWLEDGMENT

The authors are very much thankful to National Institute of Standards and Technology, USA for providing FERET database, AT and T laboratory for ORL database and Yale University for Yale database.

REFERENCES

Belhumeur, P. N., Hespanha, J. P., & Kriegman, D. J. (1997). Eigenfaces vs. Fisherfaces: Recognition using class specific linear projection. *IEEE Transactions on Pattern Analysis and Machine Intelligence, 19*(7), 711–720. doi:10.1109/34.598228

Chellappa, R., Wilson, C. L., & Sirohey, S. (1995). Human and machine recognition of faces: A survey. *Proceedings of the IEEE, 23*(5), 705–740. doi:10.1109/5.381842

Chen, W., Er, M. J., & Wu, S. (2005). PCA and LDA in DCT domain. *Pattern Recognition Letters, 26*, 2474–2482. doi:10.1016/j.patrec.2005.05.004

Cheng, Y. Q., Liu, K., Yang, J. Y., & Wang, H. F. (2002). A robust algebraic method for human face recognition. *IEEE Transactions on Pattern Analysis and Machine Intelligence, 24*(6), 764–779.

Chien, J.-T., & Wu, C.-C. (2002). Discriminant waveletfaces and nearest feature classifiers for face recognition. *IEEE Transactions on Pattern Analysis and Machine Intelligence, 24*(12), 1644–1649. doi:10.1109/TPAMI.2002.1114855

Eickler, S., Muller, S., & Rigoll, G. (2000). Recognition of JPEG compressed face images based on statistical methods. *Image and Vision Computing, 18*, 279–287. doi:10.1016/S0262-8856(99)00055-4

Eknel, H. K., & Stiefelhagen, R. (2006). Analysis of local appearance based face recognition: Effects of feature selection and feature normalization. In *Proceedings of CVPR Biometrics Workshop*, New York, USA.

Hafed, Z. M., & Levine, M. D. (2001). Face recognition using the discrete cosine transform. *Journal of Computer Vision, 43*(3), 167–188. doi:10.1023/A:1011183429707

Jadhav, D. V., & Holambe, R. S. (2007). Multi-resolution feature based kernel Fisher classifier for face recognition. In: *Proceedings of 4th IEEE international conference on Information Technology: New Generation* (pp. 848-853).

Jadhav, D. V., & Holambe, R. S. (2008). Gabor wavelet feature based fractional power polynomial kernel Fisher classifier for face recognition. In *Proceedings of 7th IEEE international conference on Computational Intelligence and Multimedia Analysis* (pp. 387-391).

Jadhav, D. V., & Holambe, R. S. (2008). Radon and discrete cosine transforms based feature extraction and dimensionality reduction approach for face recognition. *Signal Processing, 88*(10), 2604–2609. doi:10.1016/j.sigpro.2008.04.017

Jadhav, D. V., & Holambe, R. S. (2009). Feature extraction using Radon and wavelet transforms with application to face recognition. *Neurocomputing, 72*(7-9), 1950–1959. doi:10.1016/j.neucom.2008.05.001

Jafari–Khouzani, K., & Soltanian-Zadeh, H. (2005). Rotation invariant multiresolution texture analysis using Radon and wavelet transform. *IEEE Transactions on Image Processing, 14*(6), 783–794. doi:10.1109/TIP.2005.847302

Jing, X. Y., Tang, Y. Y., & Zhang, D. (2005). A Fourier – LDA approach for image recognition. *Pattern Recognition, 38*(2), 453–457. doi:10.1016/j.patcog.2003.09.020

Jing, X.-Y., Wong, H.-S., & Zhang, D. (2006). Face recognition based on discriminant fractional Fourier feature extraction. *Pattern Recognition Letters, 27*, 1465–1471. doi:10.1016/j.patrec.2006.02.020

Kadyrov, A., & Petrou, M. (2001). The Trace Transform and Its Applications. *IEEE Transactions on Pattern Analysis and Machine Intelligence, 23*(8), 811–823. doi:10.1109/34.946986

Liu, C. (2004). Gabor based kernel PCA with fractional power polynomial models for face recognition. *IEEE Transactions on Pattern Analysis and Machine Intelligence, 26*(5), 572–581. doi:10.1109/TPAMI.2004.1273927

Liu, C., & Wechsler, H. (2001). A shape and texture based enhanced Fisher classifier for face recognition. *IEEE Transactions on Image Processing, 10*(4), 598–607. doi:10.1109/83.913594

Liu, C., & Wechsler, H. (2002). Gabor feature based classification using the enhanced Fisher linear discriminant model for face recognition. *IEEE Transactions on Image Processing, 11*(4), 467–476. doi:10.1109/TIP.2002.999679

Liu, Q., Lu, H., & Ma, S. (2004). Improving kernel Fisher discriminant analysis for face recognition. *IEEE Transactions on Circuits and Systems for Video Technology, 14*(1), 42–49. doi:10.1109/TCSVT.2003.818352

Magli, E., Olmo, G., & Lo Presti, L. (1999). Pattern Recognition by means of the Radon transform and the continuous wavelet transform. *Signal Processing, 73*, 277–289. doi:10.1016/S0165-1684(98)00198-4

Mallat, S. (1989). A theory of multiresolution signal decomposition: The wavelet representation. *IEEE Transactions on Pattern Analysis and Machine Intelligence, 11*, 674–693. doi:10.1109/34.192463

Mtiller, K. R., Mika, S., Riitsch, G., Tsuda, K., & Scholopf, B. (2001). An introduction to kernel based learning algorithm. *IEEE Transactions on Neural Networks, 12*, 181–201. doi:10.1109/72.914517

ORL face database. (n.d.). Retrieved from http://www.uk.research.att.com/facedatabase

Pan, Z., Adams, R., & Bolouri, H. (2000). Image redundancy reduction for neural network classification using discrete cosine transform. In *Proceedings of IEEE International Joint Conference on Neural Networks*, Italy (pp. 149-154).

Phillips, P. J., Moon, H., Rizvi, S. A., & Rauss, P. J. (2000). The FERET evaluation methodology for face recognition algorithms. *IEEE Transactions on Pattern Analysis and Machine Intelligence, 22*(10), 1090–1104. doi:10.1109/34.879790

Ramasubramanian, D., & Venkatesh, Y. V. (2000). Encoding and recognition of faces based on the human visual model and DCT. *Pattern Recognition, 34*, 2447–2458. doi:10.1016/S0031-3203(00)00172-2

Scholof, B., Smola, A., & Muller, K. R. (1998). Nonlinear component analysis as a kernel eigenvalue problem. *Neural Computation, 10*(5), 1299–1319. doi:10.1162/089976698300017467

Srisuk, S., Petrou, M., Kurutach, W., & Kadyrov, A. (2003). Face Authentication using the Trace Transform. In *Proceedings of the IEEE Computer Society Conference on Computer Vision and Pattern Recognition* (pp. 305-312).

Turk, M., & Pentland, A. (1991). Eigenfaces for recognition. *Journal of Cognitive Neuroscience, 13*(1), 71–86. doi:10.1162/jocn.1991.3.1.71

Wang, X., Xiao, B., Ma, J. F., & Bi, X.-L. (2007). Scaling and rotation invariant approach to object recognition based on Radon and Fourier-Mellin transforms. *Pattern Recognition, 40*, 3503–3508. doi:10.1016/j.patcog.2007.04.020

Xie, X., & Lam, K.-M. (2006). Gabor based kernel PCA with doubly nonlinear mapping for face recognition with a single face image. *IEEE Transactions on Image Processing, 15*(9), 2481–2492. doi:10.1109/TIP.2006.877435

Yale face database. (n.d.). Retrieved from http://cvc.yale.edu./projects/yalefaces/yalefaces.html

Yang, M. H., Ahuja, N., & Kriegman, D. (2000). Face recognition using kernel Eigenfaces. In *Proceedings of IEEE International Conference on Image Processing* (pp. 37-40).

Yu, H., & Bennamoun, M. (2006). Complete invariants for robust face recognition. *Pattern Recognition, 40*, 1579–1591. doi:10.1016/j.patcog.2006.08.010

Zhang, B. L., Zhang, H., & Ge, S. S. (2004). Face recognition by applying wavelet subband representation and kernel associative memory. *IEEE Transactions on Neural Networks*, *15*(1), 166–177. doi:10.1109/TNN.2003.820673

Zhou, D., Yang, X., Peng, N., & Wang, Y. (2005). Improved LDA based face recognition using both global and local information. *Pattern Recognition Letters*, *27*, 536–543. doi:10.1016/j.patrec.2005.09.015

KEY TERMS AND DEFINITIONS

Face Recognition System: This system operates in verification and identification mode. In verification mode the claimed identity is to be verified whereas in identification mode the closest match of test image with the images in database is determined.

Discrimination Power: The capability of a classifier to separate the between class scatter in feature space so that correct recognition rate will be improved with minimum value of equal error rate.

Local or Detail Component: These components represent the fine detail information in face image. These high frequency components are formed because of local distortions such as changes in facial expressions.

Global Component: The coarse shape based information is represented by these low frequency components.

Nonlinear Mapping: The transformation relationship between the input space and the feature space is called

Gallery: As the FERET protocol the set of face images used for training the algorithm is called Gallery. Gallery must be of different size.

Probe: The set of face images used for testing the algorithm is called Probe. Probe must have different illumination, facial expression variations. Gallery and Probe must not be overlapping.

Chapter 8
FastNMF:
Efficient NMF Algorithm for Reducing Feature Dimension

Le Li
Tsinghua University, Beijing, China

Yu-Jin Zhang
Tsinghua University, Beijing, China

ABSTRACT

Non-negative matrix factorization (NMF) is a more and more popular method for non-negative dimensionality reduction and feature extraction of non-negative data, especially face images. Currently no NMF algorithm holds not only satisfactory efficiency for dimensionality reduction and feature extraction of face images but also high ease of use. To improve the applicability of NMF, this chapter proposes a new monotonic, fixed-point algorithm called FastNMF by implementing least squares error-based non-negative factorization essentially according to the basic properties of parabola functions. The minimization problem corresponding to an operation in FastNMF can be analytically solved just by this operation, which is far beyond existing NMF algorithms' power, and therefore FastNMF holds much higher efficiency, which is validated by a set of experimental results. For the simplicity of design philosophy, FastNMF is still one of NMF algorithms that are the easiest to use and the most comprehensible. Besides, theoretical analysis and experimental results also show that FastNMF tends to extract facial features with better representation ability than popular multiplicative update-based algorithms.

INTRODUCTION

An essential and important problem in signal processing, pattern recognition, computer vision and image engineering is how to find a suitable representation of multivariate data, which typically make latent structure in the data clear and

often reduce the dimensionality of the data so that further computation or classification can be effectively and efficiently implemented.

Principal component analysis (Jolliffe, 2002), projection pursuit (Jones, 1987), factor analysis (Reyment, 1996), redundancy reduction (Deco, 1995), and independent component analysis (Hyvärinen, 2001) are some popular data representation methods. Although they are essentially

DOI: 10.4018/978-1-61520-991-0.ch008

differentiated, they all produce negative descriptive components (that is to say, subtractive representations are allowable) and linearly implement dimensionality reduction. Different from them, a new method called non-negative matrix factorization (NMF) is proposed by Lee and Seung in *Nature* (Lee, 1999). It makes all representation components non-negative (in other words, only purely additive representations are allowable) and nonlinearly implements dimensionality reduction.

Psychological and physiological evidence for NMF is that perception of the whole is based on perception of its parts (Palmer, 1977; Wachsmuth, 1994; Logothetis, 1996), which is compatible with the intuitive notion of combining parts to form a whole (Lee, 1999), and hence it grasps the essence of intelligent or biological data representation in some degree. Besides, NMF usually produces a sparse representation for input data, which has been shown to be a useful middle ground between a completely distributed representation and a unary representation (Field, 1994).

As a effective method of non-negative dimensionality reduction and feature extraction of non-negative data, NMF has been applied in several research fields, including text analysis (Lee, 1999), document clustering (Shahnaz, 2006), digital watermarking (Liu, 2006; Ouhsain, 2009), face analysis (Chen, 2001; Lee, 1999; Guillamet, 2002; Wang, 2006a), image retrieval (Liang, 2006), image de-convolution (Kopriva, 2006), language modeling (Stouten, 2007; Stouten, 2008), sound source classification (Cho, 2003), musical signal analysis (Benetos, 2006; Holzapfel, 2008), blind source separation (Cichocki, 2006a), network security (Guan, 2009), gene (Frigyesi, 2008) and cell (Kim, 2007) analysis and many others. Among them, face analysis is one of the earliest and most widely researched applications, and besides, non-negative dimensionality reduction and feature extraction of face images has been one of the basic experiments to show the performance of NMF algorithms (Chen, 2003; Lee, 1999; Wild, 2004).

Despite these numerous applications, the algorithmic development for NMF has been relatively deficient. To our knowledge, currently no NMF algorithm holds not only satisfactory efficiency for dimensionality reduction and feature extraction of face images but also high ease of use. This causes inconvenience to the current researches on applications related to face analysis, and partly restrains the further NMF application development in this field.

To improve the applicability of NMF, this paper proposes a new monotonic, fixed-point algorithm called FastNMF by implementing least squares error-based non-negative factorization essentially according to the basic properties of parabola functions. It holds high efficiency, is easy to use, is very comprehensible, and extracts better features than the popular multiplicative update-based algorithms (Lee, 2000), as far as the ability of representation is concerned.

This chapter is structured as follows. Section 2 systematically introduces NMF. Section 3 deeply analyzes existing NMF algorithms to disclose the significance of developing FastNMF. Section 4 designs FastNMF. Section 5 discusses FastNMF's properties. Section 6 experimentally verifies high efficiency of FastNMF-based dimensionality reduction and feature extraction of face images, discloses how efficient it is, and shows the superiority of FastNMF features to the popular multiplicative update-based algorithms' ones. Finally, section 7 concludes this chapter.

For convenience of formulation in following sections, the main notations and terminologies used are listed in Table 1.

NMF

Definition 1: Denoting N observations of an M-dimensional non-negative stochastic variable $v_j, j = 1, 2, \cdots, N$, and arranging $v_j, j = 1, 2, \cdots, N$ into the columns of an $M \times N$

Table 1. Notations and terminologies used in this paper

Notations and terminologies	Descriptions
V	An $M \times N$ processed nonnegative matrix
L	Number of bases extracted by NMF
W	An $M \times L$ nonnative basis matrix extracted by NMF for **V**
H	An $L \times N$ nonnative coefficient matrix extracted by NMF for **V**
f_V	An objective function of a minimization problem for NMF, which is related to **V**
$X_{\cdot j}$	The j-th column of a matrix X
$X_{i \cdot}$	The i-th line of a matrix X
An iteration in a NMF algorithm	An update for both W and H
$\mathbf{W}(k)$	The value of W after k iterations
$\mathbf{H}(k)$	The value of H after k iterations
$\otimes$	Hadamard (element-wise) multiplication
$\odot$	Hadamard (element-wise) division
δ_{ij}	$\delta_{ij}=1$ while $i=j$, and $\delta_{ij}=0$ while $i \neq j$
$\max\{Y, a\}$	For $a \in R$ and a vector $Y \in R^n$, $\max\{Y, a\}$ makes all elements less than a in Y equal to a, and doesn't change the other elements in Y
$a \leq \mathbf{X}$	all elements of X are no less than a for $a \in R$ and a matrix or vector **X**
$\mathbf{1}_{M \times N}$	An $M \times N$ matrix with all elements equal to 1
ε	An infinitely small positive number
Z^+	The set of positive integers
Stop rule	The rule to decide whether a algorithm is stopped or not
Q.E.D.	The abbreviation for "quod erat demonstrandum" that means a mathematical proof is completed
Convergence of an iterative algorithm	The limit of any convergent subsequence of the sequence generated by the algorithm's iterative rules is a solution, according to Global Convergence Theorem.

matrix **V**, NMF solves the problem ($f_V(\mathbf{W}, \mathbf{H})$ measures the difference between **V** and **WH**)

$$\min_{0 \leq \mathbf{W}, \mathbf{H}} f_V(\mathbf{W}, \mathbf{H}) \qquad (1)$$

to find an $M \times L$ non-negative feature (basis) matrix **W** and an $L \times N$ non-negative code (coefficient) matrix **H** such that (Lee, 1999)

$$\mathbf{V} \approx \mathbf{WH} \qquad (2)$$

Usually, $L \ll \min (M, N)$ so that good approximation can only be achieved if the feature matrix **W** represents the essential structure that is latent in $v_j, j = 1, 2, \cdots, N$ (Lee, 2000).

All applicable functions for f_V are not convex in (**W, H**), and therefore, to compute the global optimum is unrealistic for the large NMF problems common in, e.g., machine learning, computer vision, or image engineering (Heiler, 2006).. Instead, to compute a local solution by performing a block coordinate optimization is a feasible, universal thought for NMF (Heiler, 2006; Lee, 1999). By the way, L is the dimension of data after dimensionality reduction by NMF, and represents the scale of the minimization problem in Equation (2) while $\mathbf{V}$ has been fixed.

From the viewpoint of geometry, NMF can be considered as a method to find a simplicial cone in the positive orthant (Donoho, 2004). From the viewpoint of algebra, NMF discloses an intrinsic factorization or representation of non-negative data. From the viewpoint of dimensionality reduction, NMF show a nonlinear approach of reducing dimension of non-negative data. The major achievements about NMF can be seen in (Chen, 2003; Cichocki, 2006a; Cichocki, 2006b; Donoho, 2004; Dhillon, 2005; Heiler, 2006; Lee, 1999; Lee, 2000; Li, 2008; Liu, 2004b; Wild, 2004; Okun, 2006; Zdunek, 2006;).

With the development of NMF, many methods of improved NMF (INMF) are proposed. INMF enforces other expected limits on $\mathbf{W}$ and $\mathbf{H}$ except non-negativity, and can be classified into three categories, sparseness-improved NMF, discriminant NMF and weighted NMF (Li, 2007), as shown in Figure 1.

Definition 2: Denoting N observations of an M-dimensional non-negative stochastic variable $v_j, j = 1, 2, \cdots, N$, and arranging $v_j, j = 1, 2, \cdots, N$ into the columns of an $M \times N$ matrix $\mathbf{V}$, sparseness-improved NMF solves the problem ($f_V(\mathbf{W,H})$ measures the difference between $\mathbf{V}$ and $\mathbf{WH}$, $S(\mathbf{W})$ and $S(\mathbf{H})$ are respectively the penalty of sparseness for $\mathbf{W}$ and $\mathbf{H}$)

$$\min_{0 \leq \mathbf{W,H}} f_V(\mathbf{W,H}) + \lambda_w S(\mathbf{W}) + \lambda_H S(\mathbf{H}) \qquad (3)$$

to find an $M \times L$ non-negative feature (basis) matrix $\mathbf{W}$ and an $L \times N$ non-negative code (coefficient) matrix $\mathbf{H}$ such that $\mathbf{V} \approx \mathbf{WH}$ and $\mathbf{W}$ or $\mathbf{H}$ is of sparseness based on the value of λ_w and λ_H.

Definition 3: Denoting N observations of an M-dimensional non-negative stochastic variable $v_j, j = 1, 2, \cdots, N$, and arranging $v_j, j = 1, 2, \cdots, N$ into the columns of an $M \times N$ matrix V, discriminant NMF solves the problem ($f_V(\mathbf{W,H})$ measures the difference between V and WH, $D(\mathbf{W})$ and $D(\mathbf{H})$ are respectively the discriminant penalty for W and H)

$$\min_{0 \leq \mathbf{W,H}} f_V(\mathbf{W,H}) + \lambda_w D(\mathbf{W}) + \lambda_H D(\mathbf{H}) \qquad (4)$$

to find an $M \times L$ non-negative feature (basis) matrix $\mathbf{W}$ and an $L \times N$ non-negative code (coefficient) matrix $\mathbf{H}$ such that $\mathbf{V} \approx \mathbf{WH}$ and $\mathbf{W}$ or $\mathbf{H}$ holds discriminant information based on the value of λ_w and λ_H.

Definition 4: Denoting N observations of an M-dimensional non-negative stochastic variable $v_j, j = 1, 2, \cdots, N$, arranging $v_j, j = 1, 2, \cdots, N$ into the columns of an $\times N$ matrix $\mathbf{V}$, and designing a weight matrix $\mathbf{B}$, **weighted NMF** solves the

Figure 1. The relationship of NMF and INMF methods

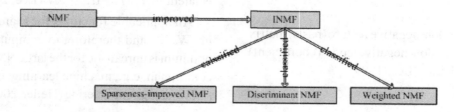

problem ($f_{\mathbf{B},\mathbf{V}}(\mathbf{W},\mathbf{H})$measures the difference between $\mathbf{B} \otimes \mathbf{V}$ and $\mathbf{B} \otimes \mathbf{WH}$)

$$\min_{0 \leq \mathbf{W},\mathbf{H}} f_{\mathbf{B},\mathbf{V}}(\mathbf{W},\mathbf{H}) \qquad (5)$$

to find an $M \times L$ non-negative feature (basis) matrix $\mathbf{W}$ and an $L \times N$ non-negative code (coefficient) matrix $\mathbf{H}$ such that

$$\mathbf{B} \otimes \mathbf{V} \approx \mathbf{B} \otimes \mathbf{WH} \qquad (6)$$

The major achievements of sparseness-improved NMF, discriminant NMF and weighted NMF can be seen in (Cichocki, 2006b; Ding, 2006; Li, 2001; Liu, 2003; Liu, 2004a; Hoyer, 2002; Hoyer, 2004; Heiler, 2006; Pascual-Montano, 2006; Xu, 2003), (Buciu, 2004; Heiler, 2006; Kotsia, 2007; Wang, 2004; Xue 2006; Zafeiriou, 2006) and (Blondel, 2009; Guillamet, 2001; Guillamet, 2003; Wang, 2006b) respectively.

ANALYSIS OF EXISTING NMF ALGORITHMS

This chapter focuses on the basic **NMF** (as shown in definition 1) model-based dimensionality reduction and feature extraction of face images, and therefore this section deeply discusses currently main NMF algorithms.

Lee and Seung consider $f_{\mathbf{V}}$ respectively as the square of the Euclidean distance and the generalized Kullback-Leibler (KL) divergence to design two monotonic multiplicative update-based algorithms by virtue of an auxiliary function analogous to that used for implementing the Expectation Maximization algorithm (Lee, 2000). They often play a role of de-facto baseline algorithms in the research of developing new algorithms. Therefore, for convenience of formulation, BaselineNMF-1 and BaselineNMF-2 respectively denote the algorithm based on the least squares error and

the one based on minimizing the generalized KL divergence in this chapter. BaselineNMF-1 and BaselineNMF-2 are the easiest to use at present and consequently are the most widely applied ones. They are the only two algorithms that hold all four following properties: (a) no dependence on any user-defined parameter, (b) simple iterative rules seeking no help from any other special algorithm, (c) no specific restriction on the initial value of iteration, and (d) high ease of deciding whether to stop or not.

Wild et al. propose a revised version of BaselineNMF-1 by using a structured initialization produced by spherical K-means clustering instead of a random initialization (Wild, 2004). According to Figure 10 in (Wild, 2004) (note that the computational load of spherical K-means clustering is not considered in this figure), the revised algorithm will be slightly more efficient than BaselineNMF-1 if a satisfactory clustering can be got by a few iterations. However, it tends to extract a set of relatively worse features than BaselineNMF-1 due to restrictions enforced on the structured initialization (Wild, 2004).

Okun et al. propose another revised version of BaselineNMF-1 by simultaneously scaling both $\mathbf{V}$ and the initial iterative values for $\mathbf{W}$ and $\mathbf{H}$ (Okun, 2006). Usually, this revision can only improve the first iteration of BaselineNMF-1 significantly.

Chen et al. put forward a least squares error-based monotonic descent NMF algorithm by the feasible direction-based optimization strategy with simulated annealing (Chen, 2003). It holds higher efficiency complexity than BaselineNMF-1 because the necessary process of one-dimensional search in the method of feasible direction and the implementation of simulated annealing are all very time-consuming. Besides, it cannot be as easy to use as BaselineNMF-1, since the parameters in the implementation of simulated annealing is user-defined. However, it can extract a set of relatively better features than BaselineNMF-1 according to the experiments in (Chen, 2003).

Liu et al. propose another least squares error-based NMF algorithm according to the relative gradient updates (Liu, 2004). Obviously, its performance is related to the choice of iterative step-size, and experiments show that it is much less efficient than BaselineNMF-1 (Liu, 2004).

Heiler et al. also design still another least squares error-based monotonic descent NMF algorithm by coordinately solving a series of convex quadric programming, and experimental results show it possesses analogous efficiency to BaselineNMF-1 while having recourse to the professional software of quadric programming in Mosek 3.2, a commercial optimization tool (Heiler, 2006).

Dhillon et al. minimize Bregman divergence between **V** and **WH** by the same optimization strategy as Lee and Seung's, and consequently put forward another monotonic NMF algorithm (Dhillon, 2005). Its efficiency has not been analyzed, but theoretically, it should hold similar efficiency to BaselineNMF-1 and BaselineNMF-2 for they are all based on the same optimization strategy. Different from BaselineNMF-1 and BaselineNMF-2, this algorithm contains a user-defined function, bad choices of which will result in the increased implementation difficulties and decreased performance of the algorithm, and vice versa.

Cichocki et al. start with applying multiplicative exponential gradient descent updates to the minimization of the dual generalized KL divergence between **V** and **WH**, and finally construct a very generic NMF algorithm that is applicable to minimize many kinds of divergences (Cichocki, 2006b). Choosing α divergence as f_V, Cichocki et al. design another NMF algorithm by using the projected (linearly transformed) gradient approach (Cichocki, 2006a), and Zdunek et al. also design a least α divergence-based algorithm which applies the quasi-Newton method followed by nonlinear projection onto positive orthant (Zdunek, 2006). Dhillon et al. deduce still another NMF algorithm to minimize the dual Bregman divergence between **V** and **WH** by use of

Karush-Kuhn-Tucker (KKT) conditions (Dhillon, 2005). These four algorithms are all somewhat heuristic; however, certain experiments have shown that some of them may be more suitable for a specific application (e.g. blind separation (Cichocki, 2006a)) than other ones. Their efficiency has not been analyzed, and to my knowledge, at least they are not designed to improve the speed of NMF. Furthermore, they are all theoretically uncertain to be monotonic. This increases the difficulty of using them, because the almost uncontrollable variation properties of $\{f_V(\mathbf{W}(k),\mathbf{H}(k))\}$ make their stop rules difficult to fix. That is to say, if a stop rule for any of the 4 algorithms is chosen, the corresponding iterative process may be stopped not until a relatively satisfactory solution (e.g. while $f_V(\mathbf{W}(k),\mathbf{H}(k)) - f_V(\mathbf{W}(k+1),\mathbf{H}(k+1)) < \varepsilon_{f_V}$ is considered as the stop rule), or a satisfactory solution may be missed (e.g. while the stop rule is to implement a fixed number of iterations). Besides, they all contain at least a user-defined parameter (or function), which may affect their performance, so they are relatively suitable for "advanced users".

All the above analysis is summarized in Table 2. It is evident that BaselineNMF-1 and BaselineNMF-2 are the easiest to use among existing algorithms and that available research achievements show no algorithm that is significantly more efficient than these two algorithms.

Then, it is very necessary to deeply analyze BaselineNMF-1's and BaselineNMF-2's efficiency to implement dimensionality reduction and feature extraction of face images. If their efficiency cannot be satisfactory, there will be urgent need for developing an algorithm that holds not only satisfactorily high efficiency for this kind of applications but also enough ease of use.

The optimization strategy of BaselineNMF-1 and BaselineNMF-2 is that an operation (an update for any of $W_{.1}, W_{.2}, \cdots, W_{.M}, H_{1.}, H_{2.}, \cdots, H_{N.}$) is based on an auxiliary function (with analytical

Table 2 Analysis on the applicability of existing NMF algorithms

Algorithm	Efficiency	Difficulty in use
BaselineNMF-1 (Lee, 2000)	Baseline	No
BaselineNMF-2 (Lee, 2000)	Baseline	No
Wild's algorithm (Wild, 2004)	According to experiments, slightly more efficient than BaselineNMF-1 at a cost of a set of worse features	A specific initial value dependent on another special algorithm
Okun's algorithm (Okun, 2006)	Just obviously improve the first iteration of BaselineNMF-1	No
Chen's algorithm (Chen, 2003)	Theoretically less efficient than BaselineNMF-1	Two user-defined parameters
Liu's algorithm (Liu, 2004)	Experimentally Less efficient than BaselineNMF-1	User-defined iterative step-size
Heiler's algorithm (Heiler, 2006)	Experimentally analogous to BaselineNMF-1	Dependence on another special algorithm
Dhillon's algorithm-1[a] (Dhillon, 2005)	Not researched but theoretically similar to BaselineNMF-1 &2	A user-defined function
Cichocki's algorithm-1[a] (Cichocki, 2006b)	Not researched in available articles	No definite stop rule, and a user-defined parameter
Cichocki's algorithm-2[a] (Cichocki, 2006a)	Not researched in available articles	No definite stop rule, and a user-defined parameter
Zdunek's algorithm (Zdunek, 2006)	Not researched in available articles	No definite stop rule, and two user-defined parameters
Dhillon's algorithm-2[a] (Dhillon, 2005)	Not researched in available articles	No definite stop rule, and a user-defined function
[a] Different algorithms of the same researchers are numbered according to their appearance order in the paper.		

non-negative minimum point) for the objective function of the current minimization problem. It focuses on the updated one of $W_{\cdot 1}, W_{\cdot 2}, \cdots, W_{\cdot M}, H_{1 \cdot}, H_{2 \cdot}, \cdots, H_{N \cdot}$ with the others fixed, and take the minimum point of the auxiliary function as its output to definitely make the objective function non-increasing. It is worth pointing out that the objective function of the current minimization problem is equivalent to the objective function of the minimization problem for **NMF** while fixing $W_{\cdot 1}, W_{\cdot 2}, \cdots, W_{\cdot M}, H_{1 \cdot}, H_{2 \cdot}, \cdots, H_{N \cdot}$ except the currently updated one of them (Lee, 2000). Hence, to alternately implement updates for $W_{\cdot 1}, W_{\cdot 2}, \cdots, W_{\cdot M}, H_{1 \cdot}, H_{2 \cdot}, \cdots, H_{N \cdot}$ by this way can produce a monotonic descent algorithm.

According to Figure 2 (cited from (Lee, 2000) where BaselineNMF-1 and BaselineNMF-2 are put forward), suppose that $F(h)$, h^t and $G(h,h^t)$ are respectively the objective function of the current minimization problem, the starting point of this operation and the current auxiliary function, and then h^{t+1} is the minimum point of $G(h,h^t)$ and the output of this operation. There is a long distance between h^{t+1} and h_{min} (the minimum point of $F(h)$), although $F(h^{t+1}) < F(h^t)$. All the above analysis qualitatively explains the defect inherent in BaselineNMF-1 and BaselineNMF-2. Therefore, in an operation, BaselineNMF-1 and BaselineNMF-2 cannot fully decrease their respective objective functions, and then the two algorithms' efficiency cannot be high.

Figure 2. An explanation for the optimization strategy used in BaselineNMF-1 and BaselineNMF-2

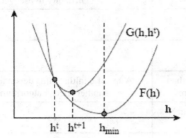

Figure 3 records the iterative process of implementing the dimensionality reduction and feature extraction of all 400 face images of ORL database (ORL face database,1992) by BaselineNMF-1 on a Pentium 4 CPU 3G Hz, 1.5G RAM computer (all experimental records will be based on this computer in this chapter), while $L=160$. Every face image of ORL database is vectorized and arranged into a column of **V**. The iterative outcome by BaselineNMF-1 is evaluated and represented by the Frobenius norm-based relative error between **V** and $\mathbf{W}(k)\mathbf{H}(k)$. Figure 3(a) portrays the curve based on the first 3000 seconds' iterative outcomes to show BaselineNMF-1's holistic iterative performance, and the iterative curve in Figure 3(b) is just based on the first 500 seconds'

iterative ones to prominently exhibit the performance in its initial iterative phase. Obviously, BaselineNMF-1 cannot approximately converge by less than 2000 seconds in this case. Therefore, to do a large amount of experiments to statistically find or validate NMF's application properties about face analysis is usually very time-consuming. It is worth noting that the 400 face images of ORL database just represent a relatively small-scale data in face analysis, which causes inconvenience to many application researches in this kind of research field. Figure 3(b) distinctly shows that the initial part of the iterative curve is very smooth, which badly restrains the efficiency of BaselineNMF-1 and is essentially caused by the problem revealed by Figure 2.

Figure 4 records the iterative process of implementing the dimensionality reduction and feature extraction of all 400 face images of ORL database(ORL face database,1992) by BaselineNMF-2, while $L=160$. The iterative outcome by BaselineNMF-2 is evaluated and represented by the generalized KL divergence between **V** and $\mathbf{W}(k)\mathbf{H}(k)$. Obviously, BaselineNMF-2 has similar efficiency to BaselineNMF-1, which is compatible with the fact that they apply the same optimization strategy.

Figure 3. The iterative process of implementing the dimensionality reduction and feature extraction of all 400 face images of ORL database by BaselineNMF-1 (L=160), in which iterative outcomes are evaluated and represented by the Frobenius norm-based relative error: (a) 3000 seconds' iteration; (b) 500 seconds' iteration.

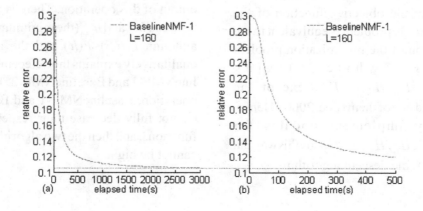

Figure 4. The iterative process of implementing the dimensionality reduction and feature extraction of all 400 face images of ORL database by BaselineNMF-2 (L=160), in which iterative outcomes are evaluated and represented by the generalized KL divergence: (a) 3000 seconds' iteration; (b) 500 seconds' iteration.

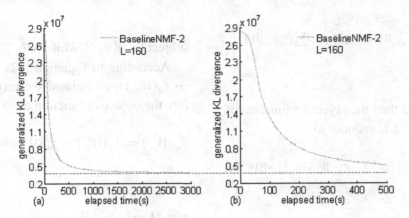

In summary, there is still no NMF algorithm that is able to hold not only satisfactory efficiency for dimensionality reduction and feature extraction of face images but also high ease of use. This causes inconvenience to the present researches on applications related to face analysis, and partly restrains the further NMF application development in this field.

FASTNMF

To improve the applicability of NMF, this section puts forward a new NMF algorithm called FastNMF.

A least squares error-based non-negative factorization is considered here, and then the corresponding minimization problem for NMF comes down to:

$$\min_{0 \leq \mathbf{W}, \mathbf{H}} \| \mathbf{V} - \mathbf{WH} \|_F^2 \tag{7}$$

Based on the minimization model in Equation (7) and the basic properties of parabola functions, it is easy to get two valuable theorems as follows.

Theorem 1. $\forall i \in \{1, 2, \cdots, L\}$, with $\mathbf{H}$ and $\{W_{\cdot 1}, W_{\cdot 2}, \cdots, W_{\cdot L}\} / W_{\cdot i}$ fixed, let

$$E_{ab} = [\mathbf{HH}^{\mathrm{T}}]_{ab}(1 - \delta_{ai}\delta_{ib}), \forall a, b \in \{1, 2, \cdots, L\} \tag{8}$$

then the objective function in Equation (7) reaches to the minimum point at

$$W_{\cdot i} = \max\{\frac{[\mathbf{VH}^{\mathrm{T}}]_{\cdot i} - \mathbf{W}E_{\cdot i})}{[\mathbf{HH}^{\mathrm{T}}]_{ii}}, \varepsilon\} \tag{9}$$

subject to $W_{\cdot i} \geq \varepsilon$ while $\| H_{i\cdot} \|_1 > 0$.

Proof: Because

$$\begin{aligned}
\| \mathbf{V} - \mathbf{WH} \|_F^2 &= trace\{(\mathbf{V} - \mathbf{WH})(\mathbf{V} - \mathbf{WH})^{\mathrm{T}}\} \\
&= trace\{\mathbf{VV}^{\mathrm{T}} - 2\mathbf{WHV}^{\mathrm{T}} + \mathbf{WHH}^{\mathrm{T}}\mathbf{W}^{\mathrm{T}}\} \\
&= trace\{\mathbf{VV}^{\mathrm{T}}\} - 2\sum_{d=1}^{M} W_{d\cdot}[\mathbf{HV}^{\mathrm{T}}]_{\cdot d} + \sum_{d=1}^{M} W_{d\cdot}\mathbf{HH}^{\mathrm{T}}W_{d\cdot}^{\mathrm{T}}
\end{aligned} \tag{10}$$

the objective function of $W_{c\cdot}, \forall c \in \{1,2,\cdots,M\}$, reduces to

$$f_{\mathbf{W}}(W_{c\cdot}) = W_{c\cdot}\mathbf{HH}^T W_{c\cdot}^T - 2W_{c\cdot}[\mathbf{HV}^T]_{\cdot c}$$
$$= \sum_{k=1}^{L}\sum_{l=1}^{L} W_{ck}[\mathbf{HH}^T]_{kl}W_{cl} - 2\sum_{h=1}^{L} W_{ch}[\mathbf{HV}^T]_{hc} \tag{11}$$

With $\mathbf{H}$ fixed, and then the objective function of $W_{ci}, \forall i \in \{1,2,\cdots,L\}$, reduces to

$$f_{\mathbf{W}}(W_{ci}) = [\mathbf{HH}^T]_{ii}W_{ci}^2 + 2W_{ci}\left(\sum_{k=1,k\neq i}^{L} W_{ck}[\mathbf{HH}^T]_{ki} - [\mathbf{HV}^T]_{ic}\right) \tag{12}$$

With $\mathbf{H}$ and $\{W_{c1}, W_{c2}, \cdots, W_{cL}\}/W_{ci}$ fixed. Based on Equation (8), $\sum_{k=1,k\neq i}^{L} W_{ck}[\mathbf{HH}^T]_{ki} = W_{c\cdot}E_{\cdot i}$.

$f_{W}(W_{ci})$ is a parabola function, and $[\mathbf{HH}^T]_{ii} > 0$ while $\|H_{i\cdot}\|_1 > 0$. To minimize $f_{W}(W_{ci})$ subject to $W_{ci} \geq \varepsilon$, W_{ci} should be equal to the minimum point $(([\mathbf{VH}^T]_{ci} - W_{c\cdot}E_{\cdot i})/[\mathbf{HH}]_{ii})$ of $f_{W}(W_{ci})$ if the minimum point $\geq \varepsilon$ (the situation shown by Figure 5 (a)) or be equal to ε if the minimum point $< \varepsilon$ (the situation shown by Figure 5 (b)). Based on the above analysis, with $\mathbf{H}$ and $\{W_{c1}, W_{c2}, \cdots, W_{cL}\}/W_{ci}$ fixed, $f_{W}(W_{ci})$ reaches to the minimum point at

$$W_{ci} = \max\left\{\frac{[\mathbf{VH}^T]_{ci} - W_{c\cdot}E_{\cdot i}}{[\mathbf{HH}]_{ii}}, \varepsilon\right\} \tag{13}$$

subject to $W_{ci} \geq \varepsilon$ while $\|H_{i\cdot}\|_1 > 0$.

According to Equation (12), $f_{W}(W_{1i}), f_{W}(W_{2i}), \cdots f_{W}(W_{Mi})$ are unrelated to each other, and therefore the objective function of $W_{\cdot i}$ reduces to

$$f_{\mathbf{W}}(W_{\cdot i}) = f_{\mathbf{W}}(W_{1i}) + f_{\mathbf{W}}(W_{2i}) + \cdots + f_{\mathbf{W}}(W_{Mi}) \tag{14}$$

with $\mathbf{H}$ and $\{W_{\cdot 1}, W_{\cdot 2}, \cdots, W_{\cdot L}\}/W_{\cdot i}$ fixed, which reaches to the minimum point at

$$W_{\cdot i} = \begin{bmatrix} \max\left\{\dfrac{[\mathbf{VH}^T]_{1i} - W_{1\cdot}E_{\cdot i}}{[\mathbf{HH}^T]_{ii}}, \varepsilon\right\} \\ \max\left\{\dfrac{[\mathbf{VH}^T]_{2i} - W_{2\cdot}E_{\cdot i}}{[\mathbf{HH}^T]_{ii}}, \varepsilon\right\} \\ \vdots \\ \max\left\{\dfrac{[\mathbf{VH}^T]_{Mi} - W_{M\cdot}E_{\cdot i}}{[\mathbf{HH}^T]_{ii}}, \varepsilon\right\} \end{bmatrix} \tag{15}$$

Figure 5. Two possible situations of $f_W(W_{ci})$ while $[\mathbf{HH}^T]_{ii} > 0$: (a) the minimum point ≥ 0; (b) the minimum point < 0

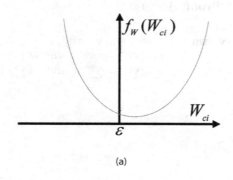

(a)

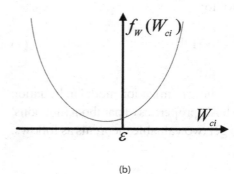

(b)

subject to $W_{\cdot i} \geq 0$ while $\| H_{i \cdot} \|_1 > 0$. Equation (15) can be expressed as Equation (9) in style that is more compact. **Q.E.D.**

Theorem 2. $\forall j \in \{1, 2, \cdots, L\}$, with $\mathbf{W}$ and $\{H_{1 \cdot}, H_{2 \cdot}, \cdots, H_{L \cdot}\} / H_{j \cdot}$ fixed, let

$$F_{ab} = [\mathbf{W}^\mathrm{T}\mathbf{W}]_{ab}(1 - \delta_{aj}\delta_{jb}), \quad \forall a, b \in \{1, 2, \cdots, L\} \tag{16}$$

then the objective function in Equation (7) reaches to the minimum point at

$$H_{j \cdot} = \max\{\frac{[\mathbf{W}^T\mathbf{V}]_{j \cdot} - F_{j \cdot}\mathbf{H}}{[\mathbf{W}^T\mathbf{W}]_{jj}}, \varepsilon\} \tag{17}$$

subject to $H_{j \cdot} \geq \varepsilon$ while $\| W_{\cdot j} \|_1 > 0$.

Proof: It is easy to find that $W_{\cdot j}$ and $H_{j \cdot}$ are dual in $\| \mathbf{V} - \mathbf{W}\mathbf{H} \|_F^2$ for $\forall j \in \{1, 2, \cdots, L\}$, and therefore, the proof for theorem 2 is very similar to that for theorem 1.

Similar to Equation (10), it is easy to get that

$$\| \mathbf{V} - \mathbf{W}\mathbf{H} \|_F^2 = trace\{\mathbf{V}\mathbf{V}^\mathrm{T}\} - 2\sum_{g=1}^{N}[\mathbf{V}^\mathrm{T}\mathbf{W}]_{g \cdot}H_{\cdot g} + \sum_{g=1}^{N}H_{\cdot g}^\mathrm{T}\mathbf{W}^\mathrm{T}\mathbf{W}H_{\cdot g} \tag{18}$$

Then, the objective function of $H_{\cdot f}$, $\forall f \in \{1, 2, \cdots, N\}$, reduces to

$$f_\mathbf{H}(H_{\cdot f}) = H_{\cdot f}^\mathrm{T}\mathbf{W}^\mathrm{T}\mathbf{W}H_{\cdot f} - 2[\mathbf{V}^\mathrm{T}\mathbf{W}]_{f \cdot}H_{\cdot f}$$
$$= \sum_{k=1}^{L}\sum_{l=1}^{L}H_{kf}[\mathbf{W}^\mathrm{T}\mathbf{W}]_{kl}H_{lf} - 2\sum_{h=1}^{L}[\mathbf{V}^\mathrm{T}\mathbf{W}]_{fh}H_{hf} \tag{19}$$

with $\mathbf{W}$ fixed. Thus, the objective function of H_{jf}, $\forall j \in \{1, 2, \cdots, L\}$, reduces to

$$f_\mathbf{H}(H_{jf}) = H_{jf}^2[\mathbf{W}^\mathrm{T}\mathbf{W}]_{jj} + 2H_{jf}(\sum_{l=1, l \neq j}^{L}[\mathbf{W}^\mathrm{T}\mathbf{W}]_{jl}H_{lf} - [\mathbf{V}^\mathrm{T}\mathbf{W}]_{fj}) \tag{20}$$

with $\mathbf{W}$ and $\{H_{1f}, H_{2f}, \cdots, H_{Lf}\} / H_{jf}$ fixed. Based on Equation (16), $\sum_{l=1, l \neq j}^{L}[\mathbf{W}^\mathrm{T}\mathbf{W}]_{jl}H_{lf} = F_{j \cdot}H_{\cdot f}$.

Still based on the analysis to get Equation (13), with $\mathbf{W}$ and $\{H_{1f}, H_{2f}, \cdots, H_{Lf}\} / H_{jf}$ fixed, $f_H(H_{jf})$ reaches to the minimum point at

$$H_{jf} = \max\{\frac{[\mathbf{W}^\mathrm{T}\mathbf{V}]_{jf} - F_{j \cdot}H_{\cdot f}}{[\mathbf{W}^\mathrm{T}\mathbf{W}]_{jj}}, \varepsilon\} \tag{21}$$

subject to $H_{jf} \geq \varepsilon$ while $\| W_{\cdot j} \|_1 > 0$.

According to Equation (20), $f_\mathbf{H}(H_{j1})$, $f_\mathbf{H}(H_{j2})$ $\cdots, f_\mathbf{H}(H_{jN})$ are unrelated to each other, and therefore the objective function of $H_{j \cdot}$ reduces to

$$f_\mathbf{H}(H_{j \cdot}) = f_\mathbf{H}(H_{j1}) + f_\mathbf{H}(H_{j2}) + \cdots + f_\mathbf{H}(H_{jN}) \tag{22}$$

with $\mathbf{W}$ and $\{H_{1 \cdot}, H_{2 \cdot}, \cdots, H_{L \cdot}\} / H_{j \cdot}$ fixed, which reaches to the minimum point at Equation (17) subject to $H_{j \cdot} \geq \varepsilon$ while $\| W_{\cdot j} \|_1 > 0$. **Q.E.D.**

For $\mathbf{W}(0) \geq \varepsilon$ and $\mathbf{H}(0) \geq \varepsilon$, it monotonically decreases the objective function in Equation (7) to alternately update $W_{\cdot 1}, W_{\cdot 2}, \cdots, W_{\cdot L}, H_{1 \cdot}, H_{2 \cdot}, \cdots, H_{L \cdot}$ according to Theorems 1~2. The pseudo-code for doing so is given in Figure 6.

It is worth noting that to prescribe $\mathbf{W}(0) \geq \varepsilon$ and $\mathbf{H}(0) \geq \varepsilon$ rather than $\mathbf{W}(0) \geq 0$ and $\mathbf{H}(0) \geq 0$ in FastNMF not only eliminates the possibility that $[\mathbf{W}^T(k)\mathbf{W}(k)]_{jj} = 0$ or $[\mathbf{H}(k)\mathbf{H}^T(k)]_{ii} = 0$ and consequently avoids the situation of mathematically no definition ("divided by 0" in line 6 and 11 of pseudo-code of FastNMF), but also hardly affects the descent speed of the algorithm (because $\varepsilon \to 0$). And in fact, if we choose the initial iterative value without any restriction, there is not any harm to FastNMF's performance, be-

Figure 6. Pseudo-code for FastNMF

FastNMF
Input: V, L
Output: W, H

---

1. Initialize $\mathbf{W}(0) \geq \varepsilon$ and $\mathbf{H}(0) \geq \varepsilon$ randomly, $k \leftarrow 0$
2. Repeat
3. $\mathbf{D}(k) = [\mathbf{H}(k)\mathbf{H}^T(k)]$, $\quad \mathbf{Q}(k) = \mathbf{V}\mathbf{H}^T(k)$
4. For i from 1 to L
5. $\quad E_{ab}(k) = [\mathbf{D}(k)]_{ab}(1 - \delta_{ai}\delta_{ib}), \forall a, b \in \{1, 2, \cdots, L\}$
6. $\quad W_{i}(k+1) \leftarrow \max\{\dfrac{[\mathbf{Q}(k)]_{.i} - [W_{.1}(k+1), \cdots, W_{.i-1}(k+1), W_{.i}(k), \cdots, W_{.L}(k)]E_{.i}(k)}{[\mathbf{D}(k)]_{ii}}, \varepsilon\}$
7. End For
8. $\mathbf{C}(k) = [\mathbf{W}^T(k+1)\mathbf{W}(k+1)]$, $\quad \mathbf{R}(k) = \mathbf{W}^T(k+1)\mathbf{V}$
9. For j from 1 to L
10. $\quad F_{ab}(k) = [\mathbf{C}(k)]_{ab}(1 - \delta_{aj}\delta_{jb}), \forall a, b \in \{1, 2, \cdots, L\}$
11. $\quad H_{j.}(k+1) \leftarrow \max\{\dfrac{[\mathbf{R}(k)]_{j.} - F_{j.}(k)[H_{1.}^T(k+1), \cdots, H_{j-1.}^T(k+1), H_{j.}^T(k), \cdots H_{L.}^T(k)]^T}{[\mathbf{C}(k)]_{jj}}, \varepsilon\}$
12. End For
13. Until $\dfrac{\|\mathbf{V} - \mathbf{W}(k)\mathbf{H}(k)\|_F - \|\mathbf{V} - \mathbf{W}(k+1)\mathbf{H}(k+1)\|_F}{\|\mathbf{V}\|_F} < 10^{-5}$

---

cause it is certain to get that $\mathbf{W}(k) \geq \varepsilon$ and $\mathbf{H}(k) \geq \varepsilon$ for $k \geq 1$ according to Equation (9) and Equation (17), and consequently that $\{\|\mathbf{V} - \mathbf{W}(k)\mathbf{H}(k)\|_F, k \geq 1\}$ is monotonically decreasing.

PROPERTIES OF FASTNMF

In this section, the efficiency, ease of use, extracted features' quality, comprehensibility, stability and convergence of **FastNMF** will be discussed.

Efficiency

According to theorems 1 and 2, the minimization problem corresponding to an operation (an update for any of $W_{.1}, W_{.2}, \cdots, W_{.L}, H_{1.}, H_{2.}, \cdots, H_{L.}$) in **FastNMF** can be analytically solved just by this operation. That is to say, in every operation **Fast-NMF** furthest decreases its objective function, which is far beyond all existing algorithms' power.

Hence, the algorithm is certain to hold much higher efficiency, which is its leading characteristic and enlightens us to coin **FastNMF** for it.

Ease of Use

Obviously, **FastNMF** is as easy to use as BaselineNMF-1 and BaselineNMF-2, because they all (a) depend on no user-defined parameter, (b) hold simple iterative rules seeking no help from any other special algorithm, (c) enforce no specific restriction on the initial value of iteration, and (d) are easy to decide whether to stop or not.

Extracted Feature's Quality

BaselineNMF-1 is implemented by coordinately doing (lee, 2000)

① j from 1 to L

$$H_{j.}(k+1) \leftarrow H_{j.}(k) \otimes [\mathbf{W}^T(k)\mathbf{V}]_{j.} \odot [\mathbf{W}^T(k)\mathbf{W}(k)\mathbf{H}(k)]_{j.} \tag{23}$$

② i from 1 to L

$$W_{\cdot i}(k+1) \leftarrow W_{\cdot i}(k) \otimes [\mathbf{VH}^T(k)]_{\cdot i} \odot [\mathbf{W}(k)\mathbf{H}(k)\mathbf{H}^T(k)]_{\cdot i}$$
(24)

BaselineNMF-2 is implemented by coordinately doing (lee, 2000)

① j from 1 to L

$$H_{j\cdot}(k+1) \leftarrow H_{j\cdot}(k) \otimes \{\mathbf{W}^T(k)\{\mathbf{V} \odot [\mathbf{W}(k)\mathbf{H}(k)]\}\}_{j\cdot} \odot [\mathbf{W}^T(k)\mathbf{1}_{M \times N}]_{j\cdot}$$
(25)

② i from 1 to L

$$W_{\cdot i}(k+1) \leftarrow W_{\cdot i}(k) \otimes \{\{\mathbf{V} \odot [\mathbf{W}(k)\mathbf{H}(k)]\}\mathbf{H}^T(k)\}_{\cdot i} \odot [\mathbf{1}_{M \times N}\mathbf{H}^T(k)]_{\cdot i}$$
(26)

$\forall i, j$, according to the multiplicative updates of BaselineNMF-1 and BaselineNMF-2, $H_{ij}(k+1)$ (or $W_{ij}(k+1)$) $\leftarrow \varepsilon$ if $H_{ij}(k)$ (or $W_{ij}(k)$) $\leftarrow \varepsilon$. So the feasible region of NMF problem becomes smaller and smaller with BaselineNMF-1 and BaselineNMF-2 implemented.

On the contrary, $\forall i, j$, even though $H_{ij}(k)$ (or $W_{ij}(k)$) $\leftarrow \varepsilon$, $H_{ij}(k+1)$ (or $W_{ij}(k+1)$) can be updated as any positive number by FastNMF's iterative rules. That is to say, the implementation of FastNMF does not change the feasible region of the corresponding NMF problem at all.

As a result, FastNMF tends to converge to better solutions than BaselineNMF-1 and BaselineNMF-2 as far as approximation accuracy is concerned.

In fact, $\mathbf{W}$ represents all of NMF solutions, because $\mathbf{H}$ can be solved according to a chosen function for $f_{\mathbf{V}}$ while $\mathbf{W}$ is fixed. Therefore, based on the discussion above, FastNMF actually tends to extract better features than BaselineNMF-1 and Baseline- NMF-2 as far as the representation ability is concerned.

Comprehensibility

According to Equation (7), Theorems 1~2, and Figure 5 (pseudo-code for FastNMF), FastNMF is just based on the most familiar objective function and the most basic properties of parabola functions.

Obviously, FastNMF seems to be more comprehensible than other algorithms mentioned in section 3.

Stability

To get the theorem to ensure the stability of Fast-NMF, it is essential to get four valuable lemmas as follows.

Lemma 1: $\forall M, L \in Z^+$, let $\mathbf{A} \in R^{M \times L}$, then $\|\mathbf{A}\|_{Abs-sum} = \sum_{i=1}^{M} \sum_{j=1}^{L} |A_{ij}|$ is a norm for it.

Proof: For $\forall \mathbf{A} \in R^{M \times L}$ and $\forall \mathbf{C} \in R^{L \times N}$,

$$\begin{aligned}
\|\mathbf{AC}\|_{Abs-sum} &= \|[\sum_{i=1}^{L} A_{\cdot i}C_{i1}, \sum_{i=1}^{L} A_{\cdot i}C_{i2}, \cdots, \sum_{i=1}^{L} A_{\cdot i}C_{iN}]\|_{Abs-sum} \\
&= \sum_{j=1}^{N} \|\sum_{i=1}^{L} A_{\cdot i}C_{ij}\|_1 \\
&\leq \sum_{j=1}^{N} \sum_{i=1}^{L} \|A_{\cdot i}\|_1 |C_{ij}| \\
&= \sum_{i=1}^{L} \|A_{\cdot i}\|_1 \|C_{i\cdot}\|_1 \\
&\leq \sum_{i=1}^{L} \|A_{\cdot i}\|_1 \sum_{i=1}^{L} \|C_{i\cdot}\|_1 \quad \text{(according to holder inequality)} \\
&= \|\mathbf{A}\|_{Abs-sum} \|\mathbf{C}\|_{Abs-sum} \quad \text{(compatibility)}
\end{aligned}$$
(27)

For $\forall \mathbf{A}, \mathbf{B} \in R^{M \times L}$ and $\forall \alpha \in R$, it is obvious that $\|\mathbf{A}\|_{Abs-sum} \geq 0$ (non-negativity), $\|\alpha \mathbf{A}\|_{Abs-sum} = |\alpha| \|\mathbf{A}\|_{Abs-sum}$ (homogeneity) and $\|\mathbf{A} + \mathbf{B}\|_{Abs-sum} \leq \|\mathbf{A}\|_{Abs-sum} + \|\mathbf{B}\|_{Abs-sum}$ (triangle inequality). **Q.E.D.**

Lemma 2: By **FastNMF**'s iterative rules, $\{(\mathbf{W}(k), \mathbf{H}(k))\}$ is bounded.

Proof: suppose that $\{(\mathbf{W}(k), \mathbf{H}(k))\}$ is unbounded. There are three possible situations as follows: (a) $\{\mathbf{H}(k)\}$ is unbounded, (b) $\{\mathbf{W}(k)\}$ is unbounded, and (c) $\{\mathbf{W}(k)\}$ and $\{\mathbf{H}(k)\}$ are all unbounded.

For $\mathbf{W}(0) \geq \varepsilon$ and $\mathbf{H}(0) \geq \varepsilon$, $\mathbf{W}(k) \geq \varepsilon$ and $\mathbf{H}(k) \geq \varepsilon$ according to corollaries 1 and 2, and therefore

$$\|\mathbf{W}(k)\mathbf{H}(k)\|_{Abs-sum} = \sum_{j=1}^{M} \|\sum_{i=1}^{L} W_{ji}(k)H_{i\cdot}(k)\|_1 = \sum_{j=1}^{M} \sum_{i=1}^{L} \sum_{l=1}^{N} W_{ji}(k)H_{il}(k)$$

.

For situation (a), $\| \mathbf{W}(k)\mathbf{H}(k) \|_{Abs-sum} \geq M\varepsilon \| \mathbf{H}(k) \|_{Abs-sum}$, so $\{\| \mathbf{W}(k)\mathbf{H}(k) \|_{Abs-sum}\}$ is unbounded. $\| \mathbf{W}(k)\mathbf{H}(k) \|_{Abs-sum} - \| \mathbf{V} \|_{Abs-sum} \leq \| \mathbf{V} - \mathbf{W}(k)\mathbf{H}(k) \|_{Abs-sum}$ and therefore, $\{\| \mathbf{V} - \mathbf{W}(k)\mathbf{H}(k) \|_{Abs-sum}\}$ is unbounded. $\{\| \mathbf{V} - \mathbf{W}(k)\mathbf{H}(k) \|_{F}\}$ is monotonically decreasing and bounded below, and thus it is bounded. According to lemma 1, $\|\bullet\|_{Abs-sum}$ is a norm, then $\|\bullet\|_{F}$ is equivalent to $\|\bullet\|_{Abs-sum}$ for $R^{M \times N}$ (Kreyszig, 1978), so that $\{\| \mathbf{W}(k)\mathbf{H}(k) \|_{Abs-sum}\}$ is bounded, a contradiction. Situation (a) is impossible.

For the same reason, situation (b) is impossible. Then obviously, situation (c) is also impossible. **Q.E.D.**

Lemma 3: $\| \mathbf{V} - \mathbf{WH} \|_{F}^{2}$ is a continuous function of $(\mathbf{W}, \mathbf{H})$.

Proof:

$$\lim_{\Delta \mathbf{W} \to 0, \Delta \mathbf{H} \to 0} \| \mathbf{V} - (\mathbf{W} + \Delta \mathbf{W})(\mathbf{H} + \Delta \mathbf{H}) \|_{F}^{2} - \| \mathbf{V} - \mathbf{WH} \|_{F}^{2}$$
$$= \lim_{\Delta \mathbf{W} \to 0, \Delta \mathbf{H} \to 0} trace\{[\mathbf{V} - (\mathbf{W} + \Delta \mathbf{W})(\mathbf{H} + \Delta \mathbf{H})] \cdot$$
$$[\mathbf{V} - (\mathbf{W} + \Delta \mathbf{W})(\mathbf{H} + \Delta \mathbf{H})]^{\mathsf{T}} - (\mathbf{V} - \mathbf{WH})(\mathbf{V} - \mathbf{WH})^{\mathsf{T}}\}$$
$$= \lim_{\Delta \mathbf{W} \to 0, \Delta \mathbf{Q} \to 0} trace\{2(-\mathbf{V} + \mathbf{WH})(\Delta \mathbf{WH} + \mathbf{W}\Delta \mathbf{H} + \Delta \mathbf{W}\Delta \mathbf{H})^{\mathsf{T}}$$
$$+ (\Delta \mathbf{WH} + \mathbf{W}\Delta \mathbf{H} + \Delta \mathbf{W}\Delta \mathbf{H})(\Delta \mathbf{WH} + \mathbf{W}\Delta \mathbf{H} + \Delta \mathbf{W}\Delta \mathbf{H})^{\mathsf{T}}\}$$
$$= 0$$

$$(28)$$

According to the definition of a continuous function in (Kreyszig, 1978), the proposition in lemma 3 is right. **Q.E.D.**

Lemma 4: $\forall i \in \{1, 2, \cdots, L\}$, $\| \mathbf{V} - \mathbf{WH} \|_{F}^{2}$ is strictly convex in $W_{\bullet i}$ with H and $\{W_{\bullet 1}, W_{\bullet 2}, \cdots, W_{\bullet L}\} / W_{\bullet i}$ fixed, while $[\mathbf{HH}^{T}]_{ii} > 0$; $\forall j \in \{1, 2, \cdots, L\}$, $\| \mathbf{V} - \mathbf{WH} \|_{F}^{2}$ is strictly convex in $H_{j \bullet}$ with W and $\{H_{1 \bullet}, H_{2 \bullet}, \cdots, H_{L \bullet}\} / H_{j \bullet}$ fixed, while $[\mathbf{W}^{T}\mathbf{W}]_{jj} > 0$.

Proof: According to Equation (12) and Equation (14), $\forall i \in \{1, 2, \cdots, L\}$, the objective function ($\| \mathbf{V} - \mathbf{W} \mathbf{H} \|_{F}^{2}$) of $W_{\bullet i}$ reduces to

$$f(W_{\bullet i}) = W_{\bullet i}^{\mathsf{T}}\{[\mathbf{HH}^{\mathsf{T}}]_{ii}\mathbf{I}\}W_{\bullet i}$$
$$+ 2\sum_{d=1}^{M} W_{di}(\sum_{k=1, k \neq i}^{L} W_{dk}[\mathbf{HH}^{\mathsf{T}}]_{ki} - [\mathbf{HV}^{\mathsf{T}}]_{id})$$

$$(29)$$

with $\mathbf{H}$ and $\{W_{\bullet 1}, W_{\bullet 2}, \cdots, W_{\bullet L}\} / W_{\bullet i}$ fixed.

Because $[\mathbf{HH}^{T}]_{ii}\mathbf{I}$ is the Hesse matrix of $f(W_{\bullet i})$ and is positive definite while $[\mathbf{HH}^{T}]_{ii} > 0$, $f(W_{\bullet i})$ is strictly convex in $W_{\bullet i}$.

$\forall j \in \{1, 2, \cdots, L\}$, $W_{\bullet i}$ and $H_{j \bullet}$ are dual in $\| \mathbf{V} - \mathbf{WH} \|_{F}^{2}$, so by the same token, $\| \mathbf{V} - \mathbf{WH} \|_{F}^{2}$ is strictly convex in $H_{j \bullet}$ with W and $\{H_{1 \bullet}, H_{2 \bullet}, \cdots, H_{L \bullet}\} / H_{j \bullet}$ fixed, while $[\mathbf{W}^{T}\mathbf{W}]_{jj} > 0$. **Q.E.D.**

Theorem 3 (Stability of FastNMF). By FastNMF's iterative rules, $\| (\mathbf{W}(k + b), \mathbf{H}(k + b)) - (\mathbf{W}(k), \mathbf{H}(k)) \| \to 0$ for $\forall b \in Z^{+}$.

Proof: suppose that $\| (\mathbf{W}(k+1), \mathbf{H}(k+1)) - (\mathbf{W}(k), \mathbf{H}(k)) \| \to 0$ is wrong. Then, there exist a subsequence $\{(\mathbf{W}(k_{l}), \mathbf{H}(k_{l}))\}$ such that $\| (\mathbf{W}(k_{l} + 1), \mathbf{H}(k_{l} + 1)) - (\mathbf{W}(k_{l}), \mathbf{H}(k_{l})) \| > \delta > 0$ $(l = 1, 2, \cdots)$.

According to Lemma 2, $\{(\mathbf{W}(k), \mathbf{H}(k))\}$ is bounded, so there is a convergent subsequence $\{(\mathbf{W}(k_{l_{h}}), \mathbf{H}(k_{l_{h}}))\}$ in $\{\mathbf{W}(k_{l}), \mathbf{H}(k_{l})\}$. Moreover, it is obviously true that $\| (\mathbf{W}(k_{l_{h}} + 1), \mathbf{H}(k_{l_{h}} + 1)) - (\mathbf{W}(k_{l_{h}}), \mathbf{H}(k_{l_{h}})) \| > \delta > 0$ $(h = 1, 2, \cdots)$.

Suppose that $\{\mathbf{W}(k_{l_{h}}), \mathbf{H}(k_{l_{h}})\} \to (\bar{\mathbf{W}}, \bar{\mathbf{H}})$. Because $\| \mathbf{V} - \mathbf{WH} \|_{F}^{2}$ is continuous for $\forall \mathbf{W} \in R^{M \times L}$ and $\forall \mathbf{H} \in R^{L \times N}$ according to Lemma 3, $\{\| \mathbf{V} - \mathbf{W}(k_{l_{h}})\mathbf{H}(k_{l_{h}}) \|_{F}^{2}\} \to \| \mathbf{V} - \bar{\mathbf{W}}\bar{\mathbf{H}} \|_{F}^{2}$. Then $\{\| \mathbf{V} - \mathbf{W}(k)\mathbf{H}(k) \|_{F}^{2}\} \to \| \mathbf{V} - \bar{\mathbf{W}}\bar{\mathbf{H}} \|_{F}^{2}$ for $\{\| \mathbf{V} - \mathbf{W}(k)\mathbf{H}(k) \|_{F}^{2}\}$ converges.

Furthermore,

$$\{\| \mathbf{V} - [W_{\bullet1}(k_{l_h}+1), W_{\bullet2}(k_{l_h}), \cdots, W_{\bullet L}(k_{l_h})]\mathbf{H} \|_F^2\} \to \| \mathbf{V} - \bar{\mathbf{W}}\bar{\mathbf{H}} \|_F^2$$

b e c a u s e $\{(W_{\bullet1}(k_{l_h}+1),$ $W_{\bullet2}(k_{l_h}), \cdots, W_{\bullet L}(k_{l_h}), \mathbf{H}(k_{l_h}))\}$ can be considered as a subsequence of $\{(\mathbf{W}(k), \mathbf{H}(k))\}$ according to **FastNMF**'s iterative rules.

There is no other choice except that $W_{\bullet1}(k_{l_h}+1) \to \bar{W}_{\bullet1}$, b e c a u s e (a) $\{(W_{\bullet2}(k_{l_h}), \cdots, W_{\bullet L}(k_{l_h})$ $, \mathbf{H}(k_{l_h}))\} \to (\bar{W}_{\bullet2}, \cdots, \bar{W}_{\bullet L}, \bar{\mathbf{H}})$,(b)$\| \mathbf{V} - \mathbf{WH} \|_F^2$ is strictly convex in $W_{\bullet1}$ with $W_{\bullet2}, \cdots, W_{\bullet L}$ and $\mathbf{H}$ fixed according to Lemma 4, and (c) there exist at least a convergent subsequence in $\{W_{\bullet1}(k_{l_h}+1)\}$ a c c o r d i n g t o lemma 2. So $\{W_{\bullet1}(k_{l_h}+1), W_{\bullet2}(k_{l_h}), \cdots, W_{\bullet L}(k_{l_h}), \mathbf{H}(k_{l_h})\} \to (\bar{W}_{\bullet1}, \bar{W}_{\bullet2}, \cdots,$ $\bar{W}_{\bullet L}, \bar{\mathbf{H}})$. F o r t h e s a m e r e a s o n , $\{(W_{\bullet1}(k_{l_h}+1), W_{\bullet2}(k_{l_h}+1), \cdots, W_{\bullet L}(k_{l_h}), \mathbf{H}(k_{l_h}))\} \to (\bar{W}_{\bullet1}, \bar{W}_{\bullet2}, \cdots, \bar{W}_{\bullet L}, \bar{\mathbf{H}})$ and then obviously, $\{(\mathbf{W}(k_{l_h}+1), \mathbf{H}(k_{l_h}))\} \to$ $(\bar{\mathbf{W}}, \bar{\mathbf{H}})$.

For the same reason, it is easy to prove that

$$\{(\mathbf{W}(k_{l_h}+1), \mathbf{H}(k_{l_h}+1))\} \to (\bar{\mathbf{W}}, \bar{\mathbf{H}}).$$

So $\| (\mathbf{W}(k_{l_h}+1), \mathbf{H}(k_{l_h}+1)) - (\mathbf{W}(k_{l_h}), \mathbf{H}(k_{l_h})) \| \to 0$ a contradiction. Then, $\| (\mathbf{W}(k+1), \mathbf{H}(k+1)) - (\mathbf{W}(k), \mathbf{H}(k)) \| \to 0$. $\| (\mathbf{W}(k+2), \mathbf{H}(k+2)) - (\mathbf{W}(k), \mathbf{H}(k)) \| \le$ $\| (\mathbf{W}(k+2), \mathbf{H}(k+2)) - (\mathbf{W}(k+1), \mathbf{H}(k+1)) \| + \| (\mathbf{W}(k+1),$ $\mathbf{H}(k+1)) - (\mathbf{W}(k), \blacklozenge(k)) \| \to 0$. By mathematical induction, $\forall b \in Z^+, \| (\mathbf{W}(k+b), \mathbf{H}(k+b)) -(\mathbf{W}(k), \mathbf{H}(k)) \| \to 0$. **Q.E.D.**

Theorem 3 theoretically ensures the stability of **FastNMF**. On one hand, $\forall \varepsilon_1 > 0, \forall b \in Z^+,$ $\exists M(\varepsilon_1, b) \in Z^+,$ $\| (\mathbf{W}(k+b), \mathbf{H}(k+b)) - (\mathbf{W}(k), \mathbf{H}(k)) \| < \varepsilon_1$ while $k > M(\varepsilon_1, b)$. That is to say, the output of **FastNMF** cannot be significantly changed by b

more iterations as long as the output has been based on enough iterations. On the other hand, $\forall M \in Z^+, \qquad \forall b \in Z^+, \qquad \exists M(\varepsilon_1, b) > 0,$ $\| (\mathbf{W}(k+b), \mathbf{H}(k+b)) - (\mathbf{W}(k), \mathbf{H}(k)) \| < \varepsilon_2(M, b)$ while $k > M$. This means that the possible change of **FastNMF**'s output by b more iterations is definitely with limits and control after a fixed number of iterations.

Convergence

Theorem 4 (Convergence of FastNMF). Let the solution set $\Omega = \{$the stationary points of the problem $\min_{\varepsilon \le \mathbf{W}, \mathbf{H}} \| \mathbf{V} - \mathbf{WH} \|_F^2 \}$, FastNMF converges in the sense that every limit point of $\{(\mathbf{W}(k), \mathbf{H}(k))\}$ generated by its iterative rules is a solution.

Proof: There exists at least a convergent subsequence $\{(\mathbf{W}(k_l), \mathbf{H}(k_l))\}$ in $\{(\mathbf{W}(k), \mathbf{H}(k))\}$, because it is bounded according to lemma 2. Suppose that $\{(\mathbf{W}(k_l), \mathbf{H}(k_l))\} \to (\bar{\mathbf{W}}, \bar{\mathbf{H}})$.

Since $\| \mathbf{V} - \mathbf{WH} \|_F^2$ is convex in $W_{\bullet i}$ with $\{W_{\bullet1}, W_{\bullet2}, \cdots, W_{\bullet L}\} / W_{\bullet i}$ and $\mathbf{H}$ fixed for $\forall i \in \{1, 2, \cdots, L\}$ according to Lemma 4, $\| \mathbf{V} - \bar{\mathbf{W}}\bar{\mathbf{H}} \|_F^2 \le \| \mathbf{V} - [\bar{W}_{\bullet1}, \cdots, \bar{W}_{\bullet i-1}, W_{\bullet i}, \bar{W}_{\bullet i+1}, \cdots, \bar{W}_{\bullet L}]\mathbf{H} \|_F^2$ for $\forall W_{\bullet i} \ge \varepsilon$. Then,

$$\left[\frac{\partial \| \mathbf{V} - \mathbf{WH} \|_F^2}{\partial W_{\bullet i}}\bigg|_{(\mathbf{W}, \mathbf{H}) = (\bar{\mathbf{W}}, \bar{\mathbf{H}})}\right]^T (W_{\bullet i} - \bar{W}_{\bullet i}) \ge 0, \forall i \in \{1, 2, \cdots, L\}$$

(30)

for $\forall W_{\bullet i} \ge \varepsilon$, because there is no decent direction from the point $\bar{W}_{\bullet i}$ in $\{W_{\bullet i} | W_{\bullet i} \ge \varepsilon\}$. By the same token,

$$\left[\frac{\partial \| \mathbf{V} - \mathbf{WH} \|_F^2}{\partial H_{j\bullet}}\bigg|_{(\mathbf{W}, \mathbf{H}) = (\bar{\mathbf{W}}, \bar{\mathbf{H}})}\right](H_{j\bullet} - \bar{H}_{j\bullet})^T \ge 0, \quad \forall j \in \{1, 2, \cdots, L\}$$

(31)

for $\forall H_j \geq \varepsilon$. The combination of Equation (30) and Equation (31) meets the sufficient condition for $(\bar{W}, \bar{H})$ to be a stationary point (Bertsekas, 1999).

Let the solution set $\Omega=\{$the stationary points of the problem $\min_{\varepsilon \leq W, H} \| V - WH \|_F^2 \}$, and then $(\bar{W}, \bar{H})$ is a solution. According to the definition for convergence of an iterative program (Luenberger, 1973), FastNMF converges. **Q.E.D.**

EXPERIMENTAL RESULTS AND DISCUSSIONS

This section experimentally validates high efficiency of FastNMF-based dimensionality reduction and feature extraction of face images, discloses how efficient it is, and shows the representation ability of FastNMF features.

As de-facto baseline, Lee and Sueng's two multiplicative update-based algorithms (BaselineNMF-1 and BaselineNMF-2) are compared with FastNMF. Experiments in this section are based on ORL (ORL face database,1992) and AR face database (Martinez, 1998), images in which, as mentioned in section 3, are vectorized and arranged into columns of **V**.

The objective function of FastNMF and BaselineNMF-1 is the square of the Euclidean distance, and therefore their iterative outcomes are customarily evaluated and represented by the Frobenius norm-based relative error. Figure 7 records the iterative curves of implementing the dimensionality reduction and feature extraction of all 400 face images of ORL database by FastNMF (green dash dot curves) and BaselineNMF-1 (blue dash curves) while $L=80$, 160 and 240, respectively.

The objective function of BaselineNMF-2 is the generalized KL divergence, and therefore its iterative outcomes are evaluated and represented just by the divergence. Figure 8 records the iterative curves of implementing the dimensionality

reduction and feature extraction of all 400 face images of ORL database by BaselineNMF-2 (red dot curves) while $L=80$, 160 and 240, respectively.

What's more, the iterative curves of the three algorithms in Figure 7 and Figure 8 are based on the same initial iterative value for a chosen value of L.

According to Figure 7 and Figure 8, especially according to Figure 7(b), (d), (f) and Figure 8(b), (d), (f), it can be seen that FastNMF make its iterative curves sharply decreasing in the initial iterative phase, which is far beyond BaselineNMF-1's and BaselineNMF-2's power. This discloses how efficient FastNMF is, and can be also vividly exhibited by Figure 9, in which the reconstructed images in the three algorithms' initial iterative phase are shown.

It is easy to compare the outcomes of FastNMF with the ones of BaselineNMF-1 by Figure7(a), (c) and (e). Obviously, FastNMF tends to extract better features than BaselineNMF-1 as far as facial representation ability is concerned, and furthermore, the larger the scale (L) of NMF problem, the bigger the difference of representation ability between FastNMF's features and BaselineNMF-1's ones.

It is difficult to directly compare FastNMF's outcomes represented in Figure 7 with BaselineNMF-2's ones represented in Figure 8, because they are evaluated and represented by different standards. In order to make a comparison between them, an approach to evaluate and represent FastNMF's iterative outcomes by the generalized KL divergence could be used, if FastNMF is willing to endure possible efficiency degradation resulted from this unnatural, altruistic standard. By this approach, according to the same iterative outcomes as in Figure 7, Figure 8 portrays another group of FastNMF's iterative curves (green dash dot curves) of implementing the dimensionality reduction and feature extraction of all 400 face images of ORL database for $L=80$, 160 and 240, respectively.

Figure 7. The iterative curves of implementing the dimensionality reduction and feature extraction of all 400 face images of ORL database by FastNMF and BaselineNMF-1. Iterative outcomes are evaluated and represented by the Frobenius norm-based relative error: (a) L=80, 3000 seconds' iteration; (b) L=80, 500 seconds' iteration; (c) L=160, 3000 seconds' iteration; (d) L=160, 500 seconds' iteration; (e) L=240, 3000 seconds' iteration; (f) L=240, 500 seconds' iteration.

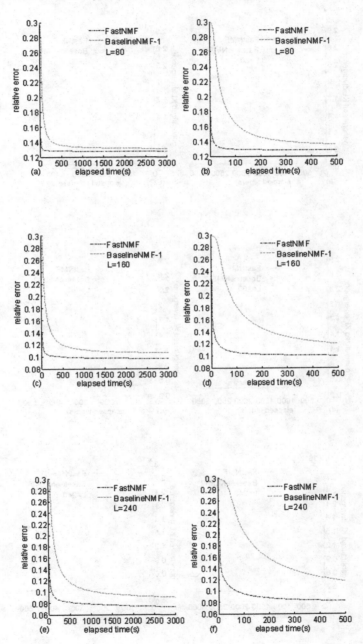

According to Figure 8(a), (c) and (e), FastNMF also tends to extract facial features with better representation ability than BaselineNMF-2, and the larger the scale (L) of NMF problem, the bigger the difference of representation ability between their features.

Figure 8. The iterative curves of implementing the dimensionality reduction and feature extraction of all 400 face images of ORL database by FastNMF and BaselineNMF-2, in which iterative outcomes are evaluated and represented by the generalized KL divergence. (a) L=80, 3000 seconds' iteration; (b) L=80, 500 seconds' iteration; (c) L=160, 3000 seconds' iteration; (d) L=160, 500 seconds' iteration; (e) L=240, 3000 seconds' iteration; (f) L=240, 500 seconds' iteration.

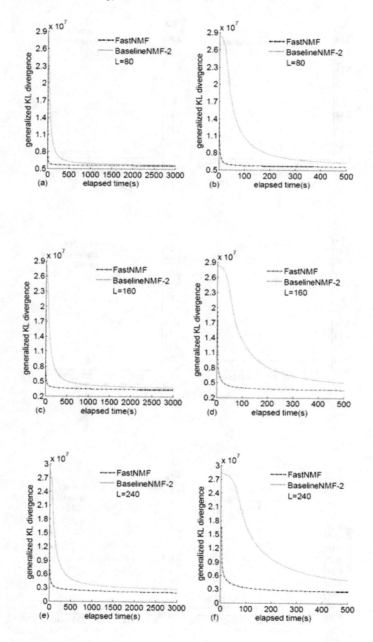

To show the experimental conclusions above are unrelated to the data used, the above experiments are repeated using 944 face images (everyone's 8 images without occlusions and expressional variations in 118 objects participating two sessions' facial image collection) of AR database.

Figure 9. Table of exhibitions of the initial iterative performance of NMF algorithms

Table of exhibitions of the initial iterative performance of NMF algorithms

Algorithm	L	Original image[a]	Reconstructed images after k iterations							
			$k=0$[b]	$k=1$[c]	$k=2$[c]	$k=3$[c]	$k=4$[c]	$k=5$[c]	$k=6$[c]	$k=7$[c]
FastNMF										
BaselineNMF-1	80									
BaselineNMF-2										
FastNMF										
BaselineNMF-1	160									
BaselineNMF-2										
FastNMF										
BaselineNMF-1	240									
BaselineNMF-2										

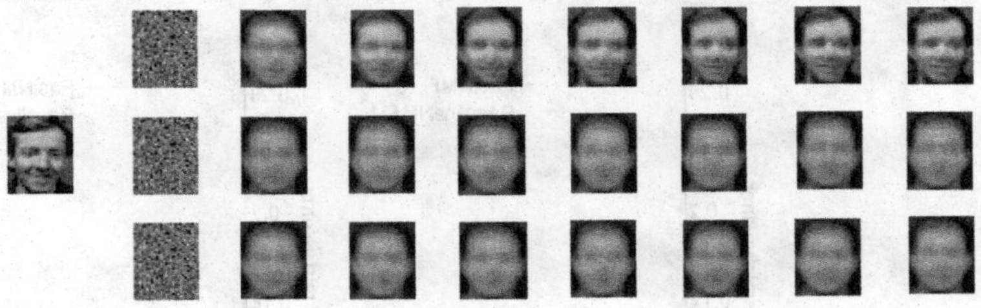

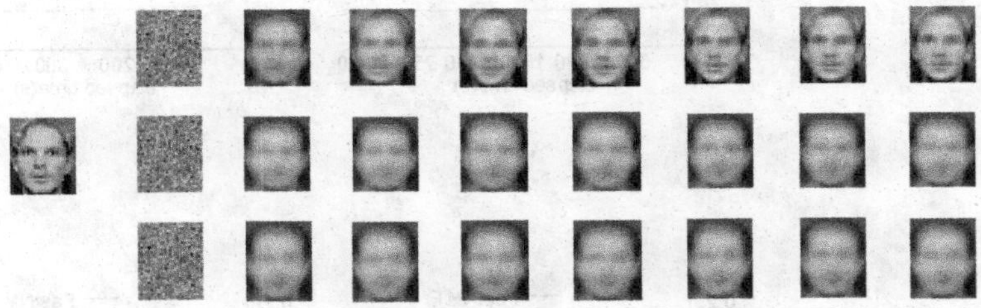

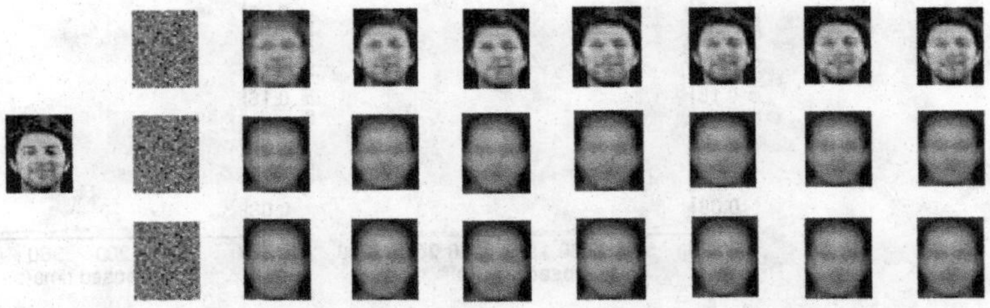

[a] The original image is one of 400 ORL images processed by NMF.

[b] There is no difference among the three algorithms' reconstructed images for k=0 because they are based on the same initial iterative value.

[c] For $\forall k \in \{1, 2, \cdots, 7\}$, any algorithm's reconstructed image is based on its $\mathbf{W}(k)$ and the column related to the original image in its $\mathbf{H}(k)$ (an algorithm's [$\mathbf{W}(k)$, $\mathbf{H}(k)$], k = 1, 2, ..., 7 are the fist 7 iterative outcomes that its iterative curve in Fig.6 or Fig.7 is based on).

CONCLUSION

NMF has been a more and more popular method of non-negative dimensionality reduction and feature extraction of non-negative data. However, there is currently no NMF algorithm that is able to hold both satisfactorily high efficiency for dimensionality reduction and feature extraction of face images and enough ease of use. This not only chapter puts forward a new monotonic fixed-point NMF algorithm called FastNMF by implementing least squares error-based non-negative factorization essentially according to the basic properties of parabola functions.

Theoretical analysis and experimental results shows FastNMF holds higher efficiency to implement dimensionality reduction and feature extraction of face images and extracts facial features

Figure 10. The iterative curves of implementing the dimensionality reduction and feature extraction of 944 face images of AR database by FastNMF and BaselineNMF-1. Iterative outcomes are evaluated and represented by the Frobenius norm-based relative error. (a) L=80, 3000 seconds' iteration; (b) L=80, 500 seconds' iteration; (c) L=160, 3000 seconds' iteration; (d) L=160, 500 seconds' iteration; (e) L=240, 3000 seconds' iteration; (f) L=240, 500 seconds' iteration.

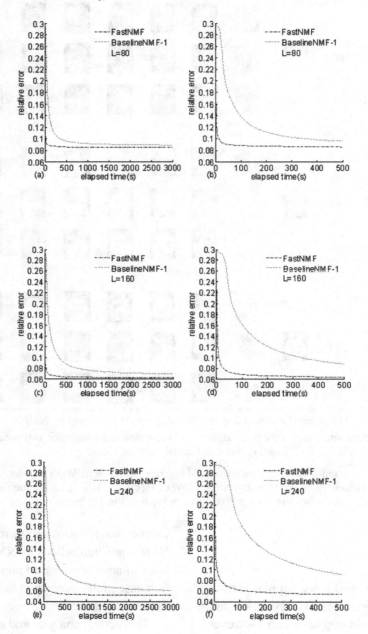

with better representation ability than the popular multiplicative update-based algorithms.

For simplicity of design philosophy, FastNMF is still one of NMF algorithms that are the easiest to use and the most comprehensible.

Figure 11. The iterative curves of implementing the dimensionality reduction and feature extraction of 944 face images of AR database by FastNMF and BaselineNMF-2. Iterative outcomes are evaluated and represented by the generalized KL divergence. (a) L=80, 3000 seconds' iteration; (b) L=80, 500 seconds' iteration; (c) L=160, 3000 seconds' iteration; (d) L=160, 500 seconds' iteration; (e) L=240, 3000 seconds' iteration; (f) L=240, 500 seconds' iteration.

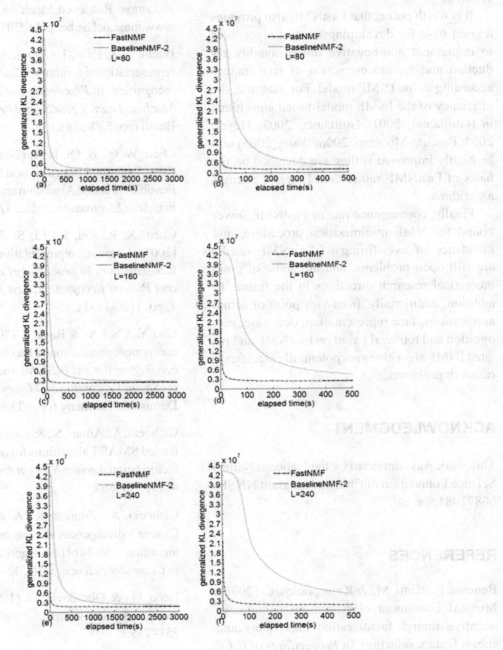

By virtue of the monotonic property of FastNMF and the boundedness of $\{\mathbf{W}(k),\mathbf{H}(k)\}$ generated by its iterative rules, the stability and convergence of FastNMF has been theoretically ensured.

It is worth noting that FastNMF also provides a good base for developing the fast algorithms to implement non-negative dimensionality reduction and feature extraction of face images according to the INMF model. For example, the efficiency of the INMF model-based algorithms in (Guillamet, 2001; Guillamet, 2003; Hoyer, 2004; Pascual-Montano, 2006; Wang, 2006) will be highly improved if they are designed on the basis of FastNMF rather than Lee and Sueng's algorithms.

Finally, convergence rate of FastNMF, lower bound for NMF minimization procedure, and avoidance of over-fitting of FastNMF results are still open problems, and are some of good theoretical research directions in the future. In addition, additionally, from viewpoint of actual applications, face representation, detection, recognition and retrieval based on FastNMF and related INMF algorithms are potentially significant research problems.

ACKNOWLEDGMENT

This work was supported by the National Nature Science Foundation of China under grant NNSF-60872084.

REFERENCES

Benetos, E., Kotti, M., & Kotropoulos, C. (2006). Musical instrument classification using non-negative matrix factorization algorithms and subset feature selection. In *Proceedings of IEEE International Conference on Acoustics, Speech and Signal Processing*, Toulouse, France (Vol. 5, pp. 14-19).

Bertsekas, D. P. (1999). *Nonlinear Programming* (2nd ed.). Belmont, MA: Athena Scientific.

Blondel, V., Ho, N. D., & Dooren, P. V. (2009). *Algorithms for weighted non-negative matrix factorization*. Retrieved Mach 26, 2009, from http://www.inma.ucl.ac.be/ publi/303209.pdf

Buciu, I., & Pitas, I. (2004). A new sparse image representation algorithm applied to facial expression recognition. In *Proceedings of IEEE Workshop on Machine Learning for Signal Processing*, Sao Luis, Brazil (pp. 539-548).

Chen, W. G., & Qi, F. H. (2003). Learning NMF Representation Using a Hybrid Method Combining Feasible Direction Algorithm and Simulated Annealing. *Acta Electronica Sinica, 31*(S1), 1290–1293.

Chen, X. R., Gu, L., Li, S. Z., & Zhang, H. J. (2001). Learning representative local features for face detection. In *proceedings of Computer Vision and Pattern Recognition*, Los Alamitos, CA (Vol. 1, pp. 1126-1131).

Cho, Y., Choi, S., & Bang, S. (2003). Non-negative component parts of sound for classification. In *Proceedings of the 3rd IEEE International Symposium on Signal Processing and Information Technology*, Darmstadt, Germany (pp. 633-636).

Cichocki, A., Amari, S., & Zdunek, R. (2006b). Extended SMART algorithms for non-negative matrix factorization. *Lecture Notes in Artificial Intelligence, 4029*, 548–562.

Cichocki, A., Zdunek, R., & Amari, S. (2006a). Csiszar's divergences for non-negative matrix factorization: Family of new algorithms. *Lecture Notes in Computer Science, 3889*, 32–39.

Deco, G., & Obradovic, D. (1995). Linear redundancy reduction learning. *Neural Networks, 8*(5), 751–755.

Dhillon, I., & Sra, S. (2005). Generalized nonnegative matrix approximations with Bregman divergences. In *Advances in Neural Information Processing Systems* (NIPS, pp. 283-290). Cambridge, MA: MIT Press.

Ding, C., Li, T., Peng, W., & Park, H. (2006). Orthogonal nonnegative matrix tri-factorization for clustering. In *Proceedings of the Twelfth ACM SIGKDD international conference on knowledge discovery and data mining*, Philadelphia, PA, USA (pp.126-135).

Donoho, D., & Stodden, V. (2004). When does non-negative matrix factorization give a correct decomposition into parts? In *Advances in Neural Information Processing Systems* (NIPS, pp. 1141-1148). Cambridge, MA: MIT Press.

Field, D. J. (1994). What is the goal of sensory coding? *Neural Computation, 6*(4), 559–601.

Frigyesi, A., & Höglund, M. (2008). Non-negative matrix factorization for the Analysis of complex and gene expression data: identification of clinically relevant tumor subtypes. *Cancer Informatics, 6*, 275–292.

Guan, X. H., Wang, W., & Zhang, X. L. (2009). Fast intrusion detection based on a non-negative matrix factorization model. *Journal of Network and Computer Applications, 32*(1), 31–44.

Guillamet, D., Bressan, M., & Vitria, J. (2001). A weighted non-negative matrix factorization for local representation. In *Proceedings of Computer Vision and Pattern Recognition*, Los Alamitos, CA (Vol. 1, pp. 942-947).

Guillamet, D., & Vitrià, J. (2002). Non-negative matrix factorization for face recognition. *Lecture Notes in Computer Science, 2504*, 336–344.

Guillamet, D., Vitrià, J., & Schiele, B. (2003). Introducing a weighted non-negative matrix factorization for image classification. *Pattern Recognition Letters, 24*(14), 2447–2454.

Heiler, M., & Schnorr, C. (2006). Learning sparse representations by non-negative matrix factorization and sequential cone programming. *Journal of Machine Learning Research, 7*(7), 1385–1407.

Holzapfel, A., & Stylianou, Y. (2008). Musical Genre classification using nonnegative matrix factorization-based features. *IEEE transactions on Audio, Speech, and Language processing, 16*(2), 424-434.

Hoyer, P. O. (2002). Non-negative sparse coding. In *Proceedings of IEEE Workshop on Neural Networks for Signal Processing*, Martigny, Switzerland (pp. 557-565).

Hoyer, P. O. (2004). Non-negative matrix factorization with sparseness constraints. *Journal of Machine Learning Research, 5*(9), 1457–1469.

Hyvärinen, A., Karhunen, J., & Oja, E. (2001). *Independent Component Analysis*. Hoboken, NJ: Wiley- Interscience.

Jolliffe, I. T. (2002). *Principal Component Analysis* (2nd ed.). New York: Springer-Verlag.

Jones, M. C., & Sibson, R. (1987). What is projection pursuit? *Journal of the Royal Statistical Society. Series A (General), 150*(1), 1–36.

Kim, H., & Park, H. (2007). Cancer class discovery using non-negative matrix factorization based on alternating non-negativity-constrained least squares. *Lecture Notes in Computer Science, 4463*, 477–487.

Kopriva, I., & Nuzillard, D. (2006). Non-negative matrix factorization approach to blind image deconvolution. *Lecture Notes in Computer Science, 3889*, 966–973.

Kotsia, I., Zafeiriou, S., & Pitas, I. (2007). A novel discriminant non-negative matrix factorization algorithm with applications to facial image characterization problems. *IEEE Transactions on Information Sorensics and Security, 2*(3), 588–595.

Kreyszig, E. (1978). *Introductory functional analysis with applications*. New York: Wiley.

Lee, D. D., & Seung, H. S. (1999). Learning the parts of objects by non-negative matrix factorization. *Nature, 401*(6755), 788–791.

Lee, D. D., & Seung, H. S. (2000). Algorithms for non-negative matrix factorization. In *Advances in Neural Information Processing Systems* (NIPS, pp. 556-562). Cambridge, MA: MIT Press.

Li, L., & Zhang, Y. J. (2007). Survey on algorithms of non-negative matrix factorization. *Acta Electronica Sinica, 36*(4), 737–743.

Li, L., & Zhang, Y. J. (2008). FastNMF: A fast monotonic fixed-point non-negative matrix factorization algorithm with high ease of use. In *Proceedings of the 19th International Conference on Pattern Recognition*, Tampa, Florida, USA.

Li, S. Z., Hou, X. W., Zhang, H. J., et al. (2001). Learning spatially localized, parts-based representation. In *Proceedings of Computer Vision and Pattern Recognition*, Los Alamitos, CA (Vol. 1, pp. 207-212).

Liang, D., Yang, J., & Chang, Y. C. (2006). Relevance feedback based on non-negative matrix factorization for image retrieval. *IEE Proceedings. Vision Image and Signal Processing, 153*(4), 436–444.

Liu, W. X., & Zheng, N. N. (2004a). Learning sparse features for classification by mixture models. *Pattern Recognition Letters, 25*(2), 155–161.

Liu, W. X., Zheng, N. N., & Li, X. (2004b). Relative gradient speeding up additive updates for nonnegative matrix factorization. *Neurocomputing, 57*, 493–499.

Liu, W. X., Zheng, N. N., & Lu, X. F. (2003). Non-negative matrix factorization for visual coding. In *Proceedings of IEEE International Conference on Acoustics, Speech and Signal Processing*, Hong Kong (Vol. 3, pp. 293-296).

Liu, W. X., Zheng, N. N., & You, Q. B. (2006). Non-negative matrix factorization and its applications in pattern recognition. *Chinese Science Bulletin, 51*(1), 7–18.

Logothetis, N. K., & Sheinberg, D. L. (1996). Visual object recognition. *Annual Review of Neuroscience, 19*(1), 577–621.

Luenberger, D. G. (1973). *Introduction to Linear and Nonlinear Programming*. Reading, MA: Addson-wesley.

Martinez, A. M., & Benavente, R. (1998). *The AR Face Database. CVC Technical Report #24*. West Lafayette, Indiana, USA: Purdue University.

Okun, O., & Priisalu, H. (2006). Fast nonnegative matrix factorization and its application for protein fold recognition. *EURASIP Journal on Applied Signal Processing*, Article ID 71817. *ORL face database*. (1992). The AT&T (Olivetti) Research Laboratory. Retrieved March 26, 2008, from http://www.cl.cam.ac.uk/Research/DTG/archive/facedata base.html

Ouhsain, M., & Hamza, A. B. (2009). Image watermarking scheme using nonnegative matrix factorization and wavelet transform. *International Journal on Expert Systems with Applications, 36*(2), 2123–2129.

Palmer, S. E. (1977). Hierarchical structure in perceptual representation. *Cognitive Psychology, 9*(3), 441–474.

Pascual-Montano, A., Carzzo, J. M., & Lochi, K. (2006). Non-smooth nonnegative matrix factorization (nsNMF). *IEEE Transactions on Pattern Analysis and Machine Intelligence, 28*(3), 403–415.

Reyment, R. A., & Jvreskog, K. G. (1996). *Applied Factor Analysis in the Natural Sciences* (2nd ed.). Cambridge, UK: Cambridge University Press.

Shahnaz, F., Berry, M. W., & Pauca, V. P., & PLemmons, R. J. (2006). Document clustering using nonnegative matrix factorization. *Journal of Information Processing and Management, 42*(3), 373–386.

Stouten, V., Demuynck, K., & Hamme, H. V. (2007). Automatically learning the units of speech by non-negative matrix factorization. In *Proceedings of European Conference on Speech Communication and Technology*, Antwerp, Belgium (pp. 1937- 1940).

Stouten, V., Demuynck, K., & Hamme, H. V. (2008). Discovering phone patterns in spoken utterances by non-negative matrix factorization. *IEEE Signal Processing Letters, 15*(1), 131–134.

Wachsmuth, E., Oram, M. W., & Perrett, D. I. (1994). Recognition of objects and their component parts: responses of single units in the temporal cortex of the macaque. *Cerebral Cortex, 4*(5), 509–522.

Wang, F. (2006a). *Research of Face Detection Technology Based on Skin Color and Non-negative Matrix Factorization*. Master dissertation, Huaqiao University, China.

Wang, G. L., Kossenkov, A. V., & Ochs, M. F. (2006b). LS-NMF: a modified non-negative matrix factorization algorithm utilizing uncertainty estimates. *BMC Bioinformatics, 7*, 175.

Wang, Y., Jia, Y. D., Hu, C. B., et al. (2004). Fisher non-negative matrix factorization for learning local features. In *Proceedings of Asian Conference on Computer Vision*, Jeju Island, Korea.

Wild, S., Curry, J., & Dougherty, A. (2004). Improving non-negative matrix factorizations through structured initialization. *Pattern Recognition, 37*(11), 2217–2232.

Xu, B. W., Lu, J. J., & Huang, G. S. (2003). A constrained non-negative matrix factorization in information retrieval. In *Proceedings of the IEEE International Conference on Information Reuse and Integration*, Nevada, USA (pp. 273-277).

Xue, Y., Tong, C. S., Chen, W. S., et al. (2006). A modified Non-negative Matrix Factorization Algorithm for Face Recognition. In *Proceedings of the 18th international conference on Pattern Recognition*, Hong Kong (Vol. 3, pp. 495- 498).

Zafeiriou, S., Tefas, A., Buciu, I., & Pitas, I. (2006). Exploiting discriminant information in nonnegative matrix factorization with application to frontal face verification. *IEEE Transactions on Neural Networks, 17*(3), 683–695.

Zdunek, R., & Cichocki, A. (2006). Non-negative matrix factorization with quasi-newton optimization. *Lecture Notes in Artificial Intelligence, 4029*, 870–879.

KEY TERMS AND DEFINITIONS

Dimensionality Reduction: One of problems with high-dimensional datasets is that, in many cases, not all the measured variables are important for understanding the underlying phenomena of interest. It is of interest in many applications to reduce the dimension of the original data prior to any modeling of the data. Dimensionality reduction is the process of reducing the number of random variables under consideration.

Feature Extraction: In pattern recognition and in image processing, feature extraction is a special form of dimensionality reduction. When the input data to an algorithm is too large to be processed and it is suspected to be notoriously redundant (much data, but not much information) then the input data will be transformed into a reduced representation set of features (also named feature vectors). Transforming the input data into the set of features is called feature extraction.

If the features extracted are carefully chosen, it is expected that the feature set will extract the relevant information from the input data in order to perform the desired task using this reduced representation instead of the full size input.

Non-Negative Matrix Factorization: Non-negative matrix factorization is an effective method of non-negative feature extraction and dimensionality reduction of face images.

Efficiency of an Algorithm: Efficiency of an algorithm means the degree of computational load required to implement the algorithm. It can be represented by time complexity or computational time to implement the algorithm under different computational scales on a chosen computational instrument (usually, PC).

FastNMF: FastNMF is an efficient NMF algorithm and is probably the fastest so far.

Section 4
Face Recognition

Chapter 9
Sparse Representation for View–Based Face Recognition

Imran Naseem
University of Western Australia, Australia

Roberto Togneri
University of Western Australia, Australia

Mohammed Bennamoun
University of Western Australia, Australia

ABSTRACT

In this chapter, the authors discuss the problem of face recognition using sparse representation classification (SRC). The SRC classifier has recently emerged as one of the latest paradigm in the context of view-based face recognition. The main aim of the chapter is to provide an insight of the SRC algorithm with thorough discussion of the underlying "Compressive Sensing" theory. Comprehensive experimental evaluation of the approach is conducted on a number of standard databases using exemplary evaluation protocols to provide a comparative index with the benchmark face recognition algorithms. The algorithm is also extended to the problem of video-based face recognition for more realistic applications.

INTRODUCTION

With the ever-increasing security threats, the problem of invulnerable authentication systems is becoming more acute. Traditional means of securing a facility essentially depend on strategies corresponding to "what you have" or "what you know", for example smart cards, keys and passwords. These systems however can easily be fooled. Passwords for example, are difficult to remember and therefore people tend to use the same password for multiple facilities making it more susceptible to hacking. Similarly, cards and keys can easily be stolen or forged. A more inalienable approach is therefore to go for strategies corresponding to "what you are" or "what you exhibit" i.e. biometrics. Although the issue of "liveliness" has recently been highlighted due to the advancement in digital media technology, biometrics arguably remain the best choice. Among the other available biometrics, such as speech, iris, fingerprints, hand geometry and gait, face seems to be the most natural choice (Li & Jain, 2005). It is nonintrusive, requires a minimum of

DOI: 10.4018/978-1-61520-991-0.ch009

user cooperation and is cheap to implement. The importance of face recognition is highlighted for widely used video surveillance systems where we typically have facial images of suspects.

It is long known that appearance-based face recognition systems critically depend on manifold learning methods. A gray-scale face image of order $a \times b$ can be represented as an ab dimensional vector in the original *image space*. However, any attempt of recognition in such a high dimensional space is vulnerable to a variety of issues often referred to as *curse of dimensionality*. Typically, in pattern recognition problems it is believed that high-dimensional data vectors are redundant measurements of an underlying source. The objective of manifold learning is therefore to uncover this "underlying source" by a suitable transformation of high-dimensional measurements to low-dimensional data vectors. View-based face recognition methods are no exception to this rule. Therefore, at the feature extraction stage, images are transformed to low dimensional vectors in *face space*. The main objective is to find a basis function for this transformation, which could distinguishably represent faces in the face space. Linear transformation from the image space to the feature space is perhaps the most traditional way of dimensionality-reduction, also called "Linear Subspace Analysis".

A number of approaches have been reported in the literature including Principle Component Analysis (PCA) (Turk & Pentland, 1991), (Jolliffe, 1986), Linear Discriminant Analysis (LDA) (Belhumeur, Hespanha, & Kriegman, 1997) and Independent Component Analysis (ICA) (Yuen & Lai, 2002). These approaches have been classified in two categories namely *reconstructive* and *discriminative* methods. Reconstructive approaches (such as PCA and ICA) are reported to be robust for the problem related to contaminated pixels, whereas discriminative approaches (such as LDA) are known to yield better results in clean conditions (Duda, Hart, & Stork, 2000). Nevertheless, the choice of the manifold learning method for a

given problem of face recognition has been a hot topic of research in the face recognition literature. These debates have recently been challenged by a new concept of "Sparse Representation Classification (SRC)" (Wright, Yang, Ganesh, Sastri, & Ma, 2009). It has been shown that unorthodox features such as down-sampled images and random projections can serve equally well. As a result, the choice of the feature space may no longer be so critical (Naseem, Togneri, & Bennamoun, 2009) (Wright, Yang, Ganesh, Sastri, & Ma, 2009). What really matters is the dimensionality of the feature space and the design of the classifier. The key factor to the success of sparse representation classification is the recent development of "Compressive Sensing" theory. In sparse representation classification, a down-sampled probe image vector is represented by a linear combination of down-sampled gallery images vectors. The ill-conditioned inverse problem is solved using the l_1-norm minimization. The sparse nature of the l_1-norm solution helps identifying the true class of a given probe.

The main objective of the chapter is to comprehensively evaluate the SRC algorithm for the problem of view-based face recognition using static and temporal images. The chapter provides an extensive evaluation on three standard face databases with a thorough discussion of the underlying compressive sensing theory. The algorithm is evaluated under a number of exemplary evaluation protocols reported in the face recognition literature, a comprehensive comparison with state of the art methods is included. The problem of varying gestures is one of the major challenges in the face recognition research.

Latest evaluations using benchmark methods have shown degraded results for severe expression conditions. In this chapter we address the problem of gesture variations by comparing the results of sparse representation classification with the most standard and successful techniques, specifically we target the Bayesian Eigenfaces (MIT) (Moghaddam & Pentland, 1997) and the FaceIT

(Visionics) algorithms. The Bayesian Eigenfaces approach was reported to be one of the best in the 1996 FERET test (Phillips, Wechsler, Huang, & Rauss, 1998)}, whereas the FaceIt algorithm (based on Local Feature Analysis) (Penev & Atick, 1996) is claimed to be one of the most successful commercial face recognition system (Gross, Shi, & Cohn, 2001). In the end, the SRC algorithm is also evaluated for the problem of video-based face recognition.

COMPRESSIVE SENSING

Most of the signals of practical interest are compressible in nature. For example, audio signals are compressible in localized Fourier domain and digital images are compressible in Discrete Cosine Transform (DCT) and wavelet domains. This concept of compressibility gives rise to the notion of transform coding so that subsequent processing of information is computationally efficient. It simply means that a signal when transformed into a specific domain becomes sparse in nature and could be approximated efficiently by say a K number of large coefficients, ignoring all the small values. However, the initial data acquisition is typically performed in accordance with the Nyquist sampling theorem, which states that a signal could only be safely recovered from the samples if and only if the samples are drawn at a sampling rate that is at least twice the maximum frequency of the signal. Consequently, the data acquisition part can be an overhead since a huge number of acquired samples will have to be further compressed for any subsequent realistic processing.

As a result, a legitimate question is whether there is any efficient way of data acquisition to remove the Nyquist overhead, yet safely recovering the signal. The new area of compressive sensing answers this question. Let us formulate the problem in the following manner (Baraniuk, 2007).

Let g be a signal vector of order $N \times 1$ Any signal in $\mathbb{R}^N$ can be represented in terms of an $N \times N$ orthonormal basis matrix Ψ and $N \times 1$ vector of weighting coefficients s such that:

$$g = \Psi s \tag{1}$$

It has to be noted here that g and s are essentially two different representations of the same signal. g is the signal expressed in the time domain while s is the signal represented in Ψ domain. Note that the transformation of the signal g in Ψ basis makes it K sparse. This means that ideally s has only K non-zero entries.

Now the aim of compressive sensing is to measure a low dimensional vector y of order $M \times 1$ (M<N) such that the original information g can be safely retrieved from y. It means that we are looking for a transformation Φ such that:

$$y_{M \times 1} = \Phi_{M \times N} \, g_{N \times 1} \tag{2}$$

$$y_{M \times 1} = \Phi_{M \times N} \, \Psi_{N \times N} s_{N \times 1} \tag{3}$$

$$y_{M \times 1} = \Theta_{M \times N} \, s_{N \times 1} \tag{4}$$

The main aim is to design a stable measurement matrix Φ that would ensure that there is no information loss in compressible signal due to the dimensionality reduction from $\mathbb{R}^N$ to $\mathbb{R}^M$ (Baraniuk, 2007). Leaving the issue of measurement matrix for a moment, we would like to emphasize that given the measurement vector y the problem is still ill-posed as we are looking for N unknowns with a system of M equations. However the issue is easily resolved due to the K-sparse nature of s which means that essentially there will only be K non-zero entries in s and hence we will be looking to find K unknowns from a system of M equations where $K \leq M$.

It has been shown that for Equation 3 to be true Θ must satisfy the Restricted Isometry Property (RIP) (E, J, & T, 2006). Alternatively it has been discussed in (E, J, & T, 2006), (Donoho, 2006) that the stability of the measurement matrix Φ could be ensured if it is incoherent with the sparsifying basis Ψ. In the framework of compressive sensing, this discussion boils down to the selection of Φ as a random matrix. This means that if, for instance, we select Φ as a Gaussian random matrix, such that the entries of the matrix Φ are independent and identically distributed (iid) then Θ will satisfy the RIP with a high probability (Donoho, 2006) (E, J, & T, 2006) (Baraniuk, Davenport, DeVore, & Wakin, 2006).

Once the RIP property of Θ is satisfied in equation 3, the recovery of vector s is merely a problem of using a suitable reconstruction algorithm. In the compressive sensing literature (Donoho, 2006) (E, J, & T, 2006) it has been shown that s can be recovered with a high probability using the l_1 optimization given that

$$M = cK \log \frac{N}{K} \tag{5}$$

c being a small constant.

SPARSE REPRESENTATION FOR FACE RECOGNITION

We now discuss the basic framework (Wright, Yang, Ganesh, Sastri, & Ma, 2009) of our face recognition system in the context of sparse representation. Let us assume that we have k distinct classes and n_i images available for training from the ith class. Each training sample is a gray scale image of order $a \times b$ The image is down-sampled to an order $w \times h$ and is converted into a 1-D vector $v_{i,j}$ by concatenating the columns of the down-sampled image such that $v_{i,j} \in \mathbb{R}^m$ $(m = w \times h)$.

Here i is the index of the class, $i=1,2,\dots,k$ and j is the index of the training sample, $j=1,2,\dots,n_i$. All this training data from the ith class is placed in a matrix A_i such that $A_i = \left[v_{i,1}, v_{i,2}, \dots\dots, v_{i,n_i} \right] \in \mathbb{R}^{m \times n_i}$. As stated in (Wright, Yang, Ganesh, Sastri, & Ma, 2009), when the training samples from the ith class are sufficient, the test sample y from the same class will approximately lie in the linear span of the columns of A_i.

$$y = \pm_{i,1} v_{i,1} + \pm_{i,2} v_{i,2} + \dots + \pm_{i,n_i} v_{i,n_i} \tag{6}$$

where $a_{i,j}$ are real scalar quantities. Now we develop a dictionary matrix A for all k classes by concatenating $A_i, i=1,2,\dots,k$ as follows:

$$A = \left[A_1, A_2, \dots\dots, A_k \right] \in \mathbb{R}^{m \times n_i k} \tag{7}$$

Now a test pattern y can be represented as a linear combination of all n training samples $(n=n_i \times k)$.

$$y = Ax \tag{8}$$

where x is an unknown vector of coefficients. Now from equation 8, it is straight forward to note that only those entries of x that are non-zeros correspond to the class of y. This means that if we are able to solve equation 8 for x we can actually find the class of the test pattern y. Recent research in compressive sensing and sparse representation (Candes, Romberg, & Tao, 2006) (Candes & Tao, 2006) (Donoho, 2006) have shown that using the sparsity of the solution of equation 8, enables us to solve the problem using l_1-norm minimization:

$$\left(l^1 \right): \hat{x}_1 = \arg \min x_1; \quad Ax = y \tag{9}$$

Once we have estimated x_1, ideally, it should have nonzero entries corresponding to the class of y and now deciding about the class of y is a simple matter of locating indices of the non-zero entries in x_1. However, due to noise and modeling limitations x_1 is commonly corrupted by some small nonzero entries belonging to different classes. To resolve this problem we define an operator δ_I for each class i so that $\delta_i(x_1)$ gives us a vector $\in \mathbb{R}^n$ where the only nonzero entries are from the ith class. This process is repeated k times for each class. Now for a given class i we can approximate $y_i = A\delta_i(x_1)$ and assign the test pattern to the class with a minimum residual between y and y_i.

$$\underset{i}{min}\, r_i(y) = \left\| y - A\delta_i(x_1) \right\|_2 \qquad (10)$$

EXPERIMENTS

Yale Database

The Yale database, maintained at Yale University, consists of 165 grayscale images from 15 individuals (Yale Univ. Face Database, 2002). Images from each subject reflect gesture variations incorporating normal, happy, sad, sleepy, surprised, and wink expressions. Luminance variation is also addressed by including images with lighting source from central, right and left directions. A couple of images with and without spectacles are also included. Figure 1 (Yale Univ. Face Database, 2002) represents 11 different images from a single subject. Experiments are conducted on the original database without any preprocessing stages of face cropping and/or normalization. Each grayscale image is down-sampled to an order of 25×25 to get a 625-d feature vector. The experiments are conducted using the leave-one-out approach as reported quite regularly in the literature (Yang, Zhang, Frangi, & Yang, 2004) (Yang M. H.) (Gao, 2002). A comprehensive comparison of various approaches is provided in Table 1. The SRC approach substantially outperformed all reported techniques showing an improvement of 5.48% over the best contestant i.e. the Fisherfaces approach. Note that the SRC approach leads the traditional PCA and ICA approaches by a margin of 22.58% and 26.66% respectively. The choice of feature space dimension is elaborated in Figure 2, the dimensionality curve is shown for a randomly selected leave-one-out experiment. Classification accuracy becomes fairly constant in an approximately 600-D feature space.

Figure 1. A typical subject from the Yale database with various poses and variations

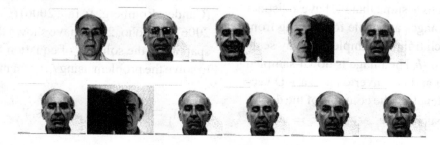

Table 1. Results for Yale database using leave-one-out method

Evaluation Method	Approach	Recognition Rate
Leave-one-out	ICA	71.52%
	Kernel Eigenfaces	72.73%
	Edge map	73.94%
	Eigenfaces	75.60%
	Correlation	76.10%
	Linear subspace	78.40%
	2DPCA	84.24%
	Eigenface w/0 1st 3	84.70%
	LEM	85.45%
	Fisherfaces	92.70%
	SRC	98.18%

AT&T Database

The AT&T database is maintained at the AT&T Laboratories, Cambridge University. Ten different images from one of the 40 subjects from the database are shown in Figure 3. The database incorporates facial gestures such as smiling or non-smiling, open or closed eyes and alterations like glasses or without glasses. It also characterizes a maximum 20-degree rotation of the face with some scale variations of about 10%.

The choice of dimensionality for the AT&T database is dilated in Figure 2 that reflects that the recognition rate becomes fairly constant above a 40-dimensional feature space. Therefore, each 112×92 grayscale image is down-sampled to an order 7×6 and is transformed to a 42 dimensional feature vector by column concatenation.

To provide a comparative value for the SRC approach we follow two evaluation strategies as proposed in the literature (Yang, Zhang, Frangi, & Yang, 2004) (Yang M. H.) (Yuen & Lai, 2002). First evaluation strategy takes the first five images of each individual as a training set, while the last five are designated as probes. Another set of experiments were conducted using the

Figure 2. Left: Recognition accuracy for Yale database. Right: Recognition accuracy for the AT&T database

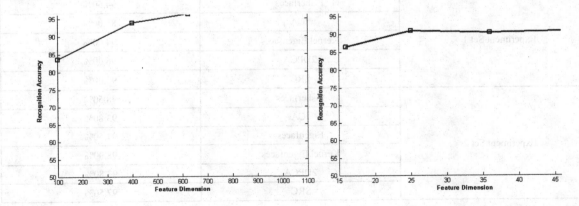

Figure 3. A typical subject from the AT&T database

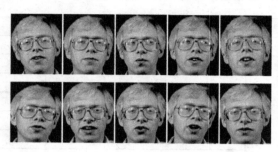

"leave-one-out" approach. A detailed comparison of the results for the two experimental setups is summarized in Table 2, all results are as reported in (Yang, Zhang, Frangi, & Yang, 2004). For first set of experiments the SRC algorithm achieves a comparable recognition accuracy of 93% in a 42-D feature space, the best results are reported for the 2DPCA approach which are 3% better than the SRC method. Also for the second set of experiments, the SRC approach attains a high recognition success of 97.5% in a 42-D feature space, it outperforms the ICA approach by 3.7% (approximately) and is comparable to Fisherfaces, Eigenfaces, Kernel Eigenfaces and 2DPCA approaches.

AR Database

The AR database consists of more than 4,000 color images of 126 subjects (70 men and 56 women) (Martinez & Benavente, 1998). The database characterizes divergence from ideal conditions by incorporating various facial expressions (neutral, smile, anger and scream), luminance alterations (left light on, right light on and all side lights on) and occlusion modes (sunglass and scarf). It also contains adverse scenarios of occlusion with luminance (sunglass with left light on, sunglass with right light on, scarf with left light on and scarf with right light on). To take care of session variability the pictures were taken in two sessions separated by two weeks and no restrictions regarding wear, make-up, hair style etc. were imposed on the

Table 2. Results for two experiment sets using the AT&T database

Evaluation Method	Approach	Recognition Rate
Experiment Set 1	Fisherfaces	94.50%
	ICA	85.00%
	Kernel Eigenfaces	94.00%
	2DPCA	96.00%
	SRC	93.00%
Experiment Set 2	Fisherfaces	98.50%
	ICA	93.80%
	Eigenfaces	97.50%
	Kernel Eigenfaces	98.00%
	2DPCA	93.80%
	SRC	97.50%

Figure 4. Gesture variations in the AR database; note the changing position of head with different poses

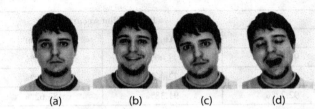

(a)   (b)   (c)   (d)

participants. Due to the large number of subjects and the substantial amount of variations, the AR database is much more challenging compared to the AT&T and Yale databases. It has been used by researchers as a test-bed to evaluate and benchmark face recognition algorithms. In this research we address the problem of varying facial expressions, see Figure 4. We evaluate the AR database under two experimental setups as proposed in literature, for all experiments the 576×768 image frames are down-sampled to an order 8×10 constituting an 80-D feature space.

For the first set of experiments, we follow the setup as designed in (Gao, 2002). A subset of AR database consisting of 112 individuals is randomly selected. The system is trained using only one image per subject that characterizes neutral expression (Figure 4 (a)), therefore we have 112 gallery images. The system is tested on the remaining three expressions shown in Figure 4 (b), (c) and (d) altogether making 336 probe images. Table 3 shows a thorough comparison of the SRC

approach and the results reported in (Gao, 2002). EM and LEM stands for Edge Map and Line Edge Map respectively while all other approaches being variants of Principle Component Analysis (PCA) (Gao, 2002).

SRC approach achieves a good recognition accuracy of 89.58% in the overall sense that outperforms the best-reported result of 75.67% (112-eigenvectors approach) by a margin of 13.91%. For the cases of smile and anger expressions, we obtained 93.75% and 91.07% respectively that are quite comparable to the best contestants i.e. 94.64% (60-eigenvectors) and 92.86% (LEM). For the screaming expression, the SRC approach outstandingly beats all the reported approaches attaining a decent recognition accuracy of 83.93%.

In the second set of experiments, we compare the proposed approach with two state of the art algorithms: Bayesian Eigenfaces (MIT) (Moghaddam & Pentland, 1997) and FaceIt (Visionics). The Bayesian Eigenfaces approach was reported

Table 3. Recognition results for gesture variations under Experiment Set 1

Approach	Recognition Accuracy			
	Smile	Anger	Scream	Overall
20-eigenvectors	87.85%	78.57%	34.82%	67.08%
60-eigenvectors	94.64%	84.82%	41.96%	73.80%
112-eigenvectors	93.97%	87.50%	45.54%	75.67%
112-eigenvectors w/o 1st 3	82.04%	73.21%	32.14%	62.46%
EM	52.68%	81.25%	20.54%	51.49%
LEM	78.57%	92.86%	31.25%	67.56%
SRC	93.75%	91.07%	83.93%	89.58%

Table 4. Recognition results for gesture variations under Experiment Set 2

Approach	Recognition Accuracy			
	Smile	**Anger**	**Scream**	**Overall**
FaceIt	96.00%	93.00%	78.00%	89.00%
MIT	94.00%	72.00%	41.00%	60.00%
SRC	92.24%	91.38%	83.62%	89.08%

to be one of the best in the 1996 FERET test (Phillips, Wechsler, Huang, & Rauss, 1998), whereas the FaceIt algorithm (based on Local Feature Analysis (Penev & Atick, 1996)) is claimed to be one of the most successful commercial face recognition system (Gross, Shi, & Cohn, 2001). A new subset of the AR database is generated by randomly selecting 116 individuals. The system is trained using the neutral expression of the first session (Figure 4 (a)) and therefore we have 116 gallery images. The system is validated for all other expressions of the same session (Figures 4 (b), (c) and (d)) making altogether 348 probe images. A comprehensive comparison of the SRC approach with these two state of the art algorithms is presented in Table 4, all the results are as reported in (Gross, Shi, & Cohn, 2001). For mild variations due to smile and anger expressions, the SRC approach yields quite competent recognition accuracies of 92.24% and 91.38% in comparison to FaceIt and MIT approaches. For the severe case of screaming expression, the SRC leads the FaceIt and MIT approaches by a margin of 5.62% and 42.62% respectively.

SPARSE REPRESENTATION FOR TEMPORAL FACE RECOGNITION

Due to ever increasing security threats, video surveillance systems have been deployed on a large scale. It is now becoming imperative to extend face recognition algorithms for the video-based applications. Video sequences are much more informative than still images as they also incorporate the temporal dimension. The most fundamental learning mode for video-based applications is called "Offline Batch Learning" in which the system is trained only once using video sequences and is not updated unless there is a need for additional enrollments. From the video surveillance perspective, this is perhaps the most important learning mode where we typically have video sequences of suspects for registration. With this understanding, we will comprehensively discuss the problem of video-based face recognition using the sparse representation classification framework. It would be quite interesting to explore if the sparse representation classification is of any added benefit when compared with the state of art SIFT feature-based approaches. For this purpose, the chapter will characterize extensive experiments on the publicly available VidTIMIT (Sanderson & Paliwal, 2004) database.

The Scale Invariant Feature Transform (SIFT) was proposed in 1999 for the extraction of unique features from images (Lowe, 1999). The idea, initially proposed for a more generic object recognition task, was later successfully applied for the problem of face recognition (Bicego, Lagorio, Grosso, & Tistarelli, 2006). Interesting characteristics of scale/rotation invariance and locality in both spatial and frequency domains have made the SIFT-based approach a pretty much standard technique in the paradigm of view-based face recognition. The first step in the derivation of the SIFT features is the identification of potential pixels of interest called "keypoints", in the face image. An efficient away of achieving this is to make use of the scale-space extremes of the Difference-of-

Gaussian (DoG) function convolved with the face image (Lowe, 1999). These potential keypoints are further refined based on the high contrasts, good localization along edges and the ratio of principal curvatures criterion. Orientation(s) are then assigned to each keypoint based on local image gradient direction(s). A gradient orientation histogram is formed using the neighboring pixels of each keypoint. Contribution from neighbors are weighted by their magnitudes and by a circular Gaussian window. Peaks in the histogram represent the dominant directions and are used to align the histogram for rotation invariance. 4×4 pixel neighborhoods are used to extract eight bin histograms resulting in 128-dimensional SIFT features. For illumination robustness, the vectors are normalized to unity, threshold to a ceiling of 0.2 and finally renormalized to unit length. Figure 5 shows a typical face from the VidTIMIT database (Sanderson, 2008) (Sanderson & Paliwal, 2004) with extracted SIFT features.

Experiments and Discussion

The problem of temporal face recognition using the SRC and SIFT feature based face recognition algorithms was evaluated on the VidTIMIT database (Sanderson, 2008) (Sanderson & Paliwal, 2004). VidTIMIT is a multimodal database consisting of video sequences and corresponding audio files from 43 distinct subjects. The video section of the database characterizes 10 different video files

Figure 5. A typical localized face from the VidTIMIT database with extracted SIFT features

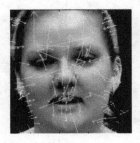

from each subject. Each video file is a sequence of 512×384 JPEG images. Two video sequences were used for training while the remaining eight were used for validation. One sequence is shown in Figure 6. Due to the high correlation between consecutive frames, training and testing were carried out on alternate frames. Off-line batch learning mode (Lee, Ho, Yang, & Kriegman, 2005) was used for these experiments and therefore probe frames did not add any information to the system.

Face localization is the first step in any face recognition system. Fully automatic face localization was carried out using a Harr-like feature based face detection algorithm (Viola & Jones, 2004) during off-line training and on-line recognition sessions. For the SIFT based face recognition, each detected face in a video frame was scale-normalized to 150×150 and histogram equalized before the extraction of the SIFT features. We achieved an identification rate of 93.83%. Verification experiments were also conducted for a more comprehensive comparison between the two approaches. An Equal Error Rate (EER) of 1.8% was achieved for the SIFT based verification. Verification rate at 0.01 False Accept Rate (FAR) was found to be 97.32%.

For the SRC classifier, each detected face in a frame is down-sampled to order 10×10. Column concatenation is carried out to generate a 100-dimensional feature vector. Off-line batch learning is carried out on alternate frames using two video sequences as discussed above. Unorthodox down-sampled images in combination with the SRC classifier yielded quite comparable recognition accuracy of 94.45%. EER dropped to 1.3% with a verification accuracy of 98.23% at 0.01 FAR. The rank profile and ROC (Receiver Operating Characteristics) curves are shown in Figure 7 (a) and (b) respectively.

We further investigated the complementary nature of the two classifiers by fusing them at the score level. The weighted sum rule is used which is perhaps the major workhorse in the field of combining classifiers (Kittler, Hatef, Duin, &

Figure 6. A sample video sequence from the VidTIMIT database

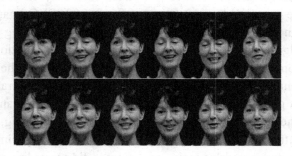

Matas, 1998). Both classifiers were equally weighted and a high recognition accuracy of 97.73% was achieved which outperforms the SIFT based classifier and the SRC classifier by a margin of 3.90% and 3.28% respectively. Verification experiments also produced superior results with an EER of 0.3% which is better than the SIFT and the SRC based classification by 1.5% and 1.0% respectively. An excellent verification of 99.90% at an FAR of 0.01 is reported. Fusion of the two classifiers substantially improved the rank profile as well achieving 100% results at rank-5 only. A detailed comparison of the results is provided in Table 5.

Apart from these appreciable results it was found that the l_1-norm minimization using a large dictionary matrix made the iterative convergence lengthy and slow. To provide a comparative value we performed computational analysis for a

randomly selected identification trail. The time required by the SRC algorithm for classifying a single frame on a typical 2.66 GHz machine with 2 GB memory was found to be 297.46 seconds (approximately 5 minutes). This duration is approximately 5 times greater than the processing time of the SIFT algorithm for the same frame which was found to be 58.18 seconds (approximately 1 minute). Typically, a video sequence consists of hundreds of frames that would suggest a rather prolonged span for the evaluation of the whole video sequence. Noteworthy is the fact that experiments were conducted using an offline learning mode (Lee, Ho, Yang, & Kriegman, 2005). The probe frames did not contribute to the dictionary information. Critically speaking, the spatiotemporal information in video sequences is best harnessed using smart online (Liu, Wang, & Tan, 2007) and hybrid (Lee, Ho, Yang, & Krieg-

Figure 7. (a) Rank profiles and (b) ROC curves for the SIFT, SRC and the combination of the two classifiers

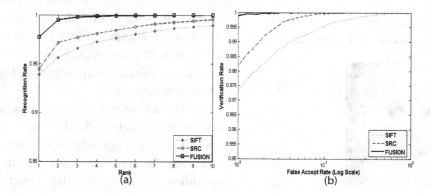

Table 5. Summary of results

Evaluation Attributes	SIFT	SRC	Fusion
Recognition Accuracy	93.83%	94.45%	97.73%
Equal Error Rate	1.80%	1.30%	0.30%
Verification rate at 0.01FAR	97.32%	98.23%	99.90%

man, 2005) learning modes. These interactive learning algorithms add useful information along the temporal dimension and therefore enhance the overall performance. However, in the context of SRC classification, this would suggest an even larger dictionary matrix and consequently a lengthier evaluation.

CONCLUSION AND FUTURE TRENDS

Sparse representation classification has recently emerged as the latest paradigm in the research of appearance-based face recognition. A comprehensive evaluation of the SRC algorithm provides a comparable index with traditional, state of the art approaches. It has also been found robust for the problem of varying facial expressions. We further extend the approach for the problem of video-based face recognition. An identification rate of 94.45% is achieved on the VidTIMIT database which is quite comparable to 93.83% accuracy using state-of-the-art SIFT features based algorithm. Verification experiments were also conducted and the SRC approach exhibited an EER of 1.30% which is 0.5% better than the SIFT method. The SRC classifier was found to nicely complement the SIFT based method, the fusion of the two methods using the weighted sum rule consistently produced superior results for identification, verification and rank-recognition experiments. However since SRC requires an iterative convergence using an l_1-norm minimization, the approach was found computationally expensive as compared to the SIFT based recognition. Typically SRC required

5 minutes (approximately) for processing a single recognition trial which is 5 times greater than the time required by the SIFT based recognition approach. To the best of our knowledge, this is the first evaluation of the SRC algorithm on a video database. From the experiments presented in the paper, it is quite safe to maintain that additional work is required before the SRC approach is declared as a standard approach for video-based applications. Computational expense is arguably an inherent issue with video processing giving rise to the emerging area of "Video Abstraction". Efficient algorithms have been proposed to cluster video sequences along the temporal dimension (for example (Chan & Vasconcelos, 2008) including others). These clusters are then portrayed by cluster-representative frame(s)/features resulting in a substantial decrease of complexity. Given the good performance of the SRC algorithm presented in this research, the evaluation of the method using state-of-the-art video abstraction methods will be the subject of future research.

REFERENCES

Baraniuk, R. (2007). *Compressive sensing*. IEEE Signal Processing Magazine.

Baraniuk, R., Davenport, M., DeVore, R., & Wakin, M. B. (2006). *The Johnson-Lindenstrauss lemma meets compressed sensing*. Retrieved from www.dsp.rice.edu/cs/jlcs-v03.pdf

Belhumeur, V., Hespanha, J., & Kriegman, D. (1997). *Eigenfaces vs Fisherfaces: Recognition Using Class Specific Linear Projection*. IEEE Tran. PAMI.

Bicego, M., Lagorio, A., Grosso, E., & Tistarelli, M. (2006). *On the use of SIFT features for face authentication*. CVPRW.

Candes, E., Romberg, J., & Tao, T. (2006). Stable signal recovery from incomplete and inaccurate measurements. *Comm. on Pure and Applied Math*, 1207-1223.

Candes, E., & Tao, T. (2006). Near-optimal signal recovery from random projections: Universal encoding strategies? *IEEE Tran. Infm. Theory*, 5406-5425.

Chan, A. B., & Vasconcelos, N. (2008). *Modeling, Clustering, and Segmenting Video with Mixtures of Dynamic Textures*. IEEE Trans. PAMI.

Donoho, D. (2006). Compressed sensing. *IEEE Transactions on Information Theory*, 1289–1306. doi:10.1109/TIT.2006.871582

Donoho, D. (2006). *For most large underdetermined systems of linear equations the minimal l1-norm solution is also the sparsest solution*. Comm. on Pure and Applied Math.

Duda, R. O., Hart, P. E., & Stork, D. G. (2000). *Pattern Classification*. New York: John Wiley & Sons, Inc.

E, C., J, R., & T, T. (2006). Robust uncertainty principles: Exact signal reconstruction from highly incomplete frequency information. *IEEE Trans. Inform. Theory*.

Gao, Y. a. (2002). Face recognition using line edge map. *IEEE Trans. on PAMI*, 764-779.

Gross, R., Shi, J., & Cohn, J. (2001). Quo Vadis Face Recognition? In *Third Workshop on Empirical Evaluation Methods in Computer Vision*.

Jolliffe, I. T. (1986). *Pricipal Component Analysis*. New York: Springer.

Kittler, J., Hatef, M., Duin, R. P., & Matas, J. (1998). *On Combining Classifiers*. IEEE Trans. on Pattern Analysis and Machine Intelligence.

Lee, K., Ho, J., Yang, M., & Kriegman, D. (2005). *Visual Tracking and Recognition using Probabilistic Appearance Manifolds*. CVIU.

Lee, K., & Kriegman, D. (2005). *Online Probabilistic Appearance Manifolds for Video-based Recognition and Tracking*. CVPR.

Li, S. Z., & Jain, A. K. (2005). *Handbook of Face Recognition*. Berlin: Springer.

Liu, L., Wang, Y., & Tan, T. (2007). *Online Appearance Model*. CVPR.

Lowe, D. (1999). Object recognition from local scale-invariant features. In *Intl. Conf. on Computer Vision* (pp. 1150-1157).

Martinez, A., & Benavente, R. (1998). *The AR Face Database*. CVC.

Moghaddam, B., & Pentland, A. P. (1997). *Probabilistic Visual Learning for Object Representation*. IEEE Trans. on PAMI.

Naseem, I., Togneri, R., & Bennamoun, M. (2008). Sparse Representation for Ear Biometrics. In *International Symposium on Visual Computing*.

Naseem, I., Togneri, R., & Bennamoun, M. (2009). *Linear Regression for Face Recognition*. IEEE Trans. on Pattern Analysis and Machine Intelligence.

Penev, P., & Atick, J. (1996). Local Feature Analysis: A General Statistical Theory for Object Representation. *Network: Computation in Neural Systems*.

Phillips, P. J., Wechsler, H., Huang, J. S., & Rauss, P. J. (1998). *The FERET Database and Evaluation Procedure for Face-recognition Algorithms*. Image and Vision Computing.

Samaria, F., & Harter, A. (1994). Parameterisation of a Stochastic Model for Human Face Identification. In *Proc. Second IEEE Workshop Applications of Computer Vision*.

Sanderson, C. (2008). *Biometric Person Recognition: Face*. Speech and Fusion.

Sanderson, C., & Paliwal, K. K. (2004). Identity Verification Using Speech and Face Information. *Digital Signal Processing*, 449–480. doi:10.1016/j.dsp.2004.05.001

Turk, M., & Pentland, A. (1991). Eigenfaces for Recognition. *Journal of Cognitive Neurosicence*.

Viola, P., & Jones, M. (2004). Robust Real-time Face Detection. *International Journal of Computer Vision*, 137–154. doi:10.1023/B:VISI.0000013087.49260.fb

Wright, J., Yang, A., Ganesh, A., Sastri, S. S., & Ma, Y. (2009). Robust face recognition via sparse representation. *IEEE Trans. PAMI*, 210-227.

Yale Univ. *Face Database*. (2002). Retrieved from http://cvc.yale.edu/projects/yalefaces

Yang, J., Zhang, D., Frangi, A. F., & Yang, J. (2004). *Two-dimensional PCA: A New Approach to Appearance-based Face Representation and Recognition*. IEEE Tans. PAMI.

Yang, M. H. (n. d.). Kernel Eignefaces vs Kernel Fisherfaces: Face Recognition using Kernel Methods. In *Proc. Fifth IEEE Int'l Conf. Automatic FAce and Gesture Recognition (RGR'02)*.

Yuen, P. C., & Lai, J. H. (2002). *Face Representation using Independent Component Analysis*. Pattern Recognition.

KEY TERMS AND DEFINITIONS

Feature Extraction: Discriminative and brief representation of patterns from various object classes, typically high dimensional data is represented a small feature vector.

Classification: Process of assigning class label to an unknown pattern.

Biometric Recognition: Identifying a person using the physiological or behavioral characteristics such as face, speech, body gait etc.

Face Recognition: Recognizing a person using facial features.

Face Identification: A face recognition scenario where a given test image is assumed to be from one of the registered users, it is also called as closed-set evaluation.

Face Verification: A face recognition scenario where a given test image is not necessarily from one of the registered users, it is also called as open-set evaluation

Temporal Face Recognition: A typical face recognition scenario based on video streams rather than static images that incorporate the temporal information.

Chapter 10
Probabilistic Methods for Face Registration and Recognition

Peng Li
University College London, UK

Simon J. D. Prince
University College London, UK

ABSTRACT

In this chapter the authors review probabilistic approaches to face recognition and present extended treatment of one particular approach. Here, the face image is decomposed into an additive sum of two parts: a deterministic component, which depends on an underlying representation of identity and a stochastic component which explains the fact that two face images from the same person are not identical. Inferences about matching are made by comparing different probabilistic models rather than comparing distance to an identity template in some projected space. The authors demonstrate that this model comparison is superior to distance comparison. Furthermore, the authors show that performance can be further improved by sampling the feature space and combining models trained using these feature subspaces. Both random sampling with and without replacement significantly improves performance. Finally, the authors illustrate how this probabilistic approach can be adapted for keypoint localization (e.g. finding the eyes, nose and mouth etc.). The keypoints can either be (1) explicitly localized by evaluating the likelihood of all the possible locations in the given image, or (2) implicitly localized by marginalizing over possible positions in a Bayesian manner. The authors show that recognition and keypoint localization performance are comparable to using manual labelling.

DOI: 10.4018/978-1-61520-991-0.ch010

INTRODUCTION

In this chapter, we present an overview of the use of probabilistic models for face recognition. In particular, we present and extended treatment of the idea of *latent identity variables* (*LIVs*). An example of LIV model is *"Probabilistic Linear Discriminant Analyzer"* (*PLDA*) model (Prince & Elder, 2007; Ioffe, 2006). In this model, the face image is decomposed into an additive sum of two parts: a deterministic component, which depends on an underlying representation of identity only and a stochastic component which explains the fact that two face images from the same person are not identical. In contrast to typical subspace algorithms, LIV models do not rely on distance measurements between representations of identity. Instead, inferences about matching are made by comparing different probabilistic models. We demonstrate that this *model comparison* is superior to distance comparison using the XM2VTS database (Matas et al., 2000).

In the next section, we show that performance of the proposed model can be further improved by sampling the feature space and combining a set of LIV models trained using these feature subspaces in an ensemble. This can relieve the curse of dimensionality problem faced by a single PLDA model. Both random sampling with or without replacement are investigated in the experiments.

Finally, we also illustrate how this probabilistic approach can be adapted to locate keypoints for *face registration*, (e.g. finding the corner of the eye, nose and mouth etc.). The keypoints can either be (1) explicitly localized by evaluating the likelihood of all the possible locations in the given image using a learned LIV model, or (2) implicitly localized by marginalizing over them in a Bayesian manner. It is shown that both the recognition and localization performance based on this probabilistic formulation are comparable to that for manual labelling.

BACKGROUND AND RELATED WORK

Automated face recognition systems can be used in access control, image search, security and other areas. However, current systems are not sufficiently accurate and reliable, which prevents the widespread deployment in the real world. One of the problems is that face recognition systems consist of a pipeline of sequential operations (Zhao, Chellappa, Phillips, & Rosenfeld, 2003): face detection, face registration and face recognition (inference). A problem at any part of the pipeline causes overall performance to degrade.

The inference stage is perhaps the most widely studied on face recognition (Turk & Pentland, 1991; Belhumeur, Hespanha, & Kriegman, 1997; Zhao et al., 2003; Yang, Frangi, Yang, & Jin, 2005; He, Yan, Hu, & Niyogi, 2005; Prince & Elder, 2007; Wang, Yan, Huang, Liu, & Tang, 2008). Many face recognition algorithms are subspace-based. The extracted image measurements are mapped to a lower dimensional feature space, in which the distance between points is used to make decisions about similarity. Proposed mappings have included linear approaches such as Principal Component Analysis (PCA) (Turk & Pentland, 1991), Linear Discriminant Analysis (LDA) (Belhumeur et al., 1997) and Laplacianfaces (He et al., 2005) as well as nonlinear approaches such as Kernel Linear Discriminant Analysis (KLDA) (Yang et al., 2005).

LDA (Belhumeur et al., 1997) is perhaps one of the most widely used approaches for face recognition: it measures the within-individual covariance and the between-individual covariance and projects the data to a subspace where the ratio of between:within variance is greatest. While this algorithm is simple and effective, it has a number of problems. First, the number of dimensions is limited by the amount of training individuals. This is known as the small sample problem (Wang & Tang, 2006). Second, there may be directions in which there no within-individual variance was observed. However, such directions cannot easily be included as the ratio of between:within variance in these directions is not defined. The null-space LDA approach (Chen, Liao, Lin, Ko, & Yu, 2000) exploited the signal in the remaining subspace. The dual-Space LDA approach (Wang & Tang, 2004) combined these two approaches.

One possible solution to the small sample problem is to learn an ensemble of single classifiers trained using different feature subsets, such as PCA subspaces (Wang & Tang, 2006), Fourier features (Su, Shan., Chen, & Gao, 2007), Gabor features (Su, Shan., Chen, & Gao, 2006; Su et al., 2007) and spatial histograms of local (Gabor) binary patterns (Shan, Zhang, Su, Chen, & Gao, 2006). Such multiple classifier ensembles are variously called mixtures of experts or combination of multiple classifiers (Kuncheva, Bezdek, & Duin, 2001). The goal is to combine a set of classifiers so that the resultant ensemble has superior classification performance to that of using each individual classifier alone. One important condition for the success of an ensemble is that the outputs of individual classifiers to the same inputs must be diverse (Kuncheva & Whitaker, 2003). Diverse individual classifiers can be obtained by using different training data sets, different feature subsets, various types of individual classifiers and fusion rules. Some attempts have been made to explain why multiple classifier ensemble outperforms individual classifiers. One explanation is based on the bias-variance decomposition of the error (Breiman, 1996). It indicates that ensembles not only reduce the variance but also the bias.

Since face recognition systems have the form of a pipeline, the achievements in the inference stage are diminished if the preceding operations are not reliable. A particular bottleneck is face registration which remains a hard problem despite much investigation (Cootes, Edwards,& Taylor, 2001;Mahoor & Abdel Mottaleb, 2006; Ilonen et al., 2008). In local approaches, data are explicitly extracted from the region around the keypoints (Cootes et al., 2001; Mahoor & Abdel Mottaleb,

2006; Ilonen et al., 2008). In global approaches, the keypoints are used to register the image to a common template (Turk & Pentland, 1991; Belhumeur et al., 1997). In either case recognition performance degrades if the keypoints are not accurately localized (Martinez, 2002; Wang et al., 2008). In order to scientifically isolate the recognition stage, it is common to use manually labelled features (Wang et al., 2008; Shan et al., 2008), while others simply do not detail how keypoints were localized.

PROBABILISTIC FACE RECOGNITION

Most approaches to face recognition rely ultimately on a distance comparison: the probe image is projected into a lower-dimensional space where its distance to each of the gallery images (templates) is calculated. The matching face is taken to be the closest gallery image. The particular choice of low-dimensional space is learned from a training data set. A good space maximizes the correlation between identity and distance while simultaneously minimizing the effect of nuisance variables such as pose or illumination on position.

These distance based models provide a hard decision of which person in the gallery matches the probe image. In practice it would be better to assign a probability to whether faces match or not and thereby possess information about the certainty of the decision. In a practical system, we could defer the final decision and collect more data if the uncertainty is too great. A probabilistic approach also allows us to combine measurements from different image regions, frames, cameras or biometrics without difficulty.

Probabilistic approaches to inference in face recognition can be divided into discriminative and generative methods. Generative models describe the probability density of the image measurements under matching and non-matching conditions. By comparing the observed data to each of these models, it is possible to calculate a posterior probability over whether the faces match using Bayes rule. In contrast, discriminative models directly take images and return a posterior distribution over matching conditions. In this chapter, we will focus on generative methods.

The most well-known example of a generative probabilistic method for face recognition is the method of Moghaddam and Pentland (Moghaddam, Jebara, & Pentland, 2000) who considers the pixelwise difference between probe and gallery images. If the two images are from the same individual, this difference will be small, whereas if they came from different individuals, it will be larger. They modelled probability distributions of "within-individual" and "between-individual" differences. For a probe image, the difference with each gallery image is considered and the one with the maximum posterior probability of being due to a "within-individual change" is selected. This is well suited to face verification, but does not provide a posterior over possible matches in face identification. Moreover, performance in uncontrolled conditions is poor (Lucey & Chen, 2006). There is no obvious way to remedy either of these problems.

An alternative approach is to assume that there are several examples of each person in the database and to build a probabilistic model for each. For example, Zhang and Martinez (Zhang & Martinez, 2006) deformed regions of the face by plausible 2-dimensional transformations and projected the results into feature space. The resulting data for each individual was described using a mixture of Gaussians model. New data is then evaluated under each of these models, and the one under which this data is most probable is declared the winner. This approach is straightforward, but is only suited to face identification where we have multiple examples of the gallery individuals. It cannot cope with face verification, and it cannot exploit training data of individuals that are not in the training database.

It should be noted that there are other approaches to face recognition that are probabilistic, but do not provide a posterior over possible matches. For example, Zhou and Chellapa (Zhou & Chellappa, 2004) presented a probabilistic framework for face recognition. They calculate a probabilistic representation of the data but subsequently measure distances between these probabilistic representations. This method is hence better characterized as a *distance-based approach*.

In recent years a series of face recognition methods have appeared that are both probabilistic and generative (Ioffe, 2006; Prince & Elder, 2007; Prince, Elder, Warrell, & Felisberti, 2008). They provide a valid posterior distribution over matches for both identification and verification tasks. They can generalize from just a single example of each gallery image and have been extended to tackle recognition under pose changes (Prince et al., 2008). In the remaining part of this chapter we review these methods and show how the probabilistic formulation can be extended to incorporate registration of the facial images.

Latent Identity Variables

We assume that there is a underlying multi-dimensional variable h which represents the identity of an individual person. Such a variable is termed a Latent Identity Variable or LIV. By definition, it is constant for an individual person regardless the effect of illumination, pose, expression or any other factors. If two LIVs differ, they describe different people. When they are identical they represent the same person.

Traditional subspace methods in face recognition such as principal component analysis (PCA) (Turk & Pentland, 1991) or linear discriminant analysis (LDA) (Belhumeur et al., 1997) attempt to find a mapping which projects an probe face image to an explicit point in a lower-dimensional space. Matching between the probe image and the gallery images is based on the distance between the mapped probe point and the mapped gallery images. In contrast to this approach, we do not assume that we can directly observe the LIVs. Instead, we consider that the observed face images were generated from the latent LIV by a noisy process (see Figure 1) as follows

$$\mathbf{x}_{ij} = f(\mathbf{h}_i, \theta, \mathbf{w}_{ij}) + \varepsilon_{ij}, \tag{1}$$

where $\mathbf{x}_{ij}$ is the feature vector from the j-th image of the i-th person. The term θ denotes the model parameters which are learned in a training stage and remains constant during testing. The term $h\mathbf{i}$ is the LIV of the ith person. This remains constant for all of the images (indexed by j) of that person which parameterizes the between-individual variance. The term $w\mathbf{i}_j$ is a latent noise variable. This parameterizes the within-individual variance due to factors such as pose and illumination. The term $\varepsilon\mathbf{i}_j$ represents additive Gaussian noise and is used to explain any remaining unexplained variation.

Probabilistic Linear Discriminant Analysis

In order to make these ideas concrete, we present an example. The "Probabilistic Linear Discriminant Analyzer" or PLDA model (Prince & Elder, 2007) is a probabilistic version of LDA (Belhumeur et al., 1997). In this particular case the function $f()$ from Equation (1) consists of an additive sum of deterministic signal and stochastic noise components:

$$\mathbf{x}_{ij} = \mu + \mathbf{F}\mathbf{h}_i + \mathbf{G}\mathbf{w}_{ij} + \varepsilon_{ij} \tag{2}$$

The first component, $\mu + \mathbf{F}\mathbf{h}_i$, represents the identity signal. It does not contain any elements that depend on the particular instance j of the given person i"s face. The term $\mathbf{h}_i$ is an LIV: an idealized representation of human identity. The second component $\mathbf{G}\mathbf{w}_{ij} + \varepsilon_{ij}$ represents within-individual noise and is different for every image.

The term μ represents the overall mean of the data. The matrix $\mathbf{F}$ defines a basis for the identity (between individual) subspace. The columns of $\mathbf{F}$ are similar to the eigenfaces of (Turk & Pentland, 1991). The term $\mathbf{h}_i$ represents the position in this subspace (similar to the weighting of eigenfaces). Similarly, the matrix $\mathbf{G}$ defines a basis for the within-individual variation, and $\mathbf{w}_{ij}$ represents the position within this subspace. The term ε_{ij} is mean zero Gaussian noise, with diagonal covariance Σ It accounts for any further image variation that is not well described by the previous components.

More formally, we can re-write the model in terms of conditional probabilities:

$$Pr(\mathbf{h}_i) = \mathbf{G}_\mathbf{h}\left[\mathbf{0}, \mathbf{I}\right] \tag{3}$$

$$Pr(\mathbf{w}_{ij}) = \mathbf{G}_\mathbf{w}\left[\mathbf{0}, \mathbf{I}\right] \tag{4}$$

$$Pr(\mathbf{x}_{ij} \mid \mathbf{h}_i, \mathbf{w}_{ij}) = \mathbf{G}_\mathbf{x}\left[\mu + \mathbf{F}\mathbf{h}_i + \mathbf{G}\mathbf{w}_{ij}, \Sigma\right] \tag{5}$$

where $\mathbf{G}_\alpha\left[\beta, \Gamma\right]$ denotes a Gaussian distribution in α with mean β and covariance Γ. We have also specified priors over the latent variables $\mathbf{h}_i, \mathbf{w}_{ij}$ to complete the model. The unknown parameters θ are learnt from training data.

Figure 1. Graphical model of typical latent identity variable model

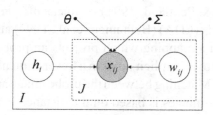

Learning the Parameters

The target of learning stage is to estimate the parameters $\theta=\{\mathbf{F},\mathbf{G},\boldsymbol{\mu},\Sigma\}$ based on training data $\mathbf{X}=\{\mathbf{x}_{ij}\in\Re^{D_x}\mid i=1\ldots N,j=1\ldots,J\}$, where D_x is the dimension of the data x. The task of learning would be easy if both observed data X and latent variables $\mathbf{H}=\{\mathbf{h}_i\in\Re^{D_h}\mid i=1\ldots N\}$ and $\mathbf{W}=\{\mathbf{w}_{ij}\in\Re^{D_w}\mid i=1\ldots N,j=1\ldots,J\}$ were known. Similarly, D_h and D_w are the dimensions of latent variables $\mathbf{h}$ and $\mathbf{w}$. Unfortunately, we only observe the original data $\mathbf{X}$. The problem is approachable using the expectation maximization (EM) algorithm (Dempster, Laird, & Rubin, 1977).

Using Equation (2), the images from the ith identity $X_i=\{\mathbf{x}_{ij}\mid j=1,2,\cdots,J\}$ form a composite system

$$\begin{pmatrix}\mathbf{x}_{i1}\\\mathbf{x}_{i2}\\\ldots\\\mathbf{x}_{iJ}\end{pmatrix}=\begin{pmatrix}\mu\\\mu\\\ldots\\\mu\end{pmatrix}+\begin{pmatrix}F & G & 0 & \cdots & 0\\F & 0 & G & \cdots & 0\\F & 0 & 0 & \cdots & 0\\\ldots & \ldots & \ldots & \ldots & \ldots\\F & 0 & 0 & \cdots & G\end{pmatrix}\begin{pmatrix}\mathbf{h}_i\\\mathbf{w}_{i1}\\\mathbf{w}_{i2}\\\ldots\\\mathbf{w}_{iJ}\end{pmatrix}+\begin{pmatrix}\varepsilon_{i1}\\\varepsilon_{i2}\\\ldots\\\varepsilon_{iJ}\end{pmatrix},$$

$$(6)$$

or

$$\tilde{\mathbf{x}}_i=\tilde{\mu}+\tilde{\mathbf{A}}\,\mathbf{y}_i+\tilde{\varepsilon}_i,\qquad(7)$$

where the covariance matrix of noise term $\tilde{\varepsilon}_i$ is

$$\tilde{\Sigma}=\begin{vmatrix}\Sigma & 0 & \cdots & 0\\0 & \Sigma & \cdots & 0\\\cdots & \cdots & \cdots & \cdots\\0 & 0 & \cdots & \Sigma\end{vmatrix}.$$ This is the form of a

standard factor analysis (FA) model (Rubin & Thayer, 1982). We can rewrite the compound model in terms of probabilities to give

$$Pr(\mathbf{y}_i)=G_{\mathbf{y}_i}\left[\mathbf{0},\mathbf{I}\right]\qquad(8)$$

$$Pr(\tilde{\mathbf{x}}_i\mid\mathbf{y}_i)=G_{\mathbf{x}_i}\left[\tilde{\mu}+\tilde{\mathbf{A}}\,\mathbf{y}_i,\tilde{\Sigma}\right]\qquad(9)$$

The joint distribution of $\tilde{\mathbf{x}}_i$ and $\mathbf{y}_i$ is

$$Pr(\mathbf{y}_i,\tilde{\mathbf{x}}_i\mid\theta)=Pr(\tilde{\mathbf{x}}_i\mid\mathbf{y}_i,\theta)Pr(\mathbf{y}_i).\qquad(10)$$

From Equations (8), (9) and (10), the joint log-likelihood of the observed data X and latent variables $Y=\{\mathbf{y}_i\mid i=1,2,\cdots,N\}$ can be written as

$$\begin{aligned}L_\theta&=\sum_{i=1}^N\log[Pr(\tilde{\mathbf{x}}_i\mid\mathbf{y}_i,\theta)Pr(\mathbf{y}_i)]\\&=-\frac{1}{2}\sum_{i=1}^N[\tilde{\mathbf{x}}_i-(\tilde{\mu}+\tilde{A}\mathbf{y}_i)]^T\tilde{\Sigma}^{-1}[\tilde{\mathbf{x}}_i-(\tilde{\mu}+\tilde{A}\mathbf{y}_i)]-\frac{N}{2}\log|\tilde{\Sigma}|-\frac{1}{2}\sum_{n=1}^N\mathbf{y}_i^T\mathbf{y}_i+Const\end{aligned}$$

$$(11)$$

The learning consists of two iterative steps: the expectation (E-Step) and maximization (M-Step) procedures. In the E-step, we compute the expected log--likelihood $Q(\theta_t\mid\theta_{t-1})=E[L_{\theta_t}\mid X,\theta_{t-1}]$ with respect to the posterior distribution over the latent variable Y, $\prod_{i=1}^N Pr(\mathbf{y}_i\mid\mathbf{x}_i,\theta_{t-1})$. Here t is the index of iteration. In the M-step, we re-estimate the parameters θ by maximizing $Q(\theta_t)$: $\theta=\arg\max_{\theta_t}Q(\theta_t\mid\theta_{t-1})$. We explain them in turn.

Expectation (E)--Step: The goal is to estimate a full posterior distribution $Pr(\mathbf{y}_i\mid\tilde{\mathbf{x}}_i,\theta)$ of LIVs $\mathbf{y}_i=(\mathbf{h}_i,w_{ij})$ for each individual separately by fixing the model parameters θ given the data $\mathbf{X}$. By Bayes rule,

$$Pr(\mathbf{y}_i\mid\tilde{\mathbf{x}}_i,\theta)\propto Pr(\tilde{\mathbf{x}}_i\mid\mathbf{y}_i,\theta)Pr(\mathbf{y}_i)\qquad(12)$$

Since the product of two Gaussians is also a Gaussian, it can be shown that the two moments of the Gaussian are:

$$E[\mathbf{y}_i \mid \tilde{\mathbf{x}}_i, \theta] = (\tilde{\mathbf{A}}^T \tilde{\Sigma}^{-1} \tilde{\mathbf{A}} + I)^{-1} \tilde{\mathbf{A}}^T \tilde{\Sigma}^{-1} (\tilde{\mathbf{x}}_i - \tilde{\mu}) \tag{13}$$

$$E[\mathbf{y}_i \mathbf{y}_i^T \mid \tilde{\mathbf{x}}_i, \theta] = (\tilde{\mathbf{A}}^T \tilde{\Sigma}^{-1} \tilde{\mathbf{A}} + I)^{-1} + E[\mathbf{y}_i \mid \tilde{\mathbf{x}}_i, \theta] E[\mathbf{y}_i \mid \tilde{\mathbf{x}}_i, \theta]^T \tag{14}$$

Maximization (M)--Step: The goal is to update the values of the parameters $\theta = \{\mu, \mathbf{F}, \mathbf{G}, \Sigma\}$. Setting the joint log--likelihood L_θ in Equation (11) to these parameters to zero respectively and re-arrange to provide the following update rules:

$$\mu = \frac{1}{NJ} \sum_{i,j} x_{ij} \tag{15}$$

$$\mathbf{A} = \left\{ \sum_{i,j} (\mathbf{x}_{ij} - \mu) E[\mathbf{y}_i]^T \right\} \left\{ \sum_{i,j} E[\mathbf{y}_i \mathbf{y}_i^T] \right\}^{-1} \tag{16}$$

$$\Sigma = \frac{1}{NJ} \sum_{i,j} diag \left[(\mathbf{x}_{ij} - \mu)(\mathbf{x}_{ij} - \mu)^T - \mathbf{A} E[\mathbf{y}_i](\mathbf{x}_{ij} - \mu)^T \right] \tag{17}$$

where $A = [\mathbf{F}\,\mathbf{G}]$ and *diag* is the operation of taking the diagonal element from a matrix.

The parameters θ can be initialized randomly. The E-step and M-step are iterated until convergence. The combination of the E-Step and M-Step is guaranteed to increase the overall likelihood of the model at every iteration. The learned parameters can then be used for the following face recognition tasks.

Inference by Model Comparison

We approach matching by comparing a set of models, each of which explains the data in a dif-

ferent way. Consider the case where we would like to match a probe image $\mathbf{x}_p$ to one of K gallery images $\mathbf{X}_G = \{\mathbf{x}_k \mid k = 1 \ldots K\}$ in a closed set identification task. We compare K models that explain the data, where model M_k describes the scenario in which the probe image $\mathbf{x}_p$ matches gallery image $\mathbf{x}_K$. The likelihood of observed data $\mathbf{x}_1 \ldots \mathbf{x}_K$ and $\mathbf{x}_p$ using Model k can be evaluated as follows

$$Pr(\mathbf{x}_{1\ldots K}, \mathbf{x}_p \mid \mathsf{M}_k) = \int \int Pr(\mathbf{x}_1 \mid \mathbf{h}_1, \mathbf{w}_1) d\mathbf{h}_1 d\mathbf{w}_1 \cdots$$

$$\int \int \int Pr(\mathbf{x}_k, \mathbf{x}_p \mid \mathbf{h}_k, \mathbf{w}_k \mathbf{w}_p) d\mathbf{h}_k d\mathbf{w}_k d\mathbf{w}_p \cdots \int \int Pr(\mathbf{x}_K \mid \mathbf{h}_K, \mathbf{w}_K) d\mathbf{h}_K \mathbf{w}_K \tag{18}$$

If the likelihood data using model M_k is the higher than all the other models, we determine that the probe image $\mathbf{x}_p$ matches gallery image $\mathbf{x}_K$. Figure 2 illustrates two models in a closed-set identification task where we have omitted the latent noise variables for clarity.

There are two types of term in Equation (18). For K-1 of the terms, the image $\mathbf{x}$ does not match any of the other images. For these terms we have:

Figure 2. Closed-set face identification by model comparison. The task is to decide which of two gallery images $\mathbf{x}_1$ and $\mathbf{x}_2$ best match a probe image $\mathbf{x}_p$. Models 1 and 2 describe the different scenarios where the probe image $\mathbf{x}_p$ matches gallery image $\mathbf{x}_1$ and $\mathbf{x}_2$ respectively. The model under which all of the observed data $\mathbf{x}_1$, $\mathbf{x}_2$ and $\mathbf{x}_p$ is most likely is selected as the final decision.

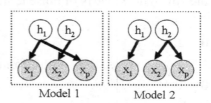

$$\mathbf{x} = \mu + \begin{bmatrix} \mathbf{F} & \mathbf{G} \end{bmatrix} \begin{bmatrix} \mathbf{h} \\ \mathbf{w} \end{bmatrix} + \varepsilon \qquad (19)$$

Let $A = [\mathbf{F}\,\mathbf{G}]$ and $z = [h\,w]^T$, which are the latent variables. Equation (19) becomes a standard factor analyzer: $\mathbf{x} = \mu + \mathbf{A}z + \varepsilon$. Thus we have

$$Pr(\mathbf{x}\mid\mathbf{z}) = \mathbf{G}_{\mathbf{x}}\left[\mu + \mathbf{A}\mathbf{z}, \Sigma\right] \qquad (20)$$

$$Pr(\mathbf{z}) = \mathbf{G}_{\mathbf{z}}\left[\mathbf{0}, \mathbf{I}\right] \qquad (21)$$

The likelihood of observing the image assuming that there was no match to any other images can be calculated by marginalizing over the hidden variables $\mathbf{z}$ to give:

$$Pr(\mathbf{x}) = \mathbf{G}_{\mathbf{x}}\left[\mu, \mathbf{A}\mathbf{A}^T + \Sigma\right] \qquad (22)$$

The second case is when the probe image $\mathbf{x}_p$ matches a gallery image $\mathbf{x}_g$. We use the generative equation:

$$\begin{bmatrix} \mathbf{x}_p \\ \mathbf{x}_g \end{bmatrix} = \begin{bmatrix} \mu \\ \mu \end{bmatrix} + \begin{bmatrix} \mathbf{F} & \mathbf{G} & \mathbf{0} \\ \mathbf{F} & \mathbf{0} & \mathbf{G} \end{bmatrix} \begin{bmatrix} \mathbf{h} \\ \mathbf{w}_p \\ \mathbf{w}_g \end{bmatrix} + \begin{bmatrix} \varepsilon_p \\ \varepsilon_g \end{bmatrix} \qquad (23)$$

or

$$\mathbf{x}' = \mu' + \mathbf{B}\mathbf{z} + \varepsilon' \qquad (24)$$

which again has the form of a standard factor analyzer. The likelihood of the data under this model is:

$$Pr(\mathbf{x}_p, \mathbf{x}_g) = \mathbf{G}_{\mathbf{x}'}\left[\mu', \mathbf{B}\mathbf{B}^T + \Sigma'\right] \qquad (25)$$

where

$$\Sigma' = \begin{bmatrix} \Sigma & 0 \\ 0 & \Sigma \end{bmatrix} \qquad (26)$$

Based on Equations (22) and (25), Equation (18) can be evaluated as

$$Pr(\mathbf{x}_{1\ldots K}, \mathbf{x}_p \mid M_k) == \frac{\prod_{i=1}^{K} \mathbf{G}_{\mathbf{x}_i}\left[\mu, \mathbf{A}\mathbf{A}^T + \Sigma\right]\mathbf{G}_{\hat{x}}\left[\mu', \mathbf{B}\mathbf{B}^T + \Sigma'\right]}{\mathbf{G}_{\mathbf{x}_k}\left[\mu, \mathbf{A}\mathbf{A}^T + \Sigma\right]} \qquad (27)$$

where $\hat{x} = \begin{bmatrix} \mathbf{x}_k & \mathbf{x}_p \end{bmatrix}^T$.

Computational Complexity

In the previous section, we showed that the matching a probe $\mathbf{x}_p$ to a set of gallery data $x_k(k = 1, 2, \cdots, K)$ can be done by comparing K models as shown in Equation (27). The likelihood of all models involves evaluating $2K$ Gaussians. To calculate this likelihood we must evaluate the quadratic term in the exponent of the Gaussian. This appears to be costly since the measurements are of high dimension. Here, we show that this is not the case - in fact the quadratic term may be calculated by projecting the data onto a subspace and calculating a dot product. To demonstrate this, we use the Woodbury matrix identity (matrix inversion lemma) to re-write the covariance matrix of the Gaussain in question:

$$\begin{aligned} \Lambda &= (\mathbf{A}\mathbf{A}^T + \tilde{\Sigma})^{-1} = \\ & \tilde{\Sigma}^{-1} - \tilde{\Sigma}^{-1}\mathbf{A}(I + \mathbf{A}^T\tilde{\Sigma}^{-1}\mathbf{A})^{-1}\mathbf{A}^T\tilde{\Sigma}^{-1} = \\ & \tilde{\Sigma}^{-1} - \Gamma\Gamma^T \end{aligned} \qquad (28)$$

where $\Gamma = \tilde{\Sigma}^{-1}\mathbf{A}(I + \mathbf{A}^T\tilde{\Sigma}^{-1}\mathbf{A})^{-1/2}$. To evaluate the Gaussian, we need to calculate a quadratic term $\mathbf{x}\Gamma\mathbf{x}$ where Γ is the top left part of the covariance matrix $\mathbf{\Gamma}$. In other words, we need to calculate part of $\mathbf{x}^T\tilde{\Sigma}^{-1}\mathbf{x} - \mathbf{x}^T\mathbf{\Gamma}\mathbf{\Gamma}^T\mathbf{x}$. The first term is efficiently calculated as $\tilde{\Sigma}$ is diagonal. The second part is also efficiently calculated as the term $\mathbf{\Gamma}$ has a number of columns that depends on the noise and signal subspace. Hence we can first calculate $\mathbf{\Gamma}^T\mathbf{x}$ and then calculate the magnitude of this vector. The final computation is of the same order as traditional LDA methods which project into a subspace and then measure a distance.

Performance Comparison

The performance of PLDA was evaluated using the XM2VTS database (Matas et al., 2000). Each color image was segmented with an iterative graph-cuts procedure. Three points were marked by hand. Faces were warped to a standard template using an affine transform. The final size was 70×70. The unprocessed RGB pixels from these images were concatenated as a feature vector to represent each face image. The training data set consists of 4 images each of the first 195 people in the database. The test set comprises 1 gallery and 1 probe image from each of the remaining 100 people. These were taken from the first and last recording sessions respectively. Note that the gallery images are not used in the training.

The PLDA model was trained using the EM algorithm. The subspace dimensions (number of columns in $\mathbf{F}$ and $\mathbf{G}$) are set to be equal although this need not necessarily be the case.

The first match identification rate is plotted as a function of the subspace dimension in Figure 3. The PLDA model is compared to our implementations of five other methods in the closed-set identification task PCA (Turk & Pentland, 1991), LDA (Belhumeur et al., 1997), the Bayesian approach (Moghaddam et al., 2000), dual-space LDA (Wang & Tang, 2004) and Ioffe's PLDA (Ioffe, 2006). It is observed that our PLDA model

outperforms all other methods on this task. The closest competing method is dual-space LDA (Wang & Tang, 2004).

Discussion

The PLDA model is closely related to factor analysis (FA) model (Rubin & Thayer, 1982). In the factor analysis model, a face image can be decomposed of a deterministic signal part F_z and a stochastic noise part ε (Prince et al., 2008): $\mathbf{x}=\boldsymbol{\mu}+\mathbf{Fz}+\varepsilon$, where the hidden variable z is defined as *factors* of a unit Gaussian distribution: $Pr(\mathbf{z}) = \mathbf{G}_z\left[\mathbf{0},\mathbf{I}\right]$ and the basis function F is defined as *factor loadings*. The stochastic noise term ε is defined as a zero-mean Gaussian $Pr(\varepsilon) = \mathbf{G}_\varepsilon\left[\mathbf{0},\Sigma\right]$.

As aforementioned, PLDA model in Equation (2) can be rewritten as the form of a standard FA model. Therefore, PLDA is a special form or a natural extension of factor analysis model. The only difference is that an extra deterministic term is introduce in PLDA to model the within individual noise.

A special case of factor analysis model is setting the noise term ε to be a spherical Gaussian $\boldsymbol{\pounds} = \tilde{\mathbf{A}}^2 I$, which means the variance of noise in each feature dimension is the same. This leads to Probabilistic Principal Component Analysis (Tipping & Bishop, 1999), a probabilistic version of PCA (Turk & Pentland, 1991).

Figure 3. Comparison of PLDA to other approaches for face recognition

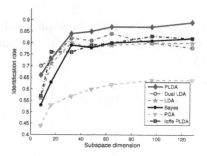

As PPCA, FA and PLDA are generative probabilistic models, their performance for face recognition depend on how well they fit to the face image data. We evaluated these three probabilistic models for face identification using the same experimental setting as in the previous section. The result is illustrated in Figure 4.

Firstly, it is observed that the performance of *PPCA* is quite similar to standard *PCA*. In fact, the PPCA model has very slightly superior performance. This is a repeatable phenomenon that results from the regularization induced by the prior over $\mathbf{h}$. When we allow Σ to have independent diagonal terms, the model takes the form of a factor analyzer. Both *PPCA* and *PCA* are outperformed by factor analysis model. This is because the assumption of same variation in each feature dimension in the PPCA model may be too rigid and it may not be in agree with the face image data. To further prove this, we can force the noise Σ to be a multiple of the identity rather than diagonal (dashed vs solid lines in Figure 4). We observed that this deteriorate the performance quite significantly which supports our hypothesis. Modelling the noise at each pixel can be seen to improve performance significantly: the algorithm has learnt which parts of the image are most variable and downweights them appropriately in the decision.

Secondly, both PPCA and factor analysis model are outperformed significantly by PLDA model in the face identification task. The reason is that PLDA model can explain the face image data better than the standard factor analysis model. All these models explain the face image data as a deterministic term which is expected to only related to identity and a stochastic Gaussian noise term. However, the within-individual variance is not explicitly modeled in factor analysis model which may pollute the latent identity term $\mathbf{h}$. The plot shows that the noise subspace $\mathbf{Gw}$ also contributes significantly to the performance.

There are several reasons why our technique outperforms other LDA based methods. First, the inclusion of the per-pixel noise term ε means we have a more sophisticated model of within-individual variation and this results in better performance. Second, our method suffers less from the small sample problem: the signal subspace $\mathbf{F}$ and noise subspace $\mathbf{G}$ may be completely parallel or completely orthogonal. There is no need for two separate procedures as in the dual-space LDA algorithm (Wang & Tang, 2004). Third, a slight benefit results from defining a reasonable prior over the identity and noise variables.

In the original design, the PLDA model can handle some illumination variation and noise. However, the variation in pose and illumination may degrade its performance. There have been some further investigation to extend PLDA model to tackle these two problems. For example, the tied PLDA model has been proposed to deal with the pose variations which is shown to outperform state of art approaches (Prince & Elder, 2007). In (Fu & Prince, 2009), multi-scale PLDA has been developed to tackle illumination variation.

Model Comparison vs. Distance Comparison

The strong performance of PLDA relative to other subspace approaches has several causes. It is possible to show that the way in which the

Figure 4. Comparison of PLDA with factor analysis (FA) and probabilistic principal xomponent analysis (PPCA) for face recognition

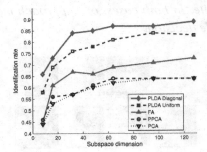

recognition decision is made is also important. The PLDA model marginalises over possible identities and uses model comparison rather than a distance comparison.

To demonstrate that this is beneficial, we re-implement a version of our method where we explicitly calculate the best values of the hidden variables **h** and **w**. This is effectively the mean of the posterior distribution found in Equation (13). Given a probe, the matching of probe image $\mathbf{x}_p$ to the gallery images $\mathbf{x}_g$ is now based on the distance between $E[\mathbf{h}_p]$ and $E[\mathbf{h}_g]$.

In Figure 5, we compare model comparison to distance comparison using the PLDA with the same experimental settings as in the previous section. The model comparison method reliably outperforms the distance comparison approach. This is because it exploits not only the estimate of the identity, but also the uncertainty on that estimate.

In fact, the decision process in the LIV framework is quite different from that in distance-based approaches. This is most easily seen by considering the resulting decision regions. Consider the case where there are different numbers of images for each gallery individual. For distance-based algorithms, there is no principled way to deal with this situation. Three possible approaches are to (1) compute the average distance from the gallery images to the probe (mean distance decision) (2)

take the smallest distance from the probe to the gallery images (nearest neighbors decision) (3) compute the distance from the mean position of the gallery images to the probe (distance to mean decision). In Figure 6 (A), (B) gallery data for two individuals is shown in the learnt subspace, together with the decision regions predicted by each of these metrics. For all three metrics, there exist situations where suboptimal decisions are made.

In Figure 6, we also show decision regions from the LIV algorithm which are all sensible. Moreover, the decision boundaries are no longer linear–a result of the quite different inference process: the predictive distributions are Gaussian. When the number of images for each gallery individual is the same, these predictive distributions will have the same variance, resulting in linear decision boundaries. When the number of images for an individual differs, the covariances of the Gaussians differ and the decision surfaces take the mathematical form of quadric surfaces.

Figure 6. Decision regions for 3 distance-based metrics and the LIV approach. Unshaded and shaded points represent data points for two gallery individuals projected into identity subspace. Gray (white) region is decision region: the subset of space where probe images would be classified as gray (white). (A) Mean distance metric always chooses the gray category. Distance to mean metric chooses a rather arbitrary decision boundary. (B) Nearest neighbor metric chooses shaded point in the exact region where there is most evidence for white. In both cases, our approach makes a sensible decision.

Figure 5. Comparison between distance-based approach and model comparison-based approach for face recognition

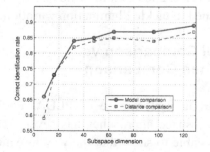

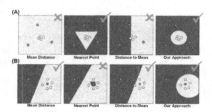

FEATURE SAMPLING

In the previous sections we have demonstrated that PLDA outperforms common subspace algorithms. However, there is still plenty of room to further improve its performance. One possible avenue for development is suggested by the work of Wang and Tang (Wang & Tang, 2006) who improved performance by using ensemble of several LDA classifiers trained on different subsets of the data.

Ensemble learning is a way to combine a set of "weak" classifiers to built up a "strong" classifier, as shown in Figure 7. These "weak" classifiers do not always make the same error so that the overall error of the combined classifier is smaller than that of each individual "weak" classifier (Wang & Tang, 2006). Sets of weak classifiers can be obtained by using different training data sets, different feature subsets, and different types of individual classifiers. They can be combined using various fusion rules. In this section we investigate building an ensemble of PLDAs trained using different feature subsets.

Decision Fusion

Since PLDA is a probabilistic model, it is natural to combine a set of PLDAs using naive Bayes' by taking the product of their likelihood under a given model configuration. Assuming an ensemble consists of a set of M individual PLDAs, each of which measures the probe image $\mathbf{x}_p$ and matches it to a gallery image $\mathbf{x}_k$ ($k=1,2,...,K$). If the likelihood of gallery image $\mathbf{x}_k$ matching the probe image $\mathbf{x}_p$ by the mth PLDA is

$Pr_m(\mathbf{x}_{1...K}, \mathbf{x}_p \mid \mathbf{M}_k)$. The overall likelihood of the ensemble is then defined to be

$$Pr(\mathbf{x}_{1...K}, \mathbf{x}_p \mid \mathbf{M}_k) = \prod_{m=1}^{M} Pr_m(\mathbf{x}_{1...K}, \mathbf{x}_p \mid \mathbf{M}_k)$$

(29)

In other words, we treat each of these individual PLDAs independently and combine them to form an overall likelihood. This is combined with a prior for each model $\mathbf{M}_{1...K}$ to calculate the posterior.

Random Feature Sampling

Similar to other learning algorithms, PLDA also suffers from the curse of dimensionality–the number of training samples is much smaller than that of the dimensionality of the data. It is possible to address this problem by training an ensemble of PLDA models each of which operates using random subset of the input dimensions. Compared to the PLDA model trained using the full feature set, the individual PLDA model here faces an easier problem: the dimensionality of the associated features space is smaller than the number of training data. The curse of dimensionality is therefore alleviated.

Performance Comparison on Raw Pixel Features

We evaluated the **random feature sampling** using the XM2VTS database. Firstly, we test it using the raw pixel data with the same setting as in previous section. An ensemble of 100 PLDAs trained using random feature subsets is compared to the best single PLDA. Figure 8 illustrates the performance of this ensemble learning technique: It is shown that an ensemble of PLDAs trained using random feature subsets outperforms the best single PLDA trained using full feature set. The best recognition rate of the ensemble is 97%, which is

Figure 7. Flowchart of ensemble learning for face recognition

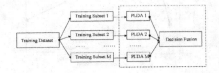

7% higher than the best individual PLDA trained using full feature set. This supports our claim that ensemble of PLDAs with random sampling the feature space is able to improve the performance.

Another way of creating diverse classifiers is bagging in which we randomly sample the training samples (Wang & Tang, 2006). Here, each individual classifier will face a more serious curse of dimensionality as its training subset has fewer training samples compared to the original data set. We do not expect performance improvement using the ensemble of bagging. We repeated the experiment as before but the PLDAs are trained using different subsets of training data, but the full feature set. The result is shown in Figure 9. No significant improvement can be observed by using the bagging-based ensemble over the best individual PLDA classifier.

Performance Comparison on Gabor Features

We also evaluate the feature sampling method using Gabor features. Similarly to previous section, we extract a 2700-dimensional Gabor feature for each of 10 keypoints at corners of eyes, nose and mouth. We treat these keypoints independently and train a single PLDA for each keypoint and

Figure 8. Percent first match correct performance on XM2VTS database using ensembles based on subsets of the features. Comparison of using single best PLDA classifier vs. using an ensemble trained on 100 random subsets of the feature data as a function of the subset size.

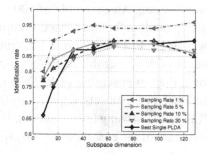

Figure 9. Percent first match correct performance on XM2VTS database using ensembles based on 100 subsets of the training data (bagging)

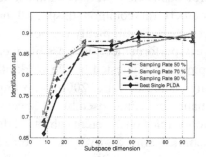

combine their result to make the final decision. For each keypoint, we randomly select several feature subsets to train a PLDA ensemble and compared this to the performance of using single PLDA model for each keypoint. The result is illustrated in Figure 10.

Similar to raw pixel data, an ensemble of PLDAs trained using random feature subsets outperforms the best single PLDA training using full feature set. Note that we use only 10 keypoints in the experiment, the performance may be further improved if more keypoints are used.

Our observation on the ensemble of PLDAs is similar to that of LDAs in (Wang & Tang, 2006). Ensembles based on feature sampling is improve the performance over individual classifiers but

Figure 10. Percent first match correct performance on XM2VTS database using ensembles based on 100 subsets of the Gabor features for each of 10 PLDA models corresponding to 10 keypoints

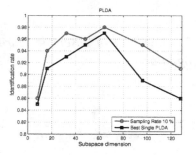

ensembles based on bagging do not improve performance.

Random Sampling With or Without Replacement

The ensemble of PLDAs are trained using random feature subsets with replacement. It is also possible to train an ensemble with random feature subsets without replacement, i.e., the whole feature set will be randomly divided into subsets with same size. The full feature set will be explored in one run. This has a more coherent probabilistic explanation than the previous models: we are simply assuming that certain (randomly chosen) features are independent to others.

We repeated the experiment using raw pixel data and compared these two settings. Firstly, we try sampling with replacement. We randomly select 1% of the feature elements to train a PLDA and repeat this 100 times. Secondly, we evaluate sampling without replacement. The whole feature set are randomly divided into 100 non-overlapping subsets and we train a PLDA for each subset. The result is plotted in Figure 11. It is shown that the performance of the two schemes are similar to each other, with sampling without replacement performing slightly better (1%).

Sampling with replacement may not explore the whole feature set in these 100 subsets and consequently, its performance may be further improved if more trials are explored. We manipulate the number of subsets and find that performance does generally increase as a function of the number of subsets, but does not significantly improve beyond the level achieved with 100 subsets.

Finally, note that a multi-scale PLDA has been proposed to deal with the illumination variance of the face images (Fu & Prince, 2009). In their work, the full images are cropped into non-overlapping grids, for each of which a specific set of parameter F or G are trained. The final decision of matching is also based on the combination of

the decisions made for each of the grids. Their work can be regarded as a specific form of our without-replacement feature sampling approach.

KEYPOINT REGISTRATION

In the previous section we have demonstrated that the LIV-based probabilistic model supports a high level of face recognition performance. In this section, the same probabilistic model is applied to face registration. In particular, we use it to find keypoints on the faces. These might include the corners of eyes, the mouth or nose. Throughout this section we shall assume that the keypoints of the gallery images are known and that our goal is to locate the keypoints in a given probe image. To simplify matters further we shall also treat each keypoint independently. The (x,y) position of the keypoint in the probe image $\mathbf{I}_p$ is denoted by $\mathbf{t}_p$.

We shall assume that we extract a feature vector containing the data surrounding each keypoint. We will model each extracted feature with a separate PLDA generative model. The feature extraction process is denoted by the function ϕ which takes the image and keypoint positions so that:

$$\mathbf{x}_p = \varphi(\mathbf{I}_p, \mathbf{t}_p) \tag{30}$$

Figure 11. Random sampling with or without replacement. The fraction of feature set used for each individual PLDA is 1%.

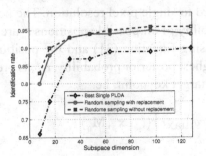

The task can be addressed in two different ways, which we term explicit and implicit registration. In the explicit approach we form a maximum a posteriori estimate of the keypoint position t_p for each keypoint. We then extract a single feature vector using Equation (30). In the implicit approach, we consider the keypoint position as a random variable that is marginalized over (integrated out).

Explicit Registration

Keypoints are usually found by a separate process from the recognition model. However, since we have described our data in terms of a generative LIV model, it is possible to exploit this to localize the keypoints: the generative model describes the probability density function of the image around the keypoint. If the keypoint position is wrong then the probability will be low. More formally, we maximize the posterior probability of the keypoint position as a function of extracted feature from this position. The posterior probability over t_p given the extracted feature on this position $\mathbf{x}_p$ can be found using Bayes' rule:

$$Pr(t_p \mid \mathbf{x}_p) \propto Pr(\mathbf{x}_p \mid t_p)Pr(t_p) \qquad (31)$$

The likelihood of the feature $\mathbf{x}_p$ at position t_p in the probe image $\mathbf{I}_p$ can be calculated using Equation (22). The prior distribution $Pr(t_p)$ of each keypoint is modeled as a two dimensional Gaussian, as shown in Figure 12. The mean and covariance are calculated using the coordinates of manually labeled keypoints of the training data. The possible locations of each keypoint are discretized to single pixel resolution. The posterior probability of all possible positions t_p are evaluated using Equation (31) and the position with the highest posterior probability, t_p^*, is predicted as the target keypoint, i.e.

$$\mathbf{t}_p^* = arg\max_{t_p} Pr(t_p \mid \mathbf{x}_p, \mathbf{M}_0) \qquad (32)$$

We use these optimal keypoint values t_p^* to calculate the features $\mathbf{x}_p$ and evaluate the model likelihoods using Equation (27) for the closed-set identification task.

Implicit Registration

Previously we estimated the keypoint positions. Now we treat each keypoint location as a hidden variable and *marginalize* over it in a Bayesian manner. Since *explicit registration* is unnecessary, we refer to this as *implicit registration*.

When we approach the identification task, we need to deal with two scenarios, *No-Match* and *Match*. For the *No-Match* scenario, the gallery image $\mathbf{x}_g$ does not match any of the other images. The related likelihood term $Pr(x_g)$ can be calculated using Equation (22) as before.

For the *Match* scenario, the probe image I_p matches a gallery image I_g. We first find a probability distribution $Pr(t_p|x_p)$ over the possible feature based on the probe image using Equation (31). Then we integrate over unknown feature positions t_p s in the probe image based on the probability distributions estimated from the probe image

Figure 12. (A) The prior distributions of the keypoints are modeled as two dimensional Guassians where the union of the discretized positions of the 9 keypoints are shown in white. The predicted distribution of a keypoint (the left corner of mouth) in a probe image (B) is illustrated in (C). The keypoint can be explicitly estimated by choosing the location with the highest posterior probability (indicated by white stars) or marginalized over all the possible locations as shown in (D). Ground truth keypoints are indicated by white crosses. The sample image is from XM2VTS database (Matas et al., 2000).

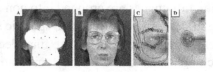

$$Pr(\mathbf{x}_p, \mathbf{x}_g) = \int Pr(\mathbf{x}_p, \mathbf{x}_g \mid \mathbf{t}_p) Pr(\mathbf{t}_p \mid \mathbf{x}_p) d\mathbf{t}_p$$

$$(33)$$

Note that the integral in the above equations is calculated over all possible positions of the keypoint. In practice, these positions are discretized and the integral can be approximated using summation over these discretized positions.

Experimental Results and Discussion

We investigate face registration and identification using the XM2VTS frontal face data set. The experimental setting is similar to previous section. The original face images are RGB color images of size 400×400. We ran a sliding window face detector over the images at several scales to identify the region of the image that is most likely to contain a face. We reshaped the resulting bounding box to 125×125 pixels using a similarity transform with bicubic interpolation. We applied histogram equalization to the resulting images.

Nine keypoints including the eye corners, nose and mouth were investigated (see Figure 12). These keypoints were manually labeled on the images of original size 400×400 by two subjects to provide ground truth for the training and test data. For the gallery images we use the manual labels, but the probe images were treated unlabelled in our experiments. We extract a feature vector by applying Gabor filters at 8 orientations and 3 scales in a 6×6 grid around each keypoint. A separate PLDA model was built for each keypoint. The keypoint positions are assumed to be independent from one another.

The prior distribution of each keypoint position is modeled as a two dimensional Gaussian whose mean and covariance are calculated using the coordinates of manually labeled keypoints of the training data. The locations of each keypoint are discretized with single pixel resolution over a region covering a Mahalanobis distance of $\leq$

2.5. This describes more than 99% of the probability density.

Recognition Performance

We compare explicit and implicit registration procedures for the face identification task. We investigate this percent first match correct as a function of the subspace dimensions (i.e. the number of columns in **F** and **G**). These are always set to be equal although this need not necessarily be the case.

First match identification rate is plotted as a function of subspace dimension in Figure 13. It shows that identification performance using implicit registration is superior to that using explicit registration. In other words, it is better to treat the probe keypoint position as a random variable and marginalize than it is to find maximum a posteriori keypoint position. The most likely explanation for this phenomenon is that there are some points where the likelihood surface over keypoint position is flat and possibly multimodal. When we are forced to choose a single estimate of position we occasionally make drastic mistakes. However, when we integrate over this distribution, the bulk of the probability may be close to the correct position, although the maximum is quite wrong.

Figure 13. Identification performance for marginalizing over keypoint position (implicit registration) is superior to using the best estimate of keypoint position (explicit registration). The identification performance of implicit registration approaches the results with manual labelling.

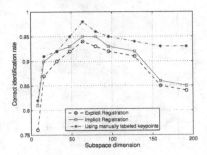

Localization Performance

We further investigate the ability of explicit registration to localize the keypoints. We assess performance in terms of the mean localization error of the 9 keypoints. This is reported in Figure 14. The localization error is described using normalized Euclidean distance (fraction of inter-ocular distance) following (Everingham & Zisserman, 2006). This metric makes the results independent of image resolution. Note that the manually labelling made use of original images with resolution of 400×400. The true labelling error may be larger if the images of resolution 125×125 had been used for manual labelling. Despite this, the localization errors of our explicit registration algorithm are very close to that of the human labeling.

An interesting observation is that smaller registration error doesn't always mean a higher identification rate. It seems that the registration is best with a small number of factors, whereas recognition is best with an intermediate number. We conjecture that low frequency components are primarily being used in the localization process and that higher frequency components which are useful for recognition, may actually impede very accurate localization.

Computational complexity

In the previous section, it has been shown that matching a probe image to a set of gallery images using PLDA model can be done quite fast. As for localizing keypoints in a probe image, we need to run the PLDA model for each possible location of a keypoint. Let S be the number of keypoints, T be the average number of possible locations for a keypoint, the computation time of finding all the keypoints in a probe image either explicitly or implicitly is $o(ST)$. Though the Gabor filter responses can be calculate quite efficiently, it may take several minutes to locate the keypoints using PLDA models. Some heuristics may be used to accelerate the processing. For example, (i) the searching space of the following keypoints can be reduced by exploiting the found keypoints. (ii) The searching over the possible locations of a keypoint can be performed in a coarse to fine manner to reduce the searching space. (iii) The dimension of feature vector (Gabor filter responses) can be reduced by exploiting parameter of Gabor filter and using some feature selection or extraction methods such as PCA. This needs to be investigated in the future work.

FUTURE TRENDS AND CONCLUSION

In this chapter, we have presented a probabilistic approach for both face registration and recognition. We model observed data as being the result of a generative process, in which some of the component variables are pure representations of identity (LIVs). We learn the parameters of this model from training data. In recognition, we calculate the probability that the probe and gallery data were generated from the same underlying identity regardless of what that identity was and match them based on model comparison. We demonstrated the advantages of LIV models using

Figure 14. Comparison of normalized registration errors for keypoints as estimated using MAP estimation to manual labelling by a second subject

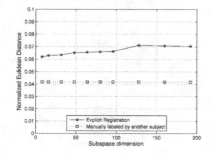

the PLDA algorithm. It outperforms contemporary algorithms in the XM2VTS database.

There are several advantages to this formulation. (1) It provides valid posterior probability over possible hypotheses in face recognition tasks. (2) There is no need to set arbitrary parameters as all components can be learnt. (3) In our method it is possible to compare face data and other biometric data captured in quite different circumstances without the need for rescaling (4) We can easily incorporate prior information about possible data hypotheses. (5) It is easy to incorporate domain specific information about the generation process. (6) There is a clear way to deal with multiple gallery and/or probe data belonging to the same person. Our method compares favorably to other decision algorithms. Distance based methods cannot always easily be adapted to have these advantages. Decisions based on frequentist statistical principles do not provide a method to incorporate prior information. Experimental results show that model comparison is better than distance comparison for face recognition.

In addition, we illustrated how to improve the performance of the LIV model by forming an ensemble of classifiers. We considered randomly splitting the whole feature set into smaller subsets or randomly selecting overlapping feature subset: the curse of dimensionality is alleviated considerably for each PLDA compared to the model trained using the whole feature set and the ensemble improves performance relative to a single classifier. In this chapter, we have combined these using naive Bayes (by assuming independence). An interesting direction for future work would be to investigate more sophisticated fusion rules.

Finally, we exploited the LIV model that was originally developed for face recognition to find keypoints in the image as well. Both explicit registration (finding the location with the highest posterior probability) and implicit registration (marginalizing over the keypoint location) work well. Performance for both registration and identification were found to be close to that with manual labelling. In this work we have assumed that the gallery keypoint positions are known and the probe positions uncertain. However, it is also possible to assume that neither gallery images or probe images are labelled. This will be investigated in the future work.

REFERENCES

Belhumeur, P. N., Hespanha, J. P., & Kriegman, D. J. (1997). Eigenfaces vs. Fisherfaces: Recognition using class specific linear projection. *IEEE Transactions on Pattern Analysis and Machine Intelligence, 19*(7), 711–720. doi:10.1109/34.598228

Breiman, L. (1996). *Bias, variance, and arcing classifiers (Tech. Rep.)*. Statistics Department, University of California.

Chen, L., Liao, H., Lin, J., Ko, M., & Yu, G. (2000). A new LDA-based face recognition system that can solve the small sample size problem. *Pattern Recognition, 33*(11), 1713–1726. doi:10.1016/S0031-3203(99)00139-9

Cootes, T., Edwards, G., & Taylor, C. (2001). Active appearance models. *IEEE Transactions on Pattern Analysis and Machine Intelligence, 23*(6), 681–685. doi:10.1109/34.927467

Dempster, A. P., Laird, N. M., & Rubin, D. B. (1977). Maximum likelihood from incomplete data via the EM algorithm. *Journal of the Royal Statistical Society. Series B. Methodological, 39*(1), 1–38.

Everingham, M., & Zisserman, A. (2006). Regression and classification approaches to eye localization in face images. In *International Conference on Automatic Face and Gesture Recognition* (pp. 441–448).

Fu, Y., & Prince, S. J. D. (2009). Investigating the spatial support of signal and noise in face recognition. In *ICCV Subspace Workshop*.

He, X., Yan, S., Hu, Y., & Niyogi, P. (2005). Face recognition using Laplacianfaces. *IEEE Transactions on Pattern Analysis and Machine Intelligence, 27*(3), 328–340. doi:10.1109/TPAMI.2005.55

Ilonen, J., Kamarainen, J., Paalanen, P., Hamouz, M., Kittler, J., & Kalviainen, H. (2008). Image feature localization by multiple hypothesis testing of Gabor features. *IEEE Transactions on Image Processing, 17*(3), 311–325. doi:10.1109/TIP.2007.916052

Ioffe, S. (2006). Probabilistic linear discriminant analysis. In *European Conference on Computer Vision* (pp. 531–542).

Kuncheva, L., Bezdek, J., & Duin, R. (2001). Decision templates for multiple classifier fusion: An experimental comparison. *Pattern Recognition, 34*(2). doi:10.1016/S0031-3203(99)00223-X

Kuncheva, L. I., & Whitaker, C. J. (2003). Measures of diversity in classifier ensembles. *Machine Learning, 51*(2), 181–207. doi:10.1023/A:1022859003006

Lucey, S., & Chen, T. (2006). Learning patch dependencies for improved pose mismatched face verification. In *IEEE Computer Society Conference on Computer Vision and Pattern Recognition* (pp. 17–22).

Mahoor, M., & Abdel Mottaleb, M. (2006). Facial features extraction in color images using enhanced active shape model. In *International Conference on Automatic Face and Gesture Recognition* (pp. 144–148).

Martinez, A. M. (2002). Recognizing imprecisely localized, partially occluded, and expression variant faces from a single sample per class. *IEEE Transactions on Pattern Analysis and Machine Intelligence, 24*(6), 748–763. doi:10.1109/TPAMI.2002.1008382

Matas, J., Hamouz, M., Jonsson, K., Kittler, J., Li, Y., Kotropoulos, C., et al. (2000). Comparison of face verification results on the XM2VTS database. In *Proceedings of the 15th International Conference on Pattern Recognition* (Vol. 4, pp. 858–863).

Moghaddam, B., Jebara, T., & Pentland, A. (2000). Bayesian face recognition. *Pattern Recognition, 33*(11), 1771–1782. doi:10.1016/S0031-3203(99)00179-X

Prince, S. J. D., & Elder, J. H. (2007). Probabilistic linear discriminant analysis for inferences about identity. In *IEEE International Conference on Computer Vision* (pp. 1–8).

Prince, S. J. D., Elder, J. H., Warrell, J., & Felisberti, F. M. (2008). Tied factor analysis for face recognition across large pose differences. *IEEE Transactions on Pattern Analysis and Machine Intelligence, 30*(6), 970–984. doi:10.1109/TPAMI.2008.48

Rubin, D., & Thayer, D. (1982). EM algorithms for ML factor analysis. *Psychometrika, 47*(1), 69–76. doi:10.1007/BF02293851

Shan, S., Cao, B., Su, Y., Qing, L., Chen, X., & Gao, W. (2008). Unified principal component analysis with generalized covariance matrix for face recognition. In *IEEE Computer Society Conference on Computer Vision and Pattern Recognition* (pp. 1–7).

Shan, S., Zhang, W., Su, Y., Chen, X., & Gao, W. (2006). Ensemble of piecewise FDA based on spatial histograms of local (Gabor) binary patterns for face recognition. In *International Conference on Pattern Recognition* (pp. 606–609).

Su, Y. Shan., S., Chen, X., & Gao, W. (2006). Hierarchical ensemble of Gabor Fisher classifier for face recognition. In *International Conference on Automatic Face and Gesture Recognition* (pp. 91–96).

Su, Y. Shan., S., Chen, X., & Gao, W. (2007). Hierarchical ensemble of global and local classifiers for face recognition. In *IEEE International Conference on Computer Vision* (pp. 1–8).

Tipping, M. E., & Bishop, C. M. (1999). Probabilistic principal component analysis. *Journal of the Royal Statistical Society. Series B. Methodological*, *61*, 611–622. doi:10.1111/1467-9868.00196

Turk, M., & Pentland, A. (1991). Face recognition using eigenfaces. In *IEEE Computer Society Conference on Computer Vision and Pattern Recognition* (pp. 586–591).

Wang, H., Yan, S., Huang, T., Liu, J., & Tang, X. (2008). Misalignment-robust face recognition. In *IEEE Computer Society Conference on Computer Vision and Pattern Recognition* (pp. 1–6).

Wang, X., & Tang, X. (2004). Dual-space linear discriminant analysis for face recognition. In *IEEE Computer Society Conference on Computer Vision and Pattern Recognition* (Vol. 2, pp. 564–569).

Wang, X., & Tang, X. (2006). Random sampling for subspace face recognition. *International Journal of Computer Vision*, *70*(1), 91–1042. doi:10.1007/s11263-006-8098-z

Yang, J., Frangi, A. F., & Yang, J. yu, & Jin, Z. (2005). KPCA plus LDA: A complete kernel fisher discriminant framework for feature extraction and recognition. *IEEE Transactions on Pattern Analysis and Machine Intelligence*, *27*(2), 230–244. doi:10.1109/TPAMI.2005.33

Zhang, Y., & Martinez, A. (2006). A weighted probabilistic approach to face recognition from multiple images and video sequences. *Image and Vision Computing*, *24*(6), 626–638. doi:10.1016/j.imavis.2005.08.004

Zhao, W., Chellappa, R., Phillips, P. J., & Rosenfeld, A. (2003). Face recognition: A literature survey. *ACM Computing Surveys*, *35*(4), 399–458. doi:10.1145/954339.954342

Zhou, S., & Chellappa, R. (2004). Probabilistic identity characterization for face recognition. In *IEEE Computer Society Conference on Computer Vision and Pattern Recognition* (pp. 805–812).

KEY TERMS AND DEFINTIONS

Probabilistic Linear Discriminant Analyzer (PLDA): A probabilistic version of Linear Discriminant Analyzer (LDA) where a face image is decomposed into an additive sum of two parts: a deterministic component, which depends on an underlying representation of identity and a stochastic component which explains the fact that two face images from the same person are not identical.

Latent Identity Variable (LIV): A underlying multi-dimensional variable which represents the identity of an individual person.

Model Comparison: Face recognition by comparing a set of models, each of which explains the data (matching a probe image to a gallery image) in a different way, and choose the model that best explains the data (with the highest likelihood).

Distance-Based Approach: The probe image is projected into a lower-dimensional space where its distance to each of the gallery images (templates) is calculated. The matching face is taken to be the closest gallery image.

Random Feature Sampling: Train an ensemble of PLDA models each of which operates using random subset of the input dimensions.

Explicit Registration: Finding the location of keypoints explicitly with the highest posterior probability.

Implicit Registration: Marginalizing over the keypoint location for face recognition so that no explicit keypoint location is necessary.

Face Registration: Locating facial keypoints such as corner of the eye, nose and mouth etc.

Chapter 11
Discriminant Learning Using Training Space Partitioning

Marios Kyperountas
Aristotle University of Thessaloniki, Greece

Anastasios Tefas
Aristotle University of Thessaloniki, Greece

Ioannis Pitas
Aristotle University of Thessaloniki, Greece

ABSTRACT

Large training databases introduce a level of complexity that often degrades the classification performance of face recognition methods. In this chapter, an overview of various approaches that are employed in order to overcome this problem is presented and, in addition, a specific discriminant learning approach that combines dynamic training and partitioning is described in detail. This face recognition methodology employs dynamic training in order to implement a person-specific iterative classification process. This process employs discriminant clustering, where, by making use of an entropy-based measure, the algorithm adapts the coordinates of the discriminant space with respect to the characteristics of the test face. As a result, the training space is dynamically reduced to smaller spaces, where linear separability among the face classes is more likely to be achieved. The process iterates until one final cluster is retained, which consists of a single face class that represents the best match to the test face. The performance of this methodology is evaluated on standard large face databases and results show that the proposed framework gives a good solution to the face recognition problem.

INTRODUCTION

During the past 30 years, machine recognition of human faces using still images and video sequences has become an active research area in the communities of video and image processing, pattern recognition, and computer vision. Face recognition (FR) technology has many practical applications, which can be categorized into the law enforcement and the commercial field. In the law enforcement area, this technology can be used to identify faces in a picture, to help, for example, police search a database of mug shots in order to identify a person shown in an incriminat-

DOI: 10.4018/978-1-61520-991-0.ch011

ing image or videotape. Moreover, surveillance cameras could interact with a FR algorithm that is performing real-time face matching operations in order to identify the presence of a person, e.g. a terrorist, who could be dangerous to the public. In commerce, FR technology can be modeled to create a new kind of key that could match photographs on credit cards, ATM cards, passports, or driver's licenses. Moreover, a simple video camera could act as a clearance security guard simply by interfacing face images with a face recognition or verification algorithm.

The automatic recognition of human faces presents a significant challenge to the aforementioned research communities. Typically, human faces are very similar in structure with minor differences from person to person. Furthermore, varying lighting conditions, facial expressions and pose orientations further complicate the FR task, making it one of the most difficult problems in pattern analysis. Several algorithms have been developed that attempted to overcome these difficulties. A central issue to all these algorithms is which features to use in order to represent a face. A second main issue is which classification scheme to implement in order to recognize a new face image, based on the chosen feature representation. Usually, a set of selected features is used to derive an optimal subset of features that would lead to high classification performance with the expectation that similar performance can also be displayed on future trials using novel test data. In addition to high recognition accuracy and robustness to various types of test data, FR methods need to have relative computational simplicity so that they can be applied to as many real-world applications as possible.

The most popular and successful FR methods usually utilize Principal Component Analysis (Kirby 1990, Turk 1991, Xudong 2008), Linear Discriminant Analysis (Lu 2003, Etemad 1997, Kyperountas 2007), Independent Component Analysis (Hyvärinen 2001, Bartlett 1998, Gao 2009), Non-negative Matrix Factorization (Lee 2001, Li 2001, Buciu 2008), Neural Networks (Lawrence 1997, Jain 2000, Wolfrum 2008), Graph Matching (Wiskott 1997, Tefas 1998, Tefas 2002), Support Vector Machines (Tefas 2001, Hotta 2008), Template Matching (Bruneli 1993, Fukunaga 1990), or Hidden Markov Models (Samaria 1993, Nefian 2000, Bevilacqua 2008). The aforementioned variations that appear in facial images limit the effectiveness of all these methods. Moreover, the FR problem becomes much more complex when large numbers of individuals are represented in a database, where more of the aforementioned variations are expected to be found. To make matters worse, it is often not the case that a sufficient number of training images are available for each individual. As a result, the intra-class variations cannot be modeled properly, making the FR problem more difficult to solve.

In this chapter, a Face Recognition methodology is presented that was designed to overcome the problems relating to large databases and insufficient numbers of training samples. Initially, state-of-the-art methods that target the problem of training a FR system using a large database are presented. Specifically, we overview divide-and-conquer and hierarchical space-tessellation methods that attempt to partition the training space in order to improve the recognition performance. Next, we present a method that dynamically partitions the training space throughout multiple classification steps. The performance of this method is evaluated experimentally and compared against other state-of-the-art solutions.

BACKGROUND AND RELATED WORK

During the last several years, great attention has been given to the active research field of face classification. For the Face Recognition (FR) problem, the true match to a test face, out of a number of *N* different training faces stored in a database, is sought. The FR problem becomes more complex when large databases, in terms of the number of different faces, or persons, are utilized. As a result, the performance of many state-of-the-art FR methods greatly deteriorates when large databases are utilized during the training phase (Lu 2002, Guo 2001). When large databases are utilized, several variations in regards to the representation of faces are more likely to be introduced. For example, differences in viewpoint, illumination, and facial expression have created fundamental problems for most FR methods. Specifically, methods that utilize a linear criterion normally require images to follow a convex distribution. Therefore, the facial feature representation that is acquired by these methods is not capable of generalizing all the introduced variations. Furthermore, the performance of methods that utilize a non-linear criterion often deteriorates due to over-fitting problems and difficulties in optimizing the involved parameters (Lu 2002). Moreover, for non-linear face representations, the associated computational complexity can be overwhelming when a large database is used during the training phase.

An additional problem that FR methods often encounter is utilizing databases that have a limited number of training samples, i.e. images, for each face. In such a case, modelling the intra-person variations often becomes an insurmountable task. For linear methods, such as the ones that utilize Linear Discriminant Analysis (LDA), this difficulty appears as the 'small sample size' (SSS) problem. The SSS problem refers to cases where the number of available training samples is smaller than the dimensionality of the samples (Swets 1999). The aforementioned problems are expected to exacerbate when large databases, meaning databases that contain samples of faces from a large number of people, do not contain sufficient numbers of training samples per person.

Recently, various methods have been proposed in order to attempt to solve the aforementioned problems. A widely used principle that has been used is the 'divide and conquer', which decomposes a database into smaller sets in order to piecewise learn the complex distribution by a mixture of local linear models. In (Lu 2002), a separability criterion is employed to partition a training set from a large database into a set of smaller maximal separability clusters (MSCs) by utilizing a variant of linear discriminant analysis (LDA). Based on these MSCs, a hierarchical classification framework that consists of two levels of nearest neighbour classifiers is employed and the match is found. The work in (Swets 1999) concentrates on the hierarchical partitioning of the feature spaces using hierarchical discriminant analysis (HDA). A space-tessellation tree is generated using the most expressive features (MEF), by employing Principal Component Analysis (PCA), and the most discriminating features (MDF), by employing LDA, at each tree level. This is done to avoid the limitations linked to global features, by deriving a recursively better-fitted set of features for each of the recursively subdivided sets of training samples.

In general, hierarchical trees have been extensively used for pattern recognition purposes. In (Liu 2004), an owner-specific LDA-subspace is developed in order to create a personalized face verification system. The training set is partitioned into a number of clusters and only a single cluster, which contains face data that is most similar to the owner face, is retained. The system assigns the owner training images to this particular cluster and this new data set is used to determine an LDA subspace that is used to compute the verification thresholds and the matching score whenever a test face claims the identity of the owner. Rather than using the LDA space that is created by processing the full training set, the authors show that verification performance is enhanced when an owner-specific subspace is utilized.

In (Lu 2007), a face recognition method based on fuzzy clustering and parallel neural networks is proposed. The face patterns are divided into several small-scale neural networks based on fuzzy clustering and they are combined to obtain the recognition result. The fuzzy c-means clustering algorithm is used for partitioning the training space in small clusters. Each cluster is used for training a neural network and all neural networks are combined in a parallel architecture. During testing, the test sample is fed to every neural network and the responses are thresholded and combined for obtaining the output of the FR system.

In (Weng 2007) incremental hierarchical discriminant regression (IHDR) which incrementally builds a decision tree or regression tree for very high-dimensional regression or decision spaces by an online, real-time learning system is proposed. At each internal node of the IHDR tree, information in the output space is used to automatically derive the local subspace spanned by the most discriminating features. Embedded in the tree is a hierarchical probability distribution model used to prune very unlikely cases during the search. An incrementally updated probability model is used to deal with large sample-size cases, small sample-size cases, and unbalanced sample-size cases, measured among different internal nodes of the IHDR tree.

In (Pang 2005) a membership authentication method by face classification using a support vector machine (SVM) classification tree, in which the size of membership group and the members in the membership group can be changed dynamically, has been proposed. The proposed method employed a divide and conquer strategy that first performs a recursive data partition by membership- based locally linear embedding (LLE) data clustering, and then does the Support Vector Machine classification in each partitioned feature subset. The partitioning of the training space is performed during the training procedure and a binary classification tree is built. The classifiers used in the decision tree are linear Support Vector Machines. The proposed technique is able to deal with large membership groups (50-60 persons) keeping the classification performance in acceptable limits.

In general, the face recognition methods, proposed thus far, that try to alleviate the large database problem are using a clustering algorithm for partitioning the training space and then they perform training inside each cluster in order to learn a discriminant classification function. The training space clusters may be further partitioned giving tree-based clustering structures and the corresponding classifiers are constructed for each sub-cluster. This procedure takes place during the training phase and the system is then ready for testing. Incremental techniques for updating the partitioned training space when new data arrive in the dataset without having to retrain all the dataset have been also proposed.

Alternatively, one can consider that for large datasets the training procedure can be performed dynamically prior to the testing procedure (Kyperountas 2008). For instance, the training set can be partitioned according to the test sample in order to produce classifiers that are test sample oriented. This discriminant learning and partitioning procedure is described in detail in the next section.

DYNAMIC PARTITION OF THE TRAINING SPACE

This section presents a novel framework, onwards referred to as Dynamic Training for Iterative Clustering (DTIC), which implements a person-specific iterative classification process. The clustering and discriminant analysis parameters of DTIC are heavily affected by the characteristics of the test face. This methodology is able to deal with any problem that fits into the same formalism; therefore, it is not restricted to FR. For clarity, two terms that are frequently used in this presentation are now defined: 'class' refers to a set of face images from the same person, whereas 'cluster' refers to a set of classes. The ith face class is denoted by Y_i whereas the ith cluster by C_i. It is noted that, during the training phase, face images of one person may be partitioned into more than one cluster. In that case, multiple clusters will contain a class that corresponds to that particular person.

Initially, facial features are extracted from both the training and the test faces using the multilevel 2-D wavelet decomposition (MWD2) algorithm (Mallat 1989, Daubechies 1992). MWD2 has been shown to be appropriate for classification purposes (Etemad 1997, Zhang 2004, Bicego 2003) and is an effective way to achieve dimensionality reduction. Then, the training and test face vectors are projected onto a LDA-space by employing the Regularized LDA (RLDA) method of (Lu 2005) that introduces a modified version of Fisher's criterion (Lu 2003). As a result, the most discriminant features (MDF) are produced. Subsequently, k-means is used to partition the training data into a set of K discriminant clusters C_i, and the distance from the test face to the cluster centroids is utilized in order to collect a subset of K' clusters, $K' < K$, that are closest to the test face. The cardinality of this subset, or K', is defined using an entropy-based measure. This measure is calculated by making use of the discrete probability histogram. Then, the training data that reside in these K' clusters are merged and a new MDF-space of the merged face classes is found by applying LDA. Next, k-means is once again used to partition the data into a new set of discriminant clusters and a new subset that is closer to the test

face is selected. This process is repeated in as many iterations as are necessary, until a single cluster is retained. Then, discriminant analysis is applied to the data contained in this cluster and the face class that is most similar to the test face is set as its identity match.

The key idea behind the DTIC methodology has to do with its ability to apply dynamic training in order to successively solve a pipeline of easier classification problems. During each iteration, the initial classification problem is redefined to a simpler one, by discarding part of the training data and applying discriminant analysis on the new subset. The way that a classification problem can become easier by doing so is illustrated by the scatter plot shown in Figure 1. Assuming that a test sample to be classified resides closer to classes 0, 1, and 2, and furthest from class 3. That is, the distances between this sample and the centroids of classes 0, 1, and 2, are smaller than the distance between this sample and the centroid of class 3. The $\mathbf{DL}_{0,1,2,3}$ solid line that is shown represents the discriminant hyper-plane that is generated by RLDA in order to separate the data of all 4 classes. This is done by projecting the data onto this hyper-plane using orthogonal projections, as is illustrated by the dotted lines in Figure 1. Conversely, $\mathbf{DL}_{0,1,2}$ is the RLDA discriminant hyper-plane that was produced in order to only

Figure 1. Retaining a subset of the classes to solve an easier classification problem

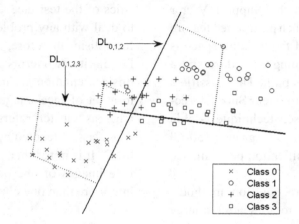

separate the data of classes 0, 1, and 2. It is clear that $\mathbf{DL}_{0,1,2,}$ produces a better separation between these three classes than $\mathbf{DL}_{0,1,2,3}$ does. Assuming that the match for the test sample can indeed be found in classes 0, 1, or 2, and then $\mathbf{DL}_{0,1,2}$ generates a larger expectation that the test sample will be classified correctly.

Computationally-wise, the proposed DTIC method is more efficient than hierarchical trees, space tessellation methods, or 'divide and conquer' techniques. DTIC applies a single discriminant analysis operation at each clustering level. The number of clustering levels is generally much smaller than the number of clusters due to the fact that at each level only a small subset of the training data is retained. On the contrary, for 'divide and conquer' techniques such as the one in (Lu 2002), multiple classification results are produced, for all clusters. Specifically, an individual discriminant analysis process and a nearest-neighbour classifier are applied to each cluster. Hierarchical tree or space tessellation methods, like the Hierarchical Discriminant Analysis (HDA) algorithm of (Swets 1999), also carry heavy computational cost. Specifically, the complete set of training samples is subdivided into smaller classification problems in order to acquire a manageable discriminant solution for each and every face class. On the contrary, DTIC only has to provide a discriminant solution for the face classes that are closer to the test face, at each clustering step. All training data that are related to the remaining face classes are discarded, thus reducing the computational complexity of each clustering step that follows.

In addition, DTIC is flexible to adding new training faces. When a new training face is added to the database, the dimension of the first MDF-space is simply increased by one. As before, the characteristics of the test face shall determine which set of clusters, which may or may not contain the new face class, will be retained at the next clustering level. On the contrary, the hierarchical tree structure requires a complete re-learning of the full training space. This is because the new MDF space at the first tree level may lead to a different decomposition result altogether.

The MDF-spaces that are created at each clustering level of DTIC are biased, with respect to the characteristics of the test face. This is not the case for the hierarchical tree or space tessellation structures since the MDF-spaces are generated in the learning phase and are not biased with respect to the characteristics of the test face. Based on the conclusions of (Tang 2003) and (Liu 2004), the fact that DTIC employs a dynamic classification structure, which utilizes a series of test-face-specific subspaces, should lead to more accurate classification results.

Dynamic Training and Iterative Clustering

The DTIC algorithm is an iterative process that, during each iteration, dynamically creates an adaptive MDF-space that is closely related to the characteristics of the test face. This MDF-space is created by utilizing dynamic training. More specifically, the set of clusters that are utilized by the training process that creates the next MDF-space, is selected based on how close the cluster centroids are to the test face in the current MDF-space. Let us assume that a sample image $\mathbf{X}$ that belongs to a test face is to be assigned to one of the Y distinct classes, $\mathcal{Y}_i$, $i = 1...Y$, that lie in the training space, T. Additionally, let us assume that each ith class in T is represented by $N_{\mathcal{Y}_i}$ images and that the total number of training images are N_Y. Hence, the face images that comprise the training set T can be represented by $\mathbf{Y}_n$, $n = 1,...,N_Y$.

MWD2 Feature Extraction

The feature extraction process that DTIC employs utilizes the MWD2 algorithm which produces a multi-resolution image representation and is described in detail in (Mallat 1989, Daubechies1992). MWD2 was selected based on the expectation that a proper wavelet transform can result in robust image representations with regard to illumination changes and be capable of capturing substantial facial features, while keeping computational complexity low (Zhang 2004). Usually, a low-pass filter, *Lo_D*, and a high-pass filter, *Hi_D*, are utilized to decompose the signal into its low frequency component and its high frequency components at three different orientations (Strang 1996).

The maximum decomposition level, J_d, of a signal is related the signal's highest resolution level, J, by $J_d = J - j$, where j is the current resolution level. The criterion that DTIC uses to define J_d requires for at least one coefficient of the convolved output to be properly calculated, considering that at each scale the convolved output is down-sampled by a factor of 2. Thus, the following should be satisfied: $2^{J_d} \left(\max\left(N_{Hi\_D}, N_{Lo\_D}\right) - 1 \right) < \min\left(N_v, N_h\right)$, where N_v and N_h are the vertical and horizontal dimensions of the 2-D signal f, and N_{Hi_D} and N_{Lo_D} are the lengths of the filter kernels *Hi_D* and *Lo_D*, respectively. As a result, J_d can be calculated by

$$J_d = floor\left(\frac{\log_2\left(\dfrac{\min\left(N_v, N_h\right)}{\max\left(N_{Hi\_D}, N_{Lo\_D}\right) - 1} \right)}{\log_2(2)} \right)$$

(1)

As earlier studies have shown, for classification purposes, the most informative components of a wavelet decomposition are low resolution components (Etemad 1997). Moreover, in (Nastar 1996), it was concluded that facial expressions and small occlusions affect the image intensity manifold locally. Under a frequency-based representation, this suggests that only the high-fre-

quency spectrum is affected. As a result, the set of features that DTIC will utilize are the wavelet coefficients that correspond to the lowest-frequency band at scale J_d (or equivalently at resolution level $J=0$), $f \prec A_0$. It is noted that the analysis filter bank (FIR) filters, *Lo_D* and *Hi_D*, are derived using the spline bi-orthogonal wavelet 'bior3.5' (Daubechies 1992).

By utilizing MWD2, the approximation wavelet coefficients $\mathbf{X} \prec A_0$ and $\mathbf{Y}_n \prec A_0$, $n = 1, \ldots, N_\Upsilon$ that are generated. Then, they are converted to 1-D vectors, by applying row concatenation, thus forming $\tilde{\mathbf{x}}$ and $\tilde{\mathbf{y}}_n$, $n = 1, \ldots, N_\Upsilon$, respectively. The training feature vectors are grouped as columns to the training feature matrix $\tilde{\mathbf{Y}}$.

RLDA MDF-spaces

In order to linearly transform the face vectors such that they become separable, they are projected onto an MDF space. Let S_W and S_B be within-class and between-class scatter matrices (Fukunaga 1990) of the training set $\tilde{\mathbf{Y}}$. A well known criterion is to find a projection that maximizes the ratio of the between-class scatter vs. the within-class scatter (Fisher's criterion) (Kyperountas 2009). In order to address the SSS problem, DTIC applies the Regularized LDA method (RLDA) of (Lu 2005) in order to produce MDF-spaces. RLDA employs a regularized Fisher's separability criterion which is particularly robust against the SSS problem, compared to the original one (Lu 2005). The purpose of regularization is to reduce the high variance related to the eigenvalue estimates of the within-class scatter matrix, at the expense of potentially increased classification bias. The regularized Fisher's discriminant criterion is defined as

$$\mathbf{W} = \arg\max_{\mathbf{w}} \frac{\left|\mathbf{W}^T S_b \mathbf{W}\right|}{\left|R(\mathbf{W}^T S_b \mathbf{W}) + (\mathbf{W}^T S_w \mathbf{W})\right|}$$

(2)

where $\mathbf{S}_w$ and $\mathbf{S}_b$ are the within-class and between-class scatter matrices, respectively, and $0 \leq \mathbf{R} \leq 1$ controls the strength of regularization. Determining the optimal value for R is based on exhaustive search (Lu 2005), making it computationally demanding. For DTIC, an approximation of this optimal value was found at each clustering level, by using data from the UMIST database. Therefore, RLDA is applied on $\tilde{\mathbf{Y}}$ and the discriminant matrix $\mathbf{W}$ of (2) is found. The training and test feature vectors are then projected to the MDF-space by

$$\tilde{\mathbf{y}}'_n = \mathbf{W}^T \tilde{\mathbf{y}}_n, \; n = 1, ..., N_\gamma \qquad (3)$$

$$\tilde{\mathbf{x}}' = \mathbf{W}^T \tilde{\mathbf{x}} \qquad (4)$$

where $\tilde{\mathbf{y}}_n$ and $\tilde{\mathbf{x}}$ are the training and test feature vectors, respectively. Each training discriminant feature vector $\tilde{\mathbf{y}}'_n$ is stored as a column in $\tilde{\mathbf{Y}}'$.

Clustering Using k-Means

The k-means algorithm is then utilized in an effort to partition the training data into the Y distinct face classes. For a given set of $\mathbf{N_T}$ data vectors in the d-dimensional space that are realized as $\tilde{\mathbf{y}}'_n, \; n = 1, ... N_\gamma$, k-means can determine a set of K vectors in $\Re^d$, called the cluster centroids, so that the sum of vector-to-centroid distances, summed over all K clusters, is minimized. The objective function of k-means that is utilized by DTIC makes use of the squared Euclidean distance and is presented in (Camastra 2005). After calculating the K cluster centroids, $\overline{\mathbf{y}}_i, \; i = 1, ..., K$, and assuming that $K=Y$, a single vector $\tilde{\mathbf{y}}'_n$ can be assigned to the cluster with the minimum vector-to-cluster-centroid distance, with respect to all Y distances that are calculated. The distance between each training feature vector and the Y

centroids, $\overline{\mathbf{y}}_i, \; i = 1, ..., Y$, can be calculated by utilizing the Euclidean distance measure:

$$D^n_i(\tilde{\mathbf{y}}'_n, \overline{\mathbf{y}}_i) = \left\| \tilde{\mathbf{y}}'_n - \overline{\mathbf{y}}_i \right\|, \; i = 1, ..., Y. \qquad (5)$$

Then, the training feature vector is assigned to the cluster associated with the minimum distance:

$$if \; D^n_i(\tilde{\mathbf{y}}'_n, \overline{\mathbf{y}}_i) = \min\{D^n_m\}, \; m = 1, ..., Y, \; then \; \tilde{\mathbf{y}}'_n \in C_i. \qquad (6)$$

Ideally, each cluster should contain all the images of only a single face class. However, this is the case only if the separation among the Y classes is sufficiently large, which is not guaranteed. Next, the Y distances between the test feature vector $\tilde{\mathbf{x}}'$ and the cluster centroids are found by using (5) and are sorted in ascending order in $D_{\tilde{\mathbf{x}}'}$:

$$D_{\tilde{\mathbf{x}}'} = \text{sort}\left(D_i\left(\tilde{\mathbf{x}}', \tilde{\mu}_i\right)\right) \qquad (7)$$

Entropy-Based Reduction of the Training Space

At this point, we would like to redefine the original classification problem to a simpler one, by discarding part of the training data. Let us consider a set of K partitions, i.e. clusters, in the T training space. Let V_i denote the surrounding *Voronoi region* of the i-th cluster. Theoretically, if the probability density function $p(\mathbf{x})$ is known, the a-priori probability for a sample feature vector, $\mathbf{x}$, to claim membership to each cluster is defined as

$$P_i = P\left(\mathbf{x} \in V_i\right) = \int_{V_i} p\left(\mathbf{x}\right) d\mathbf{x} \qquad (8)$$

For discrete data, the continuous probability density function can be replaced by the discrete probability histogram:

$$P_i = P\left(\mathbf{x} \in V_i\right) = \frac{\#\left\{j \mid \mathbf{x}_j \in V_i\right\}}{N} \qquad (9)$$

where the cardinality of a set is denoted by $\#\left\{\bullet\right\}$ and N represents the size of the training data set, whose members are $\mathbf{x}_j$, $j=1,...,N$. Similarly, the distribution of a set of K partitions in the training space can be set as $P=(P_1, P_2, ..., P_K)$. A commonly used measure that indicates the randomness of the distribution of a variable is entropy, defined as (Koskela 2004):

$$H = H\left(P\right) = -\sum_{i=1}^{K} P_i \log_2 P_i \qquad (10)$$

The result from an 'ideal' partitioning operation separates the data in a way that creates minimal overlap between the partitions. Equivalently, the expected entropy of the partitions is minimized, over all observed data.

For DTIC, the entropy-based measure is calculated in a new data space $\mathcal{T}' \subset \mathcal{T}$. This subspace consists of a subset of K' clusters, out of the K total that are generated by the k-means algorithm. Let us assume that Y' face classes, Y'_i, exist in the K' clusters that are retained. It is noted that Y'_i is used, rather than Y_i, to indicate that now a face class may be represented by a smaller number of images, than the initial number corresponding to all K clusters. This is because the face images of a person may be partitioned into more than one cluster and the subset of K' clusters may not contain all the clusters that contain all images of this particular face class.

If a true match to the test face class X does indeed exist within the T' space, then the associated entropy can be calculated. Let $P_i = p\left(Y_i' \mid X\right)$ be the probability for the i-**th** face class, Y'_i, that is now contained in T', to represent a true match for X. The discrete probability histogram of (9)

can be utilized to determine the unknown prior probabilities, $p\left(Y_i' \mid X\right)$, as such:

$$P_i = p\left(Y_i' \mid X\right) = \frac{N_{Y_i'}}{N_{Y'}} \qquad (11)$$

where N_Y is the total number of face images that are contained in T' and are stored as columns in $\tilde{\mathbf{Y}}_s' \in \mathcal{T}'$, and $N_{Y_i'}$ is the number of realizations of class i in T'. For example, $N_{Y_i'}$ different images of the person associated with class i are contained in T'. The cardinality of the new cluster set, i.e. the value K', is determined by applying a threshold T_H on the entropy value, so that the overlap between partitions is limited. In order to maintain a low computational cost, the entropy is approximated by substituting (11) to (10), so that the following is satisfied:

$$-\sum_{i=1}^{K'} \frac{N_{Y_i'}}{N_{Y'}} \log_2 \left(\frac{N_{Y_i'}}{N_{Y'}}\right) \leq T_H \qquad (12)$$

This thresholding operation on the approximated entropy values guarantees that at each step of the DTIC algorithm an easier classification problem is defined, in terms of the capability to achieve better separation among the classes. Essentially, T_H is applied to limit the number of different classes that T' will contain. Practically, this is done by limiting the number of clusters K' that comprise T'

Dynamic Selection of the Most Useful Clusters

In order to make use of the concept of breaking down the classification problem into a pipeline of easier classification problems, one must first guarantee a large expectation that the true match to the test data will reside in the $K'<K$ clusters that are retained. Equivalently, this corresponds to a high probability value $p\left(\tilde{\mathbf{x}}'\right)$. If this match does not exist, then $p\left(\tilde{\mathbf{x}}'\right)=0$. The probability that a match for the class of $\tilde{\mathbf{x}}'$ can be found in the i–th retained cluster, $p\left(\tilde{\mathbf{x}}' \mid i\right)$, is inversely proportional to the distance between $\tilde{\mathbf{x}}'$ and the cluster centroid. As a result, and as (8) indicates, the largest possible value for $p\left(\tilde{\mathbf{x}}'\right)$ is attained, if the K' clusters that are retained are associated with the smallest values of $D_{\tilde{\mathbf{x}}}$. Equivalently they are associated with the K' largest values for $p\left(\tilde{\mathbf{x}}' \mid i\right)$. This set of clusters now defines the new training space T':

$$if \quad D_i\left(\tilde{\mathbf{x}}',\tilde{\blacklozenge}_i\right) \le D_{\tilde{\mathbf{x}}}\left(K'\right) \quad then \quad C_i \in \mathcal{T}' \tag{13}$$

The training feature vector data in these K' clusters are collected by utilizing (6).

In the new training space that is comprised by the face data from the K' clusters, RLDA will attempt to discriminate the different classes found in each of the K' clusters, thus creating a new MDF-space. This enables the algorithm to formulate a clustering process that considers possible large variations in the set of images that represent each face class. For example, a portion of the set of images that corresponds to the ith training person may present this person having

facial hair, whereas others as not having facial hair. If these variations are larger than identity-related variations, then they are clustered into disjoint clusters. Thus, the match with the subset of the training images of class i whose appearance is most similar to the test face is considered, so the best match can be found. A flow-chart of the DTIC algorithm is presented in Figure 2.

Experimental Results

In this section, the classification ability of DTIC is investigated by observing FR experiments using data from the ORL, XM2VTS and FERET databases. The UMIST database was used to set the values of the threshold T_H and the regularization parameter R during each iteration of the DTIC algorithm. Essentially, as in most FR applications, the classification experiments that are carried out fall under the small sample size (SSS) problem since the dimensionality of the samples is larger than the number of available training samples per person. The performance of DTIC is presented for various degrees of how severe the SSS problem is. This is done by recording recognition rates for experiments where each face class Y_i is represented by the smallest to the largest possible number of training samples, N_T. The smallest possible value of training samples is 2, because discriminant analysis is utilized. The largest possible value of training samples relates to the number of available images per class, N_{Y_i}, and

Figure 2. Flow-chart of the DTIC algorithm

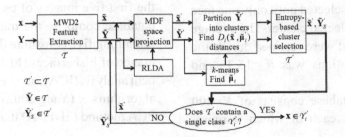

to the fact that at least one of these samples needs to be excluded in order to be used as a test sample. In fact, all remaining images that do not comprise the training set are used to test the performance of DTIC. Thus, they constitute the test set. The training and test sets are created by random selection on each set of the N_{γ_i} images of each face class. To give statistical significance to our experiments, this random selection is repeated N_R times and the N_R acquired recognition rates are then averaged in order to produce the final recognition rate, R_{rec}.

The UMIST database consists of $K=20$ different face classes, each of which is represented by at least $N_{\gamma_i}=19$ images. Consequently, 17 recognition rates were derived for training sets that contained $N_T=2,...,18$ images from each of the 20 face classes. Each corresponding rate was the average out of $N_R=20$ repetitions. In order to approximate the optimal values for T_H and R at each clustering level, exhaustive processing was utilized with the target of maximizing the overall recognition rate. For the first RLDA step, the best value was found to be $R=0$, which makes RLDA equivalent to the DLDA method of (Yu 2001), whereas for the remaining RLDA steps that followed the best value was found to be $R=0.05$. During the first and second clustering iterations, the best value for thresholding the entropy was found to be $T_H=4$, and $T_H=1.45$, respectively. For all subsequent clustering iterations, this value was found to be $T_H=1.0$. Thus, a single cluster is always selected after the second iteration. The face classes that reside in that cluster are partitioned into a new set of clusters, one per class. Then, a single cluster is again selected until only one face class remains in the selected cluster. The average number of clusters that were retained during the first and second iterations was $K'=15.35$ and $K'=2.14$.

The XM2VTS database consists of $K=200$ different face classes, each of which is represented by $N_{\gamma_i}=8$ images. The ORL database consists of $K=40$ different face classes, each of which is represented by $N_{\gamma_i}=10$ images. The number of clusters K' that are retained at each clustering level is selected by using (12). The face classes residing in the final cluster are projected to the MDF-space that is created by processing only this specific set of data. The face class that is closest to the test face in this MDF-space is selected as the true match in identity. The mean recognition rates, R_{rec}, obtained for FR experiments carried out on these face databases were averaged over $N_R=10$ independent runs. For the XM2VTS database experiments, the average number of clusters that were retained at the first and second clustering levels is $K'=9.12$ and $K'=1.51$, respectively. The corresponding results for the ORL database experiments are $K'=13.94$ and $K'=1.84$. Usually, 3 to 5 clustering iterations are required before the identity of a test face is found. The rates R_{rec} are reported in Table 1, for various numbers of training samples per face class. This table shows that DTIC is a very capable FR method that, when trained with a sufficient number of training samples per class, can achieve recognition rates of up to 99%.

The FR performance of the DTIC algorithm is now compared against the performance of a number of FR algorithms that have been recently presented in the literature. In order to derive meaningful conclusions when comparing the performance of various algorithms, the testing and evaluation methodologies, as well as the facial image databases that are used, are identical. In (Yang 2004), an experimental setup is used where the first five images of each subject in the ORL database comprise the training set, whereas the remaining five constitute the test set. The performance of Fisherfaces (FF), independent component analysis (ICA), and kernel eigenfaces (KEF) algorithms in (Yang 2002), as well as of the 2-D PCA method (2DPCA) that is proposed in (Yang

Table 1. DTIC mean recognition rates (R_{rec}) vs. for various numbers of training samples per person (N_T)

UMIST				XM2VTS		ORL	
N_T	R_{rec} (%)	N_T	R_{rec} (%)	N_T	R_{rec} (%)	N_T	R_{rec} (%)
2	59.26	11	97.03	2	31.89	2	69.44
3	82.67	12	97.04	3	93.03	3	91.96
4	90.20	13	97.38	4	96.54	4	94.73
5	92.23	14	97.95	5	97.78	5	97.03
6	92.46	15	98.13	6	97.98	6	98.06
7	94.94	16	98.42	7	99.05	7	98.50
8	95.86	17	98.63			8	98.50
9	95.85	18	100.00			9	98.75
10	96.03						

2004) is evaluated. Under the same experimental setup, DTIC achieves a recognition rate of 98.3%. As a result, DTIC shows the best FR performance, as Table 2 indicates.

In (Xiao-Jun 2004), FR rates are presented for both the ORL and the XM2VTS databases. Specifically, 4 images per person make up the training set and the remaining 6 form the test set, when ORL data is used. Results are presented for the kernel direct discriminant analysis (KDDA) method of (Lu 2003b) as well as the new KDDA (nKDDA) method that is proposed in (Xiao-Jun 2004). The same experiment is used to evaluate DTIC. DTIC outperforms these methods with a recognition rate of 94.73%, as is shown in Table 3. For the experiments done on the XM2VTS database, 4 images per person comprise the training set and the remaining 4 form the test set. DTIC is again evaluated using the same experimental

setup. Table 3 indicates that the DTIC method outperforms all other methods with a recognition rate of 96.54%.

The FERET database, which avails larger number of face classes, Y, is also used to evaluate the performance of DTIC. Once again, the 'closed universe' model (Phillips 2000) is used, where the identity that corresponds to each test image is included in the training set. We implement the testing procedure that is suggested in (Phillips 2000) where the number of different face classes in the training set, Y, is varied. This way the performance of the face recognition algorithm can be evaluated with respect to the size of the training set, or how large a database is. Additionally, results are reported as the number of training samples, N_T, also varies.

The 1199 different face classes that are available in the FERET database are represented by

Table 2. Recognition rates when training set is comprised by the first 5 images of a subject, using ORL data

Method	R_{rec} (%) for N_T=5 by selecting the first 5 images of each subject
FF (Yang 2002)	94.50
ICA (Yang 2002)	85.00
KEF (Yang 2002)	94.00
2DPCA (Yang 2004)	96.00
DTIC	98.30

Table 3. Recognition rates for 4 training samples per subject, using ORL and XM2VTS data

Method	R_{rec} (%) for $N_T=4$	
	ORL	XM2VTS
KDDA (Lu 2003b)	91.30	87.60
nKDDA (Xiao-Jun 2004)	91.30	92.50
DTIC	94.73	96.54

different number of images. In the training sets that are formed, each face class is represented by N_T=2, 3, 4, 5, 6, 7, 8, 9, and 10 images. The number of available face classes are, correspondingly, Y=480, 255, 130, 119, 103, 90, 66, 48, and 27. The average number of clusters that were retained at the first and second clustering levels is K'=10.53 and K''=1.67, respectively and, once again, 3 to 5 clustering iterations are usually required in order to determine the identity of the test face. The performance results for the DTIC

algorithm using the FERET data are presented in Table 4. This table illustrates that as N_T becomes larger, the performance of DTIC becomes less sensitive to variations in the number of face classes Y. The table also provides a comparison with the experimental results produced by applying the Hierarchical Discriminant Analysis (HDA) methodology of (Swets 1999), since HDA is considered to be a good solution to the FR problem when large databases are utilized. These results verify that the fact that DTIC iteratively selects

Table 4. Recognition rates, R_{rec} (%), for HDA (Swets 1999) and DTIC, for various number of training samples, (N_T), and face classes, Y

N_T	Method	Y=27	Y=48	Y=66	Y=90	Y=103	Y=119	Y=130	Y=255	Y=480
2	HDA	79.24	75.53	71.42	66.83	65.14	64.30	62.52	56.21	48.61
	DTIC	88.65	82.34	77.34	73.85	71.65	69.14	67.72	62.57	57.34
3	HDA	89.24	88.73	86.86	83.35	82.42	82.13	81.59	77.25	-
	DTIC	96.46	95.30	94.79	94.06	93.82	93.64	93.34	92.54	-
4	HDA	93.67	92.54	91.22	89.31	88.45	87.53	85.70	-	-
	DTIC	98.48	98.18	97.53	97.40	97.24	96.95	96.17	-	-
5	HDA	95.96	95.11	94.42	92.37	91.85	90.32	-	-	-
	DTIC	99.24	99.17	98.83	98.65	98.48	98.61	-	-	-
6	HDA	97.63	96.40	94.95	93.54	92.76	-	-	-	-
	DTIC	99.49	99.34	98.96	98.85	98.67	-	-	-	-
7	HDA	99.22	98.83	98.26	97.61	-	-	-	-	-
	DTIC	100	100	99.35	99.38	-	-	-	-	-
8	HDA	100	99.56	99.03	-	-	-	-	-	-
	DTIC	100	100	100	-	-	-	-	-	-
9	HDA	100	99.71	-	-	-	-	-	-	-
	DTIC	100	100	-	-	-	-	-	-	-
10	HDA	100	-	-	-	-	-	-	-	-
	DTIC	100	-	-	-	-	-	-	-	-

subsets of the facial classes that are closer to the test face is responsible for the algorithm being able to maintain high recognition performance when the number of face classes Y increases. In fact, the performance of DTIC is consistently superior to that of HDA.

FUTURE TRENDS AND CONCLUSION

In this chapter, a review on discriminant partitioning and learning for face recognition in large databases has been presented. Moreover, as an example, a face recognition methodology that employs dynamic training in order to implement a person-specific discriminant clustering has been described and its performance has been evaluated. By making use of an entropy-based measure, the DTIC algorithm adapts the coordinates of the MDF-space with respect to the characteristics of the test face and of the training faces that are more similar to the test face. Thus, the FR problem is broken down to multiple easier classification tasks, where linear separability is more likely to be achieved. This process iterates until one final cluster is selected that consists of a single face class, representing the best match to the test face. The algorithm is quite fast due to the gradual reduction of the training set. This reduction is quite large during the first two clustering iterations, after which only a small fraction of the original training set is usually retained. The performance DTIC was evaluated on standard face databases and results show that the proposed framework provides a good solution to the problem of FR.

As the volume of multimedia information increases, it is anticipated that a significant aspect of face recognition technology will focus on how to deal further with the problems that arise when large databases are utilized. As far as the research that is described in this chapter is concerned, the following extensions may be considered for further study: (a) When multiple images of same faces are available in the training database, a scoring system can be used during the classification/test phase of the algorithm. This system can properly weigh all results that correspond to training images of the same subject. So, rather than just utilizing the minimum distance, the weighted distances between a test face and all training images that correspond to a particular subject can be utilized to determine if this subject represents the correct match to the test face. As a result, the recognition process would become more robust, especially for 'close call' cases between two subjects in the training database. (b) The proposed algorithm can be applied to other type of pattern recognition applications such as object recognition, iris recognition, and fingerprint signature recognition. An evaluation study can be conducted in order to show that the algorithm is not limited to the face recognition problem.

The problem of classification in large databases is considered also as the biggest in data mining and information retrieval. Large databases can be only handled by combining efficient partitioning techniques and structures along with fast and accurate classification algorithms. The algorithms should be able to be trained efficiently in large datasets and to have the ability of incremental updating when the database is enriched with new content.

Discriminant learning using partitioning of the training space in order to construct classification systems with enhanced performance is an open research problem and very promising direction towards recognition in large databases. The applications vary form face/object recognition to data mining and information retrieval in large databases.

REFERENCES

Bartlett, M. S., Lades, H. M., & Sejnowski, T. J. (1998). Independent component representations for face recognition. In *Proc. of SPIE Symposium on Electronic Imaging: Science and Technology, Human Vision and Electronic Imaging III* (Vol. 3299, pp. 528-539).

Bevilacqua, V., Cariello, L., Carro, G., Daleno, D., & Mastronardi, G. (2008). A face recognition system based on Pseudo 2D HMM applied to neural network coefficients. *Journal of Soft Computing – A Fusion of Foundations . Methodologies and Applications, 12*(7), 1432–7643.

Bicego, M., Castellani, U., & Murino, V. (2003). Using Hidden Markov Models and wavelets for face recognition. In *Proc. 12th Int. Conf. on Image Analysis and Processing*, Mantova, Italy (pp. 52-56).

Bruneli, R., & Poggio, T. (1993). Face recognition: features versus templates. *IEEE Transactions on Pattern Analysis and Machine Intelligence, 15*, 1042–1052. doi:10.1109/34.254061

Buciu, I., Nikolaidis, N., & Pitas, I. (2008). Non-negative matrix factorization in polynomial feature space. *IEEE Transactions on Neural Networks, 19*(6), 1090–1100. doi:10.1109/TNN.2008.2000162

Camastra, F., & Verri, A. (2005). A novel kernel method for clustering. *IEEE Transactions on Pattern Analysis and Machine Intelligence, 27*(5), 801–805. doi:10.1109/TPAMI.2005.88

Daubechies, I. (1992). Ten lectures on wavelets. In *CBMS-NSF Conference series in Applied Mathematics* (SIAM).

Etemad, K., & Chellappa, R. (1997). Discriminant analysis for recognition of human face images. *Journal of the Optical Society of America. A, Optics, Image Science, and Vision, 14*(8), 1724–1733. doi:10.1364/JOSAA.14.001724

Fukunaga, K. (1990). *Introduction to Statistical Pattern Recognition*. New York: Academic Press.

Gao, Q., Zhang, L., & Zhang, D. (2009). Sequential row–column independent component analysis for face recognition. *Neurocomputing, 72*(4-6), 1152–1159. doi:10.1016/j.neucom.2008.02.007

Guo, G. D., Zhang, H. J., & Li, S. Z. (2001). Pairwise face recognition. In *Proc. 8th IEEE Int. Conf. on Computer Vision*, Vancouver, Canada (Vol. 2, pp. 282-287).

Hotta, K. (2008). Robust face recognition under partial occlusion based on support vector machine with local Gaussian summation kernel. *Image and Vision Computing, 26*(11), 1490–1498. doi:10.1016/j.imavis.2008.04.008

Hyvärinen, A., Kanhunen, J., & Oja, E. (2001). *Independent Component Analysis*. New York: Wiley-Intersciense. doi:10.1002/0471221317

Jain, A. K., Duin, R. P. W., & Mao, J. (2000). Statistical pattern recognition: a review. *IEEE Transactions on Pattern Analysis and Machine Intelligence, 22*(1). doi:10.1109/34.824819

Kirby, M., & Sirovich, L. (1990). Application of the Karhunen-Loève procedure for the characterization of human faces. *IEEE Transactions on Pattern Analysis and Machine Intelligence, 12*, 831–835. doi:10.1109/34.41390

Koskela, M., Laaksonen, J., & Oja, E. (2004). Entropy-based measures for clustering and SOM topology preservation applied to content-based image indexing and retrieval. In *Proc. 17th Int. Conf. on Pattern Recognition* (Vol. 2, pp. 1005-1009).

Kyperountas, M., Tefas, A., & Pitas, I. (2007). Weighted Piecewise LDA for solving the small sample size problem in face verification. *IEEE Transactions on Neural Networks, 18*(2), 506–519. doi:10.1109/TNN.2006.885038

Kyperountas, M., Tefas, A., & Pitas, I. (2008). Dynamic Training using Multistage Clustering for Face Recognition. *Pattern Recognition, Elsevier, 41*(3), 894–905. doi:10.1016/j.patcog.2007.06.017

Kyperountas, M., Tefas, A., & Pitas, I. (2010). Salient feature and reliable classifier selection for facial expression classification. *Pattern Recognition, 43*(3), 972–986. doi:10.1016/j.patcog.2009.07.007

Lawrence, S., Giles, C. L., Tsoi, A. C., & Back, A. D. (1997). Face recognition: a convolutional neural network approach. *IEEE Transactions on Neural Networks, 8*, 89–113. doi:10.1109/72.554195

Lee, D. D., & Seung, H. S. (2001). Algorithms for non-negative matrix factorization. *Advances in Neural Information Processing Systems, 13*, 556–562.

Li, S. Z., Hou, X. W., & Zhang, H. J. (2001). Learning spatially localized, parts-based representation. In *Proc. Int. Conf. Computer Vision and Pattern Recognition* (Vol.1, pp. 207–212).

Liu, H.-C., Su, C.-H., Chiang, Y.-H., & Hung, Y.-P. (2004). Personalized face verification system using owner-specific cluster-dependent LDA-subspace. In *Proc. 17th Int. Conf. on Pattern Recognition* (Vol. 4, pp. 344-347).

Lu, J., & Plataniotis, K. N. (2002). Boosting face recognition on a large-scale database. In *Proc. IEEE Int. Conf. on Image Processing*, Rochester, New York.

Lu, J., Plataniotis, K. N., & Venetsanopoulos, A. N. (2003). Face recognition using LDA based algorithms. *IEEE Transactions on Neural Networks, 14*(1), 195–200. doi:10.1109/TNN.2002.806647

Lu, J., Plataniotis, K. N., & Venetsanopoulos, A. N. (2003). Face recognition using kernel direct discriminant analysis algorithms. *IEEE Transactions on Neural Networks, 14*(1), 117–126. doi:10.1109/TNN.2002.806629

Lu, J., Plataniotis, K. N., & Venetsanopoulos, A. N. (2005). Regularization studies of linear discriminant analysis in small sample size scenarios with application to face recognition. *Pattern Recognition Letters, 26*(2), 181–191. doi:10.1016/j.patrec.2004.09.014

Lu, J., Yuan, X., & Yahagi, T. (2007). A method for face recognition based on fuzzy c-means clustering and associated sub-NNs. *IEEE Transactions on Neural Networks, 18*(1), 150–160. doi:10.1109/TNN.2006.884678

Mallat, S. G. (1989). A theory for multi-resolution signal decomposition, the wavelet representation. *IEEE Transactions on Pattern Analysis and Machine Intelligence, 11*, 674–693. doi:10.1109/34.192463

Nastar, C., & Ayach, N. (1996). Frequency-based nonrigid motion analysis. *IEEE Transactions on Pattern Analysis and Machine Intelligence, 18*(11), 1067–1079. doi:10.1109/34.544076

Nefian, A. V., & Hayes, M. H. (2000). Maximum likelihood training of the embedded HMM for face detection and recognition. In *Proc. IEEE Int. Conf. on Image Processing* (Vol. 1, pp. 33-36).

Pang, S., Kim, S., & Bang, S. Y. (2005). Face membership authentication using SVM classification tree generated by membership-based LLE data partition. *IEEE Transactions on Neural Networks, 16*(2), 436–446. doi:10.1109/TNN.2004.841776

Phillips, P. J., Moon, H., Rizvi, S. A., & Rauss, P. J. (2000). The FERET evaluation methodology for face-recognition algorithms. *IEEE Transactions on Pattern Analysis and Machine Intelligence, 22*(10), 1090–1104. doi:10.1109/34.879790

Samaria, F., & Fallside, F. (1993). Face identification and feature extraction using Hidden Markov Models. In Vernazza, G. (Ed.), *Image Processing: Theory and Application*. Amsterdam: Elsevier.

Strang, G., & Nguyen, T. (1996). *Wavelets and Filter Banks*. Wellesley, MA: Wellesley-Cambridge Press.

Swets, D. L., & Weng, J. (1999). Hierarchical discriminant analysis for image retrieval. *IEEE Transactions on Pattern Analysis and Machine Intelligence, 21*(5), 386–401. doi:10.1109/34.765652

Tang, H.-M., Lyu, M. R., & King, I. (2003). Face recognition committee machines: dynamic vs. static structures. In *Proc. 12th Int. Conf. on Image Analysis and Processing*, Mantova, Italy, Sept. 17-19 (pp. 121-126).

Tefas, A., Kotropoulos, C., & Pitas, I. (1998). Variants of Dynamic Link Architecture based on mathematical morphology for frontal face authentication. In *Proc. IEEE Computer Society Conf. on Computer Vision and Pattern Recognition*, Santa Barbara, California (pp. 814 –819).

Tefas, A., Kotropoulos, C., & Pitas, I. (2001). Using Support vector machines to enhance the performance of elastic graph matching for frontal face authentication. *IEEE Transactions on Pattern Analysis and Machine Intelligence, 23*(7), 735–746. doi:10.1109/34.935847

Tefas, A., Kotropoulos, C., & Pitas, I. (2002). Face verification using elastic graph matching based on morphological signal decomposition. *Signal Processing, 82*(6), 833–851. doi:10.1016/S0165-1684(02)00157-3

Turk, M., & Pentland, A. (1991). Eigenfaces for recognition. *Journal of Cognitive Neuroscience, 3*, 71–86. doi:10.1162/jocn.1991.3.1.71

Weng, J., & Hwang, W.-S. (2007). Incremental Hierarchical Discriminant Regression. *IEEE Transactions on Neural Networks, 18*(2), 397–415. doi:10.1109/TNN.2006.889942

Wiskott, L., Fellous, J. M., Kruger, N., & von der Malsburg, C. (1997). Face recognition by elastic bunch graph matching. *IEEE Trans. on Pattern Analysis and Machine Intelligence, 19*, 775 779.

Wolfrum, P., Wolff, C., Lucke, J., & von der Malsburg, C. (2008). A recurrent dynamic model for correspondence-based face recognition. *Journal of Vision (Charlottesville, Va.), 8*(7), 1–18. doi:10.1167/8.7.34

Xiao-Jun, W. U., Kittler, J., Jing-Yu, Y., Messer, K., & Shi-Tong, W. (2004). A new kernel direct discriminant analysis (KDDA) algorithm for face recognition. In *Conf. British Machine Vision*, Kingston University, London.

Xudong, J., Mandal, B., & Kot, A. (2008). Eigenfeature regularization and extraction in face recognition. *IEEE Transactions on Pattern Analysis and Machine Intelligence, 30*(3), 383–394. doi:10.1109/TPAMI.2007.70708

Yang, J., Zhang, D., Frangi, A. F., & Yang, J.-Y. (2004). Two-dimensional PCA: a new approach to appearance-based face representation and recognition. *IEEE Transactions on Pattern Analysis and Machine Intelligence, 26*(1), 131–137. doi:10.1109/TPAMI.2004.1261097

Yang, M. H. (2002). Kernel eigenfaces vs. kernel fisherfaces: face recognition using kernel methods. In *Proc. IEEE 5th Int. Conf. on Automatic Face and Gesture Recognition* (pp. 215-220).

Yu, H., & Yang, J. (2001). A direct LDA algorithm for high-dimensional data with application to face recognition. *Pattern Recognition, Elsevier, 34*(12), 2067–2070. doi:10.1016/S0031-3203(00)00162-X

Zhang, B., Zhang, H., & Ge, S. (2004). Face recognition by applying wavelet subband representation and Kernel Associative Memories. *IEEE Transactions on Neural Networks, 15*(1), 166–177. doi:10.1109/TNN.2003.820673

KEY TERMS AND DEFINITIONS

Dynamic Training: training whose parameters change (dynamically) based on the properties of the test data.

Face Recognition: determination of the identity of a face.

Large Database: database that contains samples of faces from a large number of people.

Partitioning: separating data in clusters

Classification: the process of assigning data to a specific class, or, classes.

Clustering: grouping similar data.

Discriminant Analysis: technique that identifies which variables or combinations of variables accurately discriminate between groups or categories.

K-Means: a (clustering) method that distributes data into k clusters.

Facial Features: facial characteristics that can be observed or extracted.

Section 5
Facial Expression Classification

Chapter 12
From Face to Facial Expression

Zakia Hammal
Université de Montréal, Canada

ABSTRACT

This chapter addresses recent advances in computer vision for facial expression classification. The authors present the different processing steps of the problem of automatic facial expression recognition. They describe the advances of each stage of the problem and review the future challenges towards the application of such systems to everyday life situations. The authors also introduce the importance of taking advantage of the human strategy by reviewing advances of research in psychology towards multi-disciplinary approach for facial expression classification. Finally, the authors describe one contribution which aims at dealing with some of the discussed challenges.

INTRODUCTION

Nowadays, computers become more and more presented in everyday life of the general population. Involved in professional as well as personal activities to perform tasks more and more complex, computer accessibility needs to be greatly improved. Notably a human-computer interaction can become more effective if the communication between computers and users mimic as much as possible the way human beings interact between each other. One way to achieve this is to provide them the ability to analyze the behavior of the user in order to give them access to other dimensions of the social communication that are unattainable through the keyboard instructions. Computers may then be able to better answer the user's expectations.

The human face is an important and complex communication channel and it is considered as one of the most ecologically relevant entities for visual perception. Expressive changes in the face are a rich source of cues about intra and interpersonal indicators and functions of emotion. Facial expressions communicate information from which we can quickly infer the state of mind of our peers, and

DOI: 10.4018/978-1-61520-991-0.ch012

adjust our behavior accordingly (Darwin, 1872). Facial expressions are a visible manifestation of the emotional state, cognitive activity, intention, personality, and psychopathology of a person (Donato et al., 1999). It is said that 55% of the communicating feeling is conveyed by the facial expressions while only 7% by the linguistic language and 38% by the paralanguage (Mehrabian, 1968). This implies that facial expressions play an important role in human communication. Human-computer interaction will then definitively benefit from automated facial expression recognition.

In this chapter, we address the issue of automatic recognition of facial expression. The development of such a system constitutes a significant challenge because of the many constraints that are imposed by its application in a real world context (Pantic & Bartlett, 2007). In particular, this system should be able to provide relevant information with great accuracy and work under harsh conditions without demanding too many interventions from the user. Based on these considerations, there have been major advances in computer vision over the past 15 years applying advanced techniques of image and video processing for the recognition of facial expressions.

This chapter introduces advances in computer vision for facial expression classification. First, we describe the most comment and useful representation of facial expressions. Then, after briefly presenting the different approaches and limits of facial feature extraction methods, we survey the state of the art of automatic facial expression systems, discussing their achievements and their limitations. In order to go beyond the computational approach, we make an original introduction to the psychology of visual perception, focusing on the most recent available data of facial expression recognition by humans and we show how research in facial expression classification may favorably take advantage of a multidisciplinary approach. Finally, we describe one of the most recently proposed contributions for the recognition of the six basic facial expressions, which deals with some

of the current challenges and limitations faced by the automatic facial expression community.

FACIAL EXPRESSION REPRESENTATION

From Emotion to Emotional Facial Expression

Emotion is one of the most controversial topics in psychology, a source of intense discussion and disagreement from the earliest philosophers and other thinkers to the present day. There is a long history of interest in the problem of recognizing emotion from facial expression in several disciplines. Since 1649 Descartes (Descartes, 1649) introduced the six "simple passions": *Wonder*; *Love*; *Hatred*; *Desire*; *Smile*; and *Sadness* and assumed that all the others are composed of some of these six. In 1872, Darwin (Darwin, 1872) argued that there are specific inborn emotions and that each emotion includes a specific pattern of activation of the facial expressions and behavior. Inspired from the works of Darwin, Ekman et al. (1972) showed that observers could agree on how to label both posed and spontaneous facial expressions in terms of emotional categories across cultures. Ekman showed pictures of facial expressions to people in the U.S., Japan, Argentina, Chile and Brazil and found that they judged the expressions in the same way. Similar facial expressions tend to occur in response to particular emotion eliciting events. However, this was not conclusive because all these people could have learned the meaning of expressions by watching TV. To be more conclusive, Ekman found visually isolated people in the highlands of Papua New Guinea. The experiment's outcome showed that subjects judged the proposed expressions in the same way; moreover, their response to a particular emotion corresponded to the same expression. Based on the results Ekman confirmed the universality of the emotional expressions and put a list of six basic emotional facial expressions named *Surprise, Surprise, Sadness, Disgust, Anger* and *Fear* (Figure 1).

However, the term "*expression*" implies the existence of something that is expressed and people can conceal their internal feelings by simulating another expression. So there is a difference between "*facial expressions*" that can be recognized only by the analysis of the facial features and "*emotions*" which correspond to an internal feeling and require more than feature deformations to be recognized. Then the recognition of one facial expression allows the gain of some information about the emotional state but is not sufficient to confirm it and may require other modalities (for example the voice (Zeng et al., 2009), and the body gesture (Gunes et al., 2008)) to be recognized. In this chapter, we only focus on the facial expression classification based on the facial appearance.

Facial Expression Representation

Each facial expression corresponds to a specific combination of facial muscle movements. The widely used method for manual labeling of facial deformations corresponding to the facial muscles motion is the Facial Action Coding System (FACS; (Ekman & Friesen, 1978)). The FACS defines the specific changes that occur with muscular contractions and how best to differentiate one from another. The FACS measurement units are Action

Units (AUs). Ekman defined 46 AUs, which represent a contraction or relaxation of one or more muscles. The FACS coding consists in describing each facial expression as a combination of one or more specific AUs (see Figure 2).

Another coding model of the facial deformation is the MPEG-4 standard (Tekalp, 1999). MPEG-4 is an object-based multimedia compression standard, which allows encoding different audiovisual objects in the scene independently. The MPEG-4 measurement units are the Facial Definition Parameters (FDP). The FDP are a set of tokens that describe minimal perceptible actions in the facial area. The distances between the FDP points allow the modeling of a set of Facial Animation Parameters (FAPs) to describe each one of the six basic facial expressions (see Figure 3).

Different coding of the facial feature behavior can be then chosen according to the extracted facial features information. Automatic facial expression classification requires a number of preprocessing steps: face and facial features detection; their representation (for example FACS or MEGP-4); their interpretation and finally the expression classification.

FACIAL FEATURES EXTRACTION: SHORT OVERVIEW

The first step for facial expression analysis is face and facial features (such as eyes, eyebrows

Figure 1. The six universal emotional facial expressions

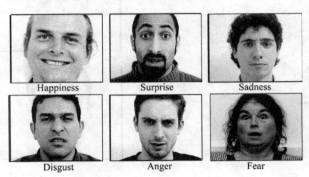

Figure 2. Examples of Action Units (AUs) defined by the FACS system. First row: upper AUs, second row: lower AUs (Ekman & Friesen, 1978).

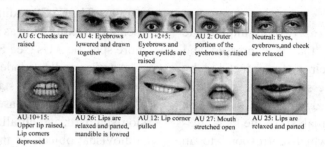

and mouth) detection and tracking. The greatest difficulties encountered in detecting permanent facial features are caused by the lighting conditions, the complexity and high variability of the face morphology; facial expressions and head pose variations. According to the extracted information and to some specific constraints, facial feature segmentation methods can be classified into four main approaches: luminance and/or chrominance based approaches, active contours, deformable templates and hybrid approaches. The first approach extracts facial features based on luminance and/or chrominance information (Tsekeridou & Pitas, 1998; Deng et al., 2004; Wang et al., 2005).

Figure 3. (a) a face model in its Neutral state and the Facial Animation Parameter Units; (b) and (c) Facial Definition Parameters used for the definition of the Facial Animation Parameters (Tekalp, 1999)

These methods allow a fast localization of the features but they do not allow obtaining an accurate and precise detection of the contours (see Figure 4.a). Moreover, based mainly on the binarization process, these approaches are highly sensitive and strongly dependent on the recording conditions and especially on the lighting conditions. The second approach is based on active contours or snakes,

Figure 4. Example of facial features segmentation: (a) illustration of luminance based localization results of (Tsekeridou & Pitas, 1998), b: illustration of snakes based method results of (Pardas & Sayrol, 2001), (c): illustration of deformable templates based approach results of (Tian et al., 2000), (d): automatic classification results based on hybrid based approach of (Hammal et al, 2006a)

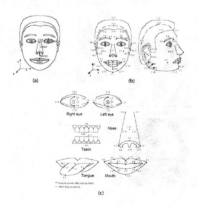

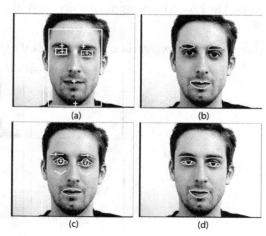

which consist in deforming curves according to a cost function to be minimized (Coots, 1998; Pardas, 2000; Pardas & Sayrol, 2001). The main advantage of the snakes is their great ability to handle deformations and adaptations on a great number of object contours (see Figure 4.b). However, the contour needs to be initialized close to the correct starting position otherwise, the algorithm may not be able to converge to the right contour. The third approach is based on deformable templates. Introducing regularity characteristics like symmetry and elasticity of the segmented contours, the active contours based approaches are more adapted than the snakes (Yuille et al., 1992; Tian et al., 2000; Malciu & Preteux, 2001; Kashima et al., 2001; Dornaika & Davoine, 2004). Using this approach, the shape of the searched features is always valid and further noise-resistant (see Figure 4.c). However, shape constraints lead sometimes to less accurate segmentation results and do not allow adapting to a great number of deformations like the ones occurring on eyes and eyebrows in the case of facial expressions. Initialization not too far from the final position is also necessary for a good detection result.

Hybrid based approach intends to take advantage of each technique. An example is the model of Hammal et al. (2006a) (see Figure 4.d) where a specific parametric model is defined for each deformable feature introducing regularization constraints. In order to fit the model with the contours to be extracted, a gradient flow (of luminance and/or chrominance) through the estimated contour is maximized (see section 6.1).

It is difficult to make an objective comparison between all these methods. The performances of each of them depend on the type of applications and the recording constraints of the used images. However, this short overview highlights the limitations of the results of the facial features segmentation methods. Indeed, based on the results of these automatic segmentation systems, an automatic facial expression classification method should be able to deal with uncertain and noisy data and to generate results so that the associated certainty varies with the certainty of facial features segmentation. One of the first models to explicitly tackle these issues was proposed by Hammal *et al.* (2005, 2007).

STATE OF THE ART OF FACIAL EXPRESSION CLASSIFICATION: ADVANCES AND CHALLENGES

The up-to-date developments in computer vision for static and dynamic facial expression recognition based on the facial features analysis can be divided into two types: Model-based approaches and fiducial-point-based approaches.

Model-Based Approach

The model-based approach either applies an image warping process to map face images into a geometrical model, or performs a local analysis where spatially localized kernels are employed to extract facial features (e.g., Gabor filters, integral image filters, and Active Appearance Models). Such systems classify new expressions as members of the expression associated with the nearest model using a suitable metric or a supervised classifier.

Kimura and Yachida (1997), for example, used a "potential net" model to track 899 positions on the face distributed in a grid pattern. The Karhunen Loeve expansion (a generalization of principal component analysis PCA) is then used to reduce the vector dimensionality. The distances of the input vector projection from three expression models and from the origin are used to estimate the type and degree of expression, respectively. However, the classification results of new subjects are described as "unsatisfactory" in the paper.

In Lyons & Akamatsu (1998), the classification process is based on the Gabor wavelet coefficients of 34 facial feature points manually initialized on the face and combined into a single vector. A linear discriminant analysis is used for the classification process. However, a manual normalization of the faces leading to a predefined distance between the eyes is required.

Oliver et al. (2000) proposed a Hidden Markov Models for facial expression recognition based on the real-time tracking of mouth shape. However, only a few facial expressions have their characteristic pattern contained in the mouth shape. For this reason, the only studied facial expressions were Open mouth, Sadness, Smile and Smile-Open mouth. Gao et al. (2003) suggested a facial expression classification that uses Line Edge Map (LEM) as the expression descriptor. The classification is based on the disparity between two line sets applied on the query face LEM and the caricature models of every expression.

Abboud et al. (2004) chose to represent each expression by an active appearance vector. The Mahalanobis distance is measured between the tested appearance vector and each estimated mean vector in Fisherspace. In order to measure the intensity of the detected facial expressions Amin et al. (2005) align and normalize an input face image, then applied a filter bank of Gabor wavelets and reduce the data's dimensionality via PCA. An unsupervised Fuzzy-C-Mean clustering algorithm is then employed to determine the principle component pairs to estimate the degree of emotion from facial expressions (for example less Happy, moderately happy, and very happy). In Dailey et al. (2002) a linear dimensionality reduction is also performed on the Gabor representation of each face via a PCA. A single layer neural network containing six outputs corresponding to the six basic facial expressions is used to classify the PCA output vector. In Barlett et al. (2005, 2006), the face is automatically detected in video streams using the method proposed by Fasel et al. (2005), rescaled, aligned, and passed through a bank of Gabor filters, leading to a collection of features. A feature selection stage based on the AdaBoost extracts a subset of the features and processes them to the Support Vector Machine (SVM) classifier, which makes a binary decision about each

of the six basic facial expressions plus Neutral. An appearance-based system was also developed by Tong et al. (2006). They applied a dynamic Bayesian model to the output of a front-end AU recognition system similar to that developed in the Bartlett laboratory.

The main limitation of model-based approach is the difficulty of designing a deterministic physical model that can represent accurately all the geometrical properties of faces, especially muscle activity in faces. The holistic approach usually involves an intensive training stage. Moreover, the trained model is sometimes unable to represent individual differences. These shortcomings led others to attack the problem differently using local facial cues, as described in the next section.

Fiducial-Points-Based Approach

The fiducial-points-based systems compare the deformation of the facial features with a reference state, i.e. the neutral facial expression. In this approach, the facial movements are quantified by measuring the geometrical displacement of facial landmarks between two frames. They are then classified into AUs or into facial expressions according to the obtained observations.

Lien et al. (1998), for example, proposed a hybrid method based on manually detected feature points (tracked by Lucas & Kanade (1981) in the remaining of the sequence) and furrows for the recognition of a set of upper and lower AUs. They used a Hidden Markov Model (HMM) for each AU or combination of AUs. The main drawback of the method is the number of HMMs required to detect a great number of AUs or combinations of AUs.

Using the same data as Lie et al. (1998), Tian et al. (2001) used a Neural Network and obtained better classification results than (Lie et al., 1998). Cohen et al. (2003) developed a system based on a non-rigid face-tracking algorithm to extract local motion features. These motion features are the inputs of a Bayesian network classifier used to recognize the six basic facial expressions. Zhang & Qiang (2005), Pantic & Patras (2006) and Hammal (2006b) described in section 6) were the firsts to take into account the temporal information in the classification process of the AUs and the facial expressions. Pantic et al. used two face models made of frontal and side views. The eyes, eyebrows and mouth are automatically segmented and transformed into AUs through the application of a set of rules; and each AU is divided into three time segments: the onset, the apex, and the offset. The classification is performed using the FACS coder (Ekman & Friesen, 1978). A limitation associated with the uses of FACS however, is that the FACS scores are only qualitative and thus provide no categorization rule. Most of the systems making use of the FACS aim at recognizing the different AUs without actually recognizing the displayed facial expression. These systems then bypass the problem of doubt between multiple expressions that can occur. Overcoming this limitation, Zhang & Qiang (2005) proposed a fusion technique based on a dynamic Bayesian network. Permanent as well as transient features are used for AUs detection. Contrary to the FACS-based methods described above, the classification results of the AUs obtained by the dynamic Bayesian network are combined using a rules table defined by the authors to associate to each combination of AUs, one of the six basic facial expressions. Rather than using the FACS coding process, (Tsapatsoulis et al., 2000; Pardas & Bonafonte, 2002; Hammal et al., 2007), proposed a description of the six basic facial expressions that employs the MPEG-4 coding model. Tsapatsoulis et al. (2000) used fuzzy inference for the classification whereas Pardas & Bonafonte (2002) used Hidden Markov Models, which offered better results.

The fiducial-points-based representation requires accurate and reliable facial feature detection and tracking to cope with variations in illumination and the non-rigid motion of facial features. Based on these considerations, the chosen classification approach should allow the modeling of the noise

and uncertainty in the segmentation results (at the end of this chapter we present a dynamic fiducial points-based approach which explicitly intends to take into account the uncertain, imprecise and noisy data (Hammal, 2006b; Hammal et al. 2007).

Limits and Future Development

This review of the state of the art in the computer vision and pattern recognition community shows that great efforts have been made to automatically recognize facial expressions. However, several challenges still need to be overcome.

Beyond the 6 Basic Emotional Facial Expressions

All the proposed models examined the facial expressions in one of the basic facial expressions proposed by Ekman and Freisen (1978) or at best classify them as a combination of a set of AUs. However, as reported in (Cohn, 2006) the list of the basic facial expressions was never intended as exhaustive of human emotion. Moreover, in everyday life human behavioral felling is not limited to the six basic facial expressions. Other emotional facial expressions can be inferred including Attentiveness (El Kaliouby & Robinson, 2004), Fatigue (Ji et al., 2006), and Pain (Littlewort et al., 2007; Ashraf et al., 2007; Hammal et al., 2008). Facial expressions include also blends and combinations of two or several expressions (Izard et al., 1983), and pure facial expressions are rarely perceived (Young et al., 1997). Based on a forced choice the proposed facial expression systems skip the problem of doubt between multiple expressions that can occur. Forced-choice designs sometimes yield consensus on the wrong answer. Then an automatic system for facial expression recognition should be able to model the set of the possible facial deformations, which do not correspond to any of the six basic facial expressions as well as the doubt between facial expressions. An example is the system proposed by Hammal et al. (2007), which explicitly models the doubt between expressions and provides an Unknown class corresponding to all the complex non-prototypic facial expressions.

Noise and Uncertainty

There are two sources of uncertainty in facial expression classification: human differences and facial feature segmentation results. Indeed, facial feature segmentation implies imprecise and partial data that should be expected in facial expression classification (see section 3). Therefore, a facial expression analyzer should facilitate the integration of a priori knowledge and should be able to deal with uncertain and imprecise data obtained from video-based segmentation algorithms (Hammal et al., 2005). Facial expression certainty should vary with the certainty of the corresponding facial features localization and tracking (Pantic & Bartlett, 2007). Another source of uncertainty is the individual differences, like, facial appearance, degree of facial elasticity, morphology and intensity of facial expressions (Tian et al., 2005). Given these considerations a logical system is not sufficient to make the classification reliable. A well-adapted model of fusion process for these considerations is the Transferable Belief Model (Smets, 2000). It decomposes the fusion process in different modeling steps where the uncertainty and imprecision is explicitly modeled at the level of the extracted data. Based on the modeling and fusion process this uncertainty is transferred as uncertainty of the expected facial expressions (see section 6 and (Hammal et al., 2007)).

Temporal Dynamic of Human Facial Behavior

Temporal dynamics of human facial behavior is a critical factor for the interpretation of the facial expressions (Cohn & Schmidt, 2004; Ambadar et al., 2005). In everyday life, facial expressions are not static, but are the result of dynamic and progres-

sive combinations of facial feature deformations. The first evidence that there are some temporal information specific to facial expressions comes from Bassili (1978). In the last 10 years, a set of subsequent research in psychology has clearly shown that dynamic information can improve the recognition of facial expressions (Harwood et al., 1999; Wehrle et al., 2000; Weyers et al., 2000; Wallraven et al., 2008; Nusseck et al., 2008). It has also been shown that dynamic behavior of human face represents a critical factor for categorization of some complex feeling like Pain and improves the perception of facial expressions compared to the static display (Ekman et al., 2005).

Neuroimaging studies have also revealed that the brain region known to be implicated in the processing of emotion, respond more to dynamic than to static emotional facial expressions (Haxby et al., 2000, 2002). Moreover, there is anatomical work suggesting that static and dynamic facial expressions possibly involve completely different brain regions (Adolphs, 2002).

Despite these findings, the vast majority of the past works on automatic facial expressions classification does not take dynamics of facial expressions into account. The main contributions are based on the combination of static classification results or, at best, only on the difference between the first and the current or the last frames. None of them takes explicitly into account the temporal dynamic of the facial features and their asynchronous deformation during a sequence of facial expression. Recent studies are proposed to explicitly model the dynamics of facial behavior for the recognition of temporal segments of AUs activation in a consecutive predefined number of frames (Pantic & Patras, 2006). However, these methods are very sensitive to the frame size and do not allow to take into account the dynamic asynchronous facial features deformation. To deal with these limitations, a recent contribution has been proposed to recognize dynamically and progressively sequences of facial expressions (Hammal, 2006b; Hammal et al., 2008, Hammal et al., 2010). The main contribution of this approach is the combination at each time of the completely permanent facial features behavior from the beginning to the end of the sequence. At the beginning of the sequence all expressions are in the set of possible expressions and, during the sequence, this set is progressively reduced by a dynamic refinement process. When reaching the end of the sequence, the decision depends on the whole set of facial feature behavior that occurred during the sequence.

Context

The existing approaches for facial expression classification are context insensitive. However, facial expressions are displayed differently in a particular context (e.g., being outdoor or indoor, the undergoing task, the other people involved, the expresser personality) (Zeng et al., 2009). Without context, even humans may misunderstand the observed facial expression. Nonetheless, a few studies (Ji et al., 2006; Kapoor et al., 2007) have investigated the influence of context on facial expressions. However, an automatic use of the context is not an easy task. Before addressing the issue of using the context one should answer several questions: context definition, detection, interpretation and finally its integration to the classification process.

Spontaneous vs. Acted Facial Expressions

Most of the past work on automatic facial expression analysis has been dedicated to the analysis of posed facial expression and could not always apply in everyday life situations. There are two main reasons: the lack of spontaneous facial expression databases and that even if these databases are available the segmentation of facial features would be difficult in this kind of data (i.e. head motion, lighting conditions, scene complexity…). With the development of few spontaneous facial expression databases the focus of the research in the field has started to shift to the analysis of the differences between the acted and the spontaneously displayed facial expressions (Cohn & Schmidt 2004; Valstar et al., 2006). It has been shown that spontaneous facial expressions are characterized by subtle changes of facial features while the acted facial expressions are characterized by exaggerated changes of facial features (Cohn & Schmidt, 2004). Moreover, there are several differences in the temporal dynamics of facial behavior between acted and spontaneous facial expressions. For example, spontaneous and deliberately displayed eyebrow actions differ by their duration, speed of the beginning of the expression and the end of the expression as well as the order and timing of facial actions occurrences (Cohn & Schmidt 2004; Valstar et al., 2006). Based on these results, few efforts have also been made for the development of automatic systems for the recognition of spontaneous facial expressions (Barlett et al., 2006; Littlewort et al., 2007; Valstar et al., 2007; Hammal et al., 2008). To go further, this advance requires new benchmark databases in order to test and compare the proposed approaches. Moreover, it requires future developments (such as described in this chapter) including: dealing with uncertainty, going beyond the 6 universal expressions, and integrating contextual information.

VISUAL PERCEPTION FOR FACIAL EXPRESSION RECOGNITION

In spite of the significant amount of research on automatic facial expression recognition, this task remains hard to achieve by computer vision systems. Human visual system remains far ahead of everything that has been done on automatic facial expressions recognition. What makes humans exceptionally capable of recognizing facial expressions? How can we take advantage of this skill to improve automatic systems?

To answer the first question, studies in visual perception show that different visual cues are used by human observers to recognize different facial expressions. Boucher and Ekman (1975) stated that the lower half of the face is mainly used by human observers to recognize Happiness and Disgust and that the whole face is used to recognize Anger and Surprise. Whereas, Gouta and Miyamoto (2000) stated that the top half of the face allows to better recognize Anger, Fear, Surprise, and Sadness, whereas the lower half is better for Disgust and Happiness. In a larger scheme, Bassili (1978, 1979) stated that the whole face leads to a better recognition of the basic facial expressions (74.4%) then lower part of the face (64.9%) or the top part of the face (55.1%). Lately, Smith et al. (2005) and Roy et al. (2008) further analyzed the importance of the facial features (such eyes, eyebrows, mouth and wrinkles) for the static and dynamic recognition of the six basic facial expressions. These experiments highlight the exact facial features used by human observers for the recognition of each one of the six basic facial expressions as well as Neutral and Pain for static and dynamic facial expressions. For example, as reported in Smith et al. (2005) humans use the mouth but not eyes for Happiness and they use the eyes but not the mouth for Fear. In other cases, humans use transient features: for example the nasolabial furrow in the case of Disgust and the wrinkles on the forehead in the case of Sadness. Given that humans easily outperform machines at recognizing facial expressions in everyday situations, it appears likely that their strategies reflect strong everyday facial expression statistics. Thus it seems promising for a future implementation of automatic facial expression recognition to take advantage of the human skills and to take into account their relative importance to improve their performances. One first modest attempt in this direction is proposed by Hammal et al. (2009), who compared their model to the human performances in the same experimental conditions as Smith et al. (2005). Their model was enhanced to deal with partially occluded facial parts. The obtained results show that the model compares favorably to human performances and reveals differences between the visual cues used by the model and the human observers. Notably they derive relative weights associated to each facial feature and according to each facial expression that may be advantageously use to further refine the classification. Such new additional processing step to the current automatic systems may be considered as one of the many fundamental improvement these systems may benefit from a multidisciplinary approach, in order to get closer to human performances.

DESCRIPTION OF ONE CONTRIBUTION

Here we describe the fiducial-based expression recognition system developed by Hammal et al. (, 2007). The described model deals with some of the previously aimed properties for the recognition of the six basic facial expression and Neutral: first, it models explicitly the doubt between facial expressions and defines the Unknown expressions (i.e. all facial deformations that cannot be categorized into one of the six basic facial expressions); Secondly, it deals with noisy and partially occluded data and compares favorably with human observers in the same experimental conditions (Hammal et al., 2009); Finally, it was recently extended to a dynamic (Hammal, 2006b), multi-cue and context depend recognition of spontaneous Pain sequences (Hammal et al., 2008). In the following, we present the main features of this model for dynamic facial expression recognition of the six basic facial expressions. For size reasons we cannot describe the extension of the dynamic model into context-dependant spontaneous Pain expressions (detail scan be found in (Hammal et al., 2008)).

Measures Extraction and Modeling

The first step in the Hammal *et al.* facial expression classification model is the extraction of the contours of the permanent facial features. In order to give the reader an overview of the data extraction limits (and then the everyday life classification limits of the proposed model) a few details on the segmentation are given here (interested reader can found more details in (Hammal et al., 2006a)).

To cope with the illumination variation problem, a preprocessing stage based on a model of the human retina (Beaudot, 1994) is first used. It enhances the contours and realizes a local correction of the illumination variations (see Figure 5.b). In each eye-bounding box (Rr and Rl areas in Figure 5.b), the iris semi-circle maximizing the normalized flow of luminance gradient is selected and is then completed by symmetry (see Figure 5.c).

A specific parametric model is then defined for each deformable feature (eyelids, eyebrows and mouth). Several characteristic points are automatically extracted to initialize each model (eyes, eyebrows and mouth corners, see Figure 6.b, 6.c). In order to fit each model with the contours to be extracted, a gradient flow (of luminance and/or chrominance) through the estimated contours is maximized. Figure 6.d shows the selection process where dashed curves (red in color) correspond to the tested curves and the white curves correspond to the selected contours (Figure 6.e). The chosen models are flexible enough to produce realistic contours. Figure 7 shows an example during Happiness, Surprise and Disgust expressions.

Intensive tests (e.g. a comparison with a manual ground truth) on several databases under various face sizes (i.e. face dimensions higher or equal to 90*90 pixels corresponding to an iris radius $4 \leq R \leq 13$ pixels and to head motion corresponding to: roll$\approx$45° and pan$\approx$40°) show the accuracy and the robustness of the method to spectacles, luminance conditions, ethnicity and facial expression deformations (Hammal et al., 2006a).

The permanent facial feature deformations that occur during facial expressions are then measured by five characteristic distances D_1 to D_5 extracted

Figure 5. Iris segmentation process: (a) input frame; (b) retinal preprocessing of detected face and zoom on the gradient of the iris semi circle area; (c) iris segmentation result (Hammal et al., 2006a)

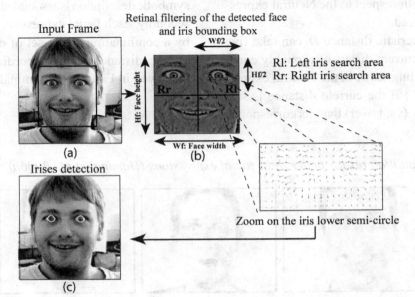

Figure 6. Example of eyelids, eyebrows and mouth segmentation process (Hammal et al., 2006a)

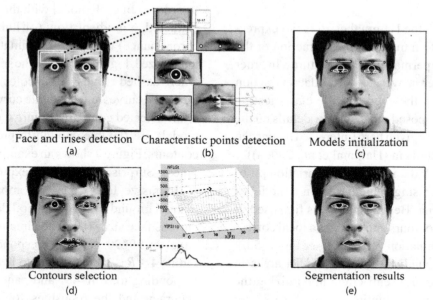

Face and irises detection   Characteristic points detection   Models initialization
(a)   (b)   (c)

Contours selection   Segmentation results
(d)   (e)

from the characteristic points corresponding to the contours of the permanent facial features (see Figure 8). To make the analysis independent of the variability of face dimensions and of the position of the face according to the camera, each distance is normalized according to the distance between the centers of both irises in the analyzed face. In addition to distance normalization, only the deformations with respect to the Neutral expression are considered.

Each characteristic distance D_i can take five states: S_i if the current distance is roughly equal to its corresponding value in the Neutral expression, C_i^+ (vs. C_i^-) if the current distance is significantly higher (vs. lower) than its correspond-

ing value in the Neutral expression, and $S_i \cup C_i^+$ (vs. $S_i \cup C_i^-$) if the current distance is neither sufficiently higher (vs. lower) to be in C_i^+ (vs. C_i^-), nor sufficiently stable to be in S_i ($\cup$ means the logical OR) (see Figure 9 for an example).

The characteristic distance states are then typically mapped to symbolic states with respect to the facial expressions in two steps: first, a symbolic description is associated to each distance; secondly, each facial expression is characterized by a combination of the set of obtained characteristic distance states according to the rules displayed in Figure 10 (Hammal et al., 2007).

Figure 7. Segmentation results under three facial expressions (Hammal et al., 2006a)

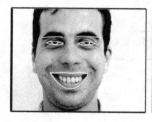 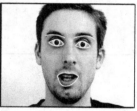 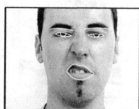

Figure 8. (Top left) facial features segmentation, (top right and bottom) characteristic distances description, (Hammal et al., 2007)

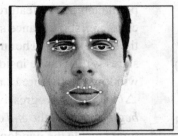 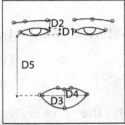

D1 Eye opening, distance between :
the center of the iris and upper eyelids
or upper and lower eyelids

D2 Distance between the interior corner of
the eye and the interior corner of the eyebrow

D3 Mouth opening width, distance between left
and right mouth corners

D4 Mouth opening height, distance between upper
and lower lips

D5 Distance between a corner of the mouth and the
corresponding external eye corner

Classification by the Transferable Belief Model

The Transferable Belief Model (TBM) is a model of representation of partial knowledge (Smets, 1998). It can deal with imprecise and uncertain information, and provides a number of tools for the combination of this information

Figure 9. Time course of the characteristic distance D2 and its corresponding state values for Surprise expression for 9 subjects from the Hammal_Caplier database (Hammal et al., 2007)

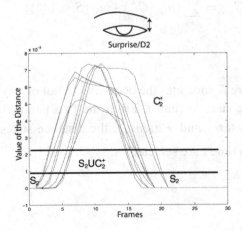

(Smets, 2000). It comprises the definition of the frame of discernment $\Omega=\{H_1,...,H_N\}$ of N exclusive and exhaustive hypotheses characterizing some situations. In the current application the hypotheses relate to the six basic facial expressions as well as Neutral characterized by a specific combination of characteristic distance states (Figure 10). Using the TBM requires then the definition of the Basic Belief Assignment (BBA)

Figure 10. Table of D_i states corresponding to each expression

		D_1	D_2	D_3	D_4	D_5
	Happiness	C_1^-	...	C_3^+	C_4^+	C_5^-
	Surprise	C_1^+	C_2^+	C_3^-	C_4^+	C_5^+
	Disgust	C_1^-	C_2^-	$S_3 \cup C_3^+$	C_4^+	S_5
	Anger	C_1^-	C_2^-	S_3	$S_4 \cup C_4^-$	S_5
	Sadness	C_1^-	C_2^+	S_3	C_4^+	S_5
	Fear	C_1^+	$S_2 \cup C_2^+$	$S_3 \cup C_3^-$	$S_4 \cup C_4^-$	$S_5 \cup C_5^-$
	Neutral	S_1	S_2	S_3	S_4	S_5

$m_{Di}^{\Omega_{Di}}$ (the belief) of each characteristic distance state $\boldsymbol{D}_i$ as:

$$m_{Di}^{\Omega_{Di}} : 2^{\Omega_{Di}} \rightarrow \begin{bmatrix} 0, & 1 \end{bmatrix} A^{\Omega_{Di}} \rightarrow m_{Di}^{\Omega_{Di}}(A),$$

$$\sum_{A \in 2^{\Omega_{Di}}} m_{Di}^{\Omega_{Di}} = 1 \qquad (1)$$

where $\boldsymbol{\Omega}_{Di} = \{\boldsymbol{C}_i^+, \boldsymbol{C}_i^-, \boldsymbol{S}_i\}$, the power set $2^{\Omega_{Di}} = \{\{C_i^+\}, \{C_i^-\}, \{S_i\}, \{S_i, C_i^+\}, \{S_i, C_i^-\}, \{S_i, C_i^+, C_i^-\}\}$ is the set of possible focal elements. $\{\boldsymbol{S}_i, \boldsymbol{C}_i^+\}$ (vs. $\{\boldsymbol{S}_i, \boldsymbol{C}_i^-\}$) corresponds to the doubt state between $\boldsymbol{C}_i^+$ (vs. $\boldsymbol{C}_i^-$) and $\boldsymbol{S}_i$. The subset corresponds to a logical proposition (for instance $\boldsymbol{C}_i^+$ is true). In the following, the notation $\{\boldsymbol{C}_i^+\}$ will be simplified to $\boldsymbol{C}_i^+$ and $\{\boldsymbol{S}_i, \boldsymbol{C}_i^+\}$ to $\boldsymbol{S}_i \cup \boldsymbol{C}_i^+$ (i.e. $\boldsymbol{S}_i$ or $\boldsymbol{C}_i^+$).

The piece of evidence (the belief) $m_{Di}^{\Omega_{Di}}$ associated with each symbolic state given that the value of the characteristic distance $\boldsymbol{D}_i$ is obtained by the function depicted in Figure 11.

Temporal Information Modeling

The dynamic and asynchronous behavior of the facial features is introduced by combining at each time t their previous deformations from the *beginning* until the *end* of the sequence to take a decision. The *beginning* of the expression corresponds to the first frame where at least one of the permanent facial features (i.e. the corresponding char-

Figure 11. Model of Basic Belief Assignment based on characteristic distance D_i. The threshold values $\{a_i, b_i, c_i, d_i, e_i, f_i, g_i, h_i\}$ have been derived by statistical analysis on the Hammal-Caplier database (Hammal et al., 2007).

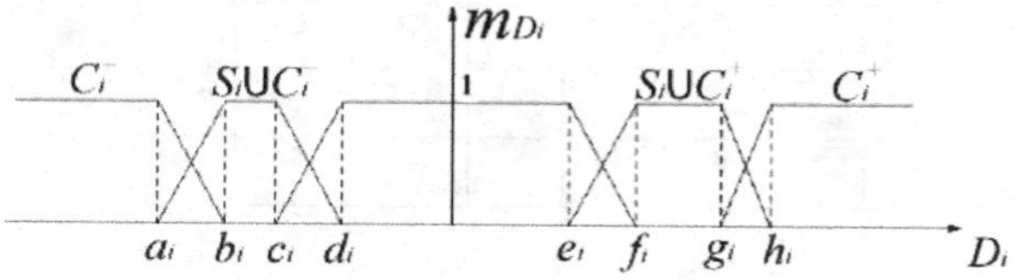

acteristic distances) is no more in the stable state $\boldsymbol{S}_i$; and the *end* to the first frame where all the permanent facial features (i.e. the corresponding characteristic distance states) have come back to the stable state $\boldsymbol{S}_i$. The analysis of the facial feature states is then made inside an increasing temporal window Δt (Figure 12.a). The size of the window Δt increases progressively at each time from the *beginning* until the *end* of the expression. At each time t inside the window Δt, the current state of each facial feature is selected by the combination of their current state at time t (i.e. current BBAs) and of the whole set of their past states since the beginning taking into account asynchronous facial feature deformations (Figure 12.b). The dynamic fusion of the BBAs is made according to the number of appearance of each symbolic states noted $\underset{\Delta t}{Nb}(state)$ and their integral (sum) of plausibility noted $\underset{\Delta t}{Pl}(state)$ (Smets, 2000) computed inside the temporal window Δt. For instance, for a characteristic distance D_i and for the $state = C_i^+$:

$$K_t(C_i^+) = \begin{cases} 1 & if \quad m_{D_i}(C_i^+) \neq 0 \\ 0 & otherwise \end{cases} \quad 1 \leq t \leq \Delta t$$

$$(2)$$

$$\underset{\Delta t}{Nb}(C_i^+) = \sum_{t=1}^{\Delta t} K_t(C_i^+) \qquad (3)$$

$$\underset{\Delta t}{Pl}(C_i^+) = \sum_{t=1}^{\Delta t} (m_{D_i}(C_i^+) + m_{D_i}(S_i \cup C_i^+)) \qquad (4)$$

where $\boldsymbol{K}_t$ indicates the occurring or not of a symbolic state at time t. From the two parameters $\underset{\Delta t}{Nb}(state)$ and $\underset{\Delta t}{Pl}(state)$, the distance states at each time t are selected as:

Figure 12. (a) example of the increasing temporal window during a sequence of Disgust expression; (b) BBAs selection process at time k based on the current BBAs and the whole set of the past BBAs; (c) example of the temporal selection of the characteristic distance states inside the increasing temporal window (C⁻ is chosen)

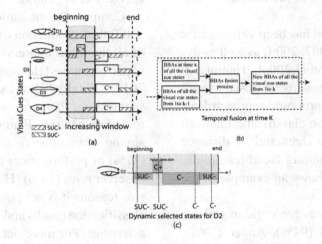

$$State(D_i) = \max_{\Delta t}(Pl(state) / Nb(state))$$
$$\quad \Delta t \quad \Delta t \qquad (5)$$

The piece of evidence associated to each chosen state for each characteristic distance corresponds to its maximum piece of evidence inside the current temporal increasing window as:

$$m_{State(D_i)_{\Delta t}} = \max(m_{D_{i,1...\Delta t}}) \qquad (6)$$

Then at time t between the *beginning* and the *end* of the expression sequence, once the BBAs of all the characteristic distances are defined, the corresponding expression or the subset of possible expressions is selected according to the rules Figure 10.

Fusion Process

The main feature of the TBM is the powerful combination operator (Smets, 2000) that integrates information from different sensors (the characteristic distance states). From the rules table and the BBAs of the states of the characteristic dis-

tances $m_{D_i}^{\Omega_{D_i}}$, a set of BBAs on facial expressions $m_{D_i}^{\Omega}$ is derived for each characteristic distance D_i. In order to combine all this information, a fusion process of the BBAs $m_{D_i}^{\Omega}$ of all the states of the characteristic distances is performed using the conjunctive combination rule (Smets, 2000) and results in m_D^{Ω} the BBA of the corresponding expressions as:

$$m_D^{\Omega} = \oplus m_{D_i}^{\Omega} \qquad (7)$$

At the end, one or more than one expression or subset of expressions with a piece of evidence different from zeros is obtained. The decision consists, then, in making a choice between various hypotheses E_e and their possible combinations. It is made using the maximum of Pignistic probability BetP (Smith, 2005) as:

$$BetP : \Omega \to [0, 1]$$
$$I \to BetP(I) =$$
$$\sum_{H \subseteq \Omega, I \in H} \frac{m^{\Omega}(H)}{(1 - m^{\Omega}(\phi)) * Card(H)}, \forall \ I \in \Omega$$
$$\qquad (8)$$

where ***BetP(I)*** corresponds to the Pignistic probability of each one of the hypothesis I of H, ɸ corresponds to the conflict between the sensors and *Card(H)* corresponds to the number of elements (hypothesis) of H.

The described method has been validated for static (Hammal et al., 2007, 2009) as well as dynamic recognition (Hammal 2006b, Hammal et al., 2008) of facial expressions for posed as well as spontaneous data. The proposed approach deals with the facial expression classification as well as the description of the characteristic distance states and their corresponding facial feature deformations (Figure 13 shows an example of the obtained results).

The performances rates for static model are obtained for Happiness (94%), Anger (79%), Surprise (94%), Disgust (76%), Fear (71%) and Neutral (96%). As found in other studies (Yacoob & Davis, 1996; Rosenblum et al., 1997) poor performance is obtained for Sadness expression (49%) (see Hammal et al., (2007, 2009) for more details). In the present case, this may reflect the fact that the classification rule used for Sadness lacks important pieces of information. Moreover, the obtained performances compare favorably to those of human observers (Hammal et al., 2009) leading to the same doubt states between confused expressions. Figure 14 shows an example for which the system remains in doubt rather than

taking the risk of making a wrong decision. Interestingly, these expressions are also notoriously difficult to discriminate for human observers (Roy et al., 2008).

Compared to the static model (Hammal et al., 2007) the introduction of the temporal modeling of all the facial expressions leads to an increase of performances (Hammal, 2006b, Hammal et al., 2010). Finally, new experimental results for spontaneous Pain sequences for an 8-alternative forced choice (i.e. Pain expression is classified among seven other facial expressions) achieved (77%) of performances compared to the human observer rates (76%) (Hammal et al., 2008). For size reasons it is not possible to describe all the classification results and the corresponding characteristics. For more details the reader can refer to the corresponding publication for static classification (Hammal et al., 2007), for dynamic classification (Hammal, 2006b, Hammal et al., 2008, Hammal et al., 2010) and for partially occluded facial parts (Hammal et al., 2009).

CONCLUSION

In the current chapter we have described the recent advance in computer vision for facial expression analysis and classification. We have described the most common and useful facial

Figure 13. User interface displaying: current frame; the BBAs of the expressions (Disgust with a piece of evidence equal to 1); the decision classification (maximum pignistic probability: MaxPigni) in this case Disgust expression; distance states estimation and the corresponding facial feature deformations with their corresponding pieces of evidence (Hammal et al., 2007)

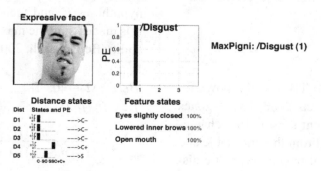

Figure 14. Example of Surprise classification. The system doubt between Surprise and Fear; based on the pignistic probability decision, the doubt yields the same probability for the two expressions (Hammal et al., 2007).

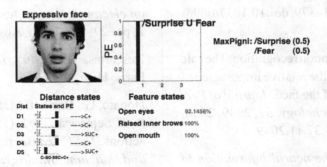

features segmentation and modeling for facial expression classification. The state of the art in facial expression classification shows that several studies have been done but still some challenges should be achieved to obtain a strong and every-day life facial expression recognition system. We have highlighted, as well, that the most important thing is to take advantage of the human skills for the recognition of facial expression in real life environment. Lastly, we have described an example of the most recent work pioneering on the future challenges that should be achieved for facial expression classification.

REFERENCES

Abboud, B., Davoine, F., & Dang, M. (2004, September). Facial expression recognition and synthesis based on appearance model. *Signal Processing Image Communication*, *19*(8), 723–740. doi:10.1016/j.image.2004.05.009

Adolphs, R. (2002). Recognizing emotion from facial expressions: psychological and neurological mechanisms. *Behavioral and Cognitive Neuroscience Reviews*, *1*, 21–61. doi:10.1177/1534582302001001003

Ambadar, Z., Schooler, W. S., & Cohn, J. (2005). The importance of facial dynamics in interpreting subtle facial expressions. *Psychological Science*, *16*(5), 403–410. doi:10.1111/j.0956-7976.2005.01548.x

Amin, M. A., Afzulpurkar, N. V., Dailey, M. N., Esichaikul, V. E., & Batanov, D. N. (2005). Fuzzy-C-Mean determines the principle component pairs to estimate the degree of emotion from facial expressions. In *Fuzzy Systems and Knowledge Discovery* (LNCS 3613, pp. 484-493).

Ashraf, A. B., Lucey, S., Chen, T., Prkachin, K., Solomon, P., Ambadar, Z., & Cohn, J. (2007). The painful face: Pain expression recognition using active appearance models. In *Proc. of the ACM International Conference on Multimodal Interfaces* (pp. 9–14).

Barlettt, M. S., Littlewort, G., Frank, M. G., Lainscsek, C., Fasel, I., & Movellan, J. (2005). Recognizing facial expression: machine learning and application to spontaneous behavior. In *Proc. IEEE Computer Vision and Pattern Recognition* (pp. 568–573).

Barlettt, M. S., Littlewort, G., Frank, M. G., Lainscsek, C., Fasel, I., & Movellan, J. (2006). Fully automatic facial action recognition in spontaneous behavior. In *Proc. IEEE Automatic Face and Gesture Recognition* (pp. 223–230).

Bassili, J. N. (1978). Facial motion in the perception of faces and of emotional expression. *Journal of Experimental Psychology. Human Perception and Performance*, *4*, 373–379. doi:10.1037/0096-1523.4.3.373

Bassili, J. N. (1979). Emotion recognition: The role of facial movement and the relative importance of upper and lower areas of the face. *Journal of Personality and Social Psychology*, *37*, 2049–2058. doi:10.1037/0022-3514.37.11.2049

Beaudot, W. (1994). *The neural information in the vertebra retina: a melting pot of ideas for artificial vision*. PhD thesis, TIRF laboratory, Grenoble, France.

Boucher, J. D., & Ekman, P. (1975). Facial areas and emotional information. *The Journal of Communication*, *25*, 21–29. doi:10.1111/j.1460-2466.1975.tb00577.x

Cohn, J. F. (2006). Foundations of Human Computing: Facial Expression and Emotion. In *Proc. Int. Conf. on Multimodal Interfaces* (pp. 233-238).

Cohn, J. F., & Schmidt, K. L. (2004). The timing of facial motion in posed and spontaneous smiles. *Journal Wavelets . Multiresolution & Information Processing*, *2*(2), 121–132. doi:10.1142/S021969130400041X

Cootes, T. F., Edwards, G. J., & Taylor, C. J. (1998). Active appearance models. *Lecture Notes in Computer Science*, 484–491. doi:10.1007/BFb0054760

Dailey, M. N., Cottrell, G. W., Padgett, C., & Adolphs, R. (2002). EMPATH: A neural network that categorizes facial expressions. *Journal of Cognitive Neuroscience*, *14*(8), 1158–1173. doi:10.1162/089892902760807177

Darwin, C. (1872). *The expression of the emotions in man and animals*. London: Murray. doi:10.1037/10001-000

Deng, X., Chang, C. H., & Brandle, E. (2004). *A new method for eye extraction from facial image. Proc. In 2nd IEEE international workshop on electronic design, test and applications* (*Vol. 2*, pp. 29–34). Perth, Australia: DELTA.

Descartes, H. (1649). *Les Passions de l'âme*. Paris: Henry Le Gras.

Donato, G., Bartlett, M. S., Hager, J. C., Ekman, P., & Sejnowski, T. J. (1999). Classifying facial actions. *IEEE Transactions on Pattern Analysis and Machine Intelligence*, *21*(10), 974–989. doi:10.1109/34.799905

Dornaika, F., & Davoine, F. (2004). Head and facial animation tracking using appearance adaptive models and particle filters . In *Workshop Real-Time Vision for Human-Computer Interaction RTV4HCI in conjunction with CVPR, 2*. DC, USA: July Washington.

Ekman, P., & Friesen, W. V. (1978). *The facial action coding system (facs), A technique for the measurement of facial action*. Palo Alto, CA: Consulting Psychologists Press.

Ekman, P., Friesen, W. V., & Ellsworth, P. (1972). *Emotion in the human face*. New York: Pergamon Press.

Ekman, P., Matsumoto, D., & Friesen, W. V. (2005). Facial Expression in Affective Disorders . In Ekman, P., & Rosenberg, E. L. (Eds.), *What the Face Reveals* (pp. 429–439).

El Kaliouby, R., & Robinson, P. (2004). Mind reading machines: automated inference of cognitive mental states from video. *SMC*, *1*, 682–688.

Fasel, I., Fortenberry, B., & Movellan, J. (2005). A generative framework for real time object detection and classification. *Computer Vision and Image Understanding*, *98*, 182–210. doi:10.1016/j.cviu.2004.07.014

Gao, Y., Leung, M. K. H, Hui, S. C., & Tananda, M. W. (2003 May). Facial expression recognition from line-based caricatures. *IEEE Transaction on System, Man and Cybernetics - PART A: System and Humans, 33*(3).

Gouta, K., & Miyamoto, M. (2000). Facial areas and emotional information. *Japanese Journal of Phycology, 71*, 211–218.

Gunes, H., Piccardi, M., & Pantic, M. (2008). From the Lab to the Real World: Affect Recognition using Multiple Cues and Modalities . In Or, J. (Ed.), *Affective Computing: Focus on Emotion Expression, Synthesis, and Recognition* (pp. 185–218). Vienna, Austria: I-Tech Education and Publishing.

Hammal, Z. (2006 February). Dynamic facial expression understanding based on temporal modeling of transferable belief model. In *Proceedings of the International Conference on Computer Vision Theory and Application*, Setubal, Portugal.

Hammal, Z., Arguin, M., & Gosselin, F. (2009). Comparing a Novel Model Based on the Transferable Belief Model with Humans During the Recognition of Partially Occluded Facial Expressions. *Journal of Vision (Charlottesville, Va.), 9*(2), 1–19. Retrieved from http://journalofvision.org/9/2/22/, doi:10.1167/9.2.22. doi:10.1167/9.2.22

Hammal, Z., Caplier, A., & Rombaut, M. (2005). A fusion process based on belief theory for classification of facial basic emotions. In *Proceedings of the 8th International Conference on Information Fusion*, Philadelphia, PA, USA.

Hammal, Z., Couvreur, L., Caplier, A., & Rombaut, M. (2007). Facial expressions classification: A new approach based on Transferable Belief Model. *International Journal of Approximate Reasoning, 46*, 542–567. doi:10.1016/j.ijar.2007.02.003

Hammal, Z., Eveno, N., Caplier, A., & Coulon, P. Y. (2006a). Parametric models for facial features segmentation. *Signal Processing, 86*, 399–413. doi:10.1016/j.sigpro.2005.06.006

Hammal, Z., Kunz, M., Arguin, M., & Gosselin, F. (2008). Spontaneous pain expression recognition in video sequences. In *BCS International Academic Conference 2008 – Visions of Computer Science* (pp. 191-210).

Hammal, Z., & Massot, C. (2010). Holistic and Feature-Based Information Towards Dynamic Multi-Expressions Recognition. In *International Conference on Computer Vision Theory and Application*, 17-21 May, Angers, France.

Harwood, N. K., Hall, L. J., & Shinkfield, A. J. (1999). Recognition of facial emotional expressions from moving and static displays by individuals with mental retardation. *American Journal of Mental Retardation, 104*(3), 270–278. doi:10.1352/0895-8017(1999)104<0270:ROFEEF>2.0.CO;2

Haxby, J., Hoffman, E., & Gobbini, M. (2000). The distributed human neural system for face perception. *Trends in Cognitive Sciences, 4*(6), 223–233. doi:10.1016/S1364-6613(00)01482-0

Haxby, J. V., Hoffman, E. A., & Gobbini, M. I. (2002). Human neural systems for face recognition and social communication. *Biological Psychiatry, 51*(1), 59–67. doi:10.1016/S0006-3223(01)01330-0

Izard, C. E., Dougherty, L. M., & Hembree, E. A. (1983). *A system for identifying affect expressions by holistic judgments*. Newark, Delaware: Instructional Resources Center, University of Delaware.

Ji, Q., Lan, P., & Looney, C. (2006). A probabilistic framework for modeling and real-time monitoring human fatigue. *IEEE System Man Cybernetic-Part A, 36*(5), 862–875. doi:10.1109/TSMCA.2005.855922

Kapoor, A., Burleson, W., & Picard, R. W. (2007). Automatic Prediction of Frustration. *International Journal of Human-Computer Studies*, *65*(8), 724–736. doi:10.1016/j.ijhcs.2007.02.003

Kashima, H., Hongo, H., Kato, K., & Yamamoto, K. (2001 June). A robust iris detection method of facial and eye movement. In *Proc. Vision Interface Annual Conference*, Ottawa, Canada.

Kimura, S., & Yachida, M. (1997). *Facial Expression Recognition and Its Degree Estimation* (pp. 295–300). Proc. Computer Vision and Pattern Recognition.

Lien, J. J., Kanade, T., Cohn, J. F., & Li, C. (1998). Subtly different facial expression recognition and expression intensity estimation. In *Proceedings of IEEE Computer Vision and Pattern Recognition*, Santa Barbara, CA (pp. 853–859).

Littlewort, G. C., Bartlett, M. S., & Kang, L. (2007 November). Faces of Pain: Automated Measurement of Spontaneous Facial Expressions of Genuine and Posed Pain. In *Proc. ICMI*, Nagoya, Aichi, Japan

Lucas, B. D., & Kanade, T. (1981). An iterative image registration technique with an application to stereo vision . In *Image Understanding Workshop* (pp. 121–130). US Defense Advanced Research Projects Agency.

Lyons, M. J., & Akamatsu, S. (1998, 14-16 Apr 1998). Coding facial expressions with gabor wavelets. In *Proc. Third IEEE International Conference on Automatic Face and Gesture Recognition*, Nara, Japan (pp. 200–205).

Malciu, M., & Preteux, F. (2001 May). Mpeg-4 compliant tracking of facial features in video sequences. In *Proc. of International Conference on Augmented, Virtual Environments and 3D Imaging*, Mykonos, Greece (pp. 108–111).

Mehrabian, A. (1968). Communication without words. *Psychology Today*, *2*(4), 53–56.

Nusseck, M., Cunningham, D. W., Wallraven, C., & Bülthoff, H. (2008). The contribution of different facial regions to the recognition of conversational expressions. *Journal of Vision (Charlottesville, Va.)*, *8*(8). doi:10.1167/8.8.1

Oliver, N., Pentland, A., & Bérard, F. (2000). Lafter: a real-time face and tracker with facial expression recognition. *Pattern Recognition*, *33*, 1369–1382. doi:10.1016/S0031-3203(99)00113-2

Pantic, M., & Bartlett, M. S. (2007). Machine analysis of facial expressions . In Delac, K., & Grgic, M. (Eds.), *Face recognition* (pp. 377–416). Vienna, Austria: I-Tech Education and Publishing.

Pantic, M., & Patras, I. (2006). Dynamics of facial expression: Recognition of facial actions and their temporal segments from face profile image sequences. *IEEE Transactions on System Systems, Man, and Cybernetics . Part B: Cybernetics*, *36*, 433–449. doi:10.1109/TSMCB.2005.859075

Pardas, M. (2000, Jun 2000). Extraction and tracking of the eyelids. In *Proc. International Conference on Acoustics, Speech and Signal Processing*, Istanbul, Turkey (Vol. 4, pp. 2357–2360).

Pardas, M., & Bonafonte, A. (2002). Facial animation parameters extraction and expression detection using hmm. *Signal Processing Image Communication*, *17*, 675–688. doi:10.1016/S0923-5965(02)00078-4

Pardas, M., & Sayrol, E. (2001, November). Motion estimation based tracking of active contours. *Pattern Recognition Letters*, *22*(13), 1447–1456. doi:10.1016/S0167-8655(01)00084-8

Rosenblum, M., Yacoob, Y., & Davis, L. S. (1996). Human expression recognition from motion using a radial basis function network architecture. *IEEE Transactions on Neural Networks*, *7*, 1121–1137. doi:10.1109/72.536309

Roy, S., Roy, C., Hammal, Z., Fiset, D., Blais, C., Jemel, B., & Gosselin, F. (2008 May). The use of Spatio-temporal Information in decoding facial expression of emotions. In *Proc. Vision Science Society*, Naples Grand Hotel, Floride.

Smets, P. (1998). The transferable belief model for quantified belief representation. In *Handbook of defeasible reasoning and uncertainty management system* (*Vol. 1*, pp. 267–301). Dordrecht: Kluwer Academic.

Smets, P. (2000 July). Data fusion in the transferable belief model. In *Proc. of International Conference on Information Fusion*, Paris, France (pp. 21–33).

Smets, P. (2005). Decision making in the TBM: the necessity of the pignistic transformation. *International Journal of Approximate Reasoning, 38*, 133–147. doi:10.1016/j.ijar.2004.05.003

Smith, M., Cottrell, G., Gosselin, F., & Schyns, P. G. (2005). Transmitting and decoding facial expressions of emotions. *Psychological Science, 16*, 184–189. doi:10.1111/j.0956-7976.2005.00801.x

Tekalp, M. (1999). *Face and 2d mesh animation in mpeg-4. Tutorial Issue on the MPEG-4 Standard*. Image Communication Journal.

Tian, Y., Kanade, T., & Cohn, J. (2000 March). Dual state parametric eye tracking. In *Proc. 4th IEEE International Conference on Automatic Face and Gesture Recognition*, Grenoble (pp. 110–115).

Tian, Y., Kanade, T., & Cohn, J. F. (2001). Recognizing action units for facial expression analysis. *IEEE Transactions on Pattern Analysis and Machine Intelligence, 23*, 97–115. doi:10.1109/34.908962

Tian, Y. L., Kanade, T., & Cohn, J. F. (2005). Facial expression analysis. In Li, S. Z., & Jain, A. K. (Eds.), *Handbook of face recognition* (pp. 247–276). New York: Springer. doi:10.1007/0-387-27257-7_12

Tong, Y., Liao, W., & Ji, Q. (2006). Inferring facial action units with causal relations. In *Proc. IEEE Computer Vision and Pattern Recognition* (pp. 1623–1630).

Tsapatsoulis, N., Karpouzis, K., Stamou, G., Piat, F., & Kollias, S. (2000 September). A fuzzy system for emotion classification based on the mpeg-4 facial definition parameter set. In *Proceedings of the 10th European Signal Processing Conference*, Tampere, Finland.

Tsekeridou, S., & Pitas, I. (1998 September). Facial feature extraction in frontal views using biometric analogies. In *Proc. 9th European Signal Processing Conference*, Island of Rhodes, Greece (Vol. 1, pp. 315–318).

Valstar, M. F., Gunes, H., & Pantic, M. (2007 November). How to Distinguish Posed from Spontaneous Smiles using Geometric Features. In *Proc. ACM Int'l Conf on Multimodal Interfaces*, Nagoya, Japan (pp. 38–45).

Valstar, M. F., Pantic, M., Ambadar, Z., & Cohn, J. F. (2006). Spontaneous vs. posed facial behavior: automatic analysis of brow actions. In *Proc. ACM Intl. Conference on Multimodal Interfaces* (pp. 162–170).

Wallraven, C., Breidt, M., Cunningham, D. W., & Bülthoff, H. (2008). Evaluating the perceptual realism of animated facial expressions. *TAP, 4*(4).

Wang, J. G., Sung, E., & Venkateswarlu, R. (2005). Estimating the eye gaze from one eye. *Computer Vision and Image Understanding, 98*, 83–103. doi:10.1016/j.cviu.2004.07.008

Wehrle, T., Kaiser, S., Schmidt, S., & Scherer, K. R. (2000). Studying the dynamics of emotional expression using synthesized facial muscle movements. *Journal of Personality and Social Psychology, 78*(1), 105–119. doi:10.1037/0022-3514.78.1.105

Weyers, P., Mühlberger, A., Hefele, C., & Pauli, P. (2006). Electromyografic responses to static and dynamic avatar emotional facial expressions. *Psychophysiology*, *43*, 450–453. doi:10.1111/j.1469-8986.2006.00451.x

Yacoob, Y., & Davis, L. S. (1996). Recognizing human facial expressions from long image sequences using optical flow. *IEEE Transactions on Pattern Analysis and Machine Intelligence*, *18*, 636–642. doi:10.1109/34.506414

Young, A. W., Rowland, D., Calder, A. J., Etcoff, N. L., Seth, A., & Perrett, D. I. (1997). Facial expression megamix: Tests of dimensional and category accounts of emotion recognition. *Cognition*, *63*, 271–313. doi:10.1016/S0010-0277(97)00003-6

Yuille, A., Hallinan, P., & Cohen, D. (1992, August). Feature extraction from faces using deformable templates. *International Journal of Computer Vision*, *8*(2), 99–111. doi:10.1007/BF00127169

Zeng, Z., Pantic, M., Roisman, G. I., & Huang, T. S. (2009, January). A Survey of Affect Recognition Methods: Audio, Visual, and Spontaneous Expressions. *IEEE Transactions on Pattern Analysis and Machine Intelligence*, *31*(1), 39–58. doi:10.1109/TPAMI.2008.52

Zhang, Y., & Qiang, J. (2005). Active and dynamic information fusion for facial expression understanding from image sequences. *IEEE Transactions on Pattern Analysis and Machine Intelligence*, *27*, 699–714. doi:10.1109/TPAMI.2005.93

KEY TERMS AND DEFINITIONS

Facial Expressions: the contraction of facial muscles, which result in temporally deformed facial features such eyes, eyebrows, lips and skin texture, often revealed by wrinkles.

Transferable Belief Model (TBM): The TBM can be seen as a generalization of the theory of probabilities. The TBM is a model of representation of partial knowledge and allows to explicitly model the doubt between several hypotheses. It can deal with imprecise and uncertain information, and provides a number of tools for the combination of this information.

Basic Belief Assignment (BBA): The (BBA) assigns an elementary piece of evidence to each proposition of the considered problem in exactly the same manner as a probability function defined on.

Piece of Evidence (PE): the piece of evidence of each proposition corresponds to the belief in the proposition.

Uncertainty and Imprecision: Uncertain data (i.e. partial information) and imprecise data (i.e. noisy information).

Facial Action Coding System (FACS): manual labeling method of facial deformations corresponding to the facial muscles motion. The FACS defines the specific changes that occur with muscular contractions and how best to differentiate one from another.

Action Units (AUs): represent a contraction or relaxation of one or more muscles.

MPEG-4 Coding Model: object based multimedia compression standard. The MPEG-4 measurement units are the Facial Definition Parameters (FDP), a set of tokens that describe minimal perceptible actions in the facial area.

Chapter 13
Facial Expression Analysis by Machine Learning

Siu-Yeung Cho
Nanyang Technological University, Singapore

Teik-Toe Teoh
Nanyang Technological University, Singapore

Yok-Yen Nguwi
Nanyang Technological University, Singapore

ABSTRACT

Facial expression recognition is a challenging task. A facial expression is formed by contracting or relaxing different facial muscles on human face that results in temporally deformed facial features like wide-open mouth, raising eyebrows or etc. The challenges of such system have to address with some issues. For instances, lighting condition is a very difficult problem to constraint and regulate. On the other hand, real-time processing is also a challenging problem since there are so many facial features to be extracted and processed and sometimes, conventional classifiers are not even effective in handling those features and produce good classification performance. This chapter discusses the issues on how the advanced feature selection techniques together with good classifiers can play a vital important role of real-time facial expression recognition. Several feature selection methods and classifiers are discussed and their evaluations for real-time facial expression recognition are presented in this chapter. The content of this chapter is a way to open-up a discussion about building a real-time system to read and respond to the emotions of people from facial expressions.

DOI: 10.4018/978-1-61520-991-0.ch013

INTRODUCTION

Given the significant role of the face in our emotional and social lives, it is not surprising that the potential benefits from efforts to automate the analysis of facial signals, in particular rapid facial signals, are varied and numerous (Ekman et al., 1993), especially when it comes to computer science and technologies brought to bear on these issues (Pantic, 2006). As far as natural interfaces between humans and computers are concerned, facial expressions provide a way to communicate basic information about needs and demands to the machine. In fact, automatic analysis of facial signals seem to have a natural place in various vision sub-systems, including automated tools for tracking gaze and focus of attention, lip reading, bimodal speech processing, face/visual speech synthesis, and face-based command issuing.

Facial Expression Analysis is a challenging task. A facial expression is formed by contracting or relaxing different facial muscles on human face that results in temporally deformed facial features like wide-open mouth, raising eyebrows or etc. The challenges of such system have to address the following issues:

Lighting conditions is a very difficult problem to constraint and regulate. The strength of the light depends on the light source (see Figure 1).

The direction of the subjects face is not always ideal which may pose difficulties when the system is implemented live that captures moving subjects' facial expression (see Figure 2).

Another difficulty is the way image is acquired by the image acquisition system. The character-istics of the image acquisition system can affect the quality of the images or videos captured.

Occlusion of subject face may tumble the hit rate of many established approaches. The experiments being carried out by most researchers do not take occlusion into account (see Figure 3).

Because of the above challenges, this chapter is going to introduce the recent advances in feature selection and classification methodologies for facial expression analysis. It first describes the background of different techniques used for facial expression analysis. Then it introduces the ideas of an automatic facial expression recognition system proposed by the authors which includes feature extraction, feature selection and classification methods. Finally, some of the future trends in terms of scientific and engineering challenges are discussed and recommendations for achieving a better facial expression technology are outlined.

BACKGROUND

The first known facial expression analysis was presented by Darwin in 1872 (Darwin, 1872). He presented the universality of human face expressions and the continuity in man and animals. He pointed out that there are specific inborn emotions, which originated in serviceable associated habits. After about a century, Ekman and Friesen (1971) postulated six primary emotions that possess each a distinctive content together with a unique facial expression. These prototypic emotional displays are also referred to as basic emotions in many of the later literature. They seem to be universal across human cultures and are namely

Figure 1. Light variations problem: face images are taken from different illumination conditions (source: Yale Face Database B http://cvc.yale.edu/projects/yalefacesB/yalefacesB.html)

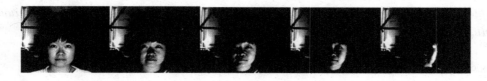

happiness, sadness, fear, disgust, surprise and anger. They developed the Facial Action Coding System (FACS) for describing facial expressions. It is appearance-based. FACS uses 44 action units (AUs) for the description of facial actions with regard to their location as well as their intensity. Individual expressions may be modeled by single action units or action unit combinations. FACS codes expression from static pictures.

In the nineties, more works emerge started from Cottrell et al. (1990) who described the use of a Multi-Layer Perceptron Neural Networks for processing face images. They presented a number of face images to the network and train it to perform various tasks such as coding, identification, gender recognition, and expression recognition. During this procedure, face images are projected onto a subspace in the hidden layers of the network; it is interesting to note that this subspace is very similar to the eigenfaces space. However, an important difference is that, in this case, the face subspace is defined according to the application for which the system is to be used. Correct identification rates of up to 97 percent were reported when the system was tested using a database of images from 11 individuals. Mase et al. (1991) then used dense optical flow to estimate the activity of 12 of the 44 facial muscles. The motion seen on the skin surface at each muscle location was compared

to a pre-determined axis of motion along which each muscle expands and contracts, allowing estimates as to the activity of each muscle to be made. Recognition rates of 86% were reported. Subsequently, Matsuno et al. (1994) presented a method of facial expressions recognition using two dimensional physical models named *Potential Net* without using feature extraction. *Potential Net* is a physical model that consists of nodes connected by springs in two dimensional grid configurations. Recognition is achieved by comparing nodal displacement vectors of a net deformed by an input image with facial expression vectors. It recognized four kinds of facial expressions, happiness, anger, surprise and sad and the hit rate is about 90%.

After that, Yacoob and Davis (1996) continues the research in optical flow computation to identify the direction of rigid and non-rigid motions that are caused by human facial expressions. The approach is based on qualitative tracking of principal regions of the face and flow computation at high intensity gradient points. Three stages of the approach are: locating and tracking prominent facial features, using optical flow at these features to construct a mid-level representation that describes spatio-temporal actions, and applying rules for classification of mid-level representation of actions into one of the six universal facial expressions. In the mean time, Rosenblum et al. (1996) proposed a

Figure 2. Pose variations problem: face images are taken from different postures of the object (source NTU Asian Emotion Database http://www3.ntu. edu.sg/SCE/labs/forse/Asian%20Emotion%20 Database.htm)

Figure 3. Occlusion problems: facial components are occluded by some artifact objects. (Source NTU Asian Emotion Database http://www3.ntu. edu.sg/SCE/labs/forse/Asian%20Emotion%20 Database.htm)

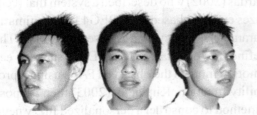

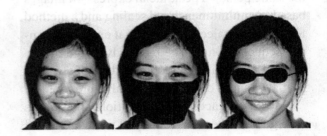

radial basis function network to learn the correlation of facial feature motion patterns and human expressions. The network was trained to recognize "smile" and "surprise" expressions. Success rate was about 83%~88%. The work explores the use of a connectionist learning architecture for identifying the motion patterns characteristic of facial expressions. Essa and Pentland (1997a) also described facial structure using optimal estimation optical flow method coupled with geometric, physical and motion-based dynamic models. It is an extension variance of FACS, called FACS+ that is a more accurate representation of human facial expressions. Another work by Lanitis's group (Lanitis, 1997) used an active shape model to locate facial features and then used shape and texture information at these locations to classify expressions, obtaining a recognition rate of 74% for expression of the basic emotions and also neutral expressions. In the following year, Otsuka and Ohya (1998) proposed a method for spotting segments displaying facial expression from image sequences. The motion of the face is modeled by HMM in such a way that each state corresponds to the conditions of facial muscles, e.g., relaxed, contracting, apex and relaxing. Off-line and on-line experiments were carried out. Off-line experiment obtains the optimum threshold values and to evaluate relation of recognition rate and frame rate. On-line experiments were used to evaluate recognition performance for sequences of multiple instances of facial expressions. Experiments showed that the segments for the six basic expressions can be spotted accurately near real time. In 1999, Chandrasiri et al. (1999) proposed a facial expression space that is made by the same person's peak facial expression images based on multidimensional scaling and a method for deriving trajectory of a facial expression image sequence on it. The main advantage of this method is that it focuses on both temporal and spatial changes of personal facial expression.

More variances of recognition approaches emerge after the year 2000, and some are tested with video sequences (Bourel, 2002; Pardas, 2002; Barlett et al, 2003). Shin et al. (2000) extract pleasure/displeasure and arousal dimension emotion features using hybrid approach. The hybrid approach used feature clustering and dynamic linking to extract sparse local features from edges on expression images. The expressions are happiness, surprise, sadness, disgust, fear, satisfaction, comfort, distress, tiredness and worry. They concluded that the arousal-sleep dimension may depend on the personal internal state more than pleasure-displeasure dimension, that is to say, the relative importance of dimension can have an effect on facial expression recognition on the two dimensional structure of emotion. Fasel and Lüttin (2000) described a system that adopts holistic approach that recognizes asymmetric FACS Action Unit activities and intensities without the use of markers. Facial expression extraction is achieved by difference images that are projected into a sub-space using either PCA or ICA, followed by nearest neighbor classification. Recognition rates are between 74~83%. Bourel (2002) investigated the representation of facial expression based on spatially-localized geometric facial model coupled to a state-based model of facial motion. The system consists of a feature point tracker, a geometric facial feature extractor, a state-based feature extractor, and a classifier. The feature extraction process uses 12 facial feature points. The spatio-temporal features are then created to form a geometric parameter. The state-based model then transforms the geometric parameter into 3 possible states: 'increase', 'stable', 'decrease'. The classifier makes use of k-nearest neighbor approach. Another work on video sequence recognition is by Pardas (2002) who described a system that recognizes emotion based on MPEG4 facial animation parameters. The system is based on HMM. They defined a four-state HMM. Each state of each emotion models the observed FAPs using a probability function. Kim et al. (2003) then proposed a method to construct a personalized fuzzy neural networks classifier based on histogram-based feature selection. Recognition rate is reported to be in the range of 91.6%~98.0%. The system proposed in (Bartlett et al., 2003) detects frontal faces in the video stream and classifies them in seven classes in real time: neutral, anger, disgust, fear, joy, sadness, and surprise. An expression recognizer receives image regions produced by a face detector and then a Gabor representation of the facial image region is formed to be later processed by a bank of SVMs classifiers.

Ji (2005) based on FACS and developed a system that adopted a dynamic and probabilistic framework based on combining Dynamic Bayesian Networks (DBM) with FACS for modeling the dynamic and stochastic behaviors of spontaneous facial expressions. The three major components of the system are facial motion measurement, facial expression representation and facial expression recognition. Wu et al. (2005) modeled uncertainty in facial expressions space for facial expression recognition using fuzzy integral. The fuzzy measure is constructed in each facial expression space. They adopted Active Appearance Models (AAM) to extract facial key points and classify based on shape feature vector. Fuzzy C-means (FCM) was used to build a set of classifiers. The recognition rates were found to be 83.2% and 91.6% on JAFFE and FGnet databases respectively. Yeasin et al. (2005) compared the performances of linear and non-linear data projection techniques in classifying six universal facial expressions. The three data projection techniques are Principal Component Analysis (PCA), Non-negative Matrix Factorization (NMF) and Local Linear Embedding (LLE). The system developed by (Anderson and McOwan, 2006) characterized monochrome frontal views of facial expression with the ability to operate in cluttered and dynamic scenes, recognizing six emotions universally associated with unique facial expressions, namely happiness, sadness, disgust, surprise, fear, and anger. Faces are located using a spatial ratio template tracker algorithm. Optical flow of face is subsequently determined using a real-time implementation of

gradient model. The expression recognition system then averages facial velocity information. The motion signatures produced are then classified using Support Vector Machines. The best recognition rate is 81.82%. Zeng et al. (2006) classified emotional and non emotional facial expressions occurred in a realistic human conversation setting-Adult Attachment Interview (AAI). The AAI is a semi-structured interview used to characterize individuals' current state of mind with respect to past parent-child experiences. Piecewise Bezier Volume Deformation (PBVD) was used to track face. They applied kernel whitening to map the data to a spherical symmetrical cluster. Then Support Vector Data Description (SVDD) was applied to directly fit a boundary with minimal volume around the target data. Experimental results suggested the system generalize better than using PCA and single Gaussian approaches. Xiang et al. (2007) utilized Fourier transform, fuzzy C means to generate a spatio-temporal model for each expression type. Unknown input expressions are matched to the models using Hausdorff distance to compute dissimilarity values for classification. The recognition rate was found to be 88.8% with expression sequences.

In general, a facial expression recognizer comprises of 3 stages, namely feature extraction, features selection, and classification. Feature extraction involves general manipulation of the image. The raw image is processed to provide a region of interest (human face without hairs and background) for the second stage to select meaningful features. Some noise reduction, clustering, labeling or cropping may be done in this stage. For some ready data that are taken off the shelf from online database, the first stage is unnecessary.

Features selection is an important module. Without good features, the effort made in the classification stage would be in vain. Fasel and Luettin (2003) provides a detailed survey on facial expression, they classified the feature extraction methods into several groups. Some of the methods were highlighted like Gabor wavelets, Active Appearance Model, Dense Flow Fields, Motion and Deformable Models, Principal Component Analysis, High Gradient Components etc. They group the facial features into 2 types: intransient facial features and transient facial features. Intransient features are like eyes, eyebrow and mouth that are always present in the face. Transient features include wrinkles and bulges.

Neural network may be a popular choice for classification. Most of them fall under supervised learning. The other classification methods underscored by Pantic and Rothkrantz (2000) are Expert System Rules, Discriminant functions by Cohn et al. (1998), Spatio-temporal motion energy templates by Essa and Pentland (1997b), Thresholded motion parameters by (Black & Yacoob, 1997), and Adaptive Facial Emotion Tree Structures by Wong and Cho (2006). In the past two decades, research has focused on how to make face recognition systems fully automated by tackling problems, such as, localization of a face in a given image or video clip and extraction of features such as eyes, mouth, etc. Meanwhile, significant advances have been made in the design of feature extractions and classifiers for successful face recognition. Both the appearance-based holistic approaches and feature-based methods have the strength and weaknesses. Compared to holistic approaches, feature-based methods are less sensitive to variations in illumination and viewpoint and to inaccuracy in face localization. Several survey papers offer more insights on facial expression systems that can be found in (Andrea et al., 2007; Kevin et al., 2006; Zhao et al., 2003; Fasel & Luettin, 2003; Lalonde & Li, 1995)

FACIAL EXPRESSION SYSTEMS

Most computer vision researchers think of motion when they consider the problem of facial expression recognition. An often cited study by Bassili (1978) showed that humans can recognize facial expressions above chance from motion, using point-light displays. In contrast to the Bassili's study in which humans were barely above chance using motion without texture, humans are nearly at ceiling for recognizing expressions from texture without motion (i.e. static photographs).

Appearance-based features include Gabor filters, integral image filters (also known as box-filters, and Haar-like filters), features based on edge-oriented histograms and those based on Active Appearance Models (Edwards et al., 1998). A common reservation about appearance-based features for expression recognition is that they are affected by lighting variation and individual difference. However, machine learning systems taking large sets of appearance-features as input, and trained on a large database of examples, are emerging as some of the most robust systems in computer vision. Machine learning combined with appearance-based features has been shown to be highly robust for tasks of face detection (Viola & Jones, 2004; Fasel et al., 2005), feature detection (Vukadionvic & Pantic, 2005; Fasel, 2006), and expression recognition (Littlewort et al., 2006). Such systems also do not suffer from issues of initialization and drift, which are major challenges for motion tracking.

Figure 4 shows an outline of the real-time expression recognition system developed by Bartlett and colleagues (Barlett et al., 2003; Littlewort et al., 2006). The system automatically detects frontal faces in the video stream and codes each frame with respect to 7 dimensions: neutral, anger, disgust, fear, joy, sadness, surprise. The system first performs automatic face and eye detection using the appearance-based method of Fasel et al. (2005). Faces are then aligned based on the automatically detected eye positions, and passed to a bank of appearance-based features. A feature selection stage extracts subsets of the features and passes them to an ensemble of classifiers that make a binary decision about each of the six basic emotions plus neutral. According to their results, they found that Gabor wavelets and ICA (Independent Component Analysis) gave better performance than PCA (Principal Component Analysis), LFA (Local Feature Analysis), Fisher's linear discriminants, and outperformed motion flow field templates. More recent comparisons included comparisons of Gabor filters, integral image filters, and edge-oriented histogram (e.g., Whitehill & Omlin, 2006), using SVMs and AdaBoost as the classifiers. They found an interaction between feature-type and classifier, where AdaBoost performs better with integral image filters, while SVMs perform better with Gabors. The difference may be attributable to the fact that the pool of integral image filters was much larger. AdaBoost performs feature selection and does well with redundancy; whereas SVMs were calculated on the full set of filters and do not do well with redundancy.

In this chapter, we will present our recent works in recognizing facial expressions. Our work attempts to use a boosting Naïve Bayes Classifier (NBC) to classify facial expressions. Both theoretical and practical studies have often been carried out to understand the predictive properties on this boosting NBC method. The Bayesian classifier is the most popular classifier among the probabilistic classifiers used in the machine learning community. Furthermore, Naive Bayesian classifier is perhaps one of the simplest yet surprisingly powerful techniques to construct predictive models from labeled training sets when comparing to other supervised machine learning methods. NBC can also provide a valuable insight to the training data by exposing the relations between attribute values and classes besides good predictive accuracy. The resulting of NBC are often robust to a degree where they match or even outperform other more complex machine learning methods despite NBC's assumption of conditional independence of attributes given in the class. The study of probabilistic classification is the study of approximating a joint distribution with a product distribution. Probabilistic classifiers operate on data sets where each example x consists of feature values $\langle a_1, a_2, ..., a_i \rangle$ and the target function y can take on any value from a pre-defined finite set $V = (v_1, v_2, ... v_j)$ Bayesian rule is used to estimate the conditional probability of a class label y, and then assumptions are made on the model, to decompose this probability into a product of conditional probabilities. The formula used by the simple Bayesian classifier is: $P(a_i|v_j)$ and $P(v_j)$ which can be calculated based on their frequency in the training data, under the assumption that features values are conditionally independent given the target value. On the other hand, one can model the component marginal distributions in a wide variety of ways for numerical features. The zero counts are another problem with this formula. Zero counts are obtained when a given class and feature value never occur together in the training set, and is problematic because the resulting zero probabilities will wipe

Figure 4. Outline of the real-time expression recognition system of Littlewort et al. (2006)

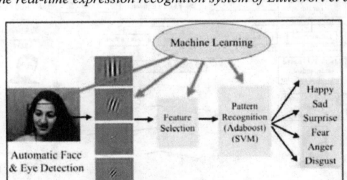

out the information in all the other probabilities when they are multiplied. Incorporating a small sample correction into all probabilities is one of the solutions to this problem. Its probability is set to 1/N, where N is the number of examples in the training set if a feature value does not occur given some class,. The assumption of independence is clearly usually wrong. However, a large scale comparison of simple Bayesian classifier with state-of-the-art algorithms for decision tree induction and instance-based learning on standard benchmark datasets found that simple Bayesian classifier sometimes is superior to each of the other learning schemes even on datasets with substantial feature dependencies. An explanation on why simple Bayesian method remains competitive, even though it provides very poor estimates of the true underlying probabilities. NBC algorithm always had the best accuracy per needed training time and it predicts the class feature in a very short time.

In this section, we outline the structure of our developed facial expression recognizer. The proposed model is going to recognize four types of facial expression, namely, neutral, joy, sad and surprise. A probabilistic based approach using the Naïve Bayesian Boost is adopted to recognize these four types of facial expressions. Figure 5 demonstrates the block diagram of the entire system.

The system is composed of three major blocks, i.e., the feature locator, the feature extractor, and the classifier. The feature locator finds crucial fiducial points for subsequent feature extraction processing. We adopted Gabor features and Gini extractions that will be discussed in the following sub-sections. Finally, the meaningful features are classified into the corresponding class.

FEATURE EXTRACTION

The first step in the system is face detection, i.e., identification of all regions in the scene that contain a human face. The problem of finding faces should be solved regardless of clutter, occlusions, and variations in head pose and lighting conditions. The presence of non-rigid movements due to facial expression and a high degree of variability in facial size, color and texture make this problem even more difficult. Numerous techniques have been developed for face detection in still images (Yang et al., 2002; Li & Jian, 2005).

In our work, we used the most commonly face detector proposed by Viola and Jones (2004) to detect the face region from either a still image or a video stream. This detector consists of a cascade of classifiers trained by AdaBoost. Each classifier employs integral image filter, also called

Figure 5. A system is proposed to recognize four types of facial expressions using Naïve Bayesian Boost

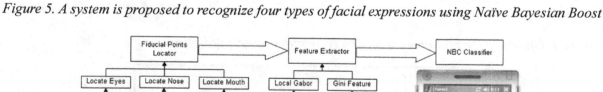
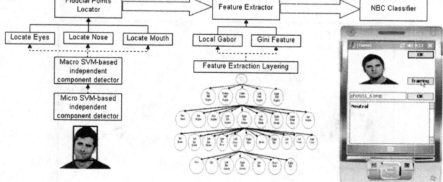

"box filters", which are reminiscent of Haar Basis functions, and can be computed very fast at any location and scale. This is essential to the speed of the detector. For each stage in the cascade, a subset of features is chosen using a feature selection procedure based on AdaBoost. After the process of face detection, we need to extract the fiducial point to locate at the facial components such as eyes, nose and mouth. The component-based feature detector is used in this stage. It has two levels, namely, the micro SVM based independent component detector and the macro SVM based independent component detector. The micro level uses linear SVM based independent component detection. Each component classifier was trained on a set of extracted facial components (the 4 key fiducial components) and on a set of randomly selected non-face patterns. The macro level uses the maximum outputs of the component classifiers within rectangular search regions as inputs to a combination SVM classifier. The macro SVM performs the final detection of the face component regions.

After the presence of a face has been detected in the observed scene, the next step is to extract the information about the displayed facial signals. Most of the existing facial expression analyzers are directed toward 2D spatiotemporal facial feature extraction. The feature extractor then adopted Gabor wavelet feature extraction. Gabor wavelet is a popular choice because of its capability to approximate mammals' visual cortex. The primary cortex of human brain interprets visual signals. It consists of neurons, which respond differently to different stimuli attributes. The receptive field of cortical cell consists of a central ON region is surrounded by 2 OFF regions, each region elongates along a preferred orientation (Daugman, 1985). According to Jones and Palmer (1987), these receptive fields can be reproduced fairly well using Daugman's Gabor function.

The Gabor wavelet function can be represented by:

$$g(x,y) = g_1(x,y) \exp(j2\grave{A}Wx) \qquad (1)$$

where

$$g_1(x,y) = \left(\frac{1}{2\pi\sigma_x\sigma_y}\right)\exp\left(-\frac{1}{2}\left(\frac{x^2}{\sigma_x^2} + \frac{y^2}{\sigma_y^2}\right)\right) \qquad (2)$$

We consider the receptive field (RF) of each cortical cell consists of a central ON region (a region excited by light) surrounded by two lateral OFF regions (excited by darkness) (La Cara et al., 2003). Spatial frequency (W) determines the width of the ON and OFF regions. σ_x^2 and σ_y^2 are spatial variances that establish the dimension of the RF in the preferred and non-preferred orientations. As shown in Figure 6a, the Gabor wavelets are represented with different orientations and frequencies. These Gabor wavelets act as stimuli to the system. Figure 6b gives an overview of the optimal stimuli for the first 48 units resulting from one typical simulation. Since the processing at the retina and LGN (Lateral Geniculate Nucleus) cortical layers are used by Gaussian kernels applying to some spectral bands to simulate local inhibition, most stimuli resemble Gabor wavelets. The input image is in HSI domain and is projected into different Gabor wavelets to generate the output signals that resemble electrical signals in visual cortex. Different orientations and special frequencies produce different wavelets. After the convolution of input and wavelets, a set of feature vectors is formed that acts like the 'hypercolumns' as described by Hubel and Wiesel (1962).

FEATURE SELECTION

Feature selection plays an important role of the automatic facial expression recognition system. The objectives of feature selection include noise reduction, regularization, relevance detection and reduction of computational effort. It is likely a learned image filters, such as, ICA, PCA and LFA that are based on unsupervised learning from the statistics of large image databases. There are two main models of feature selection, the filter model and the wrapper model. The filter model is generic, which is not optimized for any specific classifier. It is modularized and may sacrifice classification accuracy. The wrapper model is always tailored to a specific classifier and it may lead to better accuracy as a result. The strength of the wrapper model is that it differentiates irrelevance, strong and weak relevance and it improves performance significantly on some datasets. One weakness of the wrapper model is that calling the induction algorithm repeatedly may cause over-fitting. Another weakness is that its computational cost is expensive. In our work, we used the filter approach for the feature selection in the facial expression recognition. Two methods will be discussed in this section.

T-Test Feature Selection

In many existing feature selection algorithms, feature ranking is often used to show which input features are more important (Guyon and Elisseeff, 2003; Wang and Fu, 2005), especially when datasets are very large. T-test (Devore and Peck, 1997) is a common type of feature ranking measures that is often used to assess whether the means of two classes are statistically different from each other by calculating a ratio between the difference of two classes means and the variability of the two classes. The T-test has been used to rank features for micro-array data (Jaeger et al., 2003; Su et al., 2003) and for mass spectrometry data (Wu et al., 2003; Levner 2005). These uses of T-test are limited to two-class problem. For multi-class problems, a T-statistic value can be calculated as Equation (3) for each feature of each class by evaluating the difference between the mean of one class and the mean of all the classes, where the difference is standardized by the within-class standard deviation.

$$t_{ic} = \frac{\overline{x}_{ic} - \overline{x}_i}{M_C \cdot \left(S_i + S_0\right)} \tag{3}$$

$$S_i^2 = \frac{1}{N-C} \sum_{c=1}^{C} \sum_{j \in c} \left(x_{ij} - \overline{x}_{ic}\right)^2 \tag{4}$$

$$M_c = \sqrt{1/n_c + 1/N} \tag{5}$$

Here t_{ic} is the T-statistics value for the i-th feature of the c-th class; $\overline{x}_{ic}$ is the mean of the i-th feature in the c-th class, and $\overline{x}_i$ is the mean of the i-th feature for all classes; x_{ij} refers to the i-th feature of the j-th sample; N is the number of all the samples in the C classes and n_c is the number of samples in class c; S_i is the within-class

Figure 6. Gabor wavelets representation and the overview of optimal excitatory and inhibitory stimuli (S+ res. S-)

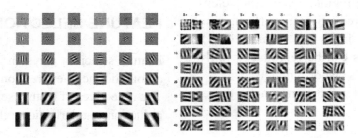

standard deviation and S_0 is set to be the median value of S_i for all the features. T-statistics is usually used to shrink class means toward the mean of all classes to constitute a nearest shrunken centriod classifier, but do not rank features regard to all the classes. In our work, another feature ranking method called GINI feature ranking for feature selection is used as discussed in the next section.

GINI Feature Selection

Apart from the statistical based feature selection likes T-test to rank the features for selection, another type of feature ranking is commonly used which is based on information theories. This type of feature ranking is normally called correlation based feature selection. It uses a correlation based heuristic to evaluate the worth of features (Hall and Simth, 1998). In order to perform the evaluation, a heuristic will be used. This heuristic takes into account of the usefulness of individual features for predicting the class label along with the level of inter-correlation among them. The hypothesis on which the heuristic can be stated as: Good feature subsets contain features highly correlated with the class, yet uncorrelated with each other.

Classification tasks in machine learning often involve learning from categorical features, as well as those are continuous or ordinal. A measure based on information theory estimates the degree of association between nominal features. If X and Y are discrete random variables, the entropy of Y before and after observing X are given as:

$$H(Y) = -\sum_{y \in Y} p(y) \log_2 p(y) \tag{6}$$

$$H(Y|X) = -\sum_{x \in X} p(x) \sum_{y \in Y} p(y|x) \log_2 p(y|x) \tag{7}$$

The amount by which the entropy of Y decreases reflects the additional information about Y provided by X and is called the information gain (Quinlan, 1993). Information gain is given by:

$$\begin{aligned}
\text{gain} &= H(Y) - H(Y|X) \\
&= H(Y) - H(X|Y) \\
&= H(Y) + H(X) - H(X,Y)
\end{aligned} \tag{8}$$

Information gain is a symmetrical measure – that is, the amount of information gained about Y after observing X is equal to the amount of information gained about X after observing Y. Unfortunately, information gain is biased in favor of features with more values, that is, attributes with greater numbers of values will appear to gain more information than those with fewer values even if they are actually no more informative. The purpose of feature selection is to decide which of the initial features to include in the final subset and which to ignore. If there are n possible features initially, then there are 2^n possible subsets. The only way to find the best subset would be to try them all – this is clearly prohibitive for all but a small number of initial features. GINI feature ranking method is a simple way to task for the feature selection even if there are many possible features to be selected.

Gini Index selects features based on information theories (Hall and Smith, 1999; Zhou and Dillion, 1988). It measures the impurity for a group of labels. Gini Index for a given set S of points assigned to, for example, two classes C_1 and C_2 is given below:

$$GINI(s) = 1 - \sum_{j=1,2} \left[p(C_j | s) \right]^2 \tag{9}$$

With $p(C_j|s)$ corresponds to the frequency of class C_j at set S. The maximum value as **1-1/nc** occurs when features are equally distributed among all classes, which implies less interesting information. On the other hand, the zero value occurs when all points belong to one class that represents the most interesting information. We then sort the n features over different classes of samples in ascending order based on their best Gini index. Low Gini index corresponds to high-ranking discriminative features.

CLASSIFICATION

After the feature components are ranked and selected, the facial expression recognition tasks are essential to make use of the feature vectors to discriminate and identify each of the expressions. Various pattern classifiers such as *Support Vector Machines (SVM)*, *K-nearest neighbors (K-NN)*, *Naïve Bayes Algorithm* and *Artificial Neural Networks* could be used for emotions recognition. SVM is a learning technique developed by Vapnik (1995) which was strongly motivated by results of statistically learning theory. SVM operates on the principle of induction, known as structural risk minimization, which minimizes the upper bound of the generalization error. K-nearest neighbor's method is a nonparametric technique in pattern recognition, which is used to generate k numbers of nearest neighbors' rules for classification. Naïve Bayes algorithm is based on the Bayesian decision theory, which is a fundamental statistical approach to the problem of pattern classification. This approach is based on quantifying the tradeoffs between various classification decisions using probability and the costs that accompany such decisions.

Naive Bayesian classifier is a simple probabilistic classifier based on applying Bayesian' theorem with strong (Naive) independence assumptions. Independent feature model is a more descriptive term for the underlying probability model. Parameter estimation for Naive Bayesian models uses the method of maximum likelihood in many practical applications; that is, one can work with the Naive Bayesian model without believing in Bayesian probability or using any Bayesian methods. Naive Bayesian classifiers can be trained very efficiently in a supervised learning setting, depending on the precise nature of the probability model. Naive Bayesian classifiers often work much better in many complex real-world situations than one might expect, in spite of their Naive design and apparently oversimplified assumptions. An advantage of the Naive Bayesian classifier is that it requires a small amount of training data to estimate the parameters (means and variances of the variables) necessary for classification. Because independent variables are assumed, only the variances of the variables for each class need to be determined and not the entire covariance matrix. Detailed analysis of the Bayesian classification problem has shown that there are some theoretical reasons for the apparently unreasonable efficacy of Naive Bayesian classifiers (Rish, 2001) recently. One should notice that the independence assumption may lead to some unexpected results in the calculation of posteriori probability. When there is a dependency between observations, the above-mentioned probability may contradict with the second axiom of probability by which any probability must be less than or equal to one. The Naive Bayesian classifier has several properties that make it surprisingly useful in practice despite the fact that the far-reaching independence assumptions are often inaccurate. For example, the decoupling of the class conditional feature distributions means that each distribution can be independently estimated as a one dimensional distribution. This will help to alleviate problems stemming from the curse of dimensionality, such as the need for data sets that scale exponentially with the number of features. It arrives at the correct classification as long as the correct class is more probable than any other class; hence class probabilities do not have to be estimated very well. In other words, the classifier is robust enough to ignore serious deficiencies in its underlying Naive probability model.

Given a set of test data X and a posteriori probability of a hypothesis H, $P(H|X)$, it may follow the Bayesian theorem (Rish 2001) as:

$$P(H|X) = \frac{P(X|H) P(H)}{P(X)} \qquad (10)$$

Informally, this can be written as posteriori $=$ likelihood $\times \dfrac{\text{prior}}{\text{evidence}}$. It predicts X belongs to C_2 iff the probability $P(C_2|X)$ is the highest among all the $P(C_k|X)$ for all the k classes. The detailed steps are as follow: Firstly, let D be a training set of tuples and their associated class labels, and a test tuple that is represented by an $n\text{-}D$ attribute vector $X = (x_1, x_2, \ldots, x_n)$. Suppose there are m classes $C_1, C_2, \ldots, C_m$. The classification is to derive the maximum posteriori, i.e., the maximal $P(C_i|X)$. Alternatively, a simplified assumption: attributes are conditionally independent (i.e., no dependence relation between attributes). This greatly reduces the computation cost: Only counts the class distribution. The formula is stated as below:

$$\begin{aligned} P(X|C_i) &= \prod_{k=1}^{n} P(X_k|C_i) \\ &= P(X_1|C_i) \times P(X_2|C_i) \times \cdots \times P(X_n|C_i) \end{aligned} \qquad (11)$$

Bayesian networks can represent joint distributions we use them to compute the posterior probability of a set of labels given the observable features, and then we classify the features with the most probable label. The idea is to use a strategy that can efficiently search through the whole space of possible structures and to extract the ones that give the best classification results.

Consider the problem of classifying facial expression by features, for example into joy and non-joy. Imagine that image are drawn from a number of classes of facial features which can be modeled as sets of words where the (independent) probability that the i-th feature of a given image occurs in a image from class C can be written as $P(W_i|C)$. For this treatment, we can simplify further by assuming that the probability of a feature in an image is independent of the total number of features, or that all image contain same number of features. Then the probability of a given image E, given a class C is

$$P(E|C) = \prod_{i}^{n} P(W_i|C) \qquad (12)$$

Bayesian' theorem manipulates these into a statement of probability in terms of likelihood given by:

$$P(C|E) = \frac{P(C)}{P(D)} \times P(E|C) \qquad (13)$$

Our proposed algorithm adopted the Naïve Bayesian with boosting. Each iteration of boosting uses the Gini reduction and selection method and to remove redundant features. Gini uses probability of separation on classes for each feature, whereas T-test uses the distance-based separation for ranking each feature. For Gini ranking, the most discriminative feature will give the lowest value. It is a measure to examine whether the data has clear discrimination between the classes. The main reason for using boosting NB approach is that the embedded feature selection technique makes the data more suitable for classification. The algorithm is summarized as below:

We assess the ability of the system to recognize different facial expressions. We have adopted the Mind Reading DVD, a computer-based guide to

Boosting Naïve Bayesian Algorithm:

GINI feature selections:
  1. Assign each training sample with weight=1.
  2. For ten iteration (ten features):
  • Sort features index S.
  • Split S.
  • Break if GINI criterion is satisfied.

BNB classification:
  1. Apply simple Bayesian to weighted data set.
  2. Compute error rate.
  3. Iterate the training examples.

  • Multiply the weight by $\dfrac{e}{1-e}$.

  • Normalize the weight

  4. Add $-\log\dfrac{e}{1-e}$ to weight of class predicted
  5. Return class with highest sum

---

emotions, developed by a team of psychologists led by Prof. Simon Baron-Cohen (2004) at the Autism Research Centre, University of Cambridge. The database contains images of approximately 100 subjects. Facial images are of size 320x240 pixels, 8-bit precision grayscale in PNG format. Subjects' age ranges from 18 to 30. Sixty-five percent were female, 15 percent were African-American, and three percent were Asian or Latino. Subjects were instructed by experimenter to perform a series of facial displays as an example shown in Figure 7. Subjects began each display from a neutral face. Before performing each display, the experimenter described and modeled the desired display. The model recognizes four types of facial expression: neutral, joy, sadness and surprise. Twenty images were used for training in which 5 images were used for representing each expression. The facial expres-

sion recognition result is shown in Figure 8. The confusion matrix is included in the figure as well where the column of the matrix represents the instances in a predicted class, in which each row represents the instances in an actual class. The system correctly recognizes 76.3% of neutral, 78.3% of joy, 74.7% of sad and 78.7% of surprise expressions amongst 100 subjects in the database, although some facial expressions do get confused by the wrong class, however at an acceptable range of less than 12%. In addition, comparisons with other approaches are necessary for us to investigate how the recognition performance of our approach can be benchmarked with others. Table 1 shows the recognition results for facial expression recognition using T-test and GINI as feature selection and Euclidean, k-nearest neighbor (kNN) as classifiers to compare our boosting Naïve Bayesian (GINI and Naïve Bayesian) approach. Gini processes 854 raw features and shrink down the dimension to 20 features to be further processed by classifier. These 20 features are used as it provides the most optimal results. According to the results in the table, the boosting Naïve Bayesian approach achieves the most optimal result. The T-test is able to assess whether the means of different groups are statistically different from each other. kNN is a classification method for classifying objects based on closest training examples in the feature space. We have used k=5 for kNN classifier based on the problem domain. These approaches are generally used for bench-marking. Our approach that combines Gini and Naïve Bayesian achieves average of 75% in which it outperforms the others. The computa-

Figure 7. Four categories of facial expressions. (a) Neutral, (b) Joy, (c) Sad, and (d) Surprise

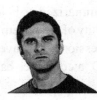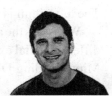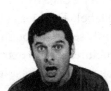

Figure 8. Facial expression recognition result of the system

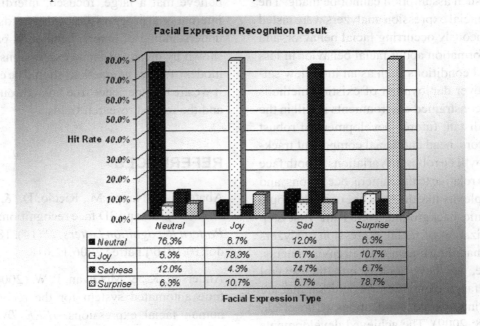

Facial Expression Recognition Result				
	Neutral	Joy	Sad	Surprise
■ Neutral	76.3%	6.7%	12.0%	6.3%
▢ Joy	5.3%	78.3%	6.7%	10.7%
▦ Sadness	12.0%	4.3%	74.7%	6.7%
▨ Surprise	6.3%	10.7%	6.7%	78.7%

tional time is recorded about 2.1 frames per second in real time implementation.

FUTURE TRENDS AND CONCLUSION

Automating the analysis of facial signals, especially rapid facial signals (facial expressions) is important to realize more natural, context-sensitive (e.g., affective) human-computer interaction, to advance studies on human emotion and affective computing, and to boost numerous applications in fields as diverse as security, medicine, and education. This chapter introduced recent work of our group in this research field.

In summary, although most of the facial expression analyzers developed so far target human facial affect analysis and attempt to recognize a small set of prototypic emotional facial expressions like happiness and anger, some progress has been made in addressing a number of other scientific challenges that are considered essential for realization of machine understanding of human facial behavior. Existing methods for machine analysis of facial expressions discussed throughout this chapter assume that the input data are near frontal-view face image sequences showing facial displays that always begin with a neutral state.

Table 1. Comparison of feature selection techniques for facial expression recognition. Three feature selection options are compared using Naïve Bayesian and kNN as the classifiers.

Feature selection	Naïve Bayesian	kNN	Euclidean
None	53%	57%	58%
T-test	57%	59%	59%
GINI	75%	57%	63%

In reality, such assumption cannot be made. The discussed facial expression analyzers were tested on spontaneously occurring facial behavior, and extract information about facial behavior in less constrained conditions such as an interview setting. However deployment of existing methods in fully unconstrained environments is still in the relatively distant future. Development of robust face detectors, head and facial component trackers, which will be robust to variations in both face orientation relative to the camera, occlusions, and scene complexity like the presence of other people and dynamic background, forms the first step in the realization of facial expression analyzers capable of handling unconstrained environments.

To date, we have looked into the several aspects of facial expression recognition that are published in separate publications (Cho et al., 2007; 2008; 2009). The achieved developments thus far include the unsupervised learning of facial emotion categorization, the tree structured model of classification and the deployment of the system in hand-held mobile devices. There are two aspects still unsolved. The first issue is how the grammar of facial behavior can be learned and how this information can be properly represented and used to handle ambiguities in the observation data. Another issue is how to include information about the context in which the observed expressive behavior was displayed so that a context-sensitive analysis of facial behavior can be achieved. Meanwhile, we will also look into explicit modeling of noise and uncertainty in the classification process. The explicit modeling may consist of the temporal dynamic of facial expressions, spontaneous facial expressions, multimodal facial expression classification (Zeng et al. 2009). These aspects of machine analysis of facial expressions form the main focus of the current and future research in the field. Yet, since the complexity of these issues concerned with the interpretation of human behavior at a deeper level is tremendous and spans several different disciplines in computer and social sciences, we believe that a large, focused, interdisciplinary, international program directed towards computer understanding of human behavioral patterns (as shown by means of facial expressions and other modes of social interaction) should be established if we are to experience true breakthroughs in this and the related research fields.

REFERENCES

Abate, A. F., Nappi, M., Riccio, D., & Sabatino, G. (2007). 2D and 3D face recognition: A survey. *Pattern Recognition Letters*, *28*(14), 1885–1906. doi:10.1016/j.patrec.2006.12.018

Anderson, K., & McOwan, P. W. (2006). A real-time automated system for the recognition of human facial expressions. *IEEE Transactions on Systems Man and Cybernetics Part B*, *36*(1), 96–105. doi:10.1109/TSMCB.2005.854502

Baron-Cohen, S., Golan, O., Wheelwright, S., & Hill, J. J. (2004). *Mind Reading: The Interactive Guide to Emotions*. London: Jessica Kingsley Publishers.

Bartlett, M. S., Littlewort, G., Fasel, I., & Movellan, J. R. (2003). *Real time face detection and facial expression recognition: Development and applications to human computer interaction*. Paper presented at the CVPR, Madison.

Bassili, J. N. (1978). Facial motion in the perception of faces and of emotional expression. *Journal of Experimental Psychology*, *4*(3), 373–379.

Black, M. J., & Yacoob, Y. (1997). Recognizing Facial Expressions in Image Sequences Using Local Parameterized Models of Image Motion. *International Journal of Computer Vision*, *25*(1), 23–48. doi:10.1023/A:1007977618277

Bourel, F. C., & Low, A. A. (2002). *Robust facial expression recognition using a state-based model of spatially-localised facial dynamics.* Paper presented at the IEEE International Conference on Automatic Face and Gesture Recognition (pp. 20-21).

Bowyer, K. W., Chang, K., & Flynn, P. (2006, January). A survey of approaches and challenges in 3D and multi-modal 3D + 2D face recognition. *Computer Vision and Image Understanding, 101*(1), 1–15. .doi:10.1016/j.cviu.2005.05.005

Chandrasiri, N. P., Park, M. C., Naemura, T., & Harashima, H. (1999). *Personal facial expression space based on multidimensional scaling for the recognition improvement.* Paper presented at the Proceedings of the Fifth International Symposium Signal Processing and Its Applications (pp. 22-25).

Cho, S. Y., & Nguwi, Y.-Y. (2007). Self-Organizing Adaptation for Facial Emotion Mapping. In *The 2007 International Conference on Artificial Intelligence*, June 2007, Las Vegas, US.

Cho, S. Y., Teoh, T.-T., & Nguwi, Y.-Y. (2009). Development of an Intelligent Facial Expression Recognizer for Mobile Applications. In *First KES International Symposium on Intelligent Decision Technologies*.

Cho, S. Y., & Wong, J.-J. (2008). Human face recognition by adaptive processing of tree structures representation. *Neural Computing & Applications, 17*(3), 201–215. doi:10.1007/s00521-007-0108-8

Cohn, J. F., Zlochower, A. J., Lien, J. J., & Kanade, A. T. (1998). *Feature-Point Tracking by Optical Flow Discriminates Subtle Differences in Facial Expression.* Paper presented at the International Conference on Face & Gesture Recognition.

Cottrell, G. W., & Fleming, M. K. (1990). *Categorization of Faces Using Unsupervised Feature Extraction.* Paper presented at the Int'l Conf. Neural Networks, San Diego.

Darwin, C. (1872). *The Expression of the Emotions in Man and Animals.* London: J. Murray. doi:10.1037/10001-000

Daugman, J. (1985). Uncertainty relation for resolution in space, spatial frequency, and orientation optimized by two-dimensional visual cortical filters. *Journal of the Optical Society of America, 2*(7), 1160–1169. doi:10.1364/JOSAA.2.001160

Devore, J., & Peck, R. (1997). *Statistics: The Exploration and Analysis of Data* (3rd ed.). Pacific Grove, CA: Duxbury Press.

Edwards, G. J., Cootes, T. F., & Taylor, C. J. (1998). Face Recognition Using Active Appearance Models. In *Proc. European Conf. Computer Vision* (Vol. 2, pp. 581-695).

Ekman, P., & Friesen, W. V. (1971). Constants across cultures in the face and emotion. *Journal of Personality and Social Psychology, 17*(2), 124–129. doi:10.1037/h0030377

Elkman, P., Huang, T. S., Sejnowski, T. J., & Hanger, J. C. (Eds.). (1993). *NSF: Understanding the Face.* Salt Lake City, UT: A Human Face eStore.

Essa, I. A., & Pentland, A. P. (1997). Coding, analysis, interpretation, and recognition of facial expressions. *IEEE Transactions on Pattern Analysis and Machine Intelligence, 19*(7), 757–763. doi:10.1109/34.598232

Fasel, B., & Luettin, J. (2003). Automatic facial expression analysis: a survey. *Pattern Recognition, 36*(1), 259–275. doi:10.1016/S0031-3203(02)00052-3

Fasel, B., & Lüttin, J. (2000). *Recognition of Asymmetric Facial Action Unit Activities and Intensities.* Paper presented at the Proceedings of the International Conference on Pattern Recognition, Barcelona, Spain.

Fasel, I. R. (2006). *Learning Real-Time Object Detectors: Probabilistic Generative Approaches.* PhD thesis, Department of Cognitive Science, University of California, San Diego, USA.

Fasel, I. R., Fortenberry, B., & Movellan, J. R. (2005). A generative framework for real time object detection and classification. *Int'l J Computer Vision and Image Understanding, 98*(1), 181–210.

Guyon, I., & Elisseeff, A. (2003). An introduction to variable and feature selection. *Journal of Machine Learning Research, 3,* 1157–1182. doi:10.1162/153244303322753616

Hall, M. A., & Smith, L. A. (1998). Practical Feature Subset Selection For Machine Learning. In *Proceedings of the 21st Australasian Computer Science Conference* (pp. 181-191). Berlin: Springer.

Hall, M. A., & Smith, L. A. (1999) Feature Selection for Machine Learning: Comparing a Correlation-Based Filter Approach to the Wrapper. In *FLAIRS Conference* (pp. 235–239).

Hubel, D., & Wiesel, T. (1962). Receptive fields, binocular interaction, and functional architecture in the cat's visual cortex. *The Journal of Physiology, 160,* 106–154.

Jaeger, J. (2003). *Improved gene selection for classification of microarrays* (pp. 53–94). Pac. Symp. Biocomput.

Ji, Y. Z. Q. (2005). Active and dynamic information fusion for facial expression understanding from image sequences. *IEEE Transactions on Pattern Analysis and Machine Intelligence, 27*(5), 699–714. doi:10.1109/TPAMI.2005.93

Jones, J. P., & Palmer, L. A. (1987). An evaluation of the Two-Dimensional Gabor Filter model of simple Receptive fields in cat striate cortex. *Journal of Neurophysiology, 58*(6), 1233–1258.

Kim, D.-J., Bien, Z., & Park, K.-H. (2003). *Fuzzy neural networks (FNN)-based approach for personalized facial expression recognition with novel feature selection method.* Paper presented at the IEEE International Conference on Fuzzy Systems.

La Cara, G. E., Ursino, M., & Bettini, M. (2003). Extraction of Salient Contours in Primary Visual Cortex: A Neural Network Model Based on Physiological Knowledge. In *Proceedings of the 25th Annual International Conference of the IEEE* (Vol. 3, pp. 2242 – 2245).

Lanitis, A. T., C.J., Cootes, T.F. (1997). Automatic interpretation and coding of face images using flexible models. *Pattern Analysis and Machine Intelligence, IEEE Transactions on, 19*(7), 743-756.

Levner, I. (2005). Feature selection and nearest centroid classification for protein mass spectrometry. *BMC Bioinformatics, 6,* 68. doi:10.1186/1471-2105-6-68

Li, S. Z., & Jain, A. K. (Eds.). (2005). *Handbook of Face Recognition.* New York: Springer.

Littlewort, G., Bartlett, M. S., Fasel, I., Susskind, J., & Movellan, J. (2006). Dynamics of facial expression extracted automatically from video. *J. Image & Vision Computing, 24*(6), 615–625. doi:10.1016/j.imavis.2005.09.011

Mase, K., & Pentland, A. (1991). Recognition of facial expression from optical flow. *IEICE Trans., 74*(10), 3474–3483.

Matsuno, K., Iee, C.-W., & Tsuji, S. (1994). *Recognition of Human Facial Expressions Without Feature Extraction.* Paper presented at the ECCV.

Otsuka, T., & Ohya, J. (1998). *Spotting segments displaying facial expression from image sequences using HMM.* Paper presented at the IEEE Proceedings of the Second International Conference on Automatic Face and Gesture Recognition, Japan.

Pantic, M. (2006). Face for Ambient Interface. In *Lecture Notes in Artificial Intelligence* (Vol. 3864, pp. 35-66).

Pantic, M., & Rothkrantz, L. J. M. (2000). Automatic analysis of facial expressions: the state of the art. *Pattern Analysis and Machine Intelligence . IEEE Transactions on, 22*(12), 1424–1445.

Pardas, M. B. A., Landabaso, J.L. (2002). *Emotion recognition based on mpeg4 facial animation parameters.* Paper presented at the IEEE International Conference on Acoustics, Speech, and Signal Processing.

Quinlan, J. R. (1993). *C4.5: Program for Machine Learning.* San Francisco: Morgan Kaufmann.

Rish I. (2001). *An empirical study of the naïve Bayes classifier.* Technical Report RC 22230.

Rosenblum, M., Yacoob, Y., & Davis, L. S. (1996). Human Expression Recognition from Motion Using a Radial Basis Function Network Architecture. *IEEE Transactions on Neural Networks, 7*(5), 1121–1138. doi:10.1109/72.536309

Sabatini, S. P. (1996). Recurrent inhibition and clustered connectivity as a basis for Gabor-like receptive fields in the visual cortex. In R. M. Joseph Sirosh, and Yoonsuck Choe (Ed.), *Lateral Interactions in the Cortex: Structure and Function.* Austin, TX: The UTCS Neural Networks Research Group.

Shin, Y., Lee, S. S., Chung, C., & Lee, Y. (2000, 21-25 Aug 2000). *Facial expression recognition based on two-dimensional structure of emotion.* Paper presented at the International Conference on Signal Processing Proceedings.

Su, Y. (2003). RankGene: identification of diagnostic genes based on expression data. *Bioinformatics (Oxford, England), 19*, 1578–1579. doi:10.1093/bioinformatics/btg179

Vapnik, V. N. (1995). *The Nature of Statistical Learning Theory.* New York: Springer-Verlag.

Viola, P., & Jones, M. (2004). Robust real-time face detection. *J. Computer Vision, 57*(2), 137–154. doi:10.1023/B:VISI.0000013087.49260.fb

Vukadinovic, D., & Pantic, M. (2005). Fully automatic facial feature point detection using Gabor feature based boosted classifiers, *Proc. IEEE Int'l Conf. Systems, Man and Cybernetics,* pp. 1692-1698.

Wang, L., & Fu, X. (2005). *Data Mining with Computational Intelligence.* Berlin: Springer.

Whitehill, J., & Omlin, C. 2006). Haar Features for FACS AU Recognition. In *Proc. IEEE Int'l Conf. Face and Gesture Recognition* (pp. 5).

Wong, J.-J., & Cho, S.-Y. (2006). *Facial emotion recognition by adaptive processing of tree structures.* Paper presented at the Proceedings the 2006 ACM symposium on Applied computing, Dijon, France.

Wu, B. (2003). Comparison of statistical methods for classification of ovarian cancer using mass spectrometry data. *Bioinformatics (Oxford, England), 19*, 1636–1643. doi:10.1093/bioinformatics/btg210

Wu, Y., Liu, H., & Zha, H. (2005). *Modeling facial expression space for recognition.* Paper presented at the IEEE/RSJ International Conference on Intelligent Robots and Systems.

Xiang, T., Leung, M. K. H., & Cho, S. Y. (2007). Expression recognition using fuzzy spatio-temporal modeling. *Pattern Recognition, 41*(1), 204–216. doi:10.1016/j.patcog.2007.04.021

Yacoob, Y., & Davis, L. S. (1996). Recognizing Human Facial Expressions from Long Image Sequences using Optical Flow. *IEEE Transactions on Pattern Analysis and Machine Intelligence, 18*(6), 636–642. doi:10.1109/34.506414

Yang, M. H., Kriegman, D. J., & Ahuja, N. (2002). Detecting faces in images: A survey. *IEEE Transactions on Pattern Analysis and Machine Intelligence, 24*(1), 34–58. doi:10.1109/34.982883

Yeasin, M., & Bullot, B. (2005). *Comparison of linear and non-linear data projection techniques in recognizing universal facial expressions.* Paper presented at the IJCNN.

Zeng, Z., Fu, Y., Roisman, G. I., Wen, Z., Hu, Y., & Huang, T. S. (2006). *One-class classification for spontaneous facial expression analysis.* Paper presented at the International Conference on Automatic Face and Gesture Recognition.

Zeng, Z., Pantic, M., Roisman, G. I., & Huang, T. S. (2009). A Survey of Affect Recognition Methods: Audio, Visual, and Spontaneous Expressions. *IEEE Transactions on Pattern Analysis and Machine Intelligence, 31*(1), 39–58. doi:10.1109/TPAMI.2008.52

Zhao, W., & Chellappa, R. (2003). A. Rosenfeld, P.J. Phillips, Face Recognition: A Literature Survey. *ACM Computing Surveys*, 399–458. doi:10.1145/954339.954342

Zhou, X. J., & Dillion, T. S. (1988). A Heuristic - Statistical Feature Selection Criterion For Inductive Machine Learning In The Real World. In *Proceedings of the 1988 IEEE International Conference on Systems, Man, and Cybernetics* (Vol. 1, pp. 548–552).

KEY TERMS AND DEFINITIONS

Facial Expression Recognition: is a computer application for automatically identifying or verifying a person's facial expression from a digital image or a video frame from a video source.

Feature Extraction: Feature extraction is a general term for methods of constructing combinations of the variables to get around these problems while still describing the data with sufficient accuracy.

Gabor Wavelet: A filter bank consisting of Gabor filters with various scales and rotations is created. The filters are convolved with the signal, resulting in a so-called Gabor space. This process is closely related to processes in the primary visual cortex.

Feature Selection: is the technique, commonly used in machine learning, of selecting a subset of relevant features for building robust learning models.

Classification: is a machine learning technique for deducing a function from training data. The training data consist of pairs of input objects (typically vectors), and desired outputs. The output of the function can predict a class label of the input object, called classification.

Naïve Bayesian Classifier: is a simple probabilistic classifier based on applying Bayes' theorem (from Bayesian statistics) with strong (naive) independence assumptions.

Human Emotion: is a mental and physiological state associated with a wide variety of feelings, thoughts, and behavior.

Affective Computing: Affective computing is a branch of the study and development of artificial intelligence that deals with the design of systems and devices that can recognize, interpret, and process human emotions.

Chapter 14
Subtle Facial Expression Recognition in Still Images and Videos

Fadi Dornaika
University of the Basque Country, Spain & IKERBASQUE, Basque Foundation for Science, Spain

Bogdan Raducanu
Computer Vision Center, Spain

ABSTRACT

This chapter addresses the recognition of basic facial expressions. It has three main contributions. First, the authors introduce a view- and texture independent schemes that exploits facial action parameters estimated by an appearance-based 3D face tracker. they represent the learned facial actions associated with different facial expressions by time series. Two dynamic recognition schemes are proposed: (1) the first is based on conditional predictive models and on an analysis-synthesis scheme, and (2) the second is based on examples allowing straightforward use of machine learning approaches. Second, the authors propose an efficient recognition scheme based on the detection of keyframes in videos. Third, the authors compare the dynamic scheme with a static one based on analyzing individual snapshots and show that in general the former performs better than the latter. The authors then provide evaluations of performance using Linear Discriminant Analysis (LDA), Non parametric Discriminant Analysis (NDA), and Support Vector Machines (SVM).

INTRODUCTION

Many researchers in the engineering and computer science communities have been developing automatic ways for machines to recognize emotional expression, as a goal towards achieving human-machine intelligent interaction. Research on emotion classification utilizes pattern recogni-

tion approaches for recognizing emotions, using different modalities as inputs to the emotion recognition models. In the vision community, still images and videos depicting faces constitute the main channel that conveys human emotion. In the last two decades many automatic facial expression recognition methods have been proposed.

In the field of Human-Computer Interaction (HCI) computers will be enabled with perceptual capabilities in order to facilitate the communica-

DOI: 10.4018/978-1-61520-991-0.ch014

tion protocols between people and machines. In other words, computers must use natural ways of communication people use in their everyday life: speech, hand and body gestures, facial expression. Recently, there is an increasing interest in non-verbal communication. Among it, affective computing plays a fundamental role: "computing that relates to, arises from, or deliberately influences emotions" (Picard, 1997). Indeed, the newest trend in computer systems aims at adapting them to the user's needs and preferences through intelligent interfaces. From the AI perspective, undergoing research emphasize the strong relationship between cognition and emotion. A central part of the human-centred paradigm is represented by affective computing, i.e. computer systems able to recognize, interpret, and react accordingly to the affective phenomena perceived. The roots of affective computing can be found in psychology, which postulates that facial expressions have a consistent and meaningful structure that can be backprojected in order to infer people inner affective state (Ekman, 1993; Ekman & Davidson, 1994).

Basic facial expressions typically recognized by psychologists are: happiness, sadness, fear, anger, disgust and surprise (Ekman, 1992). In the beginning, facial expression analysis was essentially a research topic for psychologists. However, recent progresses in image processing and pattern recognition have motivated significantly research works on automatic facial expression recognition (Fasel & Luettin, 2003; Kim et al., 2004; Yeasin et al., 2006). The automated analysis of facial expressions is a challenging task because everyone's face is unique and interpersonal differences exist in how people perform facial expressions. Numerous methodologies have been proposed to solve this problem. In the past, a lot of effort was dedicated to recognize facial expression in still images. For this purpose, many techniques have been applied: neural networks (Tian et al, 2001), Gabor wavelets (Bartlett et al., 2004) and Active Appearance Models (AAM) (Sung et al., 2006).

A very important limitation to this strategy is the fact that still images usually capture the apex of the expression, i.e., the instant at which the indicators of emotion are most marked. In their daily life, people seldom show apex of their facial expression during normal communication with their counterparts, unless for very specific cases and for very brief periods of time. In everyday life, the facial expressions observed are an interaction of emotional response and cultural convention. More recently, attention has been shifted particularly towards modeling dynamical facial expressions (Cohen et al., 2003; Shan et al., 2006; Yeasin et al., 2006).

Recent research has shown that it is not only the expression itself, but also its dynamics that are important when attempting to decipher its meaning. The dynamics of facial expression can be defined as the intensity of the Action Units coupled with the timing of their formation (Zheng, 2000). In (Ambadar et al., 2005), the authors highlighted the fact that facial expressions are frequently subtle. They found that subtle expressions that were not identifiable in individual images suddenly became apparent when viewed in a video sequence. There is now a growing body of psychological research that argues that these dynamics are a critical factor for the interpretation of the observed behavior.

This chapter describes our recent works on facial expression recognition. We proposed two frameworks for facial expression recognition given natural head motion. These frameworks are based on an appearance-based 3D face tracker (Dornaika & Davoine, 2006). The proposed frameworks can be used for both kinds of facial expression: extreme posed expressions and subtle expressions. The first framework utilizes dynamic recognition schemes. The second framework utilizes static recognition schemes. While the dynamic recognition framework implicitly models subtle facial expressions, the second framework can perform the same task provided that the training examples (still images) include such occurrences. Within the first framework, we propose two different schemes: (1) an analysis-synthesis scheme based on Markov models, and (2) example based scheme for which standard machine learning approaches can be used. Compared to existing facial expression methods our proposed frameworks have several advantages. First, unlike most expression recognition systems that require a frontal view of the face, our system is view independent since the used tracker simultaneously provides the 3D head pose and the facial actions. Second, it is texture independent since the recognition scheme relies only on the estimated facial actions—invariant geometrical parameters. Third, its learning phase is simple compared to other techniques (e.g., the HMM). As a result, even when the imaging conditions change, the learned expression dynamics need not to be recomputed.

The proposed frameworks for facial expressions are evaluated and compared using video sequences. For every framework (static and dynamic) several machine learning approaches are used and compared.

This chapter is organized as follows. Section 2 briefly presents some backgrounds in expression recognition. Section 3 briefly presents the proposed 3D face and facial action tracking. Section 4 describes the proposed dynamic recognition framework. Section 5 presents an efficient scheme for the detection and recognition of facial expression in videos. In section 6, we report method comparisons and performance evaluations for the dynamic and static recognition frameworks. Finally, section 7 presents some conclusions.

BACKGROUND AND RELATED WORK

Despite the fact that facial expressions can be either subtle or pronounced in their appearance, and fleeting or sustained in their duration, most of the studies have focused on analyzing static displays of extreme posed expressions rather than the more natural spontaneous expressions (Goneid et al., 2002; Reilly et al., 2006, Song et al., 2006). Subtle emotions are shown when an emotion is just beginning, as the muscles are not contracted very much and are at a lower intensity (Bould et al., 2008). The ability to recognize subtle facial expressions can be very useful for Human Computer Interaction applications requiring the interpretation of spontaneous facial expressions. The analysis and recognition of subtle expressions can be used for producing subtle expressivity for robots and synthetic characters (Bartneck & Reichenbach, 2005). Moreover, the usefulness of subtle facial expressions is obvious for social robots that should interact with subjects who seldom display exaggerated posed expressions.

Recognizing subtle facial expressions in still images and videos can be challenging since the facial deformations may have low intensities or appear for very short time. In (Park & Kim, 2009), the authors propose to recognize subtle facial expression using motion magnification. The magnification affects 2D motion of some facial features. The expression is inferred from the new image AAM shape and appearance parameters. In theory, dynamical classifiers can be used for recognizing subtle facial expressions since the emphasis is put on the temporal evolution of facial deformations rather than on the absolute intensities. Indeed, dynamical classifiers try to capture the temporal pattern in the sequence of feature vectors related to each frame such as the Hidden Markov Models (HMMs) and Dynamic Bayesian Networks (Zhang & Ji, 2005). Dynamical approaches can use shape deformations [Dornaika & Davoine, 2005], texture dynamics (Yang et al., 2007) or a combination of them (Cheon & Kim, 2009).

In (Black & Jacoob, 1997), parametric 2D flow models associated with the whole face as well as with the mouth, eyebrows, and eyes are first estimated. Then, mid-level predicates are inferred from these parameters. Finally, universal facial expressions are detected and recognized using the estimated predicates. In (Cheon & Kim, 2009), the authors propose a dynamic recognition based on the differential Active Appearance Model parameters. A sequence of input frames is fitted using the classical AAM then a specific frame is selected as reference frame. Then the corresponding sequence of differential AAM parameters is recognized by computing the directed Hausdorff distance and KNN classifier. In (Yeasin et al., 2006), a two-stage approach is used. Initially, a linear classification bank was applied and its output was fused to produce a characteristic signature for each universal facial expression. The signatures thus computed from the training data set were used to train discrete Hidden Markov Models to learn the underlying model for each facial expression. In (Shan et al., 2006), the authors propose a Bayesian approach to modelling temporal transitions of facial expressions represented in a manifold. In (Xiang et al., 2008), the authors propose a dynamic classifier that is based on building spatio-temporal model for each universal expression derived from Fourier transform. The recognition of unseen expression uses the Hausdorff distance to compute dissimilarity values for classification. (Dornaika & Raducanu, 2007) proposes a dynamic classifier that is based on an analysis-synthesis scheme exploiting learned predictive models given by second order Markov models. (Dornaika & Davoine, 2005) proposes a dynamic classifier based on a brute force matching of temporal signatures.

As can be seen, most proposed expression recognition schemes require a frontal view of the face. Moreover, most of them rely on the use of image raw brightness changes. The recognition of facial expressions in image sequences with significant head motion is a challenging problem. However, it is required by many applications such as human computer interaction and computer graphics animation (Cañamero & Gaussier, 2005; Pantic, 2005, Picard et al., 2001) as well as training of social robots (Breazeal, 1999; Breazeal, 2000).

3D FACIAL DYNAMICS EXTRACTION

A human face is a bumpy and mobile surface. Neither 2D dynamic data nor 3D static data may be sufficient to depict such a property. 3D static face models lacking a temporal context may be a profound handicap to recognizing facial expressions.

The first 3D dynamic facial expression database was created in 2008 by Yin et al. (Yin et al., 2008). All reported approaches were based on in-house 3D dynamic data sets. In our works, we use a common 3D deformable face model *Candide* (Ahlberg, 2002). Despite the simplicity of this 3D wireframe model, it can be used to extract a subset of 3D facial dynamics in real time using one single camera. Once the 3D facial dynamics are learned the recognition scheme should use the same 3D face model.

A Deformable 3D Face Model

The 3D shape of *Candide* model is directly recorded in coordinate form. It is given by the coordinates of the 3D vertices $\mathbf{P}_i$, $i = 1, \ldots, n$ where n is the number of vertices. Thus, the shape up to a global scale can be fully described by the $3n$-vector $\mathbf{g}$; the concatenation of the 3D coordinates of all vertices $\mathbf{P}_i$. The vector $\mathbf{g}$ is written as:

$$g = g_s + A\tau_a \qquad (1)$$

where $\mathbf{g}_s$ is the static shape of the model, τ_a is the animation control vector, and the columns of A are the Animation Units. The static shape is constant for a given person. In this study, we use six modes for the facial Animation Units (AUs) matrix A. We have chosen the following AUs: lower lip depressor, lip stretcher, lip corner depressor, upper lip raiser, eyebrow lowerer, and outer eyebrow raiser. These AUs are enough to cover most common facial animations. Moreover, they are essential for conveying emotions. Thus, for every frame in the video, the state of the 3D wireframe model is given by the 3D head pose parameters (three rotations and three translations) and the internal face animation control vector τ_a. This is given by the 12-dimensional vector **b**:

$$b = [\theta_x, \theta_y, \theta_z, t_x, t_y, t_z, \tau_a^T]^T \qquad (2)$$

where each component of the vector τ_a represents the intensity of one facial action. This belongs to the interval [0,1] where the zero value corresponds to the neutral configuration (no deformation) and the one value corresponds to the maximum deformation. In the sequel, the word "facial action" will refer to the facial action intensity.

Simultaneous Face and Facial Action Tracking

In order to recover the facial expression one has to compute the facial actions encoded by the vector τ_a which encapsulates the facial deformation. Since our recognition scheme is view-independent these facial actions together with the 3D head pose should be simultaneously estimated. In other words, the objective is to compute the state vector **b** for every video frame.

For this purpose, we use the tracker based on Online Appearance Models—described in (Dornaika & Davoine, 2006). This appearance-based tracker aims at computing the 3D head pose and the facial actions, i.e. the vector **b**, by minimizing a distance between the incoming warped frame and the current *shape-free* appearance of the face. This minimization is carried out using a gradient descent method. The statistics of the *shape-free* appearance as well as the gradient matrix are updated every frame. This scheme leads to a fast and robust tracking algorithm.

DYNAMIC RECOGNITION

In this section, we show how the time series representation of the estimated facial actions, τ_a, can be utilized for inferring the facial expression in continuous videos. The central task is to correlate movements of the face with the universal emotional states.

In order to learn the spatio-temporal structure of the facial actions associated with the universal expressions, we have used the following procedure. Video sequences have been picked up from the CMU database (Kanade et al., 2000). These sequences depict five frontal view universal expressions (surprise, sadness, joy, disgust and anger). Each expression is performed by 7 different subjects, starting from the neutral one. Altogether we select 35 video sequences composed of around 15 to 20 frames each, that is, the average duration of each sequence is about half a second. These training video sequences are tracked with the appearance-based tracker (Dornaika & Davoine, 2006) in order to get the facial action parameters τ_a (a sequence of 6-element vectors), that is, the temporal trajectories of the action parameters. Figure 1 shows some retrieved facial action parameters associated with three sequences: surprise, anger, and joy. The training video sequences have an interesting property: all performed expressions go from the neutral expression to a high magnitude expression by going through a moderate magnitude around the middle of the sequence. Therefore, using the same training set we get two kinds of trajectories: (1) an entire trajectory which models transitions from the neutral expression to a high magnitude expression, and (2) a truncated trajectory (the second half part of a given trajectory) which models the transition from small/moderate magnitudes (half apex of the expression) to high magnitudes (apex of the expression). Figure 2 shows the half apex and apex facial configurations for three expressions: surprise, anger, and joy.

In the remainder of this section, we will present two kinds of dynamic recognition schemes:

(1) the first kind is based on conditional predictive models and on an analysis-synthesis scheme, and (2) the second kind is based on examples.

An Analysis-Synthesis Scheme

Facial Action Dynamic Models

Corresponding to each basic expression class, γ, there is a stochastic dynamic model describing the temporal evolution of the facial actions $\tau_{a(t)}$, given the expression. It is assumed to be a Markov model of order K. For each basic expression γ, we associate a Gaussian Auto-Regressive Process defined by:

$$\tau_{a(t)} = \sum_{k=1}^{K} A_k^\gamma \tau_{a(t-k)} + d^\gamma + B^\gamma w_t \qquad (3)$$

in which $\mathbf{w}_t$ is a vector of 6 independent random $N(0,1)$ variables. The parameters of the dynamic model are: (1) deterministic parameters $A_1^\gamma, A_2^\gamma, ..., A_K^\gamma$ and $\mathbf{d}^\gamma$, and (2) stochastic parameters $\mathbf{B}^\gamma$ which are multipliers for the stochastic process $\mathbf{w}_t$. It is worth noting that the above model can be used in predicting the process from the previous K values. The predicted value at time t obeys a multivariate Gaussian centered at the deterministic value of (3), with $\mathbf{B}^\gamma\mathbf{B}^{\gamma T}$ being its covariance matrix. In our study, we are interested

in second-order models, i.e. $K = 2$. The reason is twofold. First, these models are easy to estimate. Second, they are able to model complex dynamics. For example, these models have been used in [6] for learning the 2D motion of talking lips (profile contours), beating heart, and writing fingers.

Given a training sequence $\tau_{a(1)},...,\tau_{a(T)}$, with $T > 2$, belonging to the same expression, it is well known that a Maximum Likelihood Estimator provides a closed-form solution for the model parameters (Blake & Isard, 2000). For a second-order model, these parameters reduce to two 6X6 matrices A_1^γ, A_2^γ, a 6-vector $\mathbf{d}^\gamma$, and a 6X6 covariance matrix $\mathbf{C}^\gamma = \mathbf{B}^\gamma\mathbf{B}^{\gamma T}$. Therefore, Equation (3) reduces to:

$$\tau_{a(t)} = A_2^\gamma \tau_{a(t-2)} + A_1^\gamma \tau_{a(t-1)} + d^\gamma + B^\gamma w_t \qquad (4)$$

The parameters of each auto-regressive model can be computed from temporal *facial action* sequences. Ideally, the temporal sequence should contain several instances of the corresponding expression.

More details about auto-regressive models and their computation can be found in (Blake & Isard, 2000; Ljung, 1987; North et al., 2000). Each universal expression has its own second-order auto-regressive model given by Equation (4). However, the dynamics of facial actions associ-

Figure 1. Three examples (sequences) of learned facial action parameters as a function of time

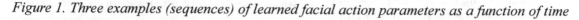

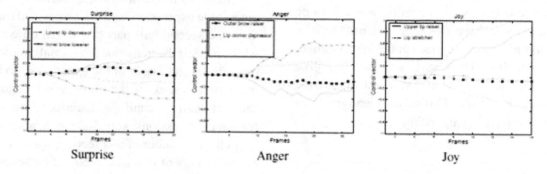

Surprise   Anger   Joy

Figure 2. Three video examples associated with the CMU database depicting surprise, anger, and joy expressions. The left frames illustrate the half apex of the expression. The right frames illustrate the apex of the expression.

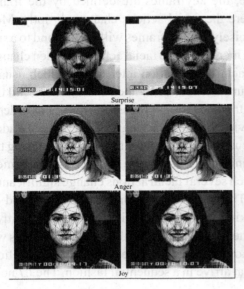

ated with the neutral expression can be simpler and are given by: $\tau_{a(t)} = \tau_{a(t-1)} + Dw_t$, where **D** is a diagonal matrix whose elements represent the variances around the ideal neutral configuration $\tau_a = 0$. The right-hand side of the above equation is constrained to belong to a predefined interval, since a neutral configuration and expression is characterized by both the lack of motion and the closeness to the ideal static configuration.

Recognition

We infer the facial expression in videos by considering the vectors $\tau_{a(t)}$ within a temporal window of size T centred at the current frame t. These vectors are provided by the 3D face tracker. The expression for frame t is recognized using the following two steps. First, we locally synthesize the facial actions, $\hat{\tau}_{a(i)}$, frame by frame using all auto-regressive models and the actual tracked facial actions. For this purpose, we utilize the deterministic part of (3) with two previous actual values. Second, the model providing the smallest prediction error over the sliding temporal window will decide the classification. In other words, we minimize the predication error

$$\sum_{i=t-\frac{T}{2}-1}^{t+\frac{T}{2}} \left\| \hat{\tau}_{a(i)} - \tau_{a(i)} \right\|^2$$ where $\hat{\tau}_{a(i)}$ are the synthesized actions and $\tau_{a(i)}$ are the actual actions.

Performance Evaluation

In order to quantify the recognition rate of the proposed approach, we have used the 35 CMU videos as test videos and have used our home made videos for building the auto-regressive models. These videos depict one subject performing several instances for each universal expression. Table 1 shows the confusion matrix associated with the 35 test videos. As can be seen, although the recognition rate was good (80%), it was not very close to 100%. This is explained by the fact that the

Table 1. Confusion matrix for the AR models based facial expression classifier associated with 35 test videos (CMU data)

	Surprise	Sadness	Joy	Disgust	Anger
Surprise	7	0	0	0	0
Sadness	0	7	0	5	0
Joy	0	0	7	0	0
Disgust	0	0	0	2	2
Anger	0	0	0	0	5

expression dynamics is highly person-dependent. The results of Table 1 were obtained when the size of the temporal window T was set to 11 frames. The conducted experiments have shown that any value belonging to the interval [9-15] has given good and similar recognition rates.

Example Based Schemes

The training temporal trajectories (the CMU sequences) can be used as examples allowing new trajectories associated with unseen persons and videos to be classified at running time. For this purpose, we use three different machine learning techniques: Linear Discriminant Analysis (LDA), Non-parametric Discriminant Analysis (NDA) and Support Vector Machines (SVM) (Shawe-Taylor & Cristianini, 2000). For LDA and NDA, the classification was based on the K Nearest Neighbor rule (KNN). We considered the following cases: K=1, 3 and 5. The SVM schemes adopts a radial basis kernel.

Since we use classic machine learning approaches that are data driven, the learned examples should have the same dimension. Therefore, all training trajectories are aligned using the Dynamic Time Warping technique by fixing a nominal duration for a facial expression. In our experiments, this nominal duration is set to 18 frames. The corresponding recognition results are given in Section 6.

EFFICIENT DETECTION AND RECOGNITION

In this section, we propose a fast and simple paradigm able to detect and recognize facial expression in continuous videos without having to apply the above recognition scheme to every frame in the video. Instead, the dynamic framework is applied only on the detected keyframes. This paradigm can also be used by a static recognition framework. This paradigm has two advantages. First, the CPU time corresponding to the recognition part will be considerably reduced. Second, since a keyframe and its surrounding frames are characterizing the expression, the discrimination performance of the recognition scheme will be boosted. In our case, the keyframes are defined by the frames where the facial actions change abruptly. More precisely, the keyframes will correspond to a sudden increase in the facial actions (sudden changes in facial deformation intensities), which usually occurs in a neutral-to-apex transition. Recall that the tracker should process all frames in order to provide the time-varying facial actions. We adopt a heuristic definition for the keyframe. Using this definition, this keyframe is forced to be a frame at which several facial actions change significantly.

Therefore, a keyframe can be detected by looking for a local maximum in the derivatives of the *facial actions*. To this end, two entities will be computed from the sequence of facial actions τ_a that arrive in a sequential fashion. The *L1* norm $\|\tau_a\|_1$ and the first derivative $\frac{\partial \tau_a}{\partial t}$. The i-th component of this vector $\frac{\partial \tau_{a(i)}}{\partial t}$ is given using the values associated with four frames:

$$\frac{\partial \tau_{a(i)}}{\partial t} = 2\left(\tau_{a(i)_{(t+1)}} - \tau_{a(i)_{(t-1)}}\right) + \tau_{a(i)_{(t+2)}} - \tau_{a(i)_{(t-2)}} \tag{5}$$

where the subscript i stands for i-th component of the **facial action** vector τ_a. Since we are interested in detecting the largest variation in the neutral-to-apex transition, we use the temporal derivative of $\|\tau_a\|_1$:

$$D_t = \frac{\partial \|\tau_a\|_1}{\partial t} \tag{6}$$

$$= \sum_{i=1}^{6} \frac{\partial \tau_{a(i)}}{\partial t} \tag{7}$$

In (7), we have used the fact that the facial actions are positive. Let W be the size of a temporal segment defining the temporal granulometry of the system. In other words, the system will detect and recognize at most one expression every W frames. The parameter W controls the rate of the recognition outputs. It does not intervene in the classification process. If one is only interested in detecting and recognizing all the subject's facial expressions, W should be small in order not to skip any displayed expression. In this case, the minimum value should correspond to the duration of the fastest expression (in our case, this was set to 15 frames ≈ 0.5 seconds). On the other hand, when a machine or a robot should react online according to the subject's facial expression W should be large so that the machine can achieve the actions before receiving a new command. In this case, skipping some expressions is allowed.

The whole scheme is depicted in Figure 3. In this figure, we can see that the system has three levels: the tracking level, the keyframe detection level, and the recognition level. The tracker provides the facial actions for every frame and

Figure 3. Efficient detection and recognition based on keyframes

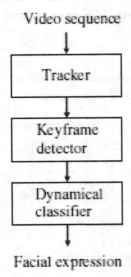

Video sequence

Tracker

Keyframe detector

Dynamical classifier

Facial expression

whenever the current video segment size reaches W frames, the keyframe detection is invoked to select a keyframe in the current segment if any. A given frame is considered as a keyframe if it meets three conditions: (1) the corresponding D_t is a positive local maximum (within the segment), (2) the corresponding norm $\left\| \tau_a \right\|_1$ is greater than a predefined threshold, (3) it's far from the previous keyframe by at least W frames. Once a keyframe is found in the current segment, the dynamical classifier (or static classifier) described in the previous sections will be invoked, that is, the temporal window will be centered on the detected keyframe. Adopting the above three conditions is justified by the following facts. The first one is to make sure that the chosen frame corresponds well to a significant facial deformation. The second one is to make sure that the chosen keyframe does not correspond to a small facial deformation (excluding quasi-neutral frames at which the derivatives can be local maxima). The third one is to avoid a large number of detected expressions per unit of time. Every facial action component $\tau_{a(i)}$ is normalized: a zero value corresponds to a neutral configuration and a one value corresponds to a maximum deformation. Thus, the $L1$ norm of the vector encoding these facial actions can be used to decide whether the current frame is a neutral frame or not. In our implementation we used a threshold of 1. A small threshold may lead to the detection of many keyframes since the derivatives have local maxima even for very small facial deformations. On the other hand, many keyframes cannot be detected if one adopts a large threshold. Based on experimental measurements, the $L1$ norm associated with the apex configurations for all universal expressions is between 2 and 3.5.

Figure 4 shows the results of applying the proposed detection scheme on a 1600-frame sequence containing 23 played expressions. For this 1600-frame test video, we asked our subject to adopt arbitrarily different facial gestures and expressions for an arbitrary duration and in an arbitrary order. In this video, there is always a neutral face between two expressions. The solid curve corresponds to the norm $\|\tau_a\|_1$, the dotted curve to the derivative D_t, and the vertical bars correspond to the detected keyframes. In this example, the value of W is set to 30 frames. As can be seen, out of 1600 frames only 23 keyframes will be processed by the expression classifier.

Figure 5 shows the results of applying the proposed scheme on a 300-frame sequence. The video contained nine arbitrary displayed expressions performed by a researcher. Some of the displayed expressions has a long duration coupled with a facial deformation. This explain why the detected keyframes are ten.

PERFORMANCE EVALUATION AND METHOD COMPARISONS

In our experiments, we used a subset from the CMU facial expression database, containing 7 persons who are displaying 5 expressions: surprise, sadness, joy, disgust and anger. For training and testing we used the truncated trajectories, that is, the temporal sequence containing 9 frames, with the first frame representing a "subtle" facial expression (corresponding more or less with a "half apex" state, see the left column of Figure 2) and the last one corresponding to the apex state

of the facial expression (see the right column of Figure 2). We decided to remove in our analysis the first few frames (from initial "neutral" state to "half-apex") since we found them irrelevant for the purposes of the current study.

In the previous section, we have described several methods for dynamic facial expression recognition. The extracted facial actions in video sequences can also be used in a *static recognition* fashion. This static recognition scheme uses the facial actions associated with only one single frame. In this case, the training examples correspond to single frames. Once again we use the classification schemes: Linear Discriminant Analysis (LDA), Non-parametric Discriminant Analysis (NDA) and Support Vector Machines (SVM).

Since we aim at studying and analyzing subtle facial expressions, we have used three kinds of training examples that are retrieved from the same training data set: (1) apex frames, (2) half apex frames, and (3) all frames associated with a given expression (trajectory).

It is worth noting that the static recognition scheme will use the facial actions associated with only one single frame, that is, the dimension of the feature vector is 6. However, the dynamic classifier use the concatenation of facial actions within a temporal window, that is, the feature vector size is $6 \times n$ where n is the number of frames within the temporal window. In the sequel, n is set to 9.

Figure 4. Keyframe detection and recognition applied on a 1600-frame sequence

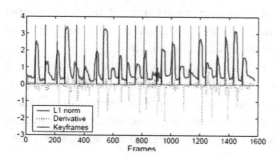

Figure 5. Keyframe detection and recognition applied on a 300-frame sequence

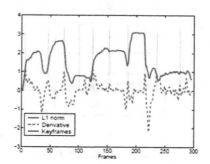

Classification Results Using the CMU Data

The results reported in this section are based on the "leave-one-out" cross-validation strategy. As mentioned earlier, several machine learning techniques have been tested: Linear Discriminant Analysis (LDA), Non-parametric Discriminant Analysis (NDA) and Support Vector Machines (SVM). For LDA and NDA, the classification was based on the K Nearest Neighbor rule (KNN) where the following cases were considered K=1, 3 and 5.

In order to assess the benefit of using temporal information, we performed also the "static" facial expression recognition. Three static classifier schemes have been adopted. In the first scheme, training and test data are associated to the apex frames. In the second scheme, training and test data are associated to the half-apex frames. In the third schemes, we considered all the training frames in the 9-frame sequence belonging to the same facial expression, but with different magnitudes. However, during testing every frame is recognized individually and the recognition rate concerns the recognition of individual frames.

The whole results (dynamic and static) for LDA and NDA are reported in Table 2 and Table 3, respectively. The SVM results for the dynamic classifier are reported in Table 4. The kernel was a radial basis function. Thus, the SVM used has two parameters to tune 'C' and 'g' (gamma). In general, gamma is taken as the inverse of the feature dimension, that is, it is set to $1/dim(vector)=1/54$ for the dynamic classifier and to $1/dim(vector)=1/6$

for the static classifier. In this case we wanted to see how the variation of the parameters 'C' (cost) affects the recognition performance. We considered 7 values for 'C'. Table 5 shows the confusion matrix associated with a given "leave-one-out" for the dynamic classifier using SVM.

To conclude this part of the experimental results, we could say that, in general, the dynamic recognition scheme has outperformed all static recognition schemes. Moreover, we found out that the SVM clearly outperforms LDA and NDA in classification accuracy. Moreover, by inspecting the recognition results obtained with SVM we can observe that the dynamic classifiers and the static classifiers based on the apex frames are slightly more accurate than the static classifiers (half-apex) and (all frame) (third and fourth columns of Table 4). This can be explained by the fact that these static classifiers are testing separately individual frames that may not contain high magnitude facial actions.

Cross-check Validation for the Static Classifier Using the CMU Data

Besides the experiments described above, we performed also a cross-check validation. In the first experiment, we trained the static classifier with the frames corresponding to half-apex expression and use the apex frames for test. We refer to this case as 'minor' static classifier. In a second experiment, we trained the classifier with the apex frames and test it using the half-apex frames ('major' static classifier). The results for LDA, NDA and SVM are presented in the Table

Table 2. LDA–Overall classification results for the dynamic and static classifiers

Classifier type	K=1	K=3	K=5
Dynamic	94.2857%	88.5714%	82.8517%
Static (apex)	91.4286%	91.4286%	88.5714%
Static (half-apex)	85.7143%	82.8571%	80.0000%
Static (all frames)	84.1270%	91.4286%	89.5238%

Table 3. NDA–Overall classification results for the dynamic and static classifiers

Classifier type	K=1	K=3	K=5
Dynamic	88.5714%	88.5714%	85.7143%
Static (apex)	85.7143%	88.5714%	91.4286%
Static (half-apex)	82.8571%	80.0000%	80.0000%
Static (all frames)	90.7937%	90.1587%	91.1111%

Table 4. SVM–Overall classification results for the dynamic and static classifiers

C	Dynamic	Apex	Half-apex	All frames
1	91.4285%	82.8571%	82.8571%	90.4761%
5	94.2857%	97.1428%	82.8571%	87.9364%
10	97.1428%	100.0000%	85.7142%	88.8888%
50	100.0000%	94.2857%	94.2857%	86.6666%
100	97.1428%	94.2857%	94.2857%	86.3491%
500	97.1428%	94.2857%	94.2857%	87.3015%
1000	97.1428%	94.2857%	91.4285%	88.5714%

Table 5. Confusion matrix for the dynamic classifier. The results correspond to the case when C=1

	Surprise	Sadness	Joy	Disgust	Anger
Surprise (7)	7	0	0	0	0
Sadness (7)	0	6	0	1	0
Joy (7)	0	0	7	0	0
Disgust (7)	0	0	0	7	0
Anger (7)	0	1	1	1	4

6, Table 7 and Table 8, respectively. By analyzing the obtained results, we could observe that the 'minor' static classifier has comparable results to the static half apex classifier. This was confirmed by the three classification methods: LDA, NDA, and SVM. This means that a learning based on data featuring half apex expressions will have very good generalization capabilities since the tests with both kinds of data (half-apex and apex expressions) have a high recognition rate. Also, one can notice that the recognition rate of the minor static classifier is higher than that of the major static classifier.

This result may have very practical implications assuming that training data contain non-apex expressions, specially for real-world applications. In human-computer interaction scenarios, for instance, we are interested in quantifying human reaction based on its natural behaviour. For this reason, we have to acquire and process data online without any external intervention. In this context, it is highly unlikely to capture automatically a person's apex of the facial expression. Most of the time we are tempted to show more subtle versions of our expressions and when we indeed show apex, this is in very specific situations and for very brief periods of time.

Table 6. LDA–Cross-check validation results for the static classifier. Minor: train with half- apex frames and test with apex. Major: train with apex frames and test with half-apex.

Static classifier	K=1	K=3	K=5
Minor	82.8571%	85.7143%	85.7143%
Major	57.1429%	65.7143%	62.8571%

Table 7. NDA–Cross-check validation results for the static classifier. Minor: train with half- apex frames and test with apex. Major: train with apex frames and test with half-apex.

Static classifier	K=1	K=3	K=5
Minor	94.2857%	88.5714%	85.7143%
Major	65.7143%	62.6571%	60.0000%

Table 8. SVM–Cross-check validation results for the static classifier. Minor: train with halfapex frames and test with apex. Major: train with apex frames and test with half-apex.

C	Minor	Major
1	80.0000%	48.5714%
5	80.0000%	60.0000%
10	85.7142%	51.4286%
50	85.7142%	45.7142%
100	80.0000%	48.5714%
500	82.8571%	48.5714%
1000	82.8571%	48.5714%

Recognition Using a Large Data Set

In order to evaluate the performance of the proposed recognition schemes with a large data set we proceed as follows. We generate 350 synthetic sequences from the existing 35 sequences by exploiting the convexity principle that states that each example can be approximated by a given linear combination of two real examples. This process is commonly used in machine learning for enlarging the size of the training data set.

In our implementation, a synthetic sequence is reconstructed by a random linear combination of two real sequences chosen at random. The sequence is then perturbed by a Gaussian noise. This will give a data set of 350 synthetic sequences. For training we used the original CMU sequences,

and for test we used the synthetic ones. The recognition results associated with LDA, NDA, and SVM are summarize in Table 9[1]. As can be seen the recognition rates are slightly better than those obtained with small data sets.

Dynamic vs. Static Recognition on Non-Aligned Videos

In order to assess the robustness of our method, we also used three arbitrary video sequences. The shortest one has 300 frames and the longest one has 1600 frames. Figure 6 shows four snapshots associated with the second test video sequence. Figure 7 shows eight snapshots associated with the third test video sequence. These sequences depicted unseen subjects displaying a variety of

Table 9. Recognition rate based on the LDA, NDA, and SVM classifiers applied to the large data set. The training was based on the CMU data and the synthetic data was used for test.

Classifier type	Recognition rate
LDA	90.5714%
NDA	91.7143%
SVM	98.0000%

different facial expressions. For training, we employed all the videos from the CMU database used in the previous sections. It is worth mentioning that the CMU videos and these three test videos are recorded at different frame rates. Moreover, the displayed expressions are not so similar to those included in the CMU data.

We compare the recognized expressions by the static and dynamic classifiers with the ground truth displayed expressions. Since the test videos are not segmented, we perform the dynamic and static recognition only at some specific frames of the test videos. These keyframes correspond to significant facial deformations and are detected using the heuristic described in Section 5. These keyframes does not correspond to a specific frame in the time domain (onset, apex, offset of the expression). As a result of this, the task of the dynamic classifier will be very hard since the temporal window of 9 frames centred at this detected keyframe will be matched against the learned aligned trajectories. The static recognizer will not be so affected since the recognition is based on comparing the attributes of the individual detected keyframe with those of a set of learned individual frames depicting several amplitudes of the expression.

In the Table 10 and Table 11, we present the results for the dynamic and static classifiers, respectively. The static scheme has outperformed the dynamic scheme for these three sequences. This confirms that the dynamic classifiers need better temporal alignment. As can be seen, the recognition rates obtained with both recognition schemes are lower than those obtained with a cross validation test based on the same database. This is due to the fact that the test was performed only on two subjects displaying arbitrary facial expressions.

DISCUSSION

This chapter provided a set of recent techniques that perform efficient facial expression recognition from video sequences. More precisely, we described two texture- and view-independent frameworks for facial expression recognition given natural head motion. While the first framework implicitly models non-apex and subtle facial expressions, the second framework can do the same provided that the training examples include such occurrences.

The chapter presented many evaluations for the case of dynamic and static classifiers, respectively.

Figure 6. Four snapshots from the second test video sequence

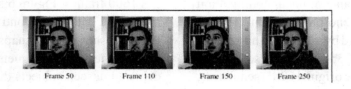

| Frame 50 | Frame 110 | Frame 150 | Frame 250 |

Figure 7. Eight snapshots from the third test video sequence (a 748-frame sequence)

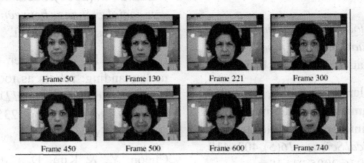

The recognition rate of the dynamic classifier is directly related to the displayed expressions. However, the recognition rate of the static classifier is related to the individual annotated frames within a video sequence. Moreover, the chapter presented an efficient scheme for dynamic facial expression recognition that relies on the detection of keyframes in video sequences.

In general, the dynamic classifier outperforms the static classifier. However, in some particular cases, the static classifier may give more accurate results than the dynamic one. One reason for this is that the generalization of the static classifier (recognizing inter-person expressions) is more significant than that of the dynamic classifier.

The proposed methods lend themselves nicely to many applications in the domain of Human Robot Interaction, in which a robot (for instance a humanoid robot) is acting according to the user's recognized facial expression. Future works can address the dynamic expression recognition by using both shape and textures dynamics.

ACKNOWLEDGMENT

B. Raducanu is supported by the CONSOLIDER-INGENIO 2010 (CSD2007-00018), Ministerio de Educación y Ciencia, Spain. The authors thank Dr. Franck Davoine from CNRS, Compiegne, France, for providing some video sequences.

Table 10. Recognition results for the dynamic classifier on extended sequences

Sequence name	LDA	NDA	SVM
Data_1	43.4783%	34.7826%	60.8696%
Data_2	60.0000%	40.0000%	60.0000%
Data_3	61.1111%	55.5556%	66.6667%

Table 11. Recognition results for the static classifier on the three arbitrary sequences. We considered only the keyframes

Sequence name	LDA	NDA	SVM
Data_1	69.5652%	65.2174%	65.2174%
Data_2	80.0000%	80.0000%	60.0000%
Data_3	66.6667%	66.6667%	72.2222%

REFERENCES

Ahlberg, J. (2002). *Model-based coding: extraction, coding and evaluation of face model parameters.* Doctoral dissertation, Linköping University.

Ambadar, Z., Schooler, J., & Cohn, J. (2005). Deciphering the enigmatic face: the importance of facial dynamics to interpreting subtle facial expressions. *Psychological Science, 16*(5), 403–410. doi:10.1111/j.0956-7976.2005.01548.x

Bartlett, M., Littlewort, G., Lainscsek, C., Fasel, I., & Movellan, J. (2004, October 10-13). Machine learning methods for fully automatic recognition of facial expressions and facial actions. In *Proceedings of IEEE. International. Conference on Systems, Man and Cybernetics (SMC 2004)*, The Hague, The Netherlands (Vol. 1, pp. 592–597). Washington, DC: IEEE Press.

Bartneck, C., & Reichenbach, J. (2005). Subtle emotional expressions of synthetic characters. *International Journal of Human-Computer Studies, 62*(2), 179–192. doi:10.1016/j.ijhcs.2004.11.006

Black, M. J., & Yacoob, Y. (1997). Recognizing facial expressions in images sequences using local parameterized models of image motion. *International Journal of Computer Vision, 25*(1), 23–48. doi:10.1023/A:1007977618277

Blake, A., & Isard, M. (2000). *Active Contours.* Berlin, Germany: Springer.

Bould, E., Morris, N., & Wink, B. (2008). Recognising subtle emotional expressions: The role of facial movements. *Cognition and Emotion, 22*(8), 1569–1587. doi:10.1080/02699930801921156

Breazeal, C. (1999, May 1). Robot in society: friend or appliance? In *Proceedings of Workshop on Emotion-Based Agent Architectures (EBAA 1999)*, Seattle, Washington, USA. New York: ACM Press.

Breazeal, C. (2000). *Sociable machines: Expressive social exchange between humans and robots.* Doctoral dissertation, MIT.

Cañamero, L., & Gaussier, P. (2005). Emotion understanding: robots as tools and models . In Nadel, J. (Eds.), *Emotional Development: Recent Research Advances* (pp. 235–258). New York: Oxford University Press.

Cheon, Y., & Kim, D. (2009). Natural facial expression recognition using differential-AAM and manifold learning. *Pattern Recognition, 42*, 1340–1350. doi:10.1016/j.patcog.2008.10.010

Cohen, I., Sebe, N., Garg, A., Chen, L., & Huang, T. S. (2003). Facial expression recognition from video sequences: temporal and static modelling. *Computer Vision and Image Understanding, 91*(1-2), 160–187. doi:10.1016/S1077-3142(03)00081-X

Dornaika, F., & Davoine, F. (2005, September 11-14). View- and texture-independent facial expression recognition in videos using dynamic programming. In *Proceedings of IEEE International Conference on Image Processing (ICIP 2005)*, Genoa, Italy (pp. 1-4). Washington DC: IEEE Press.

Dornaika, F., & Davoine, F. (2006). On appearance based face and facial action tracking. *IEEE Transactions on Circuits and Systems for Video Technology, 16*(9), 1107–1124. doi:10.1109/TCSVT.2006.881200

Dornaika, F., & Raducanu, B. (2007). Inferring facial expressions from videos: Tool and application. *Signal Processing Image Communication, 22*(9), 769–784. doi:10.1016/j.image.2007.06.006

Ekman, P. (1992). Facial expressions of emotions: an old controversy and new findings. *Philosophical Transactions of the Royal Society of London, 335*, 63–69. doi:10.1098/rstb.1992.0008

Ekman, P. (1993). Facial expression and emotion. *The American Psychologist*, *48*(4), 384–392. doi:10.1037/0003-066X.48.4.384

Ekman, P., & Davidson, R. (1994). *The nature of emotion: fundamental questions*. New York: Oxford University Press.

Fasel, B., & Luettin, J. (2003). Automatic facial expression analysis: a survey. *Pattern Recognition*, *36*(1), 259–275. doi:10.1016/S0031-3203(02)00052-3

Goneid, A., & Elkaliouby, R. (2002, September 9-12). Facial feature analysis of spontaneous facial expression. In *Proceedings of International Conference on Artificial Intelligence Applications (AIA 2002)*, Malaga, Spain. New York: ACTA Press.

Kanade, T., Cohn, J., & Tian, Y. L. (2000, March 28-30). Comprehensive database for facial expression analysis. In *Proceedings of International Conference on Automatic Face and Gesture Recognition (AFGR 2000)*, Grenoble, France (pp. 46-53). Washington, DC: IEEE Press.

Kim, Y., Lee, S., Kim, S., & Park, G. (2004, September 22-24). A fully automatic system recognizing human facial expressions. In M. Negoita et al. (Eds.), *Proceedings of the 8th International Conference on Knowledge-Based Intelligent Information and Engineering Systems (KES 2006)*, Wellington, New Zealand (LNCS 3215, pp. 203–209).

Ljung, L. (1987). *System Identification: Theory for the User*. Upper Saddle River, NJ: Prentice Hall.

North, B., Blake, A., Isard, M., & Rittscher, J. (2000). Learning and classification of complex dynamics. *IEEE Transactions on Pattern Analysis and Machine Intelligence*, *22*(9), 1016–1034. doi:10.1109/34.877523

Pantic, M. (2005). Affective computing. In Pagani, M. (Eds.), *Encyclopedia of Multimedia Technology and Networking* (*Vol. 1*, pp. 8–14). Hershey, PA: Idea Group Publishing.

Park, S., & Kim, D. (2009). Subtle facial expression recognition using motion magnification. *Pattern Recognition Letters*, *30*(7), 708–716. doi:10.1016/j.patrec.2009.02.005

Picard, R. (1997). *Affective computing*. Cambridge, MA: MIT Press.

Picard, R. W., Vyzas, E., & Healy, J. (2001). Toward machine emotional intelligence: Analysis of affective physiological state. *IEEE Transactions on Pattern Analysis and Machine Intelligence*, *23*(10), 1175–1191. doi:10.1109/34.954607

Reilly, J., Ghent, J., & McDonald, J. (2006, November 6-8). Investigating the dynamics of facial expression. In G. Bebis et al. (Eds.), *Advances in Visual Computing: Proc. of the Second International Symposium on Visual Computing (ISVC 2006)*, Lake Tahoe, Nevada, USA (LNCS 4292, pp, 334-343).

Shan, C., Gong, S., & McOwan, P. W. (2006, September 4-7). Dynamic facial expression recognition using a bayesian temporal manifold model. In *Proceedings of British Machine Vision Conference (BMVC 2006)*, Edinburgh, United Kingdom (Vol. 1, pp. 297–306). New York: BMVA Press.

Shawe-Taylor, J., & Cristianini, N. (2000). *Support Vector Machines and Other Kernel-based Learning Methods*. Cambridge, UK: Cambridge University Press.

Song, M., Wang, H., Bu, J., Chen, C., & Liu, Z. (2006, October 8-11). Subtle facial expression modelling with vector field decomposition. In *Proceedings of IEEE International Conference on Image Processing (ICIP 2006)*, Atlanta, Georgia, USA (Vol. 1, pp. 2101-2104). Washington, DC: IEEE Press

Sung, J., Lee, S., & Kim, D. (2006, August 20-24). A real-time facial expression recognition using the staam. In *Proceedings of IEEE International Conference on Pattern Recognition (ICPR 2006)*, Hong Kong, PR China (Vol. 1, pp. 275–278). Washington, DC: IEEE Press

Tian, Y., Kanade, T., & Cohn, J. F. (2001). Recognizing action units for facial expression analysis. *IEEE Transactions on Pattern Analysis and Machine Intelligence, 23*, 97–115. doi:10.1109/34.908962

Xiang, T., Leung, M. K. H., & Cho, S. Y. (2008). Expression recognition using fuzzy spatiotemporal modelling. *Pattern Recognition, 41*(1), 204–216. doi:10.1016/j.patcog.2007.04.021

Yang, P., Liu, Q., & Metaxas, D. N. (2007, July 2-5). Facial expression recognition using encoded dynamic features. In *Proceedings of IEEE International Conference on Multimedia and Expo (ICME 2007)*, Beijing, PR China (Vol. 1, pp. 1107-1110). Washington, DC: IEEE Press.

Yeasin, M., Bullot, B., & Sharma, R. (2006). Recognition of facial expressions and measurement of levels of interest from video. *IEEE Transactions on Multimedia, 8*(3), 500–508. doi:10.1109/TMM.2006.870737

Yin, L., Chen, X., Sun, Y., Worm, T., & Reale, M. (2008, September 17-19). A high-resolution 3D dynamic facial expression database. In *Proceedings of IEEE International Conference on Automatic Face and Gesture Recognition (AFGR 2008)*, Amsterdam, The Netherlands. Washington, DC: IEEE Press

Zhang, Y., & Ji, Q. (2005). Active and dynamic information fusion for facial expression understanding from image sequences. *IEEE Transactions on Pattern Analysis and Machine Intelligence, 27*(5), 699–714. doi:10.1109/TPAMI.2005.93

Zheng, A. (2000) *Deconstructing motion* (Tech. Rep.). Berkeley, CA: U. C. Berkeley EECS department.

KEY TERMS AND DEFINITIONS

Facial Expression Recognition: Computer-driven application for automatically identifying person's facial expression from a digital still or video image. It does that by comparing selected facial features in the live image and a facial database.

Subtle Facial Expression: A magnitude of facial expression different from apex

Facial Actions: Invariant geometrical parameters which define the intensity of a given facial deformation

Static Recognition: A methodology to recognize objects and activities in single (static) images (snapshots)

Dynamic Recognition: A methodology to recognize objects and activities in videos based on their time-dependent features.

Face Tracker: An estimator of facial pose/appearance/expression parameters in every frame of a video sequence.

Keyframe: corresponds to a sudden increase in the facial actions (sudden changes in facial deformation intensities), which usually occurs in a neutral-to-apex transition.

3D Deformable Model: A model which is able to modify its shape while being acted upon by an external influence. In consequence, the relative position of any point on a deformable model can change.

Machine Learning: is concerned with the design and development of algorithms that allow computers to learn based on data, such as from sensor data or databases. A major focus of machine learning research is to automatically learn to recognize complex patterns and make intelligent decisions based on data

Human–Computer Interaction (HCI): The study of interaction between people (users) and computers. It is an interdisciplinary subject, relating computer science with many other fields of study and research (Artificial Intelligence, Psychology, Computer Graphics, Design).

ENDNOTE

[1] Several parameters relative to LDA, NDA and SVM have been tested, but only the best results are shown.

Section 6
Invariance Techniques

Chapter 15
Photometric Normalization Techniques for Illumination Invariance

Vitomir Štruc
University of Ljubljana, Slovenia

Nikola Pavešić
University of Ljubljana, Slovenia

ABSTRACT

Face recognition technology has come a long way since its beginnings in the previous century. Due to its countless application possibilities, it has attracted the interest of research groups from universities and companies around the world. Thanks to this enormous research effort, the recognition rates achievable with the state-of-the-art face recognition technology are steadily growing, even though some issues still pose major challenges to the technology. Amongst these challenges, coping with illumination-induced appearance variations is one of the biggest and still not satisfactorily solved. A number of techniques have been proposed in the literature to cope with the impact of illumination ranging from simple image enhancement techniques, such as histogram equalization, to more elaborate methods, such as anisotropic smoothing or the logarithmic total variation model. This chapter presents an overview of the most popular and efficient normalization techniques that try to solve the illumination variation problem at the preprocessing level. It assesses the techniques on the YaleB and XM2VTS databases and explores their strengths and weaknesses from the theoretical and implementation point of view.

INTRODUCTION

Current face recognition technology has evolved to the point where its performance allows for its deployment in a wide variety of applications. These applications typically ensure controlled conditions for the acquisition of facial images and,

DOI: 10.4018/978-1-61520-991-0.ch015

hence, minimize the variability in the appearance of different (facial) images of a given subject. Commonly controlled external factors in the image capturing process include ambient illumination, camera distance, pose and facial expression, etc.

In these controlled conditions, state-of-the-art face recognition systems are capable of achieving the performance level which can match that of the more established biometric modalities, such as fingerprints, as shown in a recent survey (Gross et al., 2004; Phillips et al., 2007). However, the majority of the existing face recognition techniques employed in these systems deteriorate in their performance when employed in uncontrolled environments. Appearance variations caused by pose-, expression-and most of all illumination-changes pose challenging problems even to the most advanced face recognition approaches. In fact, it was empirically shown that the illumination-induced variability in facial images is often larger than the variability induced by the subject's identity (Adini et al., 1997), or, to put it differently, images of different faces appear more similar than images of the same face captured under severe illumination variations.

Due to this susceptibility to illumination variations of the existing face recognition techniques, numerous approaches to achieve illumination invariant face recognition have been proposed in the literature. As identified in a number of surveys (Heusch et al., 2005; Chen, W., et al., 2006; Zou et al., 2007), three main research directions have emerged with respect to this issue over the past decades. These directions tackle the problem of illumination variations at either:

- The pre-processing level
- The feature extraction level
- The modeling and/or classification level

When trying to achieve illumination invariant face recognition at the pre-processing level, the employed normalization techniques aim at rendering facial images in such a way that the processed images are free of illumination induced facial variations. Clearly, these approaches can be adopted for use with any face recognition technique, as they make no presumptions that could influence the choice of the feature extraction or classification procedures.

Approaches from the second group try to achieve illumination invariance by finding face representations that are stable under different illumination conditions. However, as different studies have shown, there are no representations which would ensure illumination invariance in the presence of severe illumination changes, even though some representations, such as edge maps (Gao & Leung, 2002), local binary patterns (Marcel et al., 2007) or Gabor wavelet based features (Štruc & Pavešić, 2009), are less sensitive to the influence of illumination. The inappropriateness of the feature extraction stage for compensating for the illumination variations was also formally proven in (Chen et al., 2000).

The last research direction with respect to illumination invariance focuses on the modeling or classification level. Here, assumptions regarding the effects of illumination on the face model or classification procedure are made first and then based on these assumptions counter measures are taken to obtain illumination invariant face models or illumination insensitive classification procedures. Examples of these techniques include the illumination cones technique (Georghiades et al., 2001), the spherical harmonics approach (Basri & Jacobs, 2003) and others. While these techniques are amongst the most efficient ways of achieving illumination invariant face recognition, they usually require a large training set of facial images acquired under a number of lighting conditions and are also computationally expensive.

In this chapter, we focus on the (in our opinion) most feasible way of achieving illumination invariance, namely, exploiting techniques which compensate for the illumination changes during the pre-processing level. At this level, computationally simple and effective techniques for achieving illumination invariant face recognition can easily be devised.

BACKGROUND

Before we turn our attention to different preprocessing techniques proposed in the literature for illumination invariant face recognition, we need to establish a mathematical model explaining the principles of image formation, which is capable of forming the foundation for our pre-processing. To find a suitable model, researchers commonly turn to the Retinex theory presented by Land and McCann in (Land & McCann, 1971). The theory states that the human visual system is capable of correctly perceiving colors even in difficult illumination conditions by relying on the reflectance of the scene and in a way neglecting the scenes illumination. It suggests that an image of the scene can be modeled as follows:

$$I(x,y) = R(x,y)L(x,y) \qquad (1)$$

where $I(x,y)$ denotes an image of a scene, $R(x,y)$ denotes the reflectance and $L(x,y)$ stands for the illumination (or luminance) at each of the spatial positions (x,y). Here, the reflectance $R(x,y)$ is linked to the characteristics of the objects comprising the scene of an image and is dependent upon the reflectivity of the scenes surface (Short et al., 2004). The luminance $L(x,y)$, on the other hand, is determined by the illumination source and relates to the amount of illumination falling on the scene.

To produce illumination invariant versions of facial images, researchers try to estimate the reflectance $R(x,y)$ with the goal of adopting it as an illumination invariant representation of the face. Unfortunately, it is impossible to determine the reflectance of an image using Equation (1), unless some assumptions are made regarding the factors of the presented imaging model. The most commonly made assumptions are (Park et al., 2008):

- edges in the image $I(x,y)$ represent edges in the reflectance $R(x,y)$, and
- the luminance $L(x,y)$ changes slowly with the spatial position of the image $I(x,y)$.

To determine the reflectance of an image the luminance $L(x,y)$ is commonly estimated first. This estimate is then exploited to compute the reflectance $R(x,y)$ via the manipulation of the imaging model in (1). As we have already emphasized, the luminance is considered to vary slowly with the spatial position. It can, therefore, be estimated as a smoothed (i.e., low-pass filtered) version of the original image $I(x,y)$. Various smoothing filters have been proposed in the literature resulting in different normalization procedures that were successfully applied to the problem of illumination invariant face recognition. These (Retinex-based) normalization techniques have common advantages as they exhibit low computational complexity and impose no requirements for a special (generic or user-specific) training image set (Park et al., 2008).

Of course, other pre-processing techniques used for achieving illumination invariance can also be found in the literature. Some of these techniques are not based on the Retinex theory, but can easily be linked to the imaging model in (1), while others are concerned with image characteristics not linked solely to illumination variations. While we will refer to the latter group of techniques as image enhancement techniques, we will use the term photometric normalization technique for any approach based on (or related to) the imaging model in (1).

IMAGE ENHANCEMENT TECHNIQUES

Image enhancement techniques represent a group of pre-processing techniques that try to render the input images in such a way that the resulting enhanced images exhibit some predefined characteristics. These characteristics may include the dynamic range of the intensity values of the image, the shape of the images histogram, etc. While these techniques are often deployed to ensure at least some level of robustness to illumination changes,

Figure 1. Two examples of gamma intensity corrected images for two different gamma values

their primary goal is not illumination invariance. Nevertheless, various empirical studies have proven their usefulness for robust face recognition in the presence of illumination variations. Due to these characteristics, we will in this section briefly describe four different image enhancement techniques often used as preprocessing steps for face recognition.

Gamma Intensity Correction

Let us denote an arbitrary 8-bit face image of size $a \times b$ pixels as $I(x,y)$. The gamma intensity correction transforms the pixel intensity values at each spatial position (x,y), for $x=1, 2,\ldots, a$ and $y=1, 2,\ldots, b$, in accordance with the following expression (Gonzalez & Woods, 2002):

$$I_{gam}(x, y) = I(x, y)^{\gamma} \qquad (2)$$

where $I_{gam}(x,y)$ denotes the gamma intensity corrected face image $I(x,y)$, and γ stands for the gamma value which controls the type of the mapping. An example of the effect of different gamma values on the appearance of an image is presented in Figure 1. Here, the left pair of images shows an input face image and the gamma intensity corrected one for $\gamma=0.5$, while the right pair depicts a face image and the gamma intensity corrected image for $\gamma=4$.

Logarithmic Transform

Let us adopt the same notation as above correction and denote the input image to be enhanced as $I(x,y)$. The logarithmic transform non-linearly transforms the intensity values at each spatial position (x,y), for $x=1,2,\ldots,a$ and $y=1,2,\ldots,b$, according to the following expression (Gonzalez & Woods, 2002):

$$I_{log}(x, y) = \log[I(x, y)] \qquad (3)$$

where $I_{log}(x,y)$ denotes the logarithm transformed input image $I(x,y)$.

The logarithmic transform improves the contrast of darker image regions by making them lighter and consequently ensures some level of robustness to illumination changes, as shown in Figure 2.

Histogram Equalization

Let us assume that the image $I(x,y)$ is comprised of a total of N pixels with k grey-levels. Histogram equalization aims at transforming the distribution of the pixel intensity values of the input image $I(x,y)$ into a uniform distribution and consequently at improving the image's global contrast (Gonzalez & Woods, 2002; Štruc et al., 2009).

Formally, histogram equalization can be defined as follows: given the probability $p(i)=n_i/N$ of an occurrence of a pixel with the grey level of i, where n_i denotes the number of pixels with the grey-level of i in the image, the mapping from the

Figure 2. Impact of the logarithmic transform: original images (upper row), logarithm transformed images (lower row)

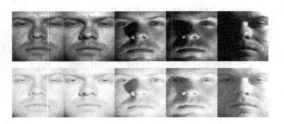

original intensity value i to the new transformed one i_{new} is given by (Heusch et al., 2005):

$$i_{new} = \sum_{j=0}^{i} \frac{n_j}{N} = \sum_{j=0}^{i} p(j) \tag{4}$$

A visual example of the effect of histogram equalization on the appearance of facial images is shown in Figure 3.

Note how applying histogram equalization improves the contrast of the facial images, but as seen on the last image of the lower row also greatly enhances the background noise contained in the image.

Histogram Remapping

More recently, Štruc et al. (Štruc et al., 2009) suggested that mapping a non-uniform distribution to facial images could also ensure robust face recognition in the presence of illumination changes. The authors' claim is based on the observation that while histogram equalization was empirically proven to provide enhanced face recognition performance when compared to unprocessed images, it still represents only a useful heuristic, which is a special case of the more general concept of histogram remapping techniques. With this class of techniques, the target distribution is not limited to the uniform distribution, but can rather represent an arbitrary one.

Figure 3. Impact of histogram equalization: original images (upper row), histogram equalized images (lower row)

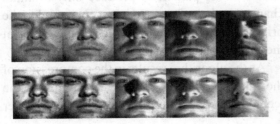

Independent of the choice of the target distribution, the procedure of mapping an arbitrary distribution to the pixel intensity values of a facial image always follows the same procedure. The first step is the transformation of the pixel intensity values using the rank transform. Here, each pixel value in the N-dimensional image $I(x,y)$ is replaced with the index (or rank) R that the pixel would correspond to if the pixel intensity values were ordered in an ascending manner. For example, the most negative pixel-value is assigned the rank of 1, while the most positive pixel-value is assigned the ranking of N. Once the rank R of each pixel is determined, the general mapping function to match the target distribution $f(x)$ may be calculated from (Gonzalez & Woods, 2002; Štruc & Pavešić, 2009):

$$\frac{N - R + 0.5}{N} = \int_{x=-\infty}^{t} f(x)dx \tag{5}$$

where the goal is to find t. Obviously, the right hand side represents the cumulative distribution function (CDF) of the target distribution. If we denote the CDF of the target distribution as $F(x)$ and the scalar value on the left as u, then the mapped value t can be determined by computing:

$$t = F^{-1}(u) \tag{6}$$

where F^{-1} denotes the inverse of the target distributions CDF.

To illustrate the effect of the histogram remapping technique on the appearance of a facial image, let us assume that our target distribution takes the following form:

$$f(x) = \frac{1}{\sigma\sqrt{2\text{Å}}} \frac{\exp(-(\ln x - \mu)^2 / 2\sigma^2)}{x} \tag{7}$$

where the parameters μ and σ>0 define the shape of the lognormal distribution. Though the parameters of the distribution can be chosen arbitrary, we choose the mean value μ=0 and standard deviation σ=0.4. These parameters result in (visually) properly normalized images as shown in Figure 4

PHOTOMETRIC NORMALIZATION TECHNIQUES

In this section, we introduce the most popular techniques based on the Retinex theory. We present their strengths and weaknesses and provide visual examples of their deployment on facial images.

The Single Scale Retinex Algorithm

The single scale Retinex technique (SR) is one of the straightforward approaches that can be derived from the imaging model defined by Equation (1). As proposed by Jobson et al. (Jobson et al., 1997a), the luminance and reflectance are first separated by taking the logarithm of the image, which results in the following expression:

$$\log I(x,y) = \log R(x,y) + \log L(x,y) \qquad (8)$$

If we denote the logarithm of the reflectance as $R'(x,y)$ and consider that the luminance $L(x,y)$ can be estimated as a blurred version of the input

Figure 4. Impact of histogram remapping using a lognormal distribution: original images (upper row), images with a remapped histogram (lower row)

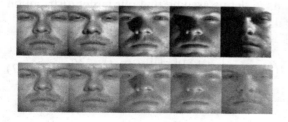

image $I(x,y)$, we can rearrange Equation (8) into the final form:

$$R'(x,y) = \log I(x,y) - \log\left[I(x,y) * K(x,y)\right] \qquad (9)$$

where "*" denotes the convolution operator, $K(x,y)$ denotes a smoothing kernel and $R'(x,y)$ stands for the illumination invariant reflectance output of the SR algorithm.

It has to be noted that, when implementing the SR algorithm, we first have to choose an appropriate smoothing kernel. Several options were presented in the literature (see, for example, (Moore et al., 1991)), one of the most prominent, however, was introduced by Jobson et al. in (Jobson et al., 1997a), where the smoothing kernel takes the form of a Gaussian:

$$K(x,y) = k \exp(-\frac{r^2}{c^2}) \qquad (10)$$

where $r=(x^2+y^2)^{1/2}$, c denotes a free parameter, and k is selected in such a way that

$$\iint K(x,y)dxdy = 1. \qquad (11)$$

Unfortunately, there are no rules on how to select the value of the parameter c. Instead, its value has to be determined through a trial and error procedure. Small values of the parameter c result in an extreme dynamic range compression of the intensity values of the images, while high values of the parameter produce only minimal changes in the reflectance when compared to the original image. Some examples of the effect of the SR algorithm are shown in Figure 5.

As the algorithm results in the compression of the images' dynamic range, the authors of the technique propose to clip the upper and lower parts of the histogram and rescale the remaining part of the histogram back to the 8-bit interval.

The Multiscale Retinex Algorithm

The multiscale Retinex algorithm (MR), proposed by Jobson et al. (Jobson et al., 1997b), is an extension of the SR approach presented in the previous section. While generally the SR technique produces good results with a properly selected Gaussian, there are still some shortcomings that limit a more extensive use of this normalization technique. The most significant issue not properly solved is halo affects, which are often visible at large illumination discontinuities. Such discontinuities are the result of strong shadows being cast over the face, which are in violation of one of the basic assumptions of the Retinex based techniques, namely, that the luminance varies slowly with the spatial position.

To avoid these difficulties, the authors of the MR technique proposed to use smoothing kernels of different sizes and combine the outputs of different SR implementations. Formally, the reflectance of a face image $I(x,y)$ using the MR technique is computed as:

$$R'(x,y) = \sum_{i=1}^{M} w_i \left(\log I(x,y) - \log\left[I(x,y) * K_i(x,y) \right] \right),$$

(12)

Figure 5. Impact of the single scale Retinex technique: original images (upper row), processed images (lower row)

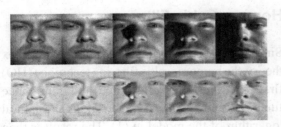

where $K_i(x,y)$ denotes a Gaussian kernel at the i-th scale, and w_i stands for the weight associated with the i-th Gaussian kernel $K_i(x,y)$. Note that the Gaussian kernels used for the smoothing are defined by the expressions (10) and (11). Some visual examples of the MR technique applied to facial images are shown in Figure 6.

The Single Scale Retinex Algorithm with Adaptive Smoothing

One of the latest modifications to the SR technique was presented by Park et al. in (Park et al., 2008). Here, the authors propose to tackle the halo effects often encountered with the original SR technique by incorporating an adaptive smoothing procedure with a discontinuity-preserving filter into the SR algorithm.

As stated by the authors, the key idea of adaptive smoothing is to iteratively convolve the input image $I(x,y)$ with the 3×3 averaging mask $w(x,y)$ whose coefficients reflect the discontinuity level of the input image at each of the spatial positions (x,y). Mathematically, the iterative smoothing procedure at the $(t+1)$-th iteration is given by

$$L^{(t+1)}(x,y) = \frac{1}{N^{(t)}(x,y)} \sum_{i=-1}^{1} \sum_{j=-1}^{1} L^{(t)}(x+i,y+j) w^{(t)}(x+i,y+j)$$

(13)

and

$$L^{(t+1)}(x,y) = \max \left\{ L^{(t+1)}(x,y), L^{(t)}(x,y) \right\},$$

(14)

where the normalizing factor $N^{(t)}(x,y)$ is defined as

$$N^{(t)}(x,y) = \sum_{i=-1}^{1} \sum_{j=-1}^{1} w^{(t)}(x+i,y+j)$$

(15)

Figure 6. Impact of the multiscale Retinex technique: original images (upper row), processed images (lower row)

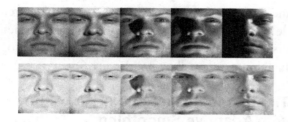

The global and the local discontinuity measures in form of the gradient magnitude and local in-homogeneity, respectively are exploited to determine the values of the adaptive averaging mask $w(x,y)$ at each of the spatial positions (x,y). First, the gradient magnitude is computed based on the following expression:

$$| \nabla I(x,y) |= \sqrt{G_x^2(x,y) + G_y^2(x,y)} \qquad (16)$$

where the partial derivatives are approximated as $G_x(x,y) = I(x+1,y) - I(x-1,y)$ and $G_y(x,y) = I(x,y+1) - I(x,y-1)$.

The second discontinuity measure, the local in-homogeneity $\tau(x,y)$, is defined as the average of local intensity differences at each spatial position (x,y):

$$\tau(x,y) = \frac{\sum\sum_{(m,n)\in\Omega} | I(x,y) - I(m,n) |}{|\Omega|} \qquad (17)$$

Here, Ω defines a 3×3 local neighborhood of the pixel location (x,y), and (m,n) indicates the locations of pixels in the local neighborhood Ω. Once the local in-homogeneity is determined, it is subjected to the following normalization procedure:

$$\tilde{\tau}(x,y) = \frac{\tau(x,y) - \tau_{min}}{\tau_{max} - \tau_{min}}, \qquad (18)$$

where τ_{max} and τ_{min} represent the maximal and minimal values of $\tau(x,y)$ across the entire face image. The final discontinuity measure is ultimately obtained by performing one last transformation that emphasizes the higher values of $\tilde{\tau}(x,y)$:

$$\hat{\tau}(x,y) = \sin[\frac{\text{Å}}{2}\tilde{\tau}(x,y)] \qquad (19)$$

The gradient magnitude and the transformed form of the local in-homogeneity are combined as $w(x,y)=\alpha(x,y)\beta(x,y)$ to produce the 3×3 averaging mask $w(x,y)$ for each spatial position (x,y). Here, $\alpha(x,y)$ and $\beta(x,y)$ denote the transformed discontinuity measures using the following conducting function:

$$g(d,k) = \frac{1}{1+\sqrt{d/k}} \qquad (20)$$

Finally, we have: $\alpha(x,y) = g(\hat{\tau}(x,y),h)$ and $\beta(x,y) = g(| \nabla I(x,y) |,S)$. Based on their empirical findings, the authors of the technique suggested to use between fifteen and twenty iterations to estimate the luminance function using equations (13) and (14) and to select the parameters of the conducting function somewhere in the range of $0\leq h\leq 0.1$ and $0\leq S\leq 10$. Similar to the SR technique, the final illumination invariant reflectance output is computed as:

$$R'(x,y) = \log I(x,y) - \log L(x,y) \qquad (21)$$

Some examples of facial images processed with the presented technique are shown in Figure 7.

Homomorphic Filtering

Similar to other techniques based on the Retinex theory, the homomorphic filtering technique (HO) first separates the reflectance and luminance functions of the image $I(x,y)$ by taking the natural logarithm of the model in (1). The result is then used as the starting point for the normalization procedure.

The second step of the technique represents the transformation of the image from the spatial to the frequency domain, which is achieved using the Fourier transform (Short et al., 2004):

$$F \{\log I(x,y)\}= F \{\log R(x,y)\}+F \{\log L(x,y)\} \tag{22}$$

The image can now be written as the sum of two functions in the frequency domain. The first contains mainly high frequency components and is the frequency equivalent of the spatial reflectance, the second function, on the other hand, is composed of low frequency components and corresponds to the spatial luminance. The Fourier transform of the input image $Z(u,v)= F \{\log I(x,y)\}$ can be filtered with the filter $H(u,v)$ that reduces the low frequencies and amplifies the high frequencies (Short et al., 2004). The final illumination invariant image $I'(x,y)$ is ultimately obtained by finding the inverse transform of the filtered image and taking its exponential, i.e.,

$$I'(x,y) =\exp\{ F^{-1}[H(u,v).Z(u,v)]\} \tag{23}$$

where ".." denotes the element-wise multiplication. Note that the result of this normalization procedure is a normalized image $I'(x,y)$ rather than the reflectance of the image since no direct subtraction of the luminance was performed. Nevertheless, the result still approximates the reflectance since the effect of the luminance was reduced and that of the reflectance emphasized through the filtering operation. Some visual examples of the effect of homomorphic filtering are shown in Figure 8.

The Self-quotient Image

Similar to the SR technique with adaptive smoothing, the self-quotient image (SQ) also represents a more recent addition to the group of photometric normalization techniques. Even though, originally not derived from the Retinex theory, the technique can be linked to the Retinex-based approaches.

The technique, proposed and presented by Wang et al. in (Wang et al., 2004), is based on a mathematical model similar to the one in Equation (1). Therefore, the illumination invariant image representation $Q(x,y)$ can be derived in the form of the quotient:

$$Q(x,y) = \frac{I(x,y)}{K(x,y) * I(x,y)} \tag{24}$$

where the nominator of the above expression denotes the original input image and the denominator represents the smoothed version of the input image. Like with the SR and MR approaches, $K(x,y)$ again represents a smoothing kernel.

The key element of the SQ technique, which distinguishes the procedure from other techniques

Figure 7. Impact of the single scale Retinex with adaptive smoothing technique: original images (upper row), processed images (lower row)

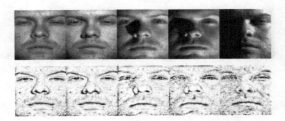

Figure 8. Impact of the homomorphic filtering technique: original images (upper row), processed images (lower row)

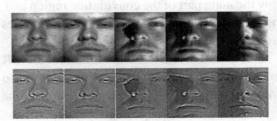

presented in the literature, is the structure of the smoothing kernel $K(x,y)$. For each convolution region, the kernel is modified using a weighting function, which is constructed as follows: first the mean value τ of the convolution region is computed, and based on this value, two non-overlapping regions (denoted as M_1 and M_2) are constructed (Heusch et al., 2005). Each pixel from the convolution region is then assigned to one of the two sub-regions M_1 and M_2 based on the following criterion (Wang et al., 2004):

$$I(x,y) \in \begin{cases} M_1, & \text{if } I(x,y) \leq \tau \\ M_2, & \text{if } I(x,y) > \tau \end{cases} \qquad (25)$$

Assuming that there are more pixels in M_1 than in M_2 then the weights of the weighting function for the Gaussian-smoothing filter $G(x,y)$ are given by:

$$W(i,j) = \begin{cases} 1, & \text{if } I(x,y) \in M_1 \\ 0, & \text{if } I(x,y) \in M_2 \end{cases} \qquad (26)$$

and the final smoothing kernel $K(x,y)$ is subject to the following condition:

$$\frac{1}{M}\sum_{\Omega} W(x,y).G(x,y) = \sum_{\Omega} K(x,y) = 1 \qquad (27)$$

In the above expressions, M denotes a normalizing factor, $G(x,y)$ represents the Gaussian kernel and Ω stands for the convolution region. As stated by the authors of the technique, the essence of the filter lies in the fact that it smoothes only the main part of the convolution region and, therefore, effectively preserves discontinuities present in the image.

Due to similar reasons as the authors of the MR technique, Wang et al. (Wang et al., 2004) also proposed to use different filter scales to produce the illumination invariant image representation. This multiscale form of the SQ technique is obtained by a simple summation of self-quotient images derived with different filter scales. As the final step, a non-linear (logarithm, sigmoid function, …) mapping is applied to the self-quotient image to compress the dynamic range. Some examples of the deployment of the SQ technique are shown in Figure 9.

DCT-Based Normalization

The discrete-cosine-transform-based (DCT) photometric normalization technique is a recently proposed technique introduced by Chen et al. in (Chen, W., at al., 2006). Like the majority of approaches presented in this chapter, the technique relies on the Retinex theory and, hence, makes similar assumptions about the characteristics of the illumination variations in the image.

The technique presumes that the illumination changes are related to the low frequency coefficients of the DCT transform and suggests discarding these low frequency coefficients before transforming the image back to the spatial domain via the inverse DCT (Chen, W., at al., 2006). To achieve illumination invariance, the DCT-based normalization takes the following steps: first, the technique takes the logarithm of the input image $I(x,y)$ to separate the reflectance and the luminance. Next, the entire image is transformed to the frequency domain via the DCT transform,

Figure 9. Impact of the self-quotient image technique: original images (upper row), processed images (lower row)

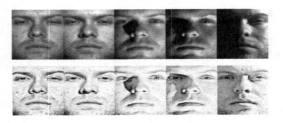

where the manipulation of the DCT coefficients takes place. Here, the first DCT coefficient $C(0,0)$ is assigned a value of:

$$C(0,0) = \log \mu \cdot \sqrt{MN} \qquad (28)$$

where M and N denote the dimensions of the input image $I(x,y)$ and μ is chosen near the mean value of $I(x,y)$.

A predefined number of DCT coefficients encoding the low-frequency information of the image are then set to zero. As the final step, the modified matrix of DCT coefficients is transformed back to the spatial domain via the inverse DCT to produce the illumination invariant representation of the image. Some examples of applying the described procedure to face images are presented in Figure 10.

It has to be noted that the authors of the technique suggest discarding between 18 and 25 DCT coefficients for the best recognition performance.

Wavelet-Based Image Denoising

A wavelet-based normalization technique was proposed by Zhang et al. in (Zhang et al., 2009). Here, the wavelet-based image denoising (WD) approach is exploited to obtain an illumination invariant representation of the facial image.

The technique starts with the imaging model of the Retinex theory given by (8). Under the

Figure 10. Impact of the DCT-based normalization technique: original images (upper row), processed images (lower row)

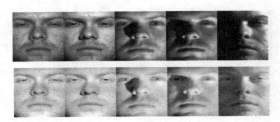

assumption that the key facial features are high frequency phenomena equivalent to "noise" in the image, the authors propose to estimate the luminance $L'(x,y)=\log L(x,y)$ by the wavelet denoising model and then to extract the illumination invariant reflectance $R'(x,y)=\log R(x,y)$ in accordance with Equation (22).

Let us denote the wavelet coefficient of the input image $I'(x,y)=\log I(x,y)$ as $X'(x,y)=W(I'(x,y))$, where W stands for the 2D DWT operator; and, similarly, let $Y(x,y)=W(L'(x,y))$ denote the matrix of wavelet coefficients of the luminance $L'(x,y)$. The estimate of the luminance in the wavelet domain $Y(x,y)$ is then obtained by modifying the detail coefficients of $X(x,y)$ using the so-called soft thresholding technique and keeping the approximation coefficients unaltered. Here, the soft thresholding procedure for each location (x,y) is defined as:

$$Y_s(x,y) = \begin{cases} X_s(x,y) - T, & \text{if } X_s(x,y) \geq T \\ X_s(x,y) + T, & \text{if } X_s(x,y) \leq T \\ 0, & \text{if } |X_s(x,y)| < T \end{cases}$$

$$(29)$$

where $X_s(x,y)$ denotes one of the three sub-bands generated by the detail DWT coefficients (either the low-high (LH), the high-low (HL) or the high-high (HH) sub-bands), $Y_s(x,y)$ stands for the corresponding soft thresholded sub-band and T represent a predefined threshold.

It is clear that for an efficient rendering of the facial images, an appropriate threshold has to be defined. The authors propose to compute the threshold T as follows:

$$T = \frac{\sigma^2}{\sigma_X} \qquad (30)$$

where the standard deviations σ and σ_X are robustly estimated from:

$$\sigma = \frac{\text{mad}(|\,X_{HH}(x,y)\,|)}{\lambda} \qquad (31)$$

In the above expressions, "mad" denotes the mean absolute deviation and "var" denotes the variance. Note that the noise variance σ^2 is estimated from the HH sub-band, while the signal standard deviation σ_x is computed based on the estimate of the variance of the processed sub-band $X_s(x,y)$ for $s \in \{LH, HL, HH\}$. For an optimal implementation of the presented WD procedure, the authors suggest using a value of λ somewhere in the range from 0.01 to 0.30.

Once, all three detail coefficient sub-bands have been thresholded, they are combined with the unaltered approximate coefficient sub-band to form the denoised wavelet coefficient matrix $Y(x,y)$. The estimate of the luminance in the spatial domain is ultimately obtained by applying the inverse DWT to the wavelet coefficients in $Y(x,y)$. Some visual examples of the effect of the presented technique are shown Figure 11.

Isotropic Smoothing

Isotropic smoothing (IS) follows a similar principle as other Retinex-based algorithms. It tries to estimate the luminance $L(x,y)$ of the imaging model in (1) as a blurred version of the original input image $I(x,y)$. However, it does not apply a simple smoothing filter to the image to produce the blurred output, but rather constructs the luminance $L(x,y)$ by minimizing the following energy-based cost function (Short et al., 2004):

$$J(L(x,y)) = \int_x \int_y (L(x,y) - I(x,y))^2\, dxdy \\ + \lambda \int_x \int_y (L_x^2(x,y) + L_y^2(x,y))dxdy \qquad (32)$$

where the first term forces the luminance to be close to the input image, and the second term

imposes a smoothing constraint on $L(x,y)$, and the parameter λ controls the relative importance of the smoothing constraint [16].

As stated in (Heusch et al., 2005), the problem in (33) can be solved by a discretized version of the Euler-Lagrange diffusion process:

$$I(x,y) = L(x,y) + \lambda\big[(L(x,y) - L(x,y-1)) + (L(x,y) - L(x,y+1)) + \\ + (L(x,y) - L(x-1,y)) + (L(x,y) - L(x+1,y))\big].$$

$$(33)$$

Once, the above equation is set up for all pixel locations (x,y) it forms a large sparse linear system of equations that can be rearranged into the following matrix form:

$$\mathbf{A} \cdot \mathbf{L}_v = \mathbf{I}_v \qquad (34)$$

where $\mathbf{I}_v$ represents the vector form of the input image $I(x,y)$, $\mathbf{L}_v$ stands for the vector form of the luminance we are trying to compute and $\mathbf{A}$ denotes the so-called differential operator. It has to be noted that the dimensionality of the operator $\mathbf{A}$ is enormous as it represents a $N{\times}N$ matrix with N being the number of pixels in $I(x,y)$. The equation given by (34), therefore, cannot be solved efficiently by a direct inversion of the matrix $\mathbf{A}$, rather multi-grid methods have to be exploited to estimate the luminance $\mathbf{L}_v$. The description of appropriate multi-grid methods to solve the problem given by (34) is beyond the scope of this chapter.

Figure 11. Impact of the wavelet-based image denoising technique: original images (upper row), processed images (lower row)

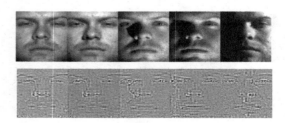

The reader should refer to (Heusch et al., 2005) for a more detailed description of these methods.

Let us assume that we have successfully estimated the luminance $L(x,y)$. Then, the illumination invariant reflectance can be computed by simply rearranging Equation (1). Some examples of the normalized images using isotropic smoothing are shown in Figure 12.

Anisotropic Smoothing

Photometric normalization using anisotropic smoothing (AN) is in general very similar to the IS technique presented in the previous section. The technique, proposed by Gross and Brajovic in (Gross & Brajovic, 2003), generalizes upon the energy-based cost function in (32) by introducing an additional weight function $\rho(x,y)$ featuring the anisotropic diffusion coefficients, which enable the penalization of the fit between the original image $I(x,y)$ and the luminance $L(x,y)$. Thus, anisotropic smoothing is based on the following cost function:

$$J(L(x,y)) = \int_x \int_y \rho(x,y)(L(x,y) \\ - I(x,y))^2 \, dxdy + \lambda \int_x \int_y (L_x^2(x,y) \\ + L_y^2(x,y)) dxdy \tag{35}$$

Figure 12. Impact of the isotropic smoothing technique: original images (upper row), processed images (lower row)

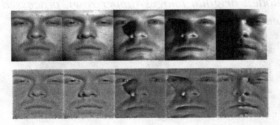

Again, the above expression is solved by a discretized version of the Euler-Lagrange diffusion process, which for the anisotropic case takes the following form:

$$I(x,y) = L(x,y) + \lambda \left[\frac{1}{\rho(x,y-1)}(L(x,y) - L(x,y-1)) + \frac{1}{\rho(x,y+1)}(L(x,y) - L(x,y+1)) \right. \\ \left. + \frac{1}{\rho(x-1,y)}(L(x,y) - L(x-1,y)) + \frac{1}{\rho(x+1,y)}(L(x,y) - L(x+1,y)) \right]. \tag{36}$$

Gross and Brajovic suggested weighing the smoothing procedure with the inverse of the local image contrast. Thus, the goodness of fit between the input image and luminance is penalized by the inverse of this local contrast. They suggested two different contrast measures between pixel locations a and b, namely, the Weber and Michelson contrasts, which are defined as:

$$\rho(b) = \frac{|I(a) - I(b)|}{\min[I(a), I(b)]} \tag{37}$$

respectively. Note that the local contrast is actually a function of two pixel locations, i.e., $\rho(b) = \rho(a,b)$; however, to be consistent with the notation in expression (36) we made a modification of the definitions of the contrast.

Like with the isotropic case, setting up Equation (36) for all pixel locations results in a large sparse linear system of equations, which is solved by a properly selected multi-grid method. Some examples of the effect of anisotropic smoothing are shown in Figure 13. Here, the value of the parameter λ of $\lambda = 7$ was used and Michelson's contrasts was exploited as the local contrast measure.

It has to be noted that the usefulness of the AN procedure heavily depends on the right choice of the parameter λ, which has to be determined empirically.

The Logarithmic Total Variation Model

The logarithmic total variation (LTV) model is based on a variant of the total variation model commonly abbreviated as TV-L[1] (Chen, T. et al., 2006). The model is capable of decomposing an image $I(x,y)$ into two distinct outputs, the first, denoted as $u(x,y)$, containing large scale facial components, and the second, denoted as $v(x,y)$, containing mainly small scale facial components.

To be consistent with the notation adopted in previous sections, we will still presume that an input image can be written as a product of two components; however, the components in the TV-L[1] model are linked to the Lambertian model and, hence, represent the surface albedos and light received at each location (x,y).

The normalization procedure starts by taking the logarithm of input image $I'(x,y)$=log $I(x,y)$, and then solves the variational problem of the following form to estimate the large scale component $u(x,y)$:

$$u(x,y) = \arg\min_u \int_\Omega |\nabla u(x,y)| + \lambda \, | \, I'(x,y) - u(x,y) \, | \, dx \tag{38}$$

where $|\nabla u(x,y)|$ denotes the total variation of $u(x,y)$ and λ stands for a scalar threshold on scale.

As noted in (Chen, T. et al., 2006), the expression in (38) can be solved by a number of tech-niques, the description of which is unfortunately beyond the scope of this chapter. The reader should refer to (Alizadeh & Goldfarb, 2003) for more information on some of these techniques.

Once the large scale component $u(x,y)$ is computed, it can be used to determine the illumination invariant small scale component $v(x,y)$ as:

$$v(x,y) = I'(x,y) - u(x,y)a \tag{39}$$

The authors of the LTV technique suggest using the following values for the threshold λ: $\lambda=0.7$ to 0.8 for images of 100×100 pixels, $\lambda=0.35$ to 0.4 for images of 200×200 pixels, and $\lambda=0.175$ to 0.2 for images of 400×400 pixels. Some examples of normalized images using the presented technique are shown in Figure 14.

EXPERIMENTAL ASSESSMENT

The Database and Experimental Setup

To assess the performance of the presented photometric normalization techniques, we conduct face recognition experiments using the YaleB and XM2VTS face databases (Georhiades et al., 2001; Messer et al., 1999).

The first, the YaleB database, contains images of 10 subjects taken under 576 different viewing conditions (9 poses × 64 illumination conditions).

Figure 13. Impact of the anisotropic smoothing technique: original images (upper row), processed images (lower row)

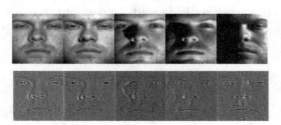

Figure 14. Impact of the logarithmic total variation model: original images (upper row), processed images (lower row)

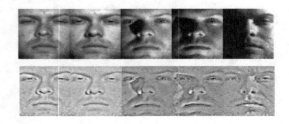

In this chapter we are only interested in the illumination induced appearance variations and their impact on the recognition performance and, therefore, employ only a subset of 640 frontal face images in our experiments.

Following the suggestion of the authors of the database, we divide the selected 640 experimental images into five image sets according to the extremity of illumination present during the image acquisition (the reader is referred to (Georhiades et al., 2001) for a detailed description of these subsets). We can see from Figure 15 that the first image set (S1) comprises images captured in "excellent" illumination conditions, while the conditions get more extreme in the image sets two (S2) to five (S5). Due to these characteristics, we employ the first image set (featuring 7 images per subject) for training and the remaining ones for testing. Such an experimental setup results in highly miss-matched conditions for the recognition stage and poses a great challenge to the photometric normalization techniques (Štruc & Pavešić, 2009).

The second, the XM2VTS database, features 2360 facial images of 295 subjects, with the images being captured in controlled conditions. For the experiments presented in the next sections, the database is divided into client and impostor groups and these groups are further partitioned into training, evaluation and test sets, as defined by the first configuration of the database's experimental protocol (Messer et al., 1999). As the XM2VTS database features only images captured in controlled conditions, it is employed as a reference database for measuring the effect that any given photometric normalization technique has not affected by illumination changes. Some sample images from the database are shown in Figure 16.

In all experiments, we use Principal Component Analysis (PCA) as the feature extractor and the nearest neighbor classifier in conjunction with the cosine similarity measure for the classification. To make the experimental setup more demanding we retain 15% of the PCA coefficients, while the remaining 85% are discarded. Note that the feature vector length is not the primary concern of our experiments and could be set differently.

Assessing the Image Enhancement Techniques

In our first series of experiments, we assess the performance of the image enhancement techniques, namely, histogram equalization (HQ), gamma intensity correction (GC) with $\gamma=4$, logarithmic transformation (LT) and remapping of the image histogram to a lognormal distribution (HL) for $\mu=0$ and $\sigma=0.4$. For baseline comparisons, experiments on unprocessed grey scale images (GR) are conducted as well. Note that the listed techniques are tested separately from other photometric normalization techniques due to their intrinsic characteristics, which make them more of

Figure 15. Sample images of two subjects from the YaleB face database drawn from (from left to right): image set 1 (S1), image set 2 (S2), image set 3 (S3), image set 4 (S4) and image set 5 (S5).

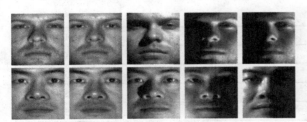

Figure 16. Sample images from the XM2VTS database

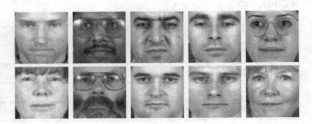

a complement than a real substitute for other, more elaborate, photometric normalization techniques - an observation supported by the following facts:

- Image enhancement techniques do not result in dynamic range compression as is the case with the photometric normalization techniques,
- Image enhancement techniques do not rely on the mathematical model given in (1), but are linked to basic image properties, such as image contrast, and
- Image enhancement techniques were shown to improve the performance of various recognition techniques even when the facial images were free of illumination variations; hence, they cannot be considered as being solely photometric normalization techniques.

The results of the assessment on the YaleB database in terms of the rank one recognition rate (in %) for all tested image sets are shown in Table 1. Here, the numbers in the brackets next to the image set labels S2 to S5 denote the number of images in each test subset. We can see that on the experimental set S5 all image enhancement techniques resulted in an increase of the recognition rate, while surprisingly only the HQ and HL improved upon the baseline recognition rate on the test sets S3 and S4.

The results of the assessment on the XM2VTS database are presented in Table 2. Note that differently from the YaleB database, images from the XM2VTS database are used in face verification experiments. Hence, the performance of the photometric normalization techniques is assessed in terms of the false rejection (FRR), the false acceptance (FAR), and the half total error rate (HTER) defined as the mean of the FAR and FRR. All errors are computed based on the threshold that ensures equal error rates on the evaluation sets.

Similar to the results presented in Table 1, we can see that only the HQ and HL techniques ensured better performance than the unprocessed grey-scale images, while the GC and LT did not improve upon the baseline error rates obtained with the unprocessed images.

It was suggested by Short et al. in (Short et al., 2004) that HQ should be used with photometric normalization techniques to further enhance their performance. However, based on the presented results, we can conclude that mapping a lognormal distribution to the pixels intensity distribution of the images might be useful as well. This issue will be further investigated in the remainder of this chapter.

Assessing the Photometric Normalization Techniques

Our second series of face recognition experiments aimed at evaluating the performance of the photometric normalization techniques presented in Section 4. In Tables 3 and 4, where the results of the assessment are presented, the following abbreviations are used for the tested techniques: SR

Table 1. Rank one recognition rates obtained on the YaleB database with the tested image enhancement techniques

Image set	GR	HQ	GC	LT	HL
S2 (120)	100	100	100	100	100
S3 (120)	93.3	99.2	73.3	67.5	95.8
S4 (140)	42.1	53.6	35.7	33.6	75.0
S5 (190)	13.7	53.2	35.8	35.3	75.0

Table 2. The verification performance of the tested image enhancement techniques on the XM2VTS database

Image set	Error (%)	GR	HQ	GC	LT	HL
Evaluation set (ES)	FRR	9.3	8.2	10.2	11.3	8.8
	FAR	9.3	8.2	10.2	11.3	8.8
	HTER	9.3	8.2	10.2	11.3	8.8
Test set (TS)	FRR	6.5	4.8	7.3	7.8	6.3
	FAR	9.7	8.4	11.3	12.5	9.2
	HTER	8.1	6.6	9.3	10.2	7.8

for the single scale Retinex, MR for the multiscale Retinex, SRA for the single scale Retinex with adaptive smoothing, HO for the homomorphic filtering, SQ for the self quotient image, DCT for the discrete cosine transformation based normalization, WD for the wavelet denoising, IS for the isotropic diffusion, AN for the anisotropic diffusion and LTV for the logarithmic total variation model.

Note that while the majority of photometric normalization techniques ensure improvements upon the baseline performance of the unprocessed

images on the YaleB database, they result in the deterioration (in most cases) in performance on images captured in controlled conditions. This result can be linked to the fact that the photometric normalization techniques remove the low frequency information, which is susceptible to illumination changes, even though it is important for recognition.

Considering the performance of the tested techniques on both databases, we can conclude that the SRA and SQ techniques resulted in the best performance with nearly 100% rank one recogni-

Table 3. Rank one recognition rates obtained with the tested photometric normalization techniques

Sets	SR	MR	SRA	HO	SQ	DCT	WD	IS	AN	LTV
S2 (120)	100	100	100	100	100	100	100	100	94.2	100
S3 (120)	99.2	94.2	100	100	100	95.0	100	94.2	97.5	100
S4 (140)	82.9	71.4	98.6	84.3	98.6	59.3	98.6	84.3	80.1	99.3
S5 (190)	81.1	66.8	99.5	81.1	100	42.6	99.5	76.8	87.4	99.5

Table 4. The verification performance of the tested photometric normalization techniques on the XM-2VTS database

Sets	Err. ()(%)	SR	MR	SRA	HO	SQ	DCT	WD	IS	AN	LTV
ES	FRR	12.7	13.0	10.0	18.7	11.8	12.0	20.8	15.8	21.3	17.8
	FAR	12.7	13.0	10.0	18.7	11.8	12.0	20.8	15.8	21.3	17.8
	HTER	12.7	13.0	10.0	18.7	11.8	12.0	20.8	15.8	21.3	17.8
TS	FRR	8.0	8.0	7.0	12.3	7.0	9.3	13.0	7.8	19.3	11.8
	FAR	13.3	13.6	10.1	18.2	12.2	13.2	20.5	15.7	21.4	17.3
	HTER	10.7	10.8	8.6	15.3	9.6	11.3	16.8	11.7	20.4	14.6

tion rates on the YaleB database and the HTER almost identical to that obtained with unprocessed images on the XM2VTS database. Note, however, that the performance of all tested techniques heavily depends on their implementation, i.e., the proper selection of their parameters. Since there is no theoretical foundation for determining these parameters, they have to be set empirically.

Based on the presented results, we can find that pure photometric normalization techniques without any pre- or post-processing of facial images cannot ensure satisfactory recognition results on images captured in controlled as well as varying illumination conditions. To this end, we assess a number of options to further improve their performance in the next section.

Combining Image Enhancement and Photometric Normalization Techniques

Several research studies have suggested that HQ successfully improves the performance of photometric normalization techniques. However, no specifics as to whether the histogram should be equalized before or after the actual deployment of the photometric normalization procedure were given, nor was a justification of why HQ improves the performance of the photometric normalization techniques ever suggested.

If we recall that the photometric normalization techniques perform a compression of the dynamic range of the intensity values of facial images and thus reduce the variability in the im-

age, it becomes evident that HQ applied after the photometric normalization increases the dynamic range of the normalized image by redistributing the pixel intensities equally across the whole 8-bit dynamic range. This procedure adds to images variability needed to successfully discriminate between different subjects. As HQ is notorious for its background noise enhancing property, applying HQ prior to the photometric normalization would result in the retention (or emphasis) of the background noise in the photometrically normalized images. Clearly, the right way to go is to use histogram equalization as a post-processing step for the photometric normalization, which is also consistent with the work presented in (Heusch et al., 2005).

Let us at this point examine the possibility of replacing the image enhancement technique HQ with HL, as proposed in Section 5.2. For a technique to be suitable to take the place of HQ, it should exhibit similar characteristics. As we have shown during the introduction of the histogram remapping techniques, HL remaps the histogram of the input image to approximate the lognormal, thus increasing the dynamic range of the processed images to the full 8-bit interval. Furthermore, as it does not force the target distribution to be uniform, it does not increase the background noise. Without a doubt, HQ and HL can both be adopted as post-processing techniques to photometric normalization.

Using HQ and HL for post-processing, we perform two types of experiments. The results of these experiments are presented in Tables 5 and

Table 5. Rank one recognition rates on all image sets of the YaleB database using histogram equalization as the post-processing step to the normalization

Sets	SR	MR	SRA	HO	SQ	DCT	WD	IS	AN	LTV
S2 (120)	100	100	100	100	100	100	100	100	100	100
S3 (120)	99.2	98.3	99.2	100	100	95.8	100	100	100	100
S4 (140)	91.4	87.1	97.1	88.6	93.6	72.9	99.3	86.4	95.7	99.3
S5 (190)	98.4	91.1	100	99.5	100	77.4	100	98.4	93.2	100

Table 6. Rank one recognition rates on all image sets of the YaleB database using remapping of the histogram to a lognormal distribution as the post-processing step to the normalization

Sets	SR	MR	SRA	HO	SQ	DCT	WD	IS	AN	LTV
S2 (120)	100	100	100	100	100	100	100	100	100	100
S3 (120)	100	100	100	100	100	97.5	100	100	100	100
S4 (140)	92.1	91.4	97.9	100	96.4	75.7	99.3	91.4	97.1	100
S5 (190)	97.4	96.3	99.5	100	100	83.2	100	95.3	100	100

6 for the YaleB database and Tables 7 and 8 for the XMVTS database.

The presented results support our suggestion that the increase of the dynamic range of the processed images governs the improvements in the recognition rates, as both HQ and HL improve upon the vast majority of the results presented in Tables 3 and 4. While the relative ranking of the assessed techniques remained similar to the one presented in the previous series of experiments, the differences in the rank one recognition rates

and HTERs are smaller in absolute terms. This again suggests that decent performance gains can be achieved when photometric normalization techniques are combined with image enhancement approaches and that photometric normalization techniques need to be combined with image enhancement methods to ensure proper performance on both images captured in controlled and uncontrolled conditions.

Table 7. The verification performance on the XM2VTS database using histogram equalization as the post-processing step to the normalization

Sets	Err. ()(%)	SR	MR	SRA	HO	SQ	DCT	WD	IS	AN	LTV
ES	FRR	9.2	9.0	7.0	13.2	8.2	8.2	17.3	12.3	12.5	12.2
	FAR	9.2	9.0	7.0	13.2	8.2	8.2	17.3	12.3	12.5	12.2
	HTER	9.2	9.0	7.0	13.2	8.2	8.2	17.3	12.3	12.5	12.2
TS	FRR	5.8	6.3	6.0	7.3	5.5	4.3	8.8	6.5	10.0	7.5
	FAR	8.9	8.9	7.0	13.3	8.4	8.4	17.0	12.2	12.4	11.8
	HTER	7.4	7.6	6.5	10.3	7.0	6.4	12.9	9.4	11.2	9.7

Table 8. The verification performance on the XM2VTS database remapping of the histogram to a lognormal distribution as the post-processing step to the normalization

Sets	Err. ()(%)	SR	MR	SRA	HO	SQ	DCT	WD	IS	AN	LTV
ES	FRR	11.3	11.3	8.2	13.7	10.2	10.0	16.8	14.2	15.7	15.3
	FAR	11.3	11.3	8.2	13.7	10.2	10.0	16.8	14.2	15.7	15.3
	HTER	11.3	11.3	8.2	13.7	10.2	10.0	16.8	14.2	15.7	15.3
TS	FRR	6.5	6.8	6.8	9.8	6.0	6.8	10.3	8.3	11.0	8.8
	FAR	11.4	11.5	8.3	13.8	10.1	10.4	16.2	14.1	15.7	14.9
	HTER	9.0	9.2	7.6	11.8	8.1	8.6	13.3	11.2	13.4	11.9

CONCLUSION

The chapter presented an overview of the most popular photometric normalization techniques for illumination invariant for face recognition. A number of techniques were presented and later on assessed on the YaleB and XM2VTS databases. The experimental results suggest that several techniques are capable of achieving state-of-the-art recognition results and that the performance of a vast majority of these techniques can be further improved when combined with image enhancement techniques, such as histogram equalization or histogram remapping.

It has to be noted that many of the photometric normalization techniques result in an extreme compression of the dynamic range of the intensities values of images and that a small dynamic range usually implies that the photometric normalization procedure has removed most of the variability from the image, albeit induced by illumination or some other factor, and that the pixel intensity distribution thus exhibits a strong peak around a specific pixel value. In such cases, recognition algorithms cannot model the variations of faces due to intrinsic factors, such as facial expression or pose, even though shadows are removed perfectly (Park et al., 2008).

Future research with respect to photometric normalization techniques will, therefore, undoubtedly focus on the development of pre-processing techniques capable of efficiently removing the influence of illumination, while still preserving the image's dynamic range. These techniques will be deployable on larger scale databases and will provide illumination invariance without the loss of subject specific information contained in the low-frequency part of the images.

To promote the future development of photometric normalization techniques we make most of the Matlab source code used in our experiments freely available. To obtain a copy of the code, the reader should follow the links given at: http://luks.fe.uni-lj.si/en/staff/vitomir/index.html.

REFERENCES

Adini, Y., Moses, Y., & Ullman, S. (1997). Face Recognition: The Problem of Compensating for Changes in Illumination Direction. *IEEE TPAMI, 19*(7), 721–732.

Alizadeh, F., & Goldfarb, D. (2003). Second-Order Cone Programming. *Mathematical Programming, 95*(1), 3–51. doi:10.1007/s10107-002-0339-5

Basri, R., & Jacobs, D. (2003). Lambertian Reflectance and Linear Subspaces. *IEEE TPAMI, 25*(2), 218–233.

Chen, H., Belhumeur, P., & Jacobs, D. (2000). In Search of Illumination Invariants. In *Proc. of the ICVPR'00* (pp. 254-261).

Chen, T., Yin, W., Zhou, X. S., Comaniciu, D., & Huang, T. S. (2006). Total Variation Models for Variable Lighting Face Recognition. *IEEE TPAMI, 28*(9), 1519–1524.

Chen, W., Er, M. J., & Wu, S. (2006). Illumination Compensation and Normalization for Robust Face Recognition Using Discrete Cosine Transform in Logarithmic Domain. *IEEE Transactions on Systems, Man and Cybernetics – part B, 36*(2), 458-466.

Gao, Y., & Leung, M. K. H. (2002). Face Recognition Using Line Edge Map. *IEEE TPAMI, 24*(6), 764–779.

Georghiades, A. G., Belhumeur, P. N., & Kriegman, D. J. (2001). From Few to Many: Illumination Cone Models for Face Recognition under Variable Lighting and Pose. *IEEE TPAMI, 23*(6), 643–660.

Gonzalez, R. C., & Woods, R. E. (2002). *Digital Image Processing* (2nd ed.). Upper Saddle River, NJ: Prentice Hall.

Gross, R., Baker, S., Matthews, I., & Kanade, T. (2004). Face Recognition Across Pose and Illumination. In Li, S. Z., & Jain, A. K. (Eds.), *Handbook of Face Recognition*. Berlin: Springer-Verlag.

Gross, R., & Brajovic, V. (2003). An Image Preprocessing Algorithm for Illumination Invariant Face Recognition. In *Proc. of AVPBA'03* (pp. 10-18).

Heusch, G., Cardinaux, F., & Marcel S. (2005, March). Lighting Normalization Algorithms for Face Verification. *IDIAP-com 05-03*.

Jabson, D. J., Rahmann, Z., & Woodell, G. A. (1997b). A Multiscale Retinex for Bridging the Gap Between Color Images and the human Observations of Scenes. *IEEE Transactions on Image Processing, 6*(7), 897–1056.

Jobson, D. J., Rahman, Z., & Woodell, G. A. (1997a). Properties and Performance of a Center/Surround Retinex. *IEEE Transactions on Image Processing, 6*(3), 451–462. doi:10.1109/83.557356

Land, E. H., & McCann, J. J. (1971). Lightness and Retinex Theory. *Journal of the Optical Society of America, 61*(1), 1–11. doi:10.1364/JOSA.61.000001

Marcel, S., Rodriguez, Y., & Heusch, G. (2007). On the Recent Use of Local Binary Patterns for Face Authentication. *International Journal of Image and Video Processing.*

Messer, K., Matas, J., Kittler, J., Luettin, J., & Maitre, G. (1999). XM2VTSDB: the extended M2VTS database. In *Proc. of AVBPA'99* (pp. 72-77).

Moore, A., Allman, J., & Goodman, R. M. (1991). A Real Time Neural System for Color Consistency. *IEEE Transactions on Neural Networks, 2*, 237–247. doi:10.1109/72.80334

Park, Y. K., Park, S. L., & Kim, J. K. (2008). Retinex Method Based on Adaptive smoothing for Illumination Invariant Face Recognition. *Signal Processing, 88*(8), 1929–1945. doi:10.1016/j.sigpro.2008.01.028

Phillips, P. J., Scruggs, W. T., O'Toole, A. J., Flynn, P. J., Bowyer, K. W., Schott, C. L., & Sharpe, M. (2007, March). FRVT 2006 and ICE 2006 Large-Scale Results. *NISTIR 7408.*

Short, J., Kittler, J., & Messer, K. (2004). A Comparison of Photometric Normalization Algorithms for Face Verification. In *Proc. of AFGR'04* (pp. 254- 259).

Štruc, V., & Pavešić, N. (2009). Gabor-Based Kernel Partial-Least-Squares Discrimination Features for Face Recognition. *Informatica, 20*(1), 115–138.

Štruc, V., Žibert, J., & Pavešić, N. (2009). Histogram Remapping as a Preprocessing Step for Robust Face Recognition. *WSEAS Transactions on Information Science and Applications, 6*(3), 520–529.

Wang, H., Li, S. Z., Wang, Y., & Zhang, J. (2004). Self Quotient Image for Face Recognition. In *Proc. of the ICPR'04* (pp. 1397- 1400).

Zhang, T., Fang, B., Yuan, Y., Tang, Y. Y., Shang, Z., Li, D., & Lang, F. (2009). Multiscale Facial Structure Representation for Face Recognition Under Varying Illumination. *Pattern Recognition, 42*(2), 252–258. doi:10.1016/j.patcog.2008.03.017

Zou, X., Kittler, J., & Messer, K. (2007). Illumination Invariant Face Recognition: A Survey. In *Proc. of BTAS'07* (pp. 1-8).

KEY TERMS AND DEFINITIONS

The Retinex Theory: (derived from the words retina and cortex) is a theory explaining the principles of scene perception and/or image formation in the human visual system. It states that the perceived sensation of color in a natural scene shows a strong correlation with reflectance, even though the amount of visible light reaching the eye depends on the product of both reflectance and illumination. Thus, the theory offers a mathematical model of images and implies that the reflectance if correctly estimated can serve as an illumination invariant representation of any given image.

Reflectance: The reflectance (or reflectance function) represents one of the two factors in the image model defined by the retinex theory. The reflectance is linked to the characteristics of the objects comprising the scene of an image and is dependent upon the reflectivity (or albedo) of the scenes surface, or, in other words, it accounts for the illumination reflected by the objects in the scene. It is usually adopted as a illumination invariant representation of the given image.

Luminance: The luminance (or luminance function) represents one of the two factors in the image model defined by the retinex theory. The luminance is determined by the illumination source and relates to the amount of illumination falling on the observed scene. The luminance is commonly considered to vary slowly with the spatial position in the image and is often estimated as a low-pass filtered version of the original image.

Image Enhancement Techniques: Image enhancement techniques represent a special class of pre-processing techniques which enhance, improve or modify image characteristics, such as the global or local contrast, the dynamic range of the intensity values, the distribution of the pixel

intensity values and others. While these techniques are not aimed directly at ensuring illumination invariance, they have been empirically shown to improve the recognition performance in difficult illuminatin conditions

Photometric Mormalization Technique: Photometrc normaliation techniques represent a class of normalization techniques, which tackle the problem of illumination invariant face recognition at the pre-processing level. Popular examples of these techniques include the single scale retinex algorithm, homomorphiv filtering or anisotropic smoothing.

Histogram Equalization: Histogram equalization is a representative of the group of image enhancement techniques, which aims at transforming the distribution of the pixel intensity values of the input image into a uniform distribution and consequently at improving the image's global. The technique is usually implemented using the rank transform.

Rank Transform: The rank transform represents a transform which replaces each pixel value in the N-dimensional image with the index (or rank) R that each pixel would correspond to if the pixel intensity values were ordered in an ascending manner. For example the most negative pixel-value is assigned the rank of 1, while the most positive pixel-value is assigned the ranking of N. Because of this procedure, the histogram of the processed image is equalized.

Chapter 16
Pose and Illumination Invariance with Compound Image Transforms

Lior Shamir
NIA/NIH, USA

ABSTRACT

While current face recognition algorithms have provided convincing performance on frontal face poses, recognition is far less effective when the pose and illumination conditions vary. Here the authors show how compound image transforms can be used for face recognition in various poses and illumination conditions. The method works by first dividing each image into four equal-sized tiles. Then, image features are extracted from the face images, transforms of the images, and transforms of transforms of the images. Finally, each image feature is assigned with a Fisher score, and test images are classified by using a simple Weighted Nearest Neighbor rule such that the Fisher scores are used as weights. Experimental results using the full color FERET dataset show that with no parameter tuning, the accuracy of rank-10 recognition for frontal, quarter-profile, and half-profile images is ~98%, ~94% and ~91%, respectively. The proposed method also achieves perfect accuracy on several other face recognition datasets such as Yale B, ORL and JAFFE. An important feature of this method is that the recognition accuracy improves as the number of subjects in the dataset gets larger.

INTRODUCTION

In the past two decades face recognition has been attracting considerable attention, and has become one of the most prominent areas in computer vision, leading to the development of numerous face recognition algorithms (Gross, Baker, Mat-

thews, & Kanade, 2004; Kong, Heo, Abidi, Paik & Abidi, 2005; Zao et al., 2003).

Established common approaches to face recognition include component-based recognition (Brunelli & Poggio, 1993; Wiskott, Fellous, Kruger, & Von Der Malsburg 1997; Ivanov, Heisele & Serre, 2004), face geometry (Samal, Taleb, & Strovoitov, 2001), elastic face matching (Gee & Haynor, 1996), eigenface (Kirby & Sirovich, 1990;

DOI: 10.4018/978-1-61520-991-0.ch016

Turk & Pentland, 1991), Hidden Markov Models (Samaria & Harter, 1994), template matching (Brunelli & Poggio, 1993), and line edge maps (Gao & Lehung, 2002).

One of the challenges in applying face recognition algorithms to forensic or CBIR (Content Based Image Retrieval) applications is the degradation of the recognition accuracy of face images taken at different poses and different illumination conditions. While previous studies reported high accuracy figures tested using the FERET dataset (Phillips, Moon, Rizvi, & Rauss, 2000), most published previous efforts focused on frontal images, and were tested using the *fa* and *fb* sets of both the color and gray FERET datasets. Attempts of classifying face in non-frontal poses (e.g., profile) have attracted less attention.

Practical application of automatic face recognition methods to forensic or surveillance purposes is dependent heavily on the ability to handle face images that are not perfectly oriented towards the camera, and in cases where the illumination conditions are not always controlled. This can be achieved by using features of the face that are less sensitive to the pose such as skin and hair textures (Singh, Vatsa, & Noore, 2005).

Here we describe a simple method of face recognition at different aspects such as facial view, profile and half profile. The method works without rendering or synthesizing the face in the image, and does not apply an estimation of the pose.

Section 2 briefly reviews previous studies of face recognition under pose and illumination variations, Section 3 describes the image features and image transforms used by the proposed method, Section 4 discusses the classification of the image features, Section 5 presents the experimental results, and in Section 6 computational complexity issues are discussed.

BACKGROUND AND RELATED WORK

One of the common approaches to face recognition under pose variations is correcting for the pose before applying a face recognition method. Beymer (1993) applied a pose estimation step before geometrically aligning the probe images to gallery images, and reported good results on a dataset with minimal pose variations. Vetter and Poggio (1997) rotated a single face image to synthesize a view at a given angle, an approach used by Lando and Edelman (1995) and Georghiades, Belhumeur, and Kriegman (2001) to perform face recognition in different poses. Pentland et al. (1994) extended the eigenface method (Turk & Pentland, 1991) to handle different views. Cottes, Wheeler, Walker, and Taylor (2002) trained separate models for several different poses, and used heuristics to select the model used for a given probe image.

Modeling the face features in different views is also a common approach to handle pose variations in face recognition. Romdhani, Psarrou, and Gong (2000) used kernel PCA to model shapes and textures in different views. Another approach is eigenspace (Murase & Nayar, 1995; Graham & Allinson, 1998), based on the observation that a sequence of face images taken at different aspects form an eigensignature. Gross et al. (2004) introduced eigen light-fields as a tool for face recognition across poses.

Testing face recognition methods under pose variations is enabled by some of the standard face datasets such as the color FERET dataset (Phillips et al., 2000), which provides face images of full, half, and quarter profiles, and allows using different poses for the probe and gallery images.

EXTRACTING IMAGE FEATURES

The described method works by first extracting a large set of image features, from which the most informative features are then selected in a systematic fashion. Image features are computed not only on the raw pixels, but also on several transforms of the image, and transforms of transforms. These compound transforms have been found highly effective in classification and similarity measurement of biological and biometric image datasets (Orlov et al., 2008; Shamir, Orlov, Eckley, Macura, & Goldberg, 2008a).

For image feature extraction, we use the following algorithms, described more thoroughly in (Shamir et al., 2008b; Orlov et al., 2008):

- **Radon transform features**, computed for angles 0, 45, 90, 135 degrees, and each of the resulting series is then convolved into a 3-bin histogram, providing a total of 12 image features.
- **Chebyshev Statistics** (Gradshtein & Ryzhik, 1994) - A 32-bin histogram of a 1×400 vector produced by Chebyshev transform of the image with order of N=20.
- **Gabor Filter,** where the kernel is in the form of a convolution with a Gaussian harmonic function (Gregorescu, Petkov, & Kruizinga, 2002), and 7 different frequencies are used (1, 2, ..., 7), providing 7 image content descriptor values.
- **Multi-scale Histograms** computed using various numbers of bins (3, 5, 7, and 9), as proposed by Hadjidementriou, Grossberg, and Nayar (2001), and providing 3+5+7+9=24 image descriptors.
- **First Four Moments**, of mean, standard deviation, skewness, and kurtosis computed on image "stripes" in four different directions (0, 45, 90, 135 degrees). Each set of stripes is then sampled into a 3-bin histogram, providing 4×4×3=48 image descriptors.
- **Tamura Texture features** of contrast, directionality and coarseness, such that the coarseness descriptors are its sum and its 3-bin histogram, providing 1+1+1+3=6 image descriptors.

- **Edge Statistics features** computed on the Prewitt gradient, and including the mean, median, variance, and 8-bin histogram of both the magnitude and the direction components. Other edge features are the total number of edge pixels (normalized to the size of the image), the direction homogeneity, and the difference amongst direction histogram bins at a certain angle α and $\alpha + \pi$, sampled into a four-bin histogram. Together, edge feature contribute 28 content descriptor values.
- **Object Statistics** computed on all 8-connected objects found in the Otsu binary mask of the image. Computed statistics include the Euler Number, and the minimum, maximum, mean, median, variance, and a 10-bin histogram of both the objects areas and distances from the to the image centroid.
- **Zernike features** (Teague, 1979) are the absolute values of the coefficients of the Zernike polynomial approximation of the image, providing 72 image descriptors.
- **Haralick features** (Haralick, Shanmugam & Dinstein, 1973) computed on the image's co-occurrence matrix, and contribute 28 image descriptor values.
- **Chebyshev-Fourier features** - 32-bin histogram of the polynomial coefficients of a Chebyshev–Fourier transform with highest polynomial order of N=23.

Image features can be informative when not only extracted from the pixels, but also when extracted from transforms and compound transforms of an image (Orlov et al., 2008; Rodenacker & Bengtsson, 2003; Gurevich & Koryabkina, 2006). Therefore, in order to extract more image content descriptors, the algorithms described above are applied not only on the raw pixels, but also on several transforms of the image and transforms of transforms. The image transforms that are used are FFT, Wavelet (Symlet 5, level 1) two-dimensional decomposition of the image, and Chebyshev transform. For the Fourier transform implementation we used the FFTW (Frigo & Johnson, 2005) open source library, the wavelet transform was implemented based on the MATLAB Wavelet Toolbox, and the Chebyshev transform was implemented by us using the description that can be found at (Gradshtein & Ryzhik, 1994).

Another transform that was used is the Edge transform, which is simply the magnitude component of the image's Prewitt gradient, binarized by Otsu global threshold. The various combinations of the compound image transforms are described in Figure 1.

According to the method described in this chapter, different image features are extracted from different image transforms or compound transforms. The image features that are extracted from all transforms are the statistics and texture features, which include the first four moments, Haralick textures, multi-scale histograms, Tamura textures, and Radon features.

Polynomial decomposition features, which include Zernike features, Chebyshev statistics, and Chebyshev-Fourier polynomial coefficients, are also extracted from all transforms, except from the Fourier and Wavelet transforms of the Chebyshev transform, and the Wavelet and Chebyshev transforms of the Fourier transform. Additionally, high contrast features (edge statistics, object statistics, and Gabor filters) are extracted from the raw pixels. The entire set of image features extracted from all image transforms described in Figure 1 consists of a total of 2633 numeric image content descriptors.

While some correlation can be expected between the features extracted from the different transforms, the different representations of the raw pixels lead to just weak correlation between the same features extracted from different image transforms. This can be evident by a feature survey (Shamir, Orlov, & Goldberg, 2009a) that showed that for different image classification problems, the informativeness of different groups of image features varied among the image transforms they were extracted from.

IMAGE CLASSIFICATION

The set of image features described in Section 3 can provide a comprehensive numeric description of the image content. However, not all image features are assumed to be equally informative, and some of these features are expected to represent noise. In order to select the most informative features while rejecting noisy features, each image feature is assigned with a Fisher score (Bishop, 2006), described by Equation 1,

$$W_f = \frac{\sum_{c=1}^{N} \left(\overline{T_f} - \overline{T_{f,c}} \right)^2}{\sum_{c=1}^{N} \sigma_{f,c}^2} \qquad (1)$$

Figure 1. Image transforms and paths of the compound image transforms

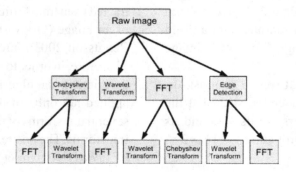

where Wf is the Fisher score, N is the total number of classes, is the mean of the values of feature f in the entire training set, and and $\sigma^2_{f,c}$ are the mean and variance of the values of feature f among all training images of class c. The Fisher score can be conceptualized as the ratio of variance of class means from the pooled mean to the mean of within-class variances. Since different image content descriptors have different numeric ranges, all variances used in the equation are computed after the values of feature f are normalized to the interval $[0, 1]$. After Fisher scores are assigned to the features, the weakest 85% of the features (with the lowest Fisher scores) are rejected, resulting in a feature space of 395 image features.

The purpose of the data-driven statistical scoring and weighing of the different features is to handle the large set of image features by applying a systematic search for the image content descriptors that are less sensitive to pose variations, and reject image features that change significantly when the pose or illumination conditions of the photo are different.

Before computing the features, each image is divided into four equal-sized tiles. Then, image features are computed on each of the four tiles, providing four feature vectors for each image. This approach was motivated by the observation of Zou, Ji & Qiang (2007), which suggested that discrimination based on just a small portion of the face is "surprisingly good". After dividing the images, each of the four feature vectors is classified using a simple weighted nearest neighbor rule, such that the feature weights are the Fisher scores.

The classification of each feature vector provides a vector of the size N (where N is the total number of persons in the dataset), such that each entry c in the vector represents the computed similarity of the feature vector to the class c, deduced using Equation 2,

$$M_{f,c} = \frac{1}{\min\left(D_{f,c}\right) \cdot \sum_{i=1}^{N} \frac{1}{\min(D_{f,i})}} \qquad (2)$$

where $M_{f,c}$ is the computed similarity of the feature vector f to the class c, and $\min(D_{f,c})$ is the shortest weighted Euclidean distance between the feature vector f and any tile in the training set that belongs to the class c. This assigns each of the four feature vectors of any image in the test set with N values within the interval $[0,1]$, representing its similarity to each class. The entire image is then classified by averaging the four feature vectors of the tiles, providing a single similarity vector. Naturally, the predicted class for each test image is the class that has the highest value in the similarity vector. Splitting each face image into four equal-sized tiles contributes significantly to the recognition accuracy of facial images taken at different aspects, as will be explained in Section 5.

EXPERIMENTAL RESULTS

The proposed method was tested using the color FERET face dataset, which consists of 11,338 images of 994 individuals. In each experiment, a maximum number of four images of each subject at different poses were used for training, and one image for testing. The training set of each subject included the *fa* (frontal view) image, and three of the five poses *fb*, *hl* (half-left profile), *hr* (half right profile), and *pr* (right profile). Not all subjects in the color FERET dataset have both *hl* and *hr* poses, and therefore some of the subjects had less than four training images.

The test set in each experiment included one image for each subject. The poses that were tested were *fa*, *hr*, *hl*, *pr*, *qr* (quarter right profile), *ql*. Not all subjects in the color FERET dataset have images for all poses, so that the sizes of the test sets for the *fb*, *hr*, *hl*, *pr*, *qr*, *ql* poses were 993, 917, 953, 994, 501, 501, respectively. In all cases, N was 994, so that random recognition would be expected to provide accuracy of ~0.001006. The rank-1 recognition accuracy for the *fb*, *hr* and *qr* poses was 90.6%, 74.1%, and 88.6%, respectively, and the rank-10 recognition accuracy was 98.1%, 91%, 93.81%, as shown in Figure 2.

As can be learned from the figure, different recognition accuracies where found for the different poses, and the recognition accuracy improves as the rotational degree of the face in the image is closer to a frontal view. The profile aspect pr performed significantly worse than the other poses. This can be explained by the fact that this pose is visually less similar to the other poses. In addition, the classification accuracy of *hr* images was significantly better than *hl*. This can be explained by the presence of right profile images, which are more similar to right half-profiles, and the absence of left profile images in the training set. The same observation also applies to left and right quarter-profiles, but the difference between the performance figures of these poses is significantly smaller, probably because the quarter profile images are more similar to the half-profiles than to the full profile images.

An interesting feature of the proposed method is that the recognition accuracy does not decrease as the number of subjects gets larger. Figure 3 shows how rank-5 recognition accuracy changes as the number of subjects in the dataset increases.

As the figure shows, the recognition accuracy drops to minimum at around 500 subjects, and then gradually increases as the number of subjects in the dataset gets larger. The improved performance when more subjects are used can be explained by the weights (determined by the Fisher

scores) that are assigned to the image features extracted from the different image transforms, as Fisher scores can normally better estimate the actual discriminative power of an image feature when more sample images are used. Apparently, in a dataset with less than 1000 subjects, the contribution of the additional subjects to the efficacy of the Fisher scores more than compensates for the additional confusion that they add to the classification. That is, adding more classes to the dataset increases the confusion of face recognition, as can be seen when less than 500 images were used, but the Fisher scores become more effective when the size of the dataset increases, which can compensate for the confusion that results from the larger number of subjects. Since the color FERET dataset does not include more than 1000 individuals, not conclusions can be made about the recognition accuracy in larger face datasets.

The effect of the number of tiles into which each face image is divided was tested by using the method on the *fb, qr, ql, hr, hl,* and *pr* datasets using different number of tiles per image. Figure 4 shows the rank-5 classification accuracy of the different poses using 1, 4, 9, and 16 tiles per face image.

Obviously, the difference between using four tiles (2×2) and one tile (the full image) is not only the number of tiles, but also the size of each tile used. In order to dismiss the possibility that the

Figure 2. Recognition accuracy for poses fb, hl, hr, pr, qr, ql of the color FERET dataset

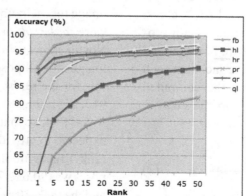

Figure 3. Rank-5 recognition accuracy as a function of the number of subjects in the dataset

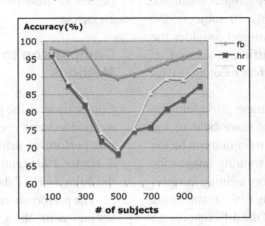

performance improves when the size of the tile gets smaller, we also tested the FERET dataset after down-sampling the images to 25% of their original sizes, making the size of each image equal to the size of a single tile when the image was divided into 2×2 tiles. Rank-1, 5, and 10 recognition accuracies of *fb* set in that case were 86.2%, 90.9%, 91.3%, respectively, which is ~5% lower than the recognition accuracy using four tiles of the full image.

Experiment Using Yale B Dataset

The proposed method was also tested for illumination variation using the Yale B dataset (Georghiades et al., 2001), which contains 5760

images of 10 subjects, taken under 576 different illumination conditions. Since a significant portion of Yale B images is background, only the 300×350 rectangle around the face in each image was used in order to reduce the computational cost and avoid computing image content descriptors for background features.

The classification accuracy was measured using different sizes of training sets. Each experiment was repeated 50 times, such that in each run the test images were selected randomly. The performance figures showed in Figure 5 are the mean classification accuracies (rank-1) of all 50 runs of each experiment.

As the figure shows, the recognition accuracy of the Yale B dataset becomes 100% when more

Figure 4. Rank-5 recognition accuracy as a function of the number of tiles per image

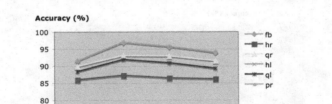

than 500 training images per subject are used. While Yale B dataset has only 10 subjects, the large number of images per subject provides the proposed method with a sufficient amount of training samples to allow perfect recognition accuracy.

In the case of Yale B dataset, dividing the image into four tiles did not contribute to the recognition accuracy. A reason for that can be the already sufficient number of training images for each subject, so that adding more training samples did not contribute significantly to the estimations of the discriminative power of the different image content descriptors, which are determined by the Fisher scores.

Experiments Using Other Datasets

In addition to the color FERET and Yale B datasets, several other publicly available face datasets have also been used for testing the efficacy of the face recognition method. In all cases, 80% of the images of each subject were used for training, while the remaining images were used for testing. Similarly, to the test using Yale B, each experiment was repeated 50 times such that each run uses a different split to training and test images. The performance of the proposed method on each of these datasets is listed in Table 1, which shows

perfect or near-perfect recognition accuracy in all cases.

Comparison to Previously Proposed Methods

Comparison of the performance of the described method to some previously proposed algorithms was performed using the ORL dataset (Samaria & Harter, 1994) and a subset of 600 subjects from the color FERET dataset.

The performance of the face recognition when testing using the ORL dataset were compared against the figures reported by (Chen, Yuen, Huang, & Dai, 2004), as listed in Table 2. In all cases, nine images per subject were used for training and one image for testing, and the average rank-1 recognition accuracies of 50 random splits are reported.

Performance using the color FERET dataset was compared by selecting 600 subjects such that only the *fa, fb, ql, qr,* and the 15°*rb, rc* poses of each individual were used. The maximum number of training images per subject was four. This relatively homogenous dataset (in terms of pose) was compared with LFA (Penev & Atick, 1996), CF (Savvides, Vijaya Kumar & Khosla, 2002) and the method of Singh, Vista & Noore, (2005), and the rank-1 recognition accuracy is specified in Table 3.

Figure 5. Recognition accuracy as a function of the size of the training set when using Yale B dataset

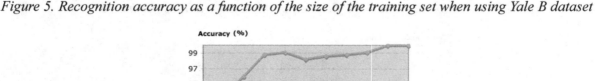
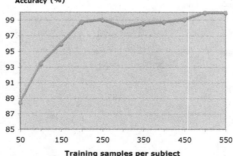

Table 1. Recognition accuracies tested using the datasets ORL, JAFFE, the Indian face dataset (females and males) and ESSEX-96

Dataset	No. of Subjects	Images per subject	Recognition accuracy (%)
ORL (Samaria & Harter, 1994)	40	10	100
JAFFE Lynos, Akamatsu, Kamachi, & Gyboa, 1998)	10	21	100
Indian Face Dataset (females) (Jain & Mukherjee, 2002)	22	11	99
Indian Face Dataset (males) (Jain & Mukherjee, 2002)	39	11	97
ESSEX-96 (Spacek, 2002)	132	20	99

As Tables 2 and 3 show the proposed algorithm performed better than existing methods also when tested using datasets with minimal variations of poses and illumination conditions such as ORL and the subset of the color FERET dataset.

The Effect of Image Transforms and Compound Transforms

In order to assess the contribution of the image features extracted from the transforms and compound transforms, we measured the recognition accuracies of the experiments with and without

using the transforms and compound transforms. The performance figures are listed in Table 4.

As the table shows, extracting image features from the transforms and compound transforms substantially improved the recognition accuracy. The only exceptions are the ORL and Indian male and female face datasets, which provided relatively high recognition accuracies when only features computed on the raw pixels were used, so that the contribution of the features extracted from transforms and compound transforms was smaller in these cases.

Table 2. Performance comparison of the proposed method to previous algorithms using the ORL face dataset

Algorithm	Recognition accuracy
Fisherface (Belhumeur, Hespanha, & Kriegman, 1997)	82.4
Direct LDA (Yu & Yang, 2001)	91.55
Huang et al. (Huang, Liu, Lu, & Ma, 2002)	95.40
Regularized LDA (Chen et al., 2004)	96.65
The proposed method	100

Table 3. Comparison of the proposed method to previous algorithms using the color FERET face dataset

Algorithm	Recognition accuracy (%)
LFA (Penev & Atick, 1996)	92.3
CF (Savvides, Vijaya Kumar & Khosla, 2002)	93.8
(Singh et al., 2005)	94
The proposed method	95.2

Table 4. Recognition accuracies (%) of face datasets when using images features extracted from raw pixels only, raw pixels and image transforms, and raw pixels, transforms and compound transforms

Dataset	Raw pixels only	Raw pixels + image transforms	Raw pixels + image transforms + compound transforms
FERET (rank-10, fb)	84	89	98
FERET (rank-10, qr)	75	84	91
FERET (rank-10, hr)	77	87	94
ORL (rank-1)	95	95	100
JAFFE (rank-1)	92	98	100
Indian Female Face Dataset (rank-1)	94	96	99
Indian Male Face Dataset (rank-1)	94	96	97

COMPUTATIONAL COMPLEXITY

A major downside of the proposed face recognition method is its computational complexity. The set of image features extracted from the raw pixels and the several transforms require significant CPU resources. The 11,338 images in the dataset produced 45,352 feature vectors (four feature vectors per image), such that each feature vector consisted of 2633 features, producing a total of 119,411,816 image features.

Feature vector of one tile (256×384 pixels) of a color FERET image can be extracted in 252 seconds using a system with a 2.6GHZ AMD Opteron and 2GB of RAM, so that the four feature vectors of each image can be processed in 1008 seconds. Practically, image features for the entire color FERET dataset (11338 images were extracted using 8 dual-core 2.6GHz AMD Opteron processors (a total of 16 cores) with 2GB of RAM per core in ~200 hours.

In order to reduce the required computational resources, the number of content descriptors extracted from the images can be reduced. However, image features are not extracted individually. For instance, in order to extract bin 12 of multi-scale histograms from the Fourier transform of an image, all multi-scale histograms bins should be computed in order to make the value of the required bin available. Therefore, if only one image content descriptor of the certain type of features is required, all features of the type should be computed. This leads to a sharp increase in computational cost when a high number of image features are used. Figure 6 shows how the time required for one processor to extract image features from one 256×384 tile increases as the

Figure 6. Processing time of one tile (256×384pixels) as a function of the percentage of extracted features (out of the total of 2633)

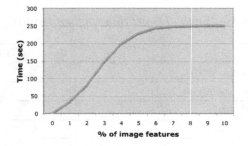

percentage of image features from the pool of 2633 image features gets higher.

As can be learned from the graph, when using more than 5% of the 2633 image content descriptors, the computational cost is as nearly as high as when computing the full set. The response time for computing a single image can be reduced significantly by using several processors, as the different groups of image features extracted from several different image transforms allow a considerable speedup when multiple processing units are used. E.g., while one processor computes the Zernike features of the raw pixels, another processor can extract Haralick features from the Fourier transform. A comprehensive mechanism for scheduling the image transforms and feature extraction algorithms and distributing the task to several processors working concurrently has been implemented as part of OME (Open Microscopy Environment) software suite (Swedlow, Goldberg, Brauner, & Peter, 2003), a platform for storing and processing microscopy images. The increase in speedup when using this platform is nearly linear to the number of processors, until a number of 20 processors is reached (Macura, 2008). OME is an open source project, and it is available for free download via the internet at http://www.openmicroscopy.org

When using multiple processors to compute the feature vector, the bottleneck of the computation of a single feature vector is the image feature that is the most computationally expensive among the image features described in Section 3. Obviously, different image features are different in their computational cost, and some features require the sacrifice of more computational resources than others do. In this case, the most expensive features are the Zernike polynomial features, which take ~14 second to compute using a 2.6 GHz Intel processor. That means that even with maximum parallelization of the code, the full feature vector cannot be computed within less than 14 seconds.

FUTURE TRENDS AND CONCLUSION

Here we described a method of automatic face recognition that makes use of a large set of image content descriptors extracted from the raw pixels, image transforms, and transforms of transforms. An important feature of this approach is that in datasets smaller than 1000 individuals, the recognition accuracy increases as the number of subjects gets larger due to the more accurate assessment of the discriminative power of the different image features determined by the Fisher scores. Since the color FERET dataset is limited to 1000 individuals, the response of the algorithm for larger face datasets was not tested. Future work will include testing more image features, image transforms, and using different types of feature selection and classification techniques.

A clear downside of this method is computational complexity. Using a 2.6 GHZ AMD Opteron processor and 2GM of RAM, one tile of 256×384 pixels can be processed in 252 seconds. However, the different image features allow parallelization to reduce the response time of a potential practical application.

The face classification method described here is the core technology of a real-life face recognition system, which has been tested successfully using a limited number of individuals. A future application of this algorithm is associating gene expressions with face similarities, which will potentially enable the mining of SNP databases (Single Nucleotide Polymorphism) of known subjects for genes that affect facial look.

The method discussed in this paper is based on extracting a very large set of image content descriptors, followed by a data-driven search for the most informative image features that are informative for face recognition but less sensitive to pose variations. Thus, no assumptions are made regarding each individual image feature, and the most informative descriptors in the feature set are selected and weighed. This approach can be used for visual biometric recognition that is not based on standard photos, or on what the human eye can easily sense.

The process of evolution "trained" the human eye to easily solve vision and cognition problems that are essential for day-to-day life, such as recognizing different persons by their faces. However, the fact that the human eye and brain can easily perform these tasks does not necessarily mean that other parts of the body are less effective for the purpose of visual biometric identification. In other words, the considerable amount of efforts invested in making identification based on facial features might be biased by the way the human eye makes the recognition of different persons. That is, other types of imaging of other parts of the body can be less trivial to the human cognition, but can still provide discriminative power when applying automatic recognition enabled by computer vision methods. These include identification based on X-rays (Shamir, Ling, Rahimi, Ferrucci, Goldberg, 2009b) and other medical imaging methods such as Computed Tomography (CT) and Magnetic Resonance Imaging (MRI). While these devices are typically expensive, and in many cases hazardous, they have the clear advantage of being robust to deception, as they image parts of the body that can be accessed and modified only by an invasive operation.

The source code (Shamir et al., 2008b) used for this experiment is available for free download at http://www.cs.mtu.edu/~lshamir/downloads/ImageClassifier, and readers are encouraged to download, replicate the experiments described in this paper, and use it for other recognition and computer vision applications.

ACKNOWLEDGMENT

This research was supported entirely by the Intramural Research Program of the NIH, National Institute on Aging. Portions of the research in this paper use the FERET database of facial images collected under the FERET program, sponsored by the DOD Counterdrug Technology Development Program Office.

REFERENCES

Belhumeur, P. N., Hespanha, J. P., & Kriegman, D. J. (1997). Eigenfaces vs. Fisherfaces: recognition using class specific linear projection. *IEEE Transactions on Pattern Analysis and Machine Intelligence, 19*, 711–720. .doi:10.1109/34.598228

Beymer, D. (1993). *Face recognition under varying poses*. Technical report 1461, MIT AI Lab. Retrieved from ftp://publications.ai.mit.edu/ai-publications/1000-1499/AIM-1461.ps.Z

Bishop, C. M. (2006). *Pattern Recognition and Machine Learning*. New York: Springer Press.

Brunelli, R., & Poggio, T. (1993). Face recognition: Features versus templates. *IEEE Transactions on Pattern Analysis and Machine Intelligence, 15*, 1042–1052. .doi:10.1109/34.254061

Chen, W., Yuen, P. C., Huang, J., & Dai, D. (2004). A novel one-parameter regularized linear discriminant analysis for solving small sample size problem in face recognition. In *Proceedings of the 5th Chinese Conference on Advances in Biometric Person Authentication* (pp. 320–329).

Cottes, T., Wheeler, G., Walker, K., & Taylor, C. (2002). View-based active appearance models. *Image and Vision Computing, 20*, 657–664. .doi:10.1016/S0262-8856(02)00055-0

Frigo, M., & Johnson, S. G. (2005). The Design and Implementation of FFTW3. *Proceedings of IEEE, 93*, 216-231. doi: 10.1.1.136.7045

Gao, Y., & Lehung, M. K. H. (2002). Face recognition using line edge map. *IEEE Transactions on Pattern Analysis and Machine Intelligence, 24*, 764–779. .doi:10.1109/TPAMI.2002.1008383

Gee, J. C., & Haynor, D. R. (1996). Rapid coarse-to-fine matching using scale-specific priors. In *Proceedings of SPIE Conference on Medical Imaging* (LNCS 2710, pp. 416–427). doi: 10.1.1.45.4826

Georghiades, A. S., Belhumeur, P. N., & Kriegman, D. J. (2001). From few to many: illumination cone models for face recognition under variable lighting and pose. *IEEE Transactions on Pattern Analysis and Machine Intelligence, 23*, 643–660. .doi:10.1109/34.927464

Gradshtein, I., & Ryzhik, I. (1994). *Table of integrals, series and products* (5th ed., p. 1054). New York: Academic Press.

Graham, D., & Allinson, N. (1998). Face recognition from unfamiliar views: subspace methods and pose dependency. In *Proceedings of the Third International Conference on Automatic Face and Gesture Recognition* (pp. 348–353). doi: AFGR.1998.670973

Gregorescu, C., Petkov, N., & Kruizinga, P. (2002). Comparison of texture features based on Gabor filters. *IEEE Transactions on Image Processing, 11*, 1160–1167. .doi:10.1109/TIP.2002.804262

Gross, R., Baker, S., Matthews, I., & Kanade, T. (2004). Face recognition across pose and illumination. In S. Z. Lin & A. K. Jain (Eds.), *Handbook of face recognition* (pp. 193-216). New York: Springer. doi: 10.1.1.3.9914

Gurevich, I. B., & Koryabkina, I. V. (2006). Comparative analysis and classification of features for image models. *Pattern Recognition and Image Analysis, 16*, 265–297. .doi:10.1134/S1054661806030023

Hadjidementriou, E., Grossberg, M., & Nayar, S. (2002). Spatial information in multi-resolution histograms. In *Proceedings of the IEEE Conference on Computer Vision and Pattern Recognition* (Vol. 1, pp. 702-709). doi: 10.1109/CVPR.2001.990544

Haralick, R. M., Shanmugam, K., & Dinstein, I. (1973). Textural features for image classification. *IEEE Transactions on Systems, Man, and Cybernetics, 6*, 269–285. doi:.doi:10.1109/TSMC.1973.4309314

Huang, R., Liu, Q., Lu, H., & Ma, S. (2002). Solving the small sample size problem of LDA. In *Proceedings of the International Conference on Pattern Recognition* (Vol. 3, pp. 29–32). doi: 10.1109/ICPR.2002.1047787

Ivanov, Y., Heisele, B., & Serre, T. (2004). Using component features for face recognition. In *Proceedings of the 6th IEEE International Conference on Automatic Face and Gesture Recognition* (pp. 421–426). doi: 10.1109/AFGR.2004.1301569

Jain, V., & Mukherjee, A. (2002). *Indian Face database*. Retrieved from http://vis-www.cs.umass.edu/%7Evidit/IndianFaceDatabase

Kirby, M., & Sirovich, L. (1990). Application of the Karhunen-Loeve procedure for the characterization of human faces. *IEEE Transactions on Pattern Analysis and Machine Intelligence, 12*, 831–835. .doi:10.1109/34.41390

Kong, S. G., Heo, J., Abidi, B. R., Paik, J., & Abidi, M. A. (2005). Recent advances in visual and infrared face recognition - a review. *Computer Vision and Image Understanding, 97*, 103–135. .doi:10.1016/j.cviu.2004.04.001

Lades, M., Vorbruggen, J. C., Buhmann, J., Lange, J., von der Malsburg, C., Wurtz, R. P., & Konen, M. (1993). Distortion invariant object recognition in the dynamic link architecture. *IEEE Transactions on Computers, 42*, 300–311. .doi:10.1109/12.210173

Lando, M., & Edelman, S. (1995). Generalization from a single view in face recognition. In *Proceedings of the International Workshop on Automatic Face and Gesture Recognition* (pp. 80-85). doi: 10.1.1.45.9570

Lynos, M., Akamatsu, S., Kamachi, M., & Gyboa, J. (1998). Coding facial expressions with Gabor wavelets. In *Proceedings of the 3rd IEEE International Conference on Automatic Face and Gesture Recognition* (pp. 200–205). doi: 10.1109/AFGR.1998.670949

Macura, T. J. (2008). *Open Microscopy Environment Analysis System: end-to-end software for high content, high throughput imaging.* Cambridge, UK: Ph.D Dissretation, University of Cambridge.

Murase, H., & Nayar, S. (1995). Visual learning and recognition of 3D objects from appearance. *International Journal of Computer Vision, 14*, 5–24. .doi:10.1007/BF01421486

Orlov, N., Shamir, L., Macura, T., Johnston, J., Eckley, D. M., & Goldberg, I. G. (2008). WND-CHARM: Multi-purpose image classification using compound image transforms. *Pattern Recognition Letters, 29*, 1684–1693. .doi:10.1016/j.patrec.2008.04.013

Penev, P. S., & Atick, J. J. (1996). Local feature analysis: a general statistical theory for object representation. *Network: Computation in Neural Systems, 7*, 477–500. doi: 10.1.1.105.4097

Phillips, P. J., Moon, H., Rizvi, S. A., & Rauss, P. J. (2000). The FERET evaluation methodology for face recognition algorithms. *IEEE Transactions on Pattern Analysis and Machine Intelligence, 22*, 1090–1104. .doi:10.1109/34.879790

Rodenacker, K., & Bengtsson, E. (2003). A feature set for cytometry on digitized microscopic images. *Annals of Cellular Pathology, 25*, 1–36. doi: 10.1.1.33.9697

Romdhani, S., Psarrou, A., & Gong, S. (2000). On utilizing templates and feature-based correspondence in multi-view appearance models. In *Proceedings of the 6th European Conference on Computer Vision* (Vol. 1, pp. 799-813). doi: 10.1.1.63.6036

Samal, D., Taleb, M., & Starovoitov, V. (2001). Experiments with preprocessing and analysis of human portraits. In *Proceedings of the 6th International Conference on Pattern Recognition and Image Processing* (Vol. 2, pp. 15–20).

Samaria, F., & Harter, A. C. (1994). Parameterization of a stochastic model for human face identification. In *Proceedings of the Second IEEE Workshop Applications of Computer Vision.* doi: 10.1109/ACV.1994.341300

Savvides, M., Vijaya Kumar, B. V. K., & Khosla, P. (2002). Face verification using correlation filters. In *Proceedings of the 3rd IEEE Conference on Automatic Identification Advanced Technologies* (pp. 56–61). doi: 10.1109/ICISIP.2004.1287684

Shamir, L., Ling, S., Rahimi, S., Ferrucci, L., & Goldberg, I. (2009b). Biometric identification using knee X-rays. *International Journal of Biometrics, 1*, 365–370. .doi:10.1504/IJBM.2009.024279

Shamir, L., Orlov, N., Eckley, D. M., Macura, T., & Goldberg, I. (2008a). IICBU-2008 - A proposed benchmark suite for biological image analysis. *Medical & Biological Engineering & Computing, 46*, 943–947. .doi:10.1007/s11517-008-0380-5

Shamir, L., Orlov, N., Eckley, D. M., Macura, T., Johnston, J., & Goldberg, I. (2008b). Wndchrm - An open source utility for biological image analysis. *BMC - . Source Code for Biology and Medicine, 3*, 13. .doi:10.1186/1751-0473-3-13

Shamir, L., Orlov, N., & Goldberg, I. (2009a). Evaluation of the informativeness of multi-order image transforms. In *International Conference on Image Processing Computer Vision and Pattern Recognition (IPCV'09)* (pp. 37-41).

Singh, R., Vasta, M., & Noore, A. (2005). Textural feature based face recognition for single training images. *Electronics Letters, 41*, 640–641. .doi:10.1049/el:20050352

Spacek, L. (2002). *University of Essex Face Database*. Retrieved from http://www.essex.ac.ukmvallfacesindex.html

Swedlow, J. R., Goldberg, I., Brauner, E., & Peter, K. S. (2003). Informatics and quantitative analysis in biological Imaging. *Science, 300*, 100–102. .doi:10.1126/science.1082602

Turk, M., & Pentland, A. (1991). Eigenfaces for Recognition. *Journal of Cognitive Neuroscience, 3*, 71–86. .doi:10.1162/jocn.1991.3.1.71

Vetter, T., & Poggio, T. (1997). Linear object classes and image synthesis from a single example image. *IEEE Transactions on Pattern Analysis and Machine Intelligence, 19*, 733–741. .doi:10.1109/34.598230

Wiskott, L., Fellous, J. M., Kruger, N., & Von Der Malsburg, C. (1997). Face recognition by elastic bunch graph matching. *IEEE Transactions on Pattern Analysis and Machine Intelligence, 19*, 775–779. .doi:10.1109/34.598235

Yu, H., & Yang, J. (2001). A direct LDA algorithm for high-dimensional data with application to face recognition. *Pattern Recognition, 34*, 2067–2070. .doi:10.1016/S0031-3203(00)00162-X

Zou, J., Ji, Q., & Nagy, G. A. (2007). A comparative study of local matching approach for face recognition. *IEEE Transactions on Image Processing, 16*, 2617–2628. .doi:10.1109/TIP.2007.904421

KEY TERMS AND DEFINITIONS

Face Recognition: Identification or verification of a person from a digital image.

Pose Variance: Differences in the rotational horizontal and vertical angles between the face and the camera.

Illumination Variance: Differences in the direction and brightness of the light sources when an image is acquired.

FERET: A standard face recognition database provided by NIST.

Compound Transforms: A chain of two or more transforms applied sequentially on a certain image.

Multi-Order Transforms: A chain of two or more transforms applied sequentially on a certain image.

Chapter 17
Configural Processing Hypothesis and Face–Inversion Effect

Sam S. Rakover
Haifa University, Israel

ABSTRACT

Perception and recognition of faces presented upright are better than Perception and recognition of faces presented inverted. The difference between upright and inverted orientations is greater in face recognition than in non-face object recognition. This Face-Inversion Effect is explained by the "Configural Processing" hypothesis that inversion disrupts configural information processing and leaves the featural information intact. The present chapter discusses two important findings that cast doubt on this hypothesis: inversion impairs recognition of isolated features (hair & forehead, and eyes), and certain facial configural information is not affected by inversion. The chapter focuses mainly on the latter finding, which reveals a new type of facial configural information, the "Eye-Illusion", which is based on certain geometrical illusions. The Eye-Illusion tended to resist inversion in experimental tasks of both perception and recognition. It resisted inversion also when its magnitude was reduced. Similar results were obtained with "Headlight-Illusion" produced on a car's front, and with "Form-Illusion" produced in geometrical forms. However, the Eye-Illusion was greater than the Headlight-Illusion, which in turn was greater than the Form-Illusion. These findings were explained by the "General Visual-Mechanism" hypothesis in terms of levels of visual information learning. The chapter proposes that a face is composed of various kinds of configural information that are differently impaired by inversion: from no effect (the Eye-Illusion) to a large effect (the Face-Inversion Effect).

DOI: 10.4018/978-1-61520-991-0.ch017

INTRODUCTION

One of the most studied effects in research on face perception and recognition is the Face-Inversion Effect. Perception and recognition of a face are better when it is presented upright than when it is presented in inverted. This effect is greater in faces than in non-face objects (buildings, cars) (e.g., Rakover, 2002; Rakover & Cahlon, 2001; Valentine, 1988; Yin, 1969) and is obtained in experimental tasks of perception and recognition alike (e.g., Freire, Lee, & Symons, 2000; Rossion & Gauthier, 2002). It is explained by the "Configural Processing" hypothesis, which proposes that inversion disrupts configural information processing (spatial relations among facial features) and/or holistic information (facial information is perceived as a whole Gestalt) and leaves the processing of featural information (eyes, nose, and mouth) comparatively intact (e.g., Bartlett, Searcy, Abdi, 2003; Diamond & Carey, 1986; Leder & Bruce, 2000; Leder & Carbon, 2006; Maurer, Le Grand & Mondloch, 2002; Rakover, 2002; Rhodes, Brake, & Atkinson, 1993; Searcy & Bartlett, 1996; Tanaka & Farah, 1993, 2003; Yovel & Kanwisher, 2008).

Facial configural information concerns the spatial relations among facial features and is usually defined as follows: "In the face perception literature, the term 'configural refers to spatial information. … The span of configural information can be small (e.g., specifying the relationship between two adjacent components) or it may be large (e.g., specifying the relationship between nonadjacent components separated by large distances, or specifying the relationship among all of the components in the face)" (see Peterson & Rhodes, 2003, p. 4). However, reviewing the pertinent literature, Maurer, Le Grand & Mondloch (2002) noted that there is no agreement on the meaning of the term 'configural processing'. They suggested distinguishing three types of configural processing: (a) detection of first-order information (eyes above nose, which is above mouth), (b)

detection of second-order information (distances among facial features), and (c) detection of holistic information (the face is perceived as a gestalt). From their analysis, they concluded that inversion affected all types of configural processing, but particularly the last two. Following these analyses, the present research conceived of configural information as consisting of all distances among facial features.

Two major popular mechanisms for explaining configural processing of faces have been proposed. The "Face-Specific Mechanism" hypothesis, which suggests a special cognitive mechanism for processing facial stimuli, and the "Expertise" hypothesis, which suggests that configural-holistic information can be learned similarly in both faces and non-face objects. (For discussions of these hypotheses, see Ashworth, Vuong, Rossion, & Tarr, 2008; Diamond & Carey, 1986; Farah, Tanaka, & Drain 1995; Gauthier & Tarr, 1997; Liu & Chaudhuri, 2003; Maurer, Le Grand & Mondloch, 2002; McKone, Crookes & Kanwisher, in press; Nachson, 1995; Rakover & Cahlon, 2001; Rossion & Gauthier, 2002; Tanaka & Farah, 2003.) Recently, however, Robbins & McKone (2007) suggested on the basis of an extensive review and their own findings that the Expertise hypothesis is unfounded (for a debate see Gauthier & Bukach, 2007, and McKone & Robbins, 2007).

The present chapter has the following major goals. First, I shall briefly discuss whether the Configural Processing hypothesis provides a necessary condition for the Face-Inversion Effect.

Second, I shall consider whether the Configural Processing hypothesis offers a sufficient condition for the Face-Inversion Effect. This section, which constitutes the main part of the chapter, is based on the results of a new series of 12 experiments conducted in my laboratory in recent years. The experiments (which used pictures of faces, cars, and geometrical forms) showed that inversion of faces with particular configural information, called the "Eye-Illusion", did not impair perception and recognition of this illusion despite its being based on a change in the facial configural information. Hence, one cannot suggest that all kinds of facial configural information are sufficient for obtaining the Face-Inversion Effect.

Third, to test the Face-Specific Mechanism hypothesis, the experimental results of Eye-Illusion will be compared with similar illusions produced on a car's front (the "Headlight-Illusion") and in geometrical forms (the "Form-Illusion"), as in Figure 1.

Finally, in an attempt to explain some of the findings reported in the literature (Face-Inversion Effect) and some of the present findings, I shall suggest a relatively new tentative hypothesis, the "General Visual-Mechanism", which is based on the idea that a general cognitive mechanism, which deals with all kinds of visual information (faces, cars, geometrical forms, and the like) is also involved in processing visual illusions.

Figure 1. Presents decreased and increased Eye-Illusion (a), Headlight-Illusion (b), and Form-Illusion (c). In each pair, the size of the inner Figure is the same.

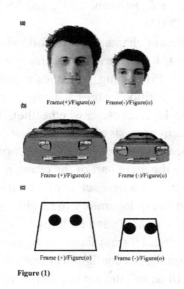

Figure (1)

BACKGROUND AND RELATED WORK

While the Configural Processing hypothesis has received wide empirical support from many studies (for reviews see Bartlett, Searcy, Abdi, 2003; Rakover, 2002; Rakover & Cahlon, 2001; Rossion, 2008; Rossion & Gauthier, 2002; Tanaka & Farah, 2003), several other cast doubt on this hypothesis.

Can an Isolated Facial Feature Show the Face-Inversion Effect?

Generally, face recognition is measured by a procedure consisting of two stages (see Rakover & Cahlon, 2001). In the first, the study stage, faces (or other forms of facial information) are presented to the participant. In the second, the test stage, the faces that were presented in the study stage (called the old faces) are mixed with new faces and are presented to the participant, who has to decide for each face whether it is old or new. (One important measure of this procedure is probability of correct recognition, p(correct).)

Given this procedure, the Configural Processing hypothesis makes the following two important predictions. If in the study stage whole faces are presented, and in the test stage isolated facial features (eyes or nose or mouth) of these faces are presented, recognition of the isolated features will be impaired since the configural information is removed in the test stage. Empirical studies have confirmed this prediction: no significant differences in p(correct) were found among upright isolated features, inverted isolated features, or inverted whole faces (e.g., Rhodes, Brake & Atkinson, 1993; Tanaka & Farah, 1993). Similarly, if in the study stage, isolated features are presented, and a whole face (composed of these features) is presented in the test stage, recognition will be impaired since the facial configural information was removed in the study stage. This prediction has also been confirmed (e.g., Farah, Tanaka & Drain, 1995).

However, one may wonder what will happen if the configural information is removed and isolated facial features are presented in both the study and the test stages? If the configural information is a necessary condition for the Face-Inversion Effect, will isolated features show this effect? Rakover & Teucher (1997) tended to propose an affirmative answer. They presented in both stages five facial features: hair & forehead, eyes, nose, mouth, and chin. The features were presented under four experimental conditions: UU-condition: the features were presented Upright in the study stage and Upright in the test stage; UI-condition: Upright and Inverted; IU-condition; and II-condition. The findings showed that (a) p(correct) in UU-condition was higher than in UI-condition and in IU-condition for all the five features, and (b) p(correct) in UU-condition was higher than in II-condition only for hair & forehead and eyes (where the difference for the latter feature was marginally significant, $p < .0526$). Hence, one may suggest that isolated features show the Face (Feature)-Inversion Effect, so configural information (the spatial relationship among facial features) is not necessary for obtaining this effect. The conclusion was challenged by Bartlett, Searcy & Abdi (2003) who suggested that finding (a) can be accounted for by certain processes that handle the change in the features' orientations (from U to I and from I to U) - a possibility that was discussed also by Rakover & Teucher. (Note though that the UU-condition and the IU-condition were used in Farah, Tanaka & Drain's (1995) study.) However, Bartlett, Searcy & Abdi (2003) admitted that with regard to finding (b), inversion might impair recognition of hair & forehead (they left out eyes). Furthermore, they pointed out that one could not account for recognition of the whole face by appeal to features' recognition, since p(correct) in the UU-condition was higher than a quantitative prediction of whole-face recognition derived from a simple feature-based mathematical model proposed by Rakover & Teucher (1997). While this comment is correct, the following

two points should be emphasized: (a) the model predicted accurately recognition of the whole face in the UI- IU- and II- conditions, and (b) the model accounted for 91% of the recognition of the whole face in the UU-condition. It therefore seems that featural information is more important than configural information, and that the Face (Feature)-Inversion Effect may occur without configural information.

One way to save the Configural Processing hypothesis is by assuming (a) that an isolated facial feature is in itself a visual form made up of basic components (for example, an eye is composed of eyebrow, eyelid, eyeball, pupil, etc.), and (b) that inversion impairs recognition of an isolated facial feature because it disrupts the spatial relations among the feature's basic components. This proposal, which may be viewed as an extension of the Configural Processing hypothesis, gives rise to the following question. Consider the comparison between two pairs of isolated eyes: a regular pair of eyes and the same eyes with a configural change such as elevated eyebrows. Would it be easier to perceive the two pairs as identical when they were presented in the upright position or in the inverted? According to the extended Configural Processing hypothesis, the answer is the inverted position, since inversion disrupts the configural information also *within* a facial feature. This prediction motivates an intriguing line of empirical research.

Does Inversion Disrupt all Kinds of Configural Information?

Several studies have showed that inversion does not impair all facial spatial relations (configural information) to the same extent. For example, inversion disrupts vertical spatial relations between features (eye height) more than horizontal spatial relations (inter-ocular distance) (e.g., Goffaux & Rossion, 2007. See also Barton, Keenan & Bass, 2001). Inversion impairs evaluations of faces as beautiful and appealing but not as interesting (e.g., Rakover, 2008). Other studies found that inversion impairs featural and configural information to a comparable degree. Sekuler, Gaspar, Gold & Bennett (2004) found that the difference between processing upright and inverted faces was quantitative rather than qualitative. Riesenhuber, Jarudi, Gilad & Sinha (2004) as well as Yovel & Kanwisher (2004) found a similar Face-Inversion Effect for facial configural and featural information. (However, see Rossion, 2008, for methodological criticism of the last three studies.)

Furthermore, Schwaninger, Ryf & Hofer (2003) found that the geometrical Horizontal-Vertical (H-V) illusion in a face resists inversion. (The H-V illusion refers to a visual form in the shape of T where the horizontal line is perceived as shorter than the vertical line although both lines are equal.) They proposed that the spatial relation between the eyes and the nose generates an illusion similar to the H-V illusion, and found that the perception of this illusion is preserved also when the face is inverted. However, they restricted this finding to perceptual tasks and the Face-Inversion Effect to recognition tasks.

Given these, one may propose that a face is composed of different kinds of configural information and that inversion impairs them differently. The aim of the present study is to show that a certain kind of configural information (the Eye-Illusion) resists inversion in perceptual tasks as well as in recognition tasks. If this is true, the Configural Processing hypothesis cannot provide a sufficient condition for the Face-Inversion Effect, since certain facial configural information resists inversion.

MAIN THRUST OF THE CHAPTER

Configural Information That Resists Inversion: An Empirical Study

The main goal of the present study was to test the Configural Processing hypothesis. A secondary goal was to test the Face-Specific Mechanism hypothesis. The tests employed two new kinds of facial configural information: the Eye-Illusions generated in faces, and the Headlight-Illusions generated on the front of cars. (The Form-Illusion will be referred to later on.) These illusions are generated by size transformations made on (1) a picture of a face: increase or decrease of the size of the Frame: the whole face except for the Figure, which is the eye-area (eyes, eyebrows and their spatial relationship), and (2) a picture of a front of car: increase or decrease of the size of the Frame: the whole front except for the Figure, which is the headlight-area (headlights and their spatial relationship, as in Figures 1a and 1b. The change in the size of the Frame alters the configural information of the visual form by altering the spatial relations of its features. A visual form composed of a Frame and an inner Figure is called "Frame/Figure".

The illusions used in the present study were generated under the inspiration of certain geometrical illusions, such as the Ebbinghaus and Delboeuf illusions, which involve spatial relations between a Frame and an inner Figure (e.g., Coren & Girgus, 1978; Robinson, 1998). For example, in the Ebbinghaus illusion the Figure, an inner circle, surrounded by a Frame made of an array of large circles, is perceived as smaller than the same Figure surrounded by a Frame made of small circles. (Note that the goal of the present study was not to conduct research on illusions per se, but only to use the present illusions to test the Configural Processing and the Face-Specific Mechanism hypotheses.)

According to the Configural Processing hypothesis, inversion should impair the Eye-Illusions generated by a change in the Frame. Since this change alters the configural information (the spatial relations among facial features), and since according to the Configural Processing hypothesis inversion impairs facial configural information, the inversion of a face is expected to impair the Eye-Illusion: there will be a significant difference between upright and inverted faces in the perceived size of the eyes. According to the Face-Specific Mechanism hypothesis, responses to the two illusions in a face and in a car should differ since the face-specific mechanism is restricted to facial information processing only.

Experiments 1-4: Faces and Cars

Method

Material
The Eye-Illusions were generated by means of the Adobe Photoshop 7.0 ME on a black-and-white picture of a face, the "origin-face", which was symbolized by Frame(o)/Figure(o), where (o) signifies that the Frame or the Figure is part of the origin-face. Frame(o)/Figure(o) has undergone the following two kinds of size transformations. The *Configural change* created new spatial relations in the origin-face, i.e., new configural information, in the following way. (1) Increase of the Frame only by 20%, a change symbolized as Frame(+)/Figure(o). The increase in the Frame only reduced the perceived size of the Figure (the origin-face's eyes), thus generating a decreased Eye-Illusion. (2) Decrease of the Frame only by 20%, a change symbolized as Frame(-)/Figure(o). The decrease in the Frame only enlarged the perceived size of the Figure (the origin-face's eyes), thus generating an increased Eye-Illusion, as in Figure 1a. As controls for the Eye-Illusion, the *Featural change* was used: increase or decrease of the Figure only (the origin-face's eyes-area) by 20%, changes symbolized as Frame(o)/Figure(+) and Frame(o)/Figure(-) respectively. The Headlight-Illusions made on a picture of the front of an "origin-car" were generated like the Eye-Illusions (by increase-decrease of the Frame or the Figure of the origin-car by 20%), as in Figure 1b.

Design, Procedure and Participants
Experiment 1: *Perception of the Eye-Illusions.* 120 pairs of faces [(6 different origin-faces) x (10 pairs per origin-face) x (2 positions – upright and inverted)] were randomly displayed on a computer monitor. The 10 pairs of faces were generated from the following five facial combinations: origin-face – Frame(o)/Figure(o); two transformations made by the Configural change – Frame(-)/Figure(o), Frame(+)/Figure(o); and two transformations made by the Featural change – Frame(o)/Figure(-), Frame(o)/Figure(+), as in Figure 1a. Conceptually, these 10 pairs can be divided into the following three categories: (a) 3 *Illusional-Pairs*, in which at least one face in a pair has undergone a Configural change only (the Frame was changed); (b) 3 *Featural-Pairs* in which at least one face in a pair has undergone a Featural change only (the Figure was changed); (c) 4 *Mixed-Pairs* in which one face in a pair has undergone a Configural change and the other face a Featural change. Each participant (n=20, mean age 23.4 years, 14 females, 6 males) was asked to choose from a given pair of faces (presented for 10 seconds maximum) the face in which the eyes were perceived as larger.

Experiment 2: *Perception of the Headlight-Illusions.* This was the same as experiment 1 except that 120 pairs of cars replaced the pairs of faces. Each participant (n=20, mean age 21.6 years, 15 females, 5 males.) was asked to choose the car on which the headlights were perceived as larger, as in Figure 1b. Note that in this as well as in the following experiments, new participants were recruited.

Experiment 3: *Recognition of the Eye-Illusions.* This was the same as experiment 1 except for the following: 120 pairs of faces were sequentially displayed on a computer monitor. Every pair included two faces shown in succession. Face A was shown first for 5 seconds and after an interval of 1.5 seconds face B was presented for 10 seconds maximum. When face B was displayed, the participants (n=20, mean age 23.0 years, 13 females, 7 males) were asked to decide which of the two faces (the remembered face A or the perceived face B) had the larger eyes.

Experiment 4: *Recognition of the Headlight-Illusions.* This was the same as experiment 3 except that 120 pairs of cars replaced the pairs of faces. Each participant (n=20, mean age 22.1 years, 14 females, 6 males) was asked to choose the car on which the headlights were remembered or perceived as larger.

Results and Discussion

The analysis of this study's results focuses on the three Illusional-Pairs and the three Featural-Pairs, since the choices in the four Mixed-Pairs were overwhelmingly determined by the Featural change (i.e., by the increase or decrease of the Figure only). Furthermore, the analyses of all 10 pairs (Illusional, Featural, and Mixed) in all the experiments reported here, showed the same order of mean p(choice) for faces, cars, and geometrical forms, which was calculated for of each of the five Frame/Figure combinations (faces, cars, geometrical forms): Frame(o)/Figure(+) > Frame(-)/Figure(o) > Frame(o)/Figure(o) > Frame(+)/Figure(o) > Frame(o)/Figure(-). (In all cases, the differences in mean p(choice) were highly significant.) Hence, the illusions reported here were bounded between two faces that had undergone featural changes: the Frame(o)/Figure(+) and the Frame(o)/Figure(-).

Analysis of the Illusional-Pairs
The results of the three Illusional-Pairs in experiments 1-4 are presented in Figure 2. The average probability of choice [p(choice)] of the perceived (or remembered) Frame(-)/Figure(o) face and the average p(choice) of the Frame(+)/Figure(o) face were calculated for each of the pairs displayed in Figure 2. Each p(choice) was tested by a t-test (df=19) to see whether it differed from chance (50%): all p(choice) were significantly different from chance, *although the size of the eye-area in all the Illusional-Pairs was the same*. Similar results were obtained for the Headlight-Illusions, except

for p(choice) in the perception upright condition in experiment 2 (see Figure 2c).

Faces

The results were handled by the following statistical analyses: *procedure* (perception-recognition) x *orientation* (upright-inverted) ANOVAs followed by post hoc comparisons with t-tests based on the appropriate ANOVA's *MSe* at α=.05. (Since these analyses were used in all the experiments reported here, they are referred to as the "Repeated Analyses"). There were no significant differences in p(choice) between the upright and inverted positions or between perception and recognition of faces in all the Illusional-Pairs in Experiment 1 (perception) and in Experiment 3 (recognition) except for the following. p(choice) with upright was higher than with inverted in the Frame(-)/Figure(o)–Frame(o)/Figure(o) pair, Experiment 1 ($t(38)$= 2.77), whereas in the Frame(+)/Figure(o)–Frame(o)/Figure(o) pair, Experiment 1, p(choice) with inverted was higher than with upright ($t(38)$=2.81) (see Figure 2b,c).

Cars

The Repeated Analyses applied to the cars' data yielded similar results with the Headlight-Illusions (Experiment 2 and Experiment 4) except for the following. p(choice) in recognition (summed over positions) was higher than in perception with the Frame(-)/Figure(o)–Frame(o)/Figure(o) pair ($F(1,38)$=5.53, p<.05) (see Figure 2b).

Faces vs. Cars

As detected by *stimuli* (faces-cars) × *procedure* (perception-recognition) × *orientation* (upright-inverted) ANOVAs, on average the p(choice) of the Frame (-)/Figure(o) face in the increased Eye-Illusions was higher than the p(choice) of the Frame(-)/Figure(o) car in the increased Headlight-Illusions: in the Frame(-)/Figure(o) –Frame(+)/Figure(o)

Figure 2. presents mean p(choice) of the Frame(-)/Figure(o) and of the Frame(+)/Figure(o) faces (without and with nose covered), cars, forms. These configurations appear in square brackets. As detected by t-tests, most of the probabilities were significantly different from chance: ^{ns} *= non-significant;* * *= p < .05;* ** *= p < .001.*

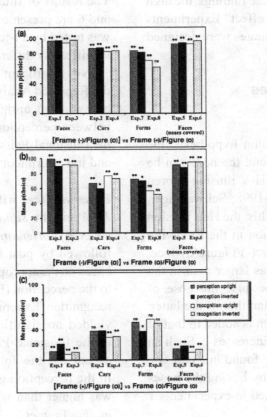

pair by 12% ($F(1,76)=20.19, p < .001$) and in the Frame(-)/Figure(o)–Frame(o)/Figure(o) pair by 24% ($F(1,76)=59.27, p < .001$) (see Figure 2a,b). In the Frame(+)/Figure(o)–Frame(o)/Figure(o) pair, p(choice) of the Frame(+)/Figure(o) car in the decreased Headlight-Illusion was higher than p(choice) of the Frame(+)/Figure(o) face in the decreased Eye-Illusion by 22% ($F(1,76)=33.70, p < .001$) (see Figure 2c).

Analysis of the Featural-Pairs

p(choice) of each facial Featural-Pair was significantly different from chance ($p < .001$, p(choice) range was .95-1.00). No significant differences emerged between upright and inverted positions or between perception and recognition. Similar results were obtained for the cars' Featural-Pairs ($p < .001$ for each pair, p(choice) range .92-1.00). Furthermore, no significant differences in p(choice) were found between faces and cars. Hence, the above "face-car" difference cannot be attributed to a general distinction in processing these visual stimuli.

Given these results, the Eye-Illusions seem greater than the Headlight-Illusions. How can this face-car difference be explained? Two explanatory hypotheses are considered: the "*Horizontal-Vertical (H-V) illusion*" hypothesis (tested in experiments 5-6) and the General Visual-Mechanism (GVM) hypothesis (tested in experiments 7-8).

Finally, the following questions were also considered. Were the findings of experiments 1-4 restricted only to the change of the Frame/Figure by 20% (20% changes)? Did these findings, the high p(choices), reflect a ceiling effect? Experiments 9-12 with 15% and 10% changes were designed to handle these questions.

Experiments 5-6: Faces with Noses Covered

According to the H-V illusion hypothesis, the spatial relation of the eyes and the nose can be viewed as analogues to the H-V illusion (Coren & Girgus, 1978; Robinson, 1998; Schwaninger, Ryf & Hofer, 2003). Given this, the H-V illusion may augment the Eye-Illusion in the following way. The eyes in the Frame(-)/Figure(o) face, for example, are perceived as larger than in the Frame(+)/Figure(o) face, because the nose of the former face is shorter than that of the latter. The effect of the H-V illusion is added to that of Eye-Illusion and as a result increases it. Such an augmenting effect cannot be found in a car. The H-V hypothesis was tested by having the noses covered in the faces presented in experiments 1 and 3.

Method

Design, Procedure and Participants
Experiment 5: *Perception of the Eye-Illusions – noses covered.* This was a replication of experiment 1, except that the noses were covered with a grey strip from below the eyes to below the nose, and from the edge of the left cheek to the edge of the right cheek. There were 20 participants, mean age 24.1, 15 females and 5 males.

Experiment 6: *Recognition of the Eye-Illusions – noses covered.* This was a replication of experiment 3, except that the noses were covered with a grey strip of the same length and width as in experiment 5. There were 20 participants, mean age 23.4, 13 females and 7 males.

Results and Discussion

Analysis of the Illusional-Pairs
The results of Illusional-Pairs in experiments 5 and 6 are presented in Figure 2. Each p(choice) was tested by a t-test (df=19): all p(choice) were significantly different from chance.

No significant differences (as detected by the Repeated Analyses) were found in p(choice) between the upright and inverted positions or between perception and recognition of faces in the Illusional-Pairs in Experiment 5 (perception) and in Experiment 6 (recognition).

Faces vs. faces with noses covered
Applying the *stimuli* (faces – faces with noses covered) x *orientation* (upright-inverted) ANOVA followed by post hoc comparisons with t-tests based on the appropriate ANOVA's *MSe* at α=.05, to the perception (Experiment 1 vs. 5) and to the recognition (Experiment 3 vs. 6) groups separately, yielded no significant differences in p(choice) in the Illusional-Pairs or in the Featural-pairs, except for the following two Illusional-Pairs. In the perception group, p(choice) with upright was higher than with inverted in Experiment 1 in the Frame(-)/Figure(o)–Frame(o)/Figure(o) pair ($t(38)= 3.01$), and p(choice) with upright was lower than with inverted in Experiment 1 in the Frame(+)/Figure(o)–Frame(o)/Figure(o) pair ($t(38)=2.54$) (see Figure 2b,c).

In conclusion, the results of the present experiments are similar to those obtained in the previous experiments. Therefore the H-V illusion hypothesis is not supported empirically.

Experiments 7-8: Geometrical Forms

The face-car difference can be accounted for by hypothesizing a General Visual-Mechanism (GVM) that deals with all kinds of visual information (faces, cars, etc.) and is involved in processing visual illusions. This visual mechanism is affected by the level of learning of the visual information in which the illusion is embedded: the higher the level of learning, the greater or more salient the illusion. The GVM hypothesis is similar to the proposal that a single visual-recognition system, which is sensitive to task demands and learning, is sufficient for the recognition of different kinds of objects (e.g., Tarr, 2003; Tarr & Cheng, 2003. See also Rakover & Cahlon's, 2001, "task-information" approach). It is assumed that the level of learned information is higher for faces than for cars, because people are exposed to faces more than to cars, and as a result they develop a prototype, a norm, or a scheme of faces, and they become expert at processing facial information (e.g., Diamond & Carey, 1986; Gauthier & Tarr, 1997; Rakover, 2002; Schwaninger, Carbon, Leder, 2003; Solso & McCarthy, 1981; Valentine, 1991). Hence, the finding that the Eye-Illusions are greater than the Headlight-Illusions can be explained by assuming that people are much more sensitive to faces than to cars.

Given the reasonable assumption that people are exposed to geometrical forms (see Figure 1c) less than to faces and cars, one can make the following prediction: the geometrical "Form-Illusions", generated from geometrical "origin-forms", will be weaker than the Eye-Illusions and Headlight-Illusions.

Method

Design, Procedure and Participants

Experiment 7: *Perception of Form-Illusions*. By means of a geometrical origin-form, the Form-Illusions were generated like the Eye-Illusions. There were six origin-forms consisting of three Frames (trapezoid, rectangle, and oval) and two Figures (two small black circles and two small black rectangles). The location of a Figure within a Frame was about one third of the length of the Frame, as in Figure 1c. Experiment 7 was the same as experiment 1, except that 120 pairs of geometrical forms replaced the pairs of faces. Each participant (n=20, mean age 23.3 years, 15

females, 5 males) was asked to choose from a pair of geometrical forms the one on which the inner Figure was perceived as larger.

Experiment 8: *Recognition of Form-Illusions*. This was the same as experiment 3 except that 120 pairs of geometrical forms replaced the pairs of faces. Each participant (n=20, mean age 25.8 years, 15 females, 5 males) was asked to choose from a pair of successive geometrical forms the one on which the inner Figure was perceived or remembered as larger.

Results and Discussion

Analysis of the Illusional-Pairs

The results of the Illusional-Pairs in experiments 7-8 are presented in Figure 2. Each p(choice) was tested by a t-test (df=19): as Figure 2 shows, several p(choice) were not significantly different from chance. In particular, note that contrary to experiment 7 (perception), p(choice) in the three Illusional-Pairs in experiment 8 (recognition) were not different from chance level (see especially Figure 2b,c).

No significant differences (as detected by the Repeated Analyses) were found in p(choice) between the upright and inverted positions in the Illusional-Pairs in Experiment 7 (perception) or in Experiment 8 (recognition) except for the following. In experiment 7, p(choice) of the Frame(+)/Figure(o) in the Frame(+)/Figure(o) - Frame(o)/Figure(o) pair was higher in the upright position than in the inverted ($t(38) = 2.26$) (see Figure 2c); and in experiment 8, p(choice) of the Frame(-)/Figure(o) in the Frame(-)/Figure(o)-Frame(+)/Figure(o) pair was higher in the upright position than in the inverted ($t(38) = 2.32$) (see Figure 2a). However, p(choice) in the perception task was higher than in the recognition task in all three pairs ($p < .05$ for all Fs), except for the Frame(+)/Figure(o)-Frame(o)/Figure(o) pair ($p > .05$). These and the above results support the hypothesis that geometrical forms were more difficult to process in the recognition than in the perception task.

Faces vs. Geometrical Forms

A comparison was made between faces and geometrical forms by employing the *stimuli* (faces (with noses)-geometrical forms) × *orientation* (upright-inverted) ANOVAs to the data of the three Illusional-Pairs (which appear in Figure 2). For both the perception and the recognition task the Eye-Illusions were greater than the Form-Illusions: for the Frame(-)/Figure(o)-Frame(+)/Figure(o) pair, perception - $F(1,38) = 12.49, p < .001$, recognition - $F(1,38) = 19.20, p < .001$; for the Frame(-)/Figure(o)-Frame(o)/Figure(o) pair, perception - $F(1,38) = 22.77, p < .001$, recognition - $F(1,38) = 39.06, p < .001$; and for the Frame(+)/Figure(o)-Frame(o)/Figure(o) pair, perception - $F(1,38) = 27.77, p < .001$, recognition - $F(1,38) = 39.99, p < .001$.

Cars vs. Geometrical Forms

A comparison was made between cars and geometrical forms by applying the *stimuli* (cars-geometrical forms) × *orientation* (upright-inverted) ANOVAs to the data of the Illusional-Pairs. For the recognition task only the Headlight-Illusions were greater than the Form-Illusions: for the Frame(−)/Figure(o) − Frame(+)/Figure(o) pair, perception − non-significant, recognition − $F(1,38) = 5.84$, $p < .05$; for the Frame(−)/Figure(o) − Frame(o)/Figure(o) pair, perception − non-significant, recognition - $F(1,38) = 10.95, p < .01$; and for the Frame(+)/Figure(o)−Frame(o)/Figure(o) pair, perception − non-significant, recognition − $F(1,38) = 9.46, p < .01$.

Analysis of the Featural-Pairs

All p(choice) of faces (with noses), cars, and forms were significantly different from chance (*p* < .001 for each pair, p(choice) range: .93-1.00). There were no significant differences in p(choice) between upright and inverted positions or between types of Frame/Figure (faces, cars, forms). However, small significant differences in p(choice) (in the range .95 - 1.00) were found in perception vs. recognition for each of the three Featural-Pairs.

These results differ strikingly from the perception vs. recognition results obtained for the three Illusional-Pairs, as in Figure 2. Therefore, the illusional differences in faces-cars-forms cannot be attributed to differential processing of the three kinds of visual stimuli.

These results seem to support the GVM hypothesis: on average, the Eye-Illusions are greater than the Form-Illusions, which are smaller (with respect to the recognition task) than the Headlight-Illusions.

Experiments 9-12: %15 and %10 Change

Given the above results, one may suggest that the Eye-Illusion tends to resist inversion. Is it possible that because the Eye-Illusion was so large and strong (it reflected a ceiling effect) it erased the effect of inversion? Will a weaker illusion allow an inversion effect? These questions suggest the "Weak Eye-Illusion" hypothesis: as the Eye-Illusion becomes weaker, the effect of inversion becomes stronger. To test this hypothesis, experiments 1 and 3 were replicated with 15% change and 10% change, which were expected to generate weaker illusions than 20% change.

Method

Design, Procedure and Participants

Experiment 9: *Perception of the Eye-Illusions – 15%Frame/Figure change*. This was a replication of experiment 1, except that the increase-decrease of the Frame/Figure was by 15% change. There were 20 participants, mean age 22.30, 15 females and 5 males.

Experiment 10: *Recognition of the Eye-Illusions – 15%Frame/Figure change*. This was a replication of experiment 3, except that the increase-decrease of the Frame/Figure was by 15% change. There were 20 participants, mean age 23.05, 13 females and 7 males.

Figure 3. presents mean p(choice) of the Frame(-)/Figure(o) and of the Frame(+)/Figure(o) faces with 20%, 15%, and 10% changes. These configurations appear in square brackets. As detected by t-tests, most of the probabilities were significantly different from chance: ns = non-significant; * = p < .05; ** = p < .001.

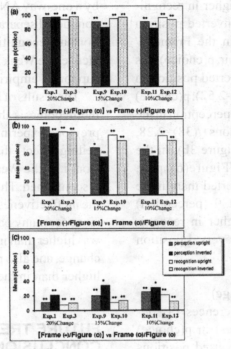

Figure (3)

Experiment 11: *Perception of the Eye-Illusions – 10%Frame/Figure change.* This was a replication of experiment 1, except that the increase-decrease of the Frame/Figure was by 10% change. There were 20 participants, mean age 21.95, 15 females and 5 males.

Experiment 12: *Recognition of the Eye-Illusions – 10%Frame/Figure change.* This was a replication of experiment 3, except that the increase-decrease of the Frame/Figure was by 10% change. There were 20 participants, mean age 22.45, 15 females and 5 males.

Results and Discussion

Analysis of the Illusional-Pairs

The results of the Illusional-Pairs in experiments 9-12 are presented in Figure 3. (For comparison, the Figure also contains the results of experiments 1 and 3.) Each p(choice) was tested by a t-test (df=19) to see whether it significantly differed from chance. Almost all the Illusional-Pairs p(choices) were significantly different from chance.

Experiments 9-10 (15% change)

There were no significant differences (as detected by the Repeated Analyses) in p(choice) between the upright and inverted positions or between perception and recognition of faces in the Illusional-Pairs in Experiment 9 (perception) and in Experiment 10 (recognition) except for the following. In the Frame(-)/Figure(o)-Frame(+)/Figure(o) pair, p(choice) was higher in recognition than in perception in the inverted position ($t(38)=2.90$) (see Figure 3a); in the Frame(-)/Figure(o)-Frame(o)/Figure(o) pair, p(choice) was higher in the upright than in inverted position in Experiment 9 (perception) ($t(38)=2.52$); p(choice) was higher in recognition than in perception in the upright and in the inverted positions ($t(38)=2.28$, $t(38)=2.90$, respectively) (see Figure 3b); in the Frame(+)/Figure(o)-Frame(o)/Figure(o) pair, p(choice) was higher in the inverted than in the upright position in Experiment 9 (perception) ($t(38)=3.05$); p(choice) was higher in recognition than in perception in the inverted position ($t(38)=3.14$) (see Figure 3c).

Experiments 11-12 (10% change)

There were no significant differences (as detected by the Repeated Analyses) in p(choice) between the upright and the inverted positions or between perception and recognition of faces in the Illusional-Pairs in Experiment 11 (perception) and in Experiment 12 (recognition) except for the following. In the Frame(-)/Figure(o)-Frame(+)/Figure(o) pair, p(choice) was higher in the upright than in the inverted position in Experiment 11 (perception) ($t(38)=2.84$); p(choice) was higher in recognition than in perception in the inverted position ($t(38)=2.79$) (see Figure 3a); in the Frame(-)/Figure(o)-Frame(o)/Figure(o) pair, p(choice) was higher in recognition than in perception in the upright and also in the inverted position ($t(38)=2.33$, $t(38)=2.64$, respectively) (see Figure 3b); finally, in the Frame(+)/Figure(o)-Frame(o)/Figure(o) pair, p(choice) was higher in recognition than in perception in the inverted position ($t(38)=3.03$) (see Figure 3c).

To test the *Weak Eye-Illusion hypothesis* (as the Eye-Illusion becomes weaker, the effect of inversion becomes stronger) the following index

was defined for each participant and for each pair of faces: UId = the difference in p(choice) between the Upright and the Inverted position. There were no significant differences [as detected by a one-way ANOVA (change: 20%, 15%, 10%) conducted separately for each pair in the perception and recognition conditions] in the UId index. Hence, the Weak Eye-Illusion hypothesis was not supported empirically.

The results of Experiments 9-12 do not support the hypothesis that the Eye-Illusion used in the previous experiments was so large (reflecting a ceiling effect) that it erased the effect of inversion, i.e., the Weak Eye-Illusion hypothesis was disconfirmed. This finding cannot be attributed to the ineffectiveness of the %change manipulation, since for many pairs p(choice) in the 20%change was higher than in the 15%change and in the 10% change, and also p(choice) in the 15%change was higher than in the 10%change.

FUTURE TRENDS AND CONCLUSION

Implications of the Present Research for Face Processing

The Configural Processing hypothesis

The foregoing results show that inversion did not impair 79% (19/24) of the cases in which the Illusional-Pairs were presented. This finding may be understood in terms of three possible methodological considerations (see Rakover, 1990).

(a) According to the strict hypothesis-testing methodology, the Configural Processing hypothesis was disconfirmed: it predicted that inversion would impair Eye-Illusions since this illusion is based on configural information, but in most cases, the prediction was not borne out.

(b) According to the hypothesis-modification methodology, if the Configural Processing hypothesis is not to be conceded because it is well entrenched both empirically and theoretically, the domain of its application may be restricted by exclusion of the configural information associated with visual geometrical illusions (for a similar idea see Schwaninger, Ryf & Hofer, 2003).

(c) According to the alternative-hypothesis methodology, an alternative hypothesis may be proposed that will provide explanations for some of the findings reported in the literature and in this study. This goal may be achieved by the GVM hypothesis discussed above. Accordingly, the GVM hypothesis may explain (a) the Face-Inversion Effect by proposing that the configural facial information, which was well learned in the upright position, becomes less discriminated, attenuated, when a face is inverted; and (b) the findings of this study (Eye-Illusions were greater than the Headlight-Illusions, which in turn were greater than Form-Illusions) by proposing that learning increases saliency in the Eye-Illusions more than in the Headlight-Illusions and in the Form-Illusions.

The Face-Specific Mechanism, the Expertise, and the GVM Hypotheses

Since the Face-Specific Mechanism is restricted to processing facial information by its very nature, it would be difficult to explain the similarity in behavioral patterns in the Eye-, the Headlight-, and the Form-Illusions: p(choices) in these illusions were significantly different from chance (except for the Form-Illusions in the recognition task); they were not affected by inversion; p(choice) in the perception task was no different from p(choice) in the recognition task (except for the Form-Illusions); the order of mean p(choice) of the five Frame/Figure combinations for faces was similar to that for cars and geometrical forms; and

the three Featural-Pairs did not differ significantly in p(choice).

These findings seem to support the Expertise hypothesis, which in contradiction to the Face-Specific Mechanism hypothesis proposes a single cognitive mechanism and emphasizes the importance of learning in explaining the Face-Inversion Effect (e.g., Ashworth, Vuong, Rossion & Tarr, 2008; Barton, Keenan & Bass, 2001; Tarr, 2003; Tarr & Cheng, 2003). In these respects, the GVM is similar to the Expertise hypothesis. Nevertheless, the two hypotheses do differ in the sense that the GVM hypothesis may be viewed as an extension of the Expertise hypothesis. It proposes a general visual mechanism that (a) deals with all kinds of visual information including illusions, and (b) interacts with learning of the visual forms in which the illusions are embedded, so that the higher the level of learning, the greater the saliency of the illusions.

Open Questions and Future Research

The present study advances our knowledge in two major points: (a) there is certain facial configural information (the Eye-Illusions) which tends to resist inversion; and (b) some of the findings of the present study and in the literature may be accounted for by appeal to the GVM hypothesis. Still, this hypothesis does not explain the nature of the illusions employed here, nor does it answer the question why these illusions resisted inversion (it explains the differences in Eye-, Headlight-, and Form-Illusions). Answers to these questions might be obtained by appeal to the theoretical mechanisms explaining the Ebbinghaus and Delboeuf illusions. However, no generally accepted theory for this kind of illusions seems to exist (see Coren & Girgus, 1978; Robinson, 1998). Whatever this theory might be, it should be emphasized that the Eye-Illusions are based on certain changes in the spatial relations among facial features (i.e., facial configural information) and are therefore of utmost relevance to research in face perception and recognition.

In view of the above, it is reasonable to propose that the Configural Processing hypothesis as presented in the literature is simplistic. First, a face seems to be composed of different kinds of information: (a) featural information, where each facial feature consists of basic components and the spatial relations among them, i.e., configural information *within* a feature; and (b) configural information, i.e., the spatial relations *between* facial features.

Second, one may conceive of inversion as a certain transformation (picture-plane rotation) which has different effects on the perception and recognition of the featural and configural information: it impairs at least some of the isolated facial features, and its impairment of the configural information varies from no effect (as in the case of the Eye-Illusions) to a great effect (as in the case of the Face-Inversion Effect).

This raises the following questions: How does inversion interact with the mechanism responsible for processing the various kinds of configural information? Why is one kind of configural information affected by inversion and another resists it? These intriguing questions require further research.

Finally, if researchers in computer vision and machine learning should wish to improve their algorithms by appeal to research in perception/recognition of human faces, the present chapter may contribute. It indicates that there are different visual information and cognitive mechanisms, which are important for processing faces presented in upright and inverted orientations.

ACKNOWLEDGMENT

I am grateful to Joel Norman, Israel Nachson and Ilan Fischer who read this chapter and made helpful suggestions. Thanks go to Hilla Kanner, Hen Maoz, Michal Kaufman, Miri Ben-Simon, Julia Kratshtein, Dadi Tal, Dan Lipner, Aviad Philipp, Alisa Bruhis, Alina Kratshtein, and Noam Mor who helped run the experiments and analyze the data. Special thanks go to Dr. Peter Peer and the CVL Face Database.

REFERENCES

Ashworth, A. R. S. III, Vuong, Q. C., Rossion, B., & Tarr, M. J. (2008). Recognizing rotated faces and Greebles: What properties drive the face inversion effect? *Visual Cognition, 16,* 754–784. doi:10.1080/13506280701381741

Bartlett, J. C., Searcy, J. H., & Abdi, H. (2003). What are the routes to face recognition? In Peterson, M. A., & Rhodes, G. (Eds.), *Perception of faces, objects, and scenes: Analytic and holistic processes.* Oxford, UK: Oxford University Press.

Barton, J. J. S., Keenan, J. P., & Bass, T. (2001). Discrimination of spatial relations and features in faces: Effects of inversion and viewing duration. *The British Journal of Psychology, 92,* 527–549. doi:10.1348/000712601162329

Coren, S., & Girgus, J. S. (1978). *Seeing is deceiving: The psychology of visual illusions.* Hillsdale, NJ: LEA.

Diamond, R., & Carey, S. (1986). Why faces are and are not special: An effect of expertise. *Journal of Experimental Psychology. General, 115,* 107–117. doi:10.1037/0096-3445.115.2.107

Farah, M. J., Tanaka, J. W., & Drain, H. M. (1995). What causes the face inversion effect? *Journal of Experimental Psychology. Human Perception and Performance, 21,* 628–634. doi:10.1037/0096-1523.21.3.628

Freire, A., Lee, K., & Symons, L. A. (2000). The face-inversion effect as a deficit in the encoding of configural information: Direct evidence. *Perception, 29,* 159–170. doi:10.1068/p3012

Gauthier, I., & Bukach, C. (2007). Should we reject the expertise hypothesis? *Cognition, 103,* 322–330. doi:10.1016/j.cognition.2006.05.003

Gauthier, I., & Tarr, M. J. (1997). Becoming a 'Greeble' expert: Exploring mechanisms for face recognition. *Vision Research, 37,* 1673–1682. doi:10.1016/S0042-6989(96)00286-6

Goffaux, V., & Rossion, B. (2007). Face inversion disproportionately impairs perception of vertical but not horizontal relations between features. *Journal of Experimental Psychology. Human Perception and Performance, 33,* 995–1001. doi:10.1037/0096-1523.33.4.995

Leder, H., & Bruce, V. (2000). When inverted faces are recognized: The role of configural information in face recognition. *Quarterly Journal of Experimental Psychology, 53A,* 513–536. doi:10.1080/027249800390583

Leder, H., & Carbon, C.-C. (2006). Face-specific configural processing of relational information. *The British Journal of Psychology, 97,* 19–29. doi:10.1348/000712605X54794

Liu, C. H., & Chaudhuri, A. (2003). What determines whether faces are special? *Visual Cognition, 10,* 385–408. doi:10.1080/13506280244000050

Maurer, D., Le Grand, R., & Mondloch, C. J. (2002). The many faces of configural processing. *Trends in Cognitive Sciences, 6,* 255–260. doi:10.1016/S1364-6613(02)01903-4

McKone, E., Crookes, K., & Kanwisher, N. (in press). The cognitive and neural development of face recognition in Humans . In Gazzaniga, M. (Ed.), *The cognitive Neurosciences.*

McKone, E., & Robbins, R. (2007). The evidence rejects the expertise hypothesis: Reply to Gauthier & Bukach. *Cognition, 103,* 331–336. doi:10.1016/j.cognition.2006.05.014

Nachson, I. (1995). On the modularity of face perception: The riddle of domain specificity. *Journal of Clinical and Experimental Neuropsychology, 9,* 353–383.

Peterson, M. A., & Rhodes, G. (2003). Introduction: analytic and holistic processing – the view through different lenses . In Peterson, M. A., & Rhodes, G. (Eds.), *Perception of faces, objects, and scenes: Analytic and holistic processes.* Oxford, UK: Oxford University Press.

Rakover, S. S. (1990). *Metapsychology: missing links in behavior, mind and science.* New York: Solomon/Paragon.

Rakover, S. S. (2002). Featural vs. configurational information in faces: A conceptual and empirical analysis. *The British Journal of Psychology, 93,* 1–30. doi:10.1348/000712602162427

Rakover, S. S. (2008). Is facial beauty an innate response to the Leonardian Proportion? *Empirical Studies of the Arts, 26,* 155–179. doi:10.2190/EM.26.2.b

Rakover, S. S., & Cahlon, B. (2001). *Face recognition: Cognitive and computational processes.* Philadelphia, PA: John Benjamins.

Rakover, S. S., & Teucher, B. (1997). Facial inversion effects: part and whole relationship. *Perception & Psychophysics, 59,* 752–761.

Rhodes, G., Brake, K., & Atkinson, A. (1993). What's lost in inverted faces? *Cognition, 47,* 25–57. doi:10.1016/0010-0277(93)90061-Y

Riesenhuber, M., Jarudi, I., Gilad, S., & Sinha, P. (2004). Face processing in humans is compatible with a simple shape-based model of vision. *Proceedings. Biological Sciences, 271*(Suppl.), S448–S450. doi:10.1098/rsbl.2004.0216

Robbins, R., & McKone, E. (2007). No face-like processing for objects-of-expertise in three behavioral tasks. *Cognition, 103,* 34–79. doi:10.1016/j.cognition.2006.02.008

Robinson, J. O. (1998). *The psychology of visual illusion*. New York: Dover Publications.

Rossion, B. (2008). Picture-plane inversion leads to qualitative changes of face perception. *Acta Psychologica, 128*, 274–289. doi:10.1016/j.actpsy.2008.02.003

Rossion, B., & Gauthier, I. (2002). How does the brain process upright and inverted faces? *Behavioral and Cognitive Neuroscience Reviews, 1*, 63–75. doi:10.1177/1534582302001001004

Schwaninger, A., Carbon, C.-C., & Leder, H. (2003). Expert face processing: Specialization and constraints . In Schwarzer, G., & Leder, H. (Eds.), *Development of face processing*. Göttingen, Germany: Hogrefe.

Schwaninger, A., Ryf, S., & Hofer, F. (2003). Configural information is processed differently in perception and recognition of faces. *Vision Research, 43*, 1501–1505. doi:10.1016/S0042-6989(03)00171-8

Searcy, J. H., & Bartlett, J. C. (1996). Inversion and processing of component and spatial-relational information in faces. *Journal of Experimental Psychology. Human Perception and Performance, 22*, 904–915. doi:10.1037/0096-1523.22.4.904

Sekuler, A. B., Gaspar, C. M., Gold, J. M., & Bennett, P. J. (2004). Inversion leads to quantitative, not qualitative, changes in face processing. *Current Biology, 14*, 391–396. doi:10.1016/j.cub.2004.02.028

Solso, R. L., & McCarthy, J. E. (1981). Prototype formation of faces: A case of pseudo-memory. *The British Journal of Psychology, 72*, 499–503.

Tanaka, J. W., & Farah, M. J. (1993). Parts and their configuration in face recognition. *Quarterly Journal of Experimental Psychology, 46A*, 225–245.

Tanaka, J. W., & Farah, M. J. (2003). The holistic representation of faces . In Peterson, M. A., & Rhodes, G. (Eds.), *Perception of faces, objects, and scenes: Analytic and holistic processes*. Oxford, UK: Oxford University Press.

Tarr, M. J. (2003). Visual object recognition: Can a single mechanism suffice? In Peterson, M. A., & Rhodes, G. (Eds.), *Perception of faces, objects, and scenes: Analytic and holistic processes*. Oxford, UK: Oxford University Press.

Tarr, M. J., & Cheng, Y. D. (2003). Learning to see faces and objects. *Trends in Cognitive Sciences, 7*, 23–30. doi:10.1016/S1364-6613(02)00010-4

Valentine, T. (1988). Upside-down faces: A review of the effect of inversion on face recognition. *The British Journal of Psychology, 79*, 471–491.

Valentine, T. (1991). A unified account of the effects of distinctiveness, inversion and race in face recognition. *Quarterly Journal of Experimental Psychology, 43A*, 161–204.

Yin, R. K. (1969). Looking at upside-down faces. *Journal of Experimental Psychology, 81*, 141–145. doi:10.1037/h0027474

Yovel, G., & Kanwisher, N. (2004). Face perception: Domain specific not process specific. *Neuron, 44*, 889–898.

Yovel, G., & Kanwisher, N. (2008). The representations of spacing and part-based information are associated for upright faces but dissociated for objects: Evidence from individual differences. *Psychonomic Bulletin & Review, 15*, 933–939. doi:10.3758/PBR.15.5.933

KEY TERMS AND DEFINITIONS

Face Perception and Recognition: Face perception is a concept that describes and explains how we come to know the face presented before us. Face recognition is a concept that describes and explains how we come to know that we saw the face presented before us.

Configural-Processing Hypothesis: suggests that inversion of a face disrupts configural information (the spatial relations among facial features) and leaves relatively intact featural information (eyes, nose, and mouth).

Face-Inversion Effect: is a phenomenon according to which perception and recognition of a face is better when the face is in upright position than when in inverted position. This kind of relation is greater in faces than in objects.

Compilation of References

Abate, A. F., Nappi, M., Riccio, D., & Sabatino, G. (2007). 2D and 3D face recognition: A survey. *Pattern Recognition Letters*, *28*(14), 1885–1906. doi:10.1016/j.patrec.2006.12.018

Abboud, B., Davoine, F., & Dang, M. (2004, September). Facial expression recognition and synthesis based on appearance model. *Signal Processing Image Communication*, *19*(8), 723–740. doi:10.1016/j.image.2004.05.009

Adini, Y., Moses, Y., & Ullman, S. (1997). Face recognition: The problem of compensating for changes in illumination direction. *IEEE Transactions on Pattern Analysis and Machine Intelligence*, *19*(7), 721–732. doi:10.1109/34.598229

Adini, Y., Moses, Y., & Ullman, S. (1997). Face Recognition: The Problem of Compensating for Changes in Illumination Direction. *IEEE TPAMI*, *19*(7), 721–732.

Adolphs, R. (2002). Recognizing emotion from facial expressions: psychological and neurological mechanisms. *Behavioral and Cognitive Neuroscience Reviews*, *1*, 21–61. doi:10.1177/1534582302001001003

Ahlberg, J. (2002). *Model-based coding: extraction, coding and evaluation of face model parameters*. Doctoral dissertation, Linköping University.

Ahonen, T., Hadid, A., & Pietikainen, M. (2006). *Face description with local binary patterns: Application to face recognition* (pp. 2037–2041). IEEE Trans. on PAMI.

Ajmal, S., Mian, M. B., & Robyn, O. (2007). An Efficient Multimodal 2D-3D Hybrid Approach to Automatic Face Recognition. *IEEE Transactions on Pattern Analysis and Machine Intelligence*, *29*(11), 1927–1943. doi:10.1109/TPAMI.2007.1105

Alizadeh, F., & Goldfarb, D. (2003). Second-Order Cone Programming. *Mathematical Programming*, *95*(1), 3–51. doi:10.1007/s10107-002-0339-5

Amaldi, E., & Kann, V. (1998). On the approximability of minimizing non zero variables or unsatisfied relations in linear systems. *Theoretical Computer Science*, *209*, 237–260. doi:10.1016/S0304-3975(97)00115-1

Ambadar, Z., Schooler, W. S., & Cohn, J. (2005). The importance of facial dynamics in interpreting subtle facial expressions. *Psychological Science*, *16*(5), 403–410. doi:10.1111/j.0956-7976.2005.01548.x

Ambadar, Z., Schooler, J., & Cohn, J. (2005). Deciphering the enigmatic face: the importance of facial dynamics to interpreting subtle facial expressions. *Psychological Science*, *16*(5), 403–410. doi:10.1111/j.0956-7976.2005.01548.x

Amin, M. A., Afzulpurkar, N. V., Dailey, M. N., Esichaikul, V., & Batanov, D. N. (2005). Fuzzy-C-Mean Determines the Principle Component Pairs to Estimate the Degree of Emotion from Facial Expressions. *FSKD*, 484-493.

Amit, Y., & Geman, D. (1997). Shape quantization and recognition with randomized trees. *Neural Computation*, *9*, 1545–1588. doi:10.1162/neco.1997.9.7.1545

Anderson, K., & McOwan, P. W. (2006). A real-time automated system for the recognition of human facial expressions. *IEEE Transactions on Systems Man and Cybernetics Part B*, *36*(1), 96–105. doi:10.1109/TSMCB.2005.854502

Ashraf, A. B., Lucey, S., Chen, T., Prkachin, K., Solomon, P., Ambadar, Z., & Cohn, J. (2007). The painful face: Pain expression recognition using active appearance models. In *Proc. of the ACM International Conference on Multimodal Interfaces* (pp. 9–14).

Ashworth, A. R. S. III, Vuong, Q. C., Rossion, B., & Tarr, M. J. (2008). Recognizing rotated faces and Greebles: What properties drive the face inversion effect? *Visual Cognition*, *16*, 754–784. doi:10.1080/13506280701381741

Asteriadis, S., Nikolaidis, N., & Pitas, I. (2009). Facial feature detection using distance vector fields. *Pattern Recognition*, *42*(7), 1388–1398. doi:10.1016/j.patcog.2009.01.009

Asteriadis, S., Nikolaidis, N., Hajdu, A., & Pitas, I. (2006). A novel eye detection algorithm utilizing edge-related geometrical information. In *14th European Signal Processing Conference (EUSIPCO)*.

Baraniuk, R. (2007). *Compressive sensing*. IEEE Signal Processing Magazine.

Baraniuk, R., Davenport, M., DeVore, R., & Wakin, M. B. (2006). *The Johnson-Lindenstrauss lemma meets compressed sensing*. Retrieved from www.dsp.rice.edu/cs/jlcs-v03.pdf

Baron, R. (1981). Mechanisms of human facial recognition. *International Journal of Man-Machine Studies*, *15*, 137–178. doi:10.1016/S0020-7373(81)80001-6

Baron-Cohen, S., Golan, O., Wheelwright, S., & Hill, J. J. (2004). *Mind Reading: The Interactive Guide to Emotions*. London: Jessica Kingsley Publishers.

Barrett, W. A. (1997). A survey of face recognition algorithms and testing results. *Proc. Asilomar Conference on Signals, Systems & Computers, 1*, 301-305.

Bartlett, M. S. (2001). *Face Image Analysis by Unsupervised Learning*. Amsterdam: Kluwer Academic Publishers.

Bartlett, M. S., Movellan, J. R., & Sejnowski, T. J. (2002). Face recognition by independent component analysis. *IEEE Trans. NN*, *13*(6), 1450–1464.

Bartlett, M., Stewart, M., Javier, R., & Sejnowski, T. J. (2002). Face recognition by independent component analysis. *IEEE Transactions on Neural Networks*, *13*(6), 1450–1464. doi:10.1109/TNN.2002.804287

Bartlett, M. S., Movellan, J. R., & Sejnowski, T. J. (2002). Face recognition by independent component analysis. *IEEE Transactions on Neural Networks*, 1450–1464. doi:10.1109/TNN.2002.804287

Bartlett, J. C., Searcy, J. H., & Abdi, H. (2003). What are the routes to face recognition? In Peterson, M. A., & Rhodes, G. (Eds.), *Perception of faces, objects, and scenes: Analytic and holistic processes*. Oxford, UK: Oxford University Press.

Bartlett, M. S., Littlewort, G., Fasel, I., & Movellan, J. R. (2003). *Real time face detection and facial expression recognition: Development and applications to human computer interaction*. Paper presented at the CVPR, Madison.

Bartlett, M., Littlewort, G., Lainscsek, C., Fasel, I., & Movellan, J. (2004, October 10-13). Machine learning methods for fully automatic recognition of facial expressions and facial actions. In *Proceedings of IEEE. International. Conference on Systems, Man and Cybernetics (SMC 2004)*, The Hague, The Netherlands (Vol. 1, pp. 592–597). Washington, DC: IEEE Press.

Bartneck, C., & Reichenbach, J. (2005). Subtle emotional expressions of synthetic characters. *International Journal of Human-Computer Studies*, *62*(2), 179–192. doi:10.1016/j.ijhcs.2004.11.006

Barton, J. J. S., Keenan, J. P., & Bass, T. (2001). Discrimination of spatial relations and features in faces: Effects of inversion and viewing duration. *The British Journal of Psychology*, *92*, 527–549. doi:10.1348/000712601162329

Basri, R., & Jacobs, D. (2003). Lambertian Reflectance and Linear Subspaces. *IEEE TPAMI*, *25*(2), 218–233.

Bassili, J. N. (1978). Facial motion in the perception of faces and of emotional expression. *Journal of Experimental Psychology. Human Perception and Performance, 4*, 373–379. doi:10.1037/0096-1523.4.3.373

Bassili, J. N. (1979). Emotion recognition: The role of facial movement and the relative importance of upper and lower areas of the face. *Journal of Personality and Social Psychology, 37*, 2049–2058. doi:10.1037/0022-3514.37.11.2049

Bassili, J. N. (1978). Facial motion in the perception of faces and of emotional expression. *Journal of Experimental Psychology, 4*(3), 373–379.

Beaudet, P. R. (1978). Rotationally Invariant Image Operators. *IJCPR*, 579-583.

Beaudot, W. (1994). *The neural information in the vertebra retina: a melting pot of ideas for artificial vision.* PhD thesis, TIRF laboratory, Grenoble, France.

Belhumeur, P. N., Hespanha, J. P., & Kriegman, D. J. (1997). Eigenfaces vs. Fisherfaces: Recognition using class specific linear projection. *IEEE Trans. PAMI, 19*(7), 711–720.

Belhumeur, Peter N., Hespanha, J. P., Kriegman, David. (1997). Eigenfaces vs. fisherfaces: Using class specific linear projection. *IEEE Transactions on Pattern Analysis and Machine Intelligence, 19*(7), 711–720. doi:10.1109/34.598228

Belhumeur, P. N., Hespanha, J. P., & Kriegman, D. J. (1997). Eigenfaces vs Fisherfaces: Recognition using class specific linear projection. *IEEE Transactions on Pattern Analysis and Machine Intelligence, 19*(7), 711–720. doi:10.1109/34.598228

Belhumeur, P. N., Hespanha, J. P., & Kriegman, D. J. (1997). Eigenfaces vs. Fisherfaces: Recognition using class specific linear projection. *IEEE Transactions on Pattern Analysis and Machine Intelligence, 19*(7), 711–720. doi:10.1109/34.598228

Belhumeur, V., Hespanha, J., & Kriegman, D. (1997). *Eigenfaces vs Fisherfaces: Recognition Using Class Specific Linear Projection.* IEEE Tran. PAMI.

Belhumeur, P. N., Hespanha, J. P., & Kriegman, D. J. (1997). Eigenfaces vs. Fisherfaces: Recognition using class specific linear projection. *IEEE Transactions on Pattern Analysis and Machine Intelligence, 19*(7), 711–720. doi:10.1109/34.598228

Belhumeur, P. N., Hespanha, J. P., & Kriegman, D. J. (1997). Eigenfaces vs. Fisherfaces: recognition using class specific linear projection. *IEEE Transactions on Pattern Analysis and Machine Intelligence, 19*, 711–720. .doi:10.1109/34.598228

Belhumeur, P. N., Hespanha, J. P., & Kriegman, D. J. (1997). Eigenfaces vs. Fisherfaces: Recognition using class specific linear projection. *IEEE Trans. PAMI*, 711–720.

Bellman, R. (1961). *Adaptive control processes: A guided tour.* Princeton, NJ: Princeton University Press.

Belongie, S., Malik, J., & Puzicha, J. (2002). *Shape Matching and Object Recognition Using Shape Contexts.* Pattern Analysis and Machine Intelligence PAMI.

Benaïm, M. (2000). Convergence with probability one of stochastic approximation algorithms whose average is cooperative. *Nonlinearity, 13*(3), 601–616. doi:10.1088/0951-7715/13/3/305

Bertsekas, D. P. (1999). *Nonlinear Programming* (2nd ed.). Belmont, MA: Athena Scientific.

Besl, P. J., & McKay, N. D. (1992). A method for registration of 3-d shapes. *IEEE Transactions on Pattern Analysis and Machine Intelligence, 14*(2), 239–256. doi:10.1109/34.121791

Bevilacqua, V., Cariello, L., Carro, G., Daleno, D., & Mastronardi, G. (2008). A face recognition system based on Pseudo 2D HMM applied to neural network coefficients. *Journal of Soft Computing – A Fusion of Foundations . Methodologies and Applications, 12*(7), 1432–7643.

Beymer, D. (1993). *Face recognition under varying poses.* Technical report 1461, MIT AI Lab. Retrieved from ftp://publications.ai.mit.edu/ai-publications/1000-1499/AIM-1461.ps.Z

Bhuiyan, M. A., Ampornaramveth, V., Muto, S., & Ueno, H. (2003). Face detection and facial feature localization for human-machine interface. *National Institute of Informatics Journal, 5*, 25–39.

Bicego, M., Lagorio, A., Grosso, E., & Tistarelli, M. (2006). *On the use of SIFT features for face authentication*. CVPRW.

Bicego, M., Lagorio, A., Grosso, E., & Tistarelli, M. (2006). On the Use of SIFT Features for Face Authentication. In *Conference on Computer Vision and Pattern Recognition Workshop*.

Bigun, J. (1997). Retinal vision applied to facial features detection and face authentication. *Pattern Recognition Letters, 23*, 463–475.

Bishop, C. M. (2006). *Pattern Recognition and Machine Learning*. New York: Springer Press.

Black, M. J., & Yacoob, Y. (1997). Recognizing Facial Expressions in Image Sequences Using Local Parameterized Models of Image Motion. *International Journal of Computer Vision, 25*(1), 23–48. doi:10.1023/A:1007977618277

Black, M. J., & Yacoob, Y. (1997). Recognizing facial expressions in images sequences using local parameterized models of image motion. *International Journal of Computer Vision, 25*(1), 23–48. doi:10.1023/A:1007977618277

Blake, A., & Isard, M. (2000). *Active Contours*. Berlin, Germany: Springer.

Blanz, V., & Vetter, T. (2003). Face recognition based on fitting a 3D morphable model. *IEEE Transactions on Pattern Analysis and Machine Intelligence, 25*(9), 1063–1074. doi:10.1109/TPAMI.2003.1227983

Blum, A., & Langley, P. (1997). Selection of relevant features and examples in machine learning. *Artificial Intelligence, 97*(1-2), 245–271. doi:10.1016/S0004-3702(97)00063-5

Boucher, J. D., & Ekman, P. (1975). Facial areas and emotional information. *The Journal of Communication, 25*, 21–29. doi:10.1111/j.1460-2466.1975.tb00577.x

Bould, E., Morris, N., & Wink, B. (2008). Recognising subtle emotional expressions: The role of facial movements. *Cognition and Emotion, 22*(8), 1569–1587. doi:10.1080/02699930801921156

Bowyer, K. W., Chang, K., & Flynn, P. (2006, January). A survey of approaches and challenges in 3D and multimodal 3D + 2D face recognition. *Computer Vision and Image Understanding, 101*(1), 1–15. .doi:10.1016/j.cviu.2005.05.005

Bowyer, K. W., Chang, K., & Flynn, P. (2004). A survey of approaches to three-dimensional face recognition. *Proc. ICPR, 1*, 358-361.

Breazeal, C. (1999, May 1). Robot in society: friend or appliance? In *Proceedings of Workshop on Emotion-Based Agent Architectures (EBAA 1999)*, Seattle, Washington, USA. New York: ACM Press.

Breazeal, C. (2000). *Sociable machines: Expressive social exchange between humans and robots*. Doctoral dissertation, MIT.

Breiman, L. (2001). Random forests. *Machine Learning, 45*(1), 5–32. doi:10.1023/A:1010933404324

Breiman, L., Friedman, J., Stone, C., & Olshen, R. (1984). *Classification and regression tree*. San Francisco: Wadsworth International.

Breiman, L. (1996). *Bias, variance, and arcing classifiers (Tech. Rep.)*. Statistics Department, University of California.

Bronstein, A. M., Bronstein, M. M., & Kimmel, R. (2005). Three-dimensional face recognition. *IJCV, 64*(1), 5–30. doi:10.1007/s11263-005-1085-y

Bruce, V. (1988). *Recognizing Faces*. London: Erlbaum.

Bruce, V. (1990). Perceiving and Recognizing Faces. *Mind & Language*, 342–364. doi:10.1111/j.1468-0017.1990.tb00168.x

Bruneli, R., & Poggio, T. (1993). Face recognition: features versus templates. *IEEE Transactions on Pattern Analysis and Machine Intelligence, 15*, 1042–1052. doi:10.1109/34.254061

Brunelli, R., & Poggio, T. (1993). Face recognition: Features versus templates. *IEEE Transactions on Pattern Analysis and Machine Intelligence, 15,* 1042–1052. .doi:10.1109/34.254061

Buciu, I., Nikolaidis, N., & Pitas, I. (2008). Non-negative matrix factorization in polynomial feature space. *IEEE Transactions on Neural Networks, 19*(6), 1090–1100. doi:10.1109/TNN.2008.2000162

Buddharaju, P., & Pavlidis, I. (2009). Physiological Face Recognition Is Coming of Age. *IEEE Trans. PAMI, 29*(4), 613–626.

Buhmann, J., Lades, M., & von der Malsburg, C. (1990). Size and distortion invariant object recognition by hierarchical graph matching. *IJCNN,* 411-416.

Camastra, F., & Verri, A. (2005). A novel kernel method for clustering. *IEEE Transactions on Pattern Analysis and Machine Intelligence, 27*(5), 801–805. doi:10.1109/TPAMI.2005.88

Campadelli, S. P., & Lanzarotti, R. (2004). An efficient method to detect facial fiducial points for face recognition. In *17th International Conference on Pattern Recognition* (Vol. 1, pp. 532-525).

Cañamero, L., & Gaussier, P. (2005). Emotion understanding: robots as tools and models . In Nadel, J. (Eds.), *Emotional Development: Recent Research Advances* (pp. 235–258). New York: Oxford University Press.

Candès, E., & Tao, T. (2005). The dantzig selector: statistical estimation when p is much larger than n. *Annals of Statistics, 35,* 2313–2351. doi:10.1214/009053606000001523

Candes, E., & Tao, T. (2006). Near-optimal signal recovery from random projections: Universal encoding strategies? *IEEE Tran. Infm. Theory,* 5406-5425.

Candes, E., Romberg, J., & Tao, T. (2006). Stable signal recovery from incomplete and inaccurate measurements. *Comm. on Pure and Applied Math,* 1207-1223.

Canny, J. (1986). A Computational Approach to Edge Detection. *IEEE Transactions on Pattern Analysis and Machine Intelligence, 8,* 679–714. doi:10.1109/TPAMI.1986.4767851

Cao, W., Lu, F., Yuan, Y., & Wang, S. (2004). Face Recognition Technique Based on Modular ICA Approach. *Intelligent Information Processing,* 291-297.

Carneiro, G., & Jepson, A. D. (2004). *Flexible Spatial Models for Grouping Local Image Features.* Computer Vision and Pattern Recognition.

Castleman, K. R. (1979). *Digital image processing.* Englewood Cliffs, NJ: Prentice Hall.

Cevikalp, H., Neamtu, M., Wilkes, M., & Barkana, A. (2005). Discriminative common vectors for face recognition. *IEEE Transactions on Pattern Analysis and Machine Intelligence, 27*(1), 4–13. doi:10.1109/TPAMI.2005.9

Chalmond, B., & Girard, S. C. (1999). Nonlinear modeling of scattered multivariate data and its application to shape change. *IEEE Transactions on Pattern Analysis and Machine Intelligence, 5*(21), 422–432. doi:10.1109/34.765654

Chan, A. B., & Vasconcelos, N. (2008). *Modeling, Clustering, and Segmenting Video with Mixtures of Dynamic Textures.* IEEE Trans. PAMI.

Chan, S. C. Y., & Lewis, P. H. (1999). A pre-filter enabling fast frontal face detection. In *3rd International Conference on Visual Information and Information Systems* (pp. 777-784)

Chandrasiri, N. P., Park, M. C., Naemura, T., & Harashima, H. (1999). *Personal facial expression space based on multidimensional scaling for the recognition improvement.* Paper presented at the Proceedings of the Fifth International Symposium Signal Processing and Its Applications (pp. 22-25).

Chellappa, R., Wilson, C. L., & Sirohey, S. (1995). Human and machine recognition of faces: A survey. *Proceedings of the IEEE, 83*(5), 705–741. doi:10.1109/5.381842

Chellappa, R., Wilson, C. L., & Sirohey, S. (1995). Human and machine recognition of faces: A survey. *Proceedings of the IEEE*, *23*(5), 705–740. doi:10.1109/5.381842

Chen, W., Er, M. J., & Wu, S. (2005). PCA and LDA in DCT domain. *Pattern Recognition Letters*, *26*, 2474–2482. doi:10.1016/j.patrec.2005.05.004

Chen, W. G., & Qi, F. H. (2003). Learning NMF Representation Using a Hybrid Method Combining Feasible Direction Algorithm and Simulated Annealing. *Acta Electronica Sinica*, *31*(S1), 1290–1293.

Chen, L., Liao, H., Lin, J., Ko, M., & Yu, G. (2000). A new LDA-based face recognition system that can solve the small sample size problem. *Pattern Recognition*, *33*(11), 1713–1726. doi:10.1016/S0031-3203(99)00139-9

Chen, T., Yin, W., Zhou, X. S., Comaniciu, D., & Huang, T. S. (2006). Total Variation Models for Variable Lighting Face Recognition. *IEEE TPAMI*, *28*(9), 1519–1524.

Chen, H., Belhumeur, P., & Jacobs, D. (2000). In Search of Illumination Invariants. In *Proc. of the ICVPR'00* (pp. 254-261).

Chen, L. F., Liao, H. Y., Ko, M. T., et al. (2000). A new LDA-based face recognition system which can solve the small sample size problem. *PR, 33*, 1713-1726.

Chen, W., Yuen, P. C., Huang, J., & Dai, D. (2004). A novel one-parameter regularized linear discriminant analysis for solving small sample size problem in face recognition. In *Proceedings of the 5th Chinese Conference on Advances in Biometric Person Authentication* (pp. 320–329).

Cheng, Y. Q., Liu, K., Yang, J. Y., & Wang, H. F. (2002). A robust algebraic method for human face recognition. *IEEE Transactions on Pattern Analysis and Machine Intelligence*, *24*(6), 764–779.

Cheon, Y., & Kim, D. (2009). Natural facial expression recognition using differential-AAM and manifold learning. *Pattern Recognition*, *42*, 1340–1350. doi:10.1016/j.patcog.2008.10.010

Chien, J.-T., & Wu, C.-C. (2002). Discriminant wavelet-faces and nearest feature classifiers for face recognition. *IEEE Transactions on Pattern Analysis and Machine Intelligence*, *24*(12), 1644–1649. doi:10.1109/TPAMI.2002.1114855

Cho, S. Y., & Wong, J.-J. (2008). Human face recognition by adaptive processing of tree structures representation. *Neural Computing & Applications*, *17*(3), 201–215. doi:10.1007/s00521-007-0108-8

Cho, S. Y., Teoh, T.-T., & Nguwi, Y.-Y. (2009). Development of an Intelligent Facial Expression Recognizer for Mobile Applications. In *First KES International Symposium on Intelligent Decision Technologies*.

Chua, C. S., Han, F., & Ho, Y. K. (2000). 3D human face recognition using point signature. In *IEEE Internat. Conf. on Automatic Face and Gesture Recognition (FG 2000)*, France, March, pp. 233–238.

Cichocki, A., Amari, S., & Zdunek, R. (2006b). Extended SMART algorithms for non-negative matrix factorization. *Lecture Notes in Artificial Intelligence*, *4029*, 548–562.

Cichocki, A., Zdunek, R., & Amari, S. (2006a). Csiszar's divergences for non-negative matrix factorization: Family of new algorithms. *Lecture Notes in Computer Science*, *3889*, 32–39.

Cohen, I., Sebe, N., Garg, A., Chen, L., & Huang, T. S. (2003). Facial expression recognition from video sequences: temporal and static modelling. *Computer Vision and Image Understanding*, *91*(1-2), 160–187. doi:10.1016/S1077-3142(03)00081-X

Cohn, J. F., & Schmidt, K. L. (2004). The timing of facial motion in posed and spontaneous smiles. *Journal Wavelets . Multiresolution & Information Processing*, *2*(2), 121–132. doi:10.1142/S021969130400041X

Cohn, J. F. (2006). Foundations of Human Computing: Facial Expression and Emotion. In *Proc. Int. Conf. on Multimodal Interfaces* (pp. 233-238).

Cohn, J. F., Zlochower, A. J., Lien, J. J., & Kanade, A. T. (1998). *Feature-Point Tracking by Optical Flow Discriminates Subtle Differences in Facial Expression*. Paper presented at the International Conference on Face & Gesture Recognition.

Cook, J., Chandran, V., Sridharan, S., & Fookes, C. (2004). Face recognition from 3D data using iterative closest point algorithm and Gaussian mixture models. In *Internat. Symposium on 3D Data Processing, Visualization and Transmission (3DPVT 2004)*, Thessaloniki, Greece, 6–9 September.

Cootes, T., Edwards, G., & Taylor, C. (2001). Active appearance models. *IEEE Transactions on Pattern Analysis and Machine Intelligence, 23*(6), 681–685. doi:10.1109/34.927467

Cootes, T. F., Edwards, G. J., & Taylor, C. J. (1998). Active appearance models. *Lecture Notes in Computer Science*, 484–491. doi:10.1007/BFb0054760

Cootes, T. F., Edwards, G. J., & Taylor, C. (1998). Active appearance models. In *5th European Conference on Computer Vision* (Vol. 2, pp. 484-498).

Coren, S., & Girgus, J. S. (1978). *Seeing is deceiving: The psychology of visual illusions*. Hillsdale, NJ: LEA.

Cottes, T., Wheeler, G., Walker, K., & Taylor, C. (2002). View-based active appearance models. *Image and Vision Computing, 20*, 657–664. .doi:10.1016/S0262-8856(02)00055-0

Cottrell, G. W., & Fleming, M. (1990). Face Recognition using unsupervised feature extraction. In *International Neural Networks Conference* (pp. 322-325).

Cristinacce, D., Cootes, T., & Scott, I. (2004). A multi-stage approach to facial feature detection. In *15th British Machine Vision Conference* (pp. 231-240).

D'Orazio, T., Leo, M., Cicirelli, G., & Distante, A. (2004). An algorithm for real time eye detection in face images. In *17th International Conference on Pattern Recognition* (Vol. 3, pp. 278-281).

Dailey, M. N., Cottrell, G. W., Padgett, C., & Adolphs, R. (2002). EMPATH: A neural network that categorizes facial expressions. *Journal of Cognitive Neuroscience*, 1158–1173. doi:10.1162/089892902760807177

Dailey, M. N., Cottrell, G. W., Padgett, C., & Adolphs, R. (2002). EMPATH: A neural network that categorizes facial expressions. *Journal of Cognitive Neuroscience, 14*(8), 1158–1173. doi:10.1162/089892902760807177

Darwin, C. (1872). *The Expression of the Emotions in Man and Animals*. London: J. Murray. doi:10.1037/10001-000

Datta, R., Li, J., & Wang, Z. (2005). Content-based image retrieval: approaches and trends of the new age. In *Proceedings of the 7th ACM SIGMM international workshop on Multimedia information retrieval* (pp. 253 - 262).

Daubechies, I. (1992). Ten lectures on wavelets. In *CBMS-NSF Conference series in Applied Mathematics* (SIAM).

Daugman, J. G. (1980). Two-Dimensional Spectral Analysis of Cortical Receptive Field Profiles. *Vision Research*, 847–856. doi:10.1016/0042-6989(80)90065-6

Daugman, J. G. (1985). Uncertainty Relation for Resolution in Space, Spatial Frequency, and Orientation Optimized by Two-Dimensional Cortical Filters. *Journal of the Optical Society of America*, 1160–1169.

Daugman, J. G. (1988). Complete Discrete 2D Gabor Transforms by Neural Networks for Image Analysis and Compression. *IEEE Trans. PAMI.*, 1169-1179.

Deco, G., & Obradovic, D. (1995). Linear redundancy reduction learning. *Neural Networks, 8*(5), 751–755.

Delac, K., Grgic, M., & Grgic, S. (2007). Image Compression Effects in Face Recognition Systems. In Delac, K., & Grgic, M. (Eds.), *Face Recognition* (pp. 75–92).

Dempster, A. P., Laird, N. M., & Rubin, D. B. (1977). Maximum likelihood from incomplete data via the EM algorithm. *Journal of the Royal Statistical Society. Series B. Methodological, 39*(1), 1–38.

Deng, X., Chang, C. H., & Brandle, E. (2004). *A new method for eye extraction from facial image. Proc. In 2nd IEEE international workshop on electronic design, test and applications* (*Vol. 2*, pp. 29–34). Perth, Australia: DELTA.

Descartes, H. (1649). *Les Passions de l'âme*. Paris: Henry Le Gras.

Devore, J., & Peck, R. (1997). *Statistics: The Exploration and Analysis of Data* (3rd ed.). Pacific Grove, CA: Duxbury Press.

Diamond, R., & Carey, S. (1986). Why faces are and are not special: An effect of expertise. *Journal of Experimental Psychology. General*, *115*, 107–117. doi:10.1037/0096-3445.115.2.107

Dibeklioglu, H., Salah, A. A., & Akarun, L. (2008). 3D facial landmarking under expression, pose, and occlusion variations. In *IEEE Second International Conference on Biometrics: Theory, Applications and Systems*.

Ding, L., & Martinez, A. M. (2008). Precise detailed detection of faces and facial features. In *IEEE Conference on Computer Vision and Pattern Recognition* (CVPR) (pp. 1-7).

Donato, G., Bartlett, M. S., Hager, J. C., Ekman, P., & Sejnowski, T. J. (1999). Classifying facial actions. *IEEE Transactions on Pattern Analysis and Machine Intelligence*, *21*(10), 974–989. doi:10.1109/34.799905

Donato, G., Bartlett, M. S., Hager, J. C., Ekman, P., & Sejnowski, T. J. (1999). Classifying Facial Actions. *IEEE Trans. PAMI*, 974-989.

Donoho, D. (2006). Compressed sensing. *IEEE Transactions on Information Theory*, 1289–1306. doi:10.1109/TIT.2006.871582

Donoho, D. (2006). *For most large underdetermined systems of linear equations the minimal l1-norm solution is also the sparsest solution*. Comm. on Pure and Applied Math.

Dornaika, F., & Davoine, F. (2004). Head and facial animation tracking using appearance adaptive models and particle filters . In *Workshop Real-Time Vision for Human-Computer Interaction RTV4HCI in conjunction with CVPR*, 2. DC, USA: July Washington.

Dornaika, F., & Davoine, F. (2006). On appearance based face and facial action tracking. *IEEE Transactions on Circuits and Systems for Video Technology*, *16*(9), 1107–1124. doi:10.1109/TCSVT.2006.881200

Dornaika, F., & Raducanu, B. (2007). Inferring facial expressions from videos: Tool and application. *Signal Processing Image Communication*, *22*(9), 769–784. doi:10.1016/j.image.2007.06.006

Dornaika, F., & Davoine, F. (2005, September 11-14). View- and texture-independent facial expression recognition in videos using dynamic programming. In *Proceedings of IEEE International Conference on Image Processing (ICIP 2005)*, Genoa, Italy (pp. 1-4). Washington DC: IEEE Press.

Dubuisson, M. P., & Jain, A. K. (1994). A modified Hausdorff distance for object matching. In *12th International Conference on Pattern Recognition* (pp. 566-568).

Duda, R. O., Hart, P. E., & Stork, D. G. (2000). *Pattern Classification*. New York: John Wiley & Sons, Inc.

Duflo, M. (1996). *Algorithms stochastiques*. Berlin: Springer-Verlag.

Dupuis, P., & Ishii, H. (1991). On Lipschitz continuity of the solution mapping to the Skorokhod problem, with applications. *Stochastics and Stochastics Reports*, *35*(1), 31–62.

Dupuis, P., & Ramanan, K. (1999). Convex duality and the Skorokhod problem (Part I & II). *Probability Theory and Related Fields*, *115*(2), 153–236. doi:10.1007/s004400050269

Edwards, G. J., Cootes, T. F., & Taylor, C. J. (1998). Face Recognition Using Active Appearance Models. In *Proc. European Conf. Computer Vision* (Vol. 2, pp. 581-695).

Eickler, S., Muller, S., & Rigoll, G. (2000). Recognition of JPEG compressed face images based on statistical methods. *Image and Vision Computing*, *18*, 279–287. doi:10.1016/S0262-8856(99)00055-4

Ekman, P., & Friesen, W. V. (1978). *The facial action coding system (facs), A technique for the measurement of facial action*. Palo Alto, CA: Consulting Psychologists Press.

Ekman, P., Friesen, W. V., & Ellsworth, P. (1972). *Emotion in the human face*. New York: Pergamon Press.

Ekman, P., & Friesen, W. V. (1971). Constants across cultures in the face and emotion. *Journal of Personality and Social Psychology*, *17*(2), 124–129. doi:10.1037/h0030377

Ekman, P. (1992). Facial expressions of emotions: an old controversy and new findings. *Philosophical Transactions of the Royal Society of London*, *335*, 63–69. doi:10.1098/rstb.1992.0008

Ekman, P. (1993). Facial expression and emotion. *The American Psychologist*, *48*(4), 384–392. doi:10.1037/0003-066X.48.4.384

Ekman, P., & Davidson, R. (1994). *The nature of emotion: fundamental questions*. New York: Oxford University Press.

Ekman, P., Matsumoto, D., & Friesen, W. V. (2005). Facial Expression in Affective Disorders . In Ekman, P., & Rosenberg, E. L. (Eds.), *What the Face Reveals* (pp. 429–439).

El Kaliouby, R., & Robinson, P. (2004). Mind reading machines: automated inference of cognitive mental states from video. *SMC*, *1*, 682–688.

Elisseeff, A., Weston, J., & Schölkopf, B. (2003). Use of the zero-norm with linear models and kernel methods. *Journal of Machine Learning Research*, *3*, 1439–1461. doi:10.1162/153244303322753751

Ellis, H. D. (1986). Introduction to aspects of face processing: Ten questions in need of answers. *Aspects of Face Processing*, 3-13.

Erik, M. C., & Trivedi, M. M. (2009). Head pose estimation in computer vision: A survey. *IEEE Trans. PAMI*, *31*(4), 607–626.

Essa, I. A., & Pentland, A. P. (1997). Coding, analysis, interpretation, and recognition of facial expressions. *IEEE Transactions on Pattern Analysis and Machine Intelligence*, *19*(7), 757–763. doi:10.1109/34.598232

Etemad, K., & Chellappa, R. (1997). Discriminant analysis for recognition of human face images. *Journal of the Optical Society of America. A, Optics, Image Science, and Vision*, *14*(8), 1724–1733. doi:10.1364/JOSAA.14.001724

Everingham, M., & Zisserman, A. (2006). Regression and classification approaches to eye localization in face images. In *International Conference on Automatic Face and Gesture Recognition* (pp. 441–448).

Farah, M. J., Tanaka, J. W., & Drain, H. M. (1995). What causes the face inversion effect? *Journal of Experimental Psychology. Human Perception and Performance*, *21*, 628–634. doi:10.1037/0096-1523.21.3.628

Fasel, I. R., Fortenberry, B., & Movellan, J. R. (2005). Gboost: A generative framework for boosting with applications to realtime eye coding. *Computer Vision and Image Understanding*, *98*(1), 182–210. doi:10.1016/j.cviu.2004.07.014

Fasel, I., Fortenberry, B., & Movellan, J. (2005). A generative framework for real time object detection and classification. *Computer Vision and Image Understanding*, *98*, 182–210. doi:10.1016/j.cviu.2004.07.014

Fasel, B., & Luettin, J. (2003). Automatic facial expression analysis: a survey. *Pattern Recognition*, *36*(1), 259–275. doi:10.1016/S0031-3203(02)00052-3

Fasel, B., & Luettin, J. (2003). Automatic facial expression analysis: a survey. *Pattern Recognition*, *36*(1), 259–275. doi:10.1016/S0031-3203(02)00052-3

Fasel, B., & Lüttin, J. (2000). *Recognition of Asymmetric Facial Action Unit Activities and Intensities*. Paper presented at the Proceedings of the International Conference on Pattern Recognition, Barcelona, Spain.

Fasel, I. R. (2006). *Learning Real-Time Object Detectors: Probabilistic Generative Approaches*. PhD thesis, Department of Cognitive Science, University of California, San Diego, USA.

Fasel, I. R., Smith, E. C., Bartlett, M. S., & Movellan, J. R. (2002). A comparison of Gabor filter methods for automatic detection of facial landmarks. In *IEEE International Conference on Automatic Face and Gesture Recognition* (pp. 231-235).

Feris, R. S., Gemmell, J., Toyama, K., & Kruger, V. (2002). Hierarchical wavelet networks for facial feature localization. In *5th International Conference on Automatic Face and Gesture Recognition* (pp. 125-130).

Field, D. J. (1987). Relations between the statistics of natural images and the response properties of cortical cells. *Journal of the Optical Society of America*, 2379–2394.

Field, D. J. (1994). What is the goal of sensory coding? *Neural Computation*, 6(4), 559–601.

Fleuret, F., & Geman, D. (2001). Coarse-to-fine face detection. *International Journal of Computer Vision*, 41, 85–107. doi:10.1023/A:1011113216584

Freeman, W., & Adelson, E. (1991). The design and use of steerable filters. *Pattern Analysis and Machine Intelligence*, 13, 891–906. doi:10.1109/34.93808

Freire, A., Lee, K., & Symons, L. A. (2000). The face-inversion effect as a deficit in the encoding of configural information: Direct evidence. *Perception*, 29, 159–170. doi:10.1068/p3012

Friedman, J., Hastie, T., & Tibshirani, R. (2000). Additive logistic regression: a statistical view of boosting. *Annals of Statistics*, 28, 337–374. doi:10.1214/aos/1016218223

Frigo, M., & Johnson, S. G. (2005). The Design and Implementation of FFTW3. *Proceedings of IEEE*, 93, 216-231. doi: 10.1.1.136.7045

Frigyesi, A., & Höglund, M. (2008). Non-negative matrix factorization for the Analysis of complex and gene expression data: identification of clinically relevant tumor subtypes. *Cancer Informatics*, 6, 275–292.

Fukunaga, K. (1990). *Introduction to Statistical Pattern Recognition*. New York: Academic Press.

Gabor, D. (1946). Theory of communication. *Journal of Institute of Electronic Engineers*, 429-457.

Gadat, S. (2008). Jump diffusion over feature space for object recognition. *SIAM Journal on Control and Optimization*, 47(2), 904–935. doi:10.1137/060656759

Gadat, S., & Younes, L. (2007). A stochastic algorithm for feature selection in pattern recognition. *Journal of Machine Learning Research*, 8, 509–547.

Gao, Y., & Leung, M. K. H. (2002). Face recognition using line edge map. *IEEE Transactions on Pattern Analysis and Machine Intelligence*, 24(6), 764–779. doi:10.1109/TPAMI.2002.1008383

Gao, Q., Zhang, L., & Zhang, D. (2009). Sequential row–column independent component analysis for face recognition. *Neurocomputing*, 72(4-6), 1152–1159. doi:10.1016/j.neucom.2008.02.007

Gao, Y., & Leung, M. K. H. (2002). Face Recognition Using Line Edge Map. *IEEE TPAMI*, 24(6), 764–779.

Gao, Y., & Lehung, M. K. H. (2002). Face recognition using line edge map. *IEEE Transactions on Pattern Analysis and Machine Intelligence*, 24, 764–779. .doi:10.1109/TPAMI.2002.1008383

Gao, Y. a. (2002). Face recognition using line edge map. *IEEE Trans. on PAMI*, 764-779.

Gao, Y., Leung, M. K. H, Hui, S. C., & Tananda, M. W. (2003 May). Facial expression recognition from line-based caricatures. *IEEE Transaction on System, Man and Cybernetics - PART A: System and Humans*, 33(3).

Garcia, C., Zikos, G., & Tziritas, G. (2000). Wavelet packet analysis for face recognition. *Image and Vision Computing*, 18, 289–297. doi:10.1016/S0262-8856(99)00056-6

Gargesha, M., & Panchanathan, S. (2002). A hybrid technique for facial feature point detection. In *5th IEEE Southwest Symposium on Image Analysis and Interpretation* (pp. 134-138).

Gauthier, I., & Bukach, C. (2007). Should we reject the expertise hypothesis? *Cognition*, *103*, 322–330. doi:10.1016/j.cognition.2006.05.003

Gauthier, I., & Tarr, M. J. (1997). Becoming a 'Greeble' expert: Exploring mechanisms for face recognition. *Vision Research*, *37*, 1673–1682. doi:10.1016/S0042-6989(96)00286-6

Gee, J. C., & Haynor, D. R. (1996). Rapid coarse-to-fine matching using scale-specific priors. In *Proceedings of SPIE Conference on Medical Imaging* (LNCS 2710, pp. 416–427). doi: 10.1.1.45.4826

Geman, S., Bienenstock, E., & Doursat, R. (1992). Neural networks and the bias/variance dilemma. *Neural Computation*, *4*, 1–58. doi:10.1162/neco.1992.4.1.1

Georghiades, A. S., Belhumeur, P. N., & Kriegman, D. J. (2001). From few to many: illumination cone models for face recognition under variable lighting and pose. *IEEE Transactions on Pattern Analysis and Machine Intelligence*, *23*, 643–660. .doi:10.1109/34.927464

Goffaux, V., & Rossion, B. (2007). Face inversion disproportionately impairs perception of vertical but not horizontal relations between features. *Journal of Experimental Psychology. Human Perception and Performance*, *33*, 995–1001. doi:10.1037/0096-1523.33.4.995

Gonzalez, R. C., & Woods, R. E. (2002). *Digital Image Processing* (2nd ed.). Upper Saddle River, NJ: Prentice Hall.

Gordon, G. (1991). Face recognition based on depth maps and surface curvature . In *Geometric Methods in Computer Vision* (pp. 1–12). SPIE.

Gourier, N., Hall, D., & Crowley, J. L. (2004). Facial features detection robust to pose, illumination and identity. In *International Conference on Systems Man and Cybernetics* (pp. 617-622).

Gouta, K., & Miyamoto, M. (2000). Facial areas and emotional information. *Japanese Journal of Phycology*, *71*, 211–218.

Gradshtein, I., & Ryzhik, I. (1994). *Table of integrals, series and products* (5th ed., p. 1054). New York: Academic Press.

Graham, D., & Allinson, N. (1998). Face recognition from unfamiliar views: subspace methods and pose dependency. In *Proceedings of the Third International Conference on Automatic Face and Gesture Recognition* (pp. 348–353). doi: AFGR.1998.670973

Gregorescu, C., Petkov, N., & Kruizinga, P. (2002). Comparison of texture features based on Gabor filters. *IEEE Transactions on Image Processing*, *11*, 1160–1167. .doi:10.1109/TIP.2002.804262

Gross, R., Baker, S., Matthews, I., & Kanade, T. (2004). Face Recognition Across Pose and Illumination . In Li, S. Z., & Jain, A. K. (Eds.), *Handbook of Face Recognition*. Berlin: Springer-Verlag.

Gross, R., & Brajovic, V. (2003). An Image Preprocessing Algorithm for Illumination Invariant Face Recognition. In *Proc. of AVPBA '03* (pp. 10-18).

Gross, R., Matthews, I., & Baker, S. (2002). Eigen light-fields and face recognition across pose. In *IEEE Internat. Conf. on Automatic Face and Gesture Recognition*, May (pp. 1–7).

Gross, R., Shi, J., & Cohn, J. (2001). Quo Vadis Face Recognition? In *Third Workshop on Empirical Evaluation Methods in Computer Vision*.

Guan, X. H., Wang, W., & Zhang, X. L. (2009). Fast intrusion detection based on a non-negative matrix factorization model. *Journal of Network and Computer Applications*, *32*(1), 31–44.

Guillamet, D., & Vitrià, J. (2002). Non-negative matrix factorization for face recognition. *Lecture Notes in Computer Science*, *2504*, 336–344.

Guillamet, D., Vitrià, J., & Schiele, B. (2003). Introducing a weighted non-negative matrix factorization for image classification. *Pattern Recognition Letters*, *24*(14), 2447–2454.

Gunes, H., Piccardi, M., & Pantic, M. (2008). From the Lab to the Real World: Affect Recognition using Multiple Cues and Modalities . In Or, J. (Ed.), *Affective Computing: Focus on Emotion Expression, Synthesis, and Recognition* (pp. 185–218). Vienna, Austria: I-Tech Education and Publishing.

Gurevich, I. B., & Koryabkina, I. V. (2006). Comparative analysis and classification of features for image models. *Pattern Recognition and Image Analysis*, *16*, 265–297. .doi:10.1134/S1054661806030023

Guyon, I., & Elisseeff, A. (2003). An introduction to variable and feature selection. *Journal of Machine Learning Research*, *3*, 1157–1182. doi:10.1162/153244303322753616

Guyon, I., Weston, J., Barnhill, S., & Vapnik, V. (2002). Gene selection for cancer classification using support vector machines. *Machine Learning*, *46*(1-3), 389–422. doi:10.1023/A:1012487302797

Guyon, I., & Elisseeff, A. (2003). An introduction to variable and feature selection. *Journal of Machine Learning Research*, *3*, 1157–1182. doi:10.1162/153244303322753616

Hafed, Z. M., & Levine, M. D. (2001). Face recognition using the discrete cosine transform. *Journal of Computer Vision*, *43*(3), 167–188. doi:10.1023/A:1011183429707

Haifeng, H. (2008). ICA-based neighborhood preserving analysis for face recognition . *Computer Vision and Image Understanding*, *3*(112), 286–295.

Hall, M. A., & Smith, L. A. (1999) Feature Selection for Machine Learning: Comparing a Correlation-Based Filter Approach to the Wrapper. In *FLAIRS Conference* (pp. 235–239).

Hammal, Z., Arguin, M., & Gosselin, F. (2009). Comparing a Novel Model Based on the Transferable Belief Model with Humans During the Recognition of Partially Occluded Facial Expressions. *Journal of Vision (Charlottesville, Va.)*, *9*(2), 1–19. Retrieved from http://journalofvision.org/9/2/22/, doi:10.1167/9.2.22. doi:10.1167/9.2.22

Hammal, Z., Couvreur, L., Caplier, A., & Rombaut, M. (2007). Facial expressions classification: A new approach based on Transferable Belief Model. *International Journal of Approximate Reasoning*, *46*, 542–567. doi:10.1016/j.ijar.2007.02.003

Hammal, Z., Eveno, N., Caplier, A., & Coulon, P. Y. (2006a). Parametric models for facial features segmentation. *Signal Processing*, *86*, 399–413. doi:10.1016/j.sigpro.2005.06.006

Hammal, Z., Caplier, A., & Rombaut, M. (2005). A fusion process based on belief theory for classification of facial basic emotions. In *Proceedings of the 8th International Conference on Information Fusion*, Philadelphia, PA, USA.

Hammal, Z., Kunz, M., Arguin, M., & Gosselin, F. (2008). Spontaneous pain expression recognition in video sequences. In *BCS International Academic Conference 2008 – Visions of Computer Science* (pp. 191-210).

Han, J., Cai, D., He, X., & Zhang, H.-J. (2006). Orthogonal laplacianfaces for face recognition. *IEEE Transactions on Image Processing*, *15*, 3608–3614. doi:10.1109/TIP.2006.881945

Han, C. C., Liao, H. Y. M., Yu, G. J., & Chen, L. H. (2000). Fast face detection via morphology-based pre-processing. *Pattern Recognition*, *33*, 1701–1712. doi:10.1016/S0031-3203(99)00141-7

Hansen, B. C., & Hess, R. F. (2006). The role of spatial phase in texture segmentation and contour integration. *Journal of Vision (Charlottesville, Va.)*, 595–615.

Haralick, R. M., Shanmugam, K., & Dinstein, I. (1973). Textural features for image classification. *IEEE Transactions on Systems, Man, and Cybernetics*, *6*, 269–285. doi:.doi:10.1109/TSMC.1973.4309314

Harris, C., & Stephens, M. (1988). A combined corner and edge detector. In *Proceedings of the 4th Alvey Vision Conference* (pp. 147-151).

Harwood, N. K., Hall, L. J., & Shinkfield, A. J. (1999). Recognition of facial emotional expressions from moving and static displays by individuals with mental retardation. *American Journal of Mental Retardation, 104*(3), 270–278. doi:10.1352/0895-8017(1999)104<0270:ROFEEF>2.0.CO;2

Haxby, J., Hoffman, E., & Gobbini, M. (2000). The distributed human neural system for face perception. *Trends in Cognitive Sciences, 4*(6), 223–233. doi:10.1016/S1364-6613(00)01482-0

Haxby, J. V., Hoffman, E. A., & Gobbini, M. I. (2002). Human neural systems for face recognition and social communication. *Biological Psychiatry, 51*(1), 59–67. doi:10.1016/S0006-3223(01)01330-0

He, X., Yan, S., Hu, Y., & Niyogi, P. (2005). Face recognition using Laplacianfaces. *IEEE Transactions on Pattern Analysis and Machine Intelligence, 27*(3), 328–340. doi:10.1109/TPAMI.2005.55

He, X., Yan, S., Hu, Y., Niyogi, P., & Zhang, H. (2005). Face recognition using Laplacianfaces. *IEEE Trans. on PAMI*, 328–340.

Heiler, M., & Schnorr, C. (2006). Learning sparse representations by non-negative matrix factorization and sequential cone programming. *Journal of Machine Learning Research, 7*(7), 1385–1407.

Hesher, C., Srivastava, A., & Erlebacher, G. (2002). Principal component analysis of range images for facial recognition. *Internat. Conf. on Imaging Science, Systems and Technology* (*CISST 2002*).

Heusch, G., Cardinaux, F., & Marcel S. (2005, March). Lighting Normalization Algorithms for Face Verification. *IDIAP-com 05-03*.

Hjelmaas, E. (2000). Feature-based face recognition. In *Norwegian Image Processing and Pattern Recognition Conference*.

Ho, T. K. (1998). The random subspace method for constructing decision forests. *IEEE Transactions on Pattern Analysis and Machine Intelligence, 20*(8), 832–844. doi:10.1109/34.709601

Holub, A., Liu, Y. H., & Perona, P. (2007). On constructing facial similarity maps. *Proc. CVPR*, 1-8.

Hong, Z. (1991). Algebraic feature extraction of image for recognition. *PR, 24,* 211-219.

Hotta, K. (2008). Robust face recognition under partial occlusion based on support vector machine with local Gaussian summation kernel. *Image and Vision Computing, 26*(11), 1490–1498. doi:10.1016/j.imavis.2008.04.008

Howland, P., & Park, H. (2004). Generalizing discriminant analysis using the generalized singular value decomposition. *IEEE Trans. PAMI, 26*(8), 995–1006.

Hoyer, P. O. (2004). Non-negative matrix factorization with sparseness constraints. *Journal of Machine Learning Research, 5*(9), 1457–1469.

Hoyer, P. O. (2002). Non-negative sparse coding. In *Proceedings of IEEE Workshop on Neural Networks for Signal Processing*, Martigny, Switzerland (pp. 557-565).

Hsu, R. L., Abdel-Mottaleb, M., & Jain, A. K. (2001). Face detection in color images. In *IEEE International Conference on Image Processing* (Vol. 1, pp. 1046-1049).

Hu, Y. X., Jiang, D. L., Yan, S. C., & Zhang, H. J. (2004). Automatic 3D Reconstruction for Face Recognition. In *IEEE International Conf. on Automatic Face and Gesture Recognition (FGR 2004)*, Seoul . *Korea & World Affairs*, (May): 843–850.

Huang, J., Chen, W.-S., Yuen, P. C., & Dai, D.-Q. (2005). Kernel machine-based one-parameter regularized Fisher discriminant method for face recognition. *IEEE Trans. Syst. Man Cybern. B, 35*(4), 659–669. doi:10.1109/TSMCB.2005.844596

Huang, W., & Yin, H. (2009). *Comparison of PCA and Nonlinear PCA for Face Recognition*. Signal Processing, Pattern Recognition and Applications.

Huang, R., Liu, Q., Lu, H., & Ma, S. (2002). Solving the small sample size problem of LDA. In *Proceedings of the International Conference on Pattern Recognition* (Vol. 3, pp. 29–32). doi: 10.1109/ICPR.2002.1047787

Huanga, K., Wanga, L., Tana, T., & Maybank, S. (2008). A real-time object detecting and tracking system for outdoor night surveillance. *Pattern Recognition*, 432–444. doi:10.1016/j.patcog.2007.05.017

Hubel, D., & Wiesel, T. (1962). Receptive fields, binocular interaction, and functional architecture in the cat's visual cortex. *The Journal of Physiology, 160*, 106–154.

Huppler, K. (2009). The art of building a good benchmark. *LNCS, 5895*, 18–30.

Hyvärinen, A., Karhunen, J., & Oja, E. (2001). *Independent Component Analysis*. Hoboken, NJ: Wiley- Interscience.

Hyvärinen, A., Kanhunen, J., & Oja, E. (2001). *Independent Component Analysis*. New York: Wiley-Intersciense. doi:10.1002/0471221317

Iancu, C., Corcoran, P., & Costache, G. (2007). A review of face recognition techniques for in-camera applications. *Proc. International Symposium on Signals, Circuits and Systems, 1*, 1-4.

Ilonen, J., Kamarainen, J., Paalanen, P., Hamouz, M., Kittler, J., & Kalviainen, H. (2008). Image feature localization by multiple hypothesis testing of Gabor features. *IEEE Transactions on Image Processing, 17*(3), 311–325. doi:10.1109/TIP.2007.916052

Ioannou, S., Karidakis, G., Kollias, S., & Karpouzis, K. (2007). Robust feature detection for facial expression recognition. *EURASIP Journal On Image and Video Processing, 2007*. IST-2000-29319. (n.d.). *ERMIS, Emotionally Rich Man-machine Intelligent System*. Retrieved from http://www.image.ntua.gr/ermis

Ioffe, S. (2006). Probabilistic linear discriminant analysis. In *European Conference on Computer Vision* (pp. 531–542).

Iordanis, M., Sotiris, M., & Michael, G. S. (2008). Bilinear Models for 3-D Face and Facial Expression Recognition. *IEEE Transactions on Information Forensics and Security, 3*(3), 498–511. doi:10.1109/TIFS.2008.924598

Irfanoglu, M. O., Gokberk, B., & Akarun, L. (2004). 3D shape-based face recognition using automatically registered facial surfaces. In *Internat. Conf. on Pattern Recognition (ICPR2004)*, Cambridge (pp. 183–186).

Ivanov, Y., Heisele, B., & Serre, T. (2004). Using component features for face recognition. In *Proceedings of the 6th IEEE International Conference on Automatic Face and Gesture Recognition* (pp. 421–426). doi: 10.1109/AFGR.2004.1301569

Izard, C. E., Dougherty, L. M., & Hembree, E. A. (1983). *A system for identifying affect expressions by holistic judgments*. Newark, Delaware: Instructional Resources Center, University of Delaware.

Jabson, D. J., Rahmann, Z., & Woodell, G. A. (1997b). A Multiscale Retinex for Bridging the Gap Between Color Images and the human Observations of Scenes. *IEEE Transactions on Image Processing, 6*(7), 897–1056.

Jadhav, D. V., & Holambe, R. S. (2008). Radon and discrete cosine transforms based feature extraction and dimensionality reduction approach for face recognition. *Signal Processing, 88*(10), 2604–2609. doi:10.1016/j.sigpro.2008.04.017

Jadhav, D. V., & Holambe, R. S. (2009). Feature extraction using Radon and wavelet transforms with application to face recognition. *Neurocomputing, 72*(7-9), 1950–1959. doi:10.1016/j.neucom.2008.05.001

Jaeger, J. (2003). *Improved gene selection for classification of microarrays* (pp. 53–94). Pac. Symp. Biocomput.

Jafari–Khouzani, K., & Soltanian-Zadeh, H. (2005). Rotation invariant multiresolution texture analysis using Radon and wavelet transform. *IEEE Transactions on Image Processing, 14*(6), 783–794. doi:10.1109/TIP.2005.847302

Jain, A. K., Duin, R. P. W., & Mao, J. (2000). Statistical pattern recognition: a review. *IEEE Transactions on Pattern Analysis and Machine Intelligence, 22*(1). doi:10.1109/34.824819

Jain, V., & Mukherjee, A. (2002). *Indian Face database.* Retrieved from http://vis-www.cs.umass.edu/%7Evidit/IndianFaceDatabase

Jesorsky, O., Kirchberg, K. J., & Frischholz, R. W. (2001). Robust face detection using the Hausdorff distance. In *3rd International Conference on Audio and Video-based Biometric Person Authentication* (pp. 90-95).

Ji, Q., Lan, P., & Looney, C. (2006). A probabilistic framework for modeling and real-time monitoring human fatigue. *IEEE System Man Cybernetic-Part A, 36*(5), 862–875. doi:10.1109/TSMCA.2005.855922

Ji, Y. Z. Q. (2005). Active and dynamic information fusion for facial expression understanding from image sequences. *IEEE Transactions on Pattern Analysis and Machine Intelligence, 27*(5), 699–714. doi:10.1109/TPAMI.2005.93

Jia, H. X., & Zhang, Y. J. (2008). Human detection in static images. *Pattern Recognition Technologies and Applications: Recent Advances,* 227-243.

Jing, X. Y., Tang, Y. Y., & Zhang, D. (2005). A Fourier–LDA approach for image recognition. *Pattern Recognition, 38*(2), 453–457. doi:10.1016/j.patcog.2003.09.020

Jing, X.-Y., Wong, H.-S., & Zhang, D. (2006). Face recognition based on discriminant fractional Fourier feature extraction. *Pattern Recognition Letters, 27,* 1465–1471. doi:10.1016/j.patrec.2006.02.020

Jobson, D. J., Rahman, Z., & Woodell, G. A. (1997a). Properties and Performance of a Center/Surround Retinex. *IEEE Transactions on Image Processing, 6*(3), 451–462. doi:10.1109/83.557356

Johnson, M. L. (2004). Biometrics and the threat to civil liberties. *Computer, 37*(4), 90–92. doi:10.1109/MC.2004.1297317

Jolliffe, I. T. (2002). *Principal component analysis.* New York: Springer.

Jolliffe, I. T. (2002). *Principal Component Analysis* (2nd ed.). New York: Springer-Verlag.

Jolliffe, I. T. (1986). *Pricipal Component Analysis.* New York: Springer.

Jones, J., & Palmer, L. (1987). An Evaluation of the Two-Dimensional Gabor Filter Model of Simple Receptive Fields in Cat Striate Cortex. *Journal of Neurophysiology,* 1233–1258.

Jones, M. C., & Sibson, R. (1987). What is projection pursuit? *Journal of the Royal Statistical Society. Series A (General), 150*(1), 1–36.

Jones, J. P., & Palmer, L. A. (1987). An evaluation of the Two-Dimensional Gabor Filter model of simple Receptive fields in cat striate cortex. *Journal of Neurophysiology, 58*(6), 1233–1258.

Jutten, C., & Herault, J. (1991). Blind separation of sources, part i: An adaptive algorithm based on neuromimetic architecture. *Signal Processing, 24*(1), 1–10. doi:10.1016/0165-1684(91)90079-X

Kadir, T., Zisserman, A., & Brady, M. (2004). An Affine Invariant Salient Region Detector. In *Conference of European Computer Vision* (pp. 228-241).

Kadyrov, A., & Petrou, M. (2001). The Trace Transform and Its Applications. *IEEE Transactions on Pattern Analysis and Machine Intelligence, 23*(8), 811–823. doi:10.1109/34.946986

Kanade, T., Cohn, J., & Tian, Y. L. (2000, March 28-30). Comprehensive database for facial expression analysis. In *Proceedings of International Conference on Automatic Face and Gesture Recognition (AFGR 2000),* Grenoble, France (pp. 46-53). Washington, DC: IEEE Press.

Kanade, T., Cohn, J., & Tian, Y.-L. (2000). Comprehensive database for facial expression analysis. In *International Conference on Automatic Face and Gesture Recognition* (pp. 46- 53).

Kapoor, A., Burleson, W., & Picard, R. W. (2007). Automatic Prediction of Frustration. *International Journal of Human-Computer Studies, 65*(8), 724–736. doi:10.1016/j.ijhcs.2007.02.003

Karungaru, S., Fukumi, M., & Akamatsu, N. (2004). Face recognition using genetic algorithm based template matching. In *IEEE International Symposium on Communications and Information Technology* (pp. 1252-1257).

Kashima, H., Hongo, H., Kato, K., & Yamamoto, K. (2001 June). A robust iris detection method of facial and eye movement. In *Proc. Vision Interface Annual Conference*, Ottawa, Canada.

Kawaguchi, T., & Rizon, M. (2003). Iris detection using intensity and edge information. *Pattern Recognition*, *36*(2), 549–562. doi:10.1016/S0031-3203(02)00066-3

Kawato, S., & Tetsutani, N. (2004). Detection and tracking of eyes for gaze-camera control. *Image and Vision Computing*, *22*(12), 1031–1038. doi:10.1016/j.imavis.2004.03.013

Kazuhiro, H. (2008). Robust face recognition under partial occlusion based on support vector machine with local Gaussian summation kernel. *Image and Vision Computing*, *26*, 1490–1498. doi:10.1016/j.imavis.2008.04.008

Ke, Y., & Sukthankar, R. (2004). *PCA-SIFT: A More Distinctive Representation for Local Image Descriptors*. Computer Vision and Pattern Recognition.

Kim, K. I., Jung, K., & Kim, H. J. (2002). Face recognition using kernel principal component analysis. *IEEE Signal Processing Letters*, *9*(2), 40–42. doi:10.1109/97.991133

Kim, H., & Park, H. (2007). Cancer class discovery using non-negative matrix factorization based on alternating non-negativity-constrained least squares. *Lecture Notes in Computer Science*, *4463*, 477–487.

Kim, D.-J., Bien, Z., & Park, K.-H. (2003). *Fuzzy neural networks(FNN)-based approach for personalized facial expression recognition with novel feature selection method*. Paper presented at the IEEE International Conference on Fuzzy Systems.

Kim, J., Choi, J., Yi, J., & Turk, M. (2005). Effective representation using ICA for face recognition robust to local distortion and partial occlusion. *IEEE Trans. on PAMI*, 1977–1981.

Kim, T.-K., Kim, H., Hwang, W., Kee, S.-C., & Kittler, J. (2003). Independent component analysis in a facial local residue space. In *IEEE Computer Society Conference on Computer Vision and Pattern Recognition* (Vol. 1, pp. 579–586).

Kim, Y., Lee, S., Kim, S., & Park, G. (2004, September 22-24). A fully automatic system recognizing human facial expressions. In M. Negoita et al. (Eds.), *Proceedings of the 8th International Conference on Knowledge-Based Intelligent Information and Engineering Systems (KES 2006)*, Wellington, New Zealand (LNCS 3215, pp. 203–209).

Kimura, S., & Yachida, M. (1997). *Facial Expression Recognition and Its Degree Estimation* (pp. 295–300). Proc. Computer Vision and Pattern Recognition.

Kira, K., & Rendell, L. A. (1992). A practical approach to feature selection. In *Proceedings of 9th International Conference on Machine Learning* (pp. 249–256).

Kirby, M., & Sirovich, L. (1990). Application of the Karhunen-Loeve procedure for the characterization of human faces. *IEEE Trans. PAMI*, *12*, 103–108.

Kirby, M., & Sirovich, L. (1990). Application of the Karhunen-Loeve procedure for the characterization of human faces. *IEEE Transactions on Pattern Analysis and Machine Intelligence*, *12*(1), 103–108. doi:10.1109/34.41390

Kirby, M., & Sirovich, L. (1990). Application of the Karhunen-Loève procedure for the characterization of human faces. *IEEE Transactions on Pattern Analysis and Machine Intelligence*, *12*, 831–835. doi:10.1109/34.41390

Kittler, J., Hatef, M., Duin, R. P., & Matas, J. (1998). *On Combining Classifiers*. IEEE Trans. on Pattern Analysis and Machine Intelligence.

Kjeldsen, R., & Kender, J. (1996). Finding skin in color images. In *2nd International Conference on Automatic Face and Gesture Recognition* (pp. 312-317).

Kong, S. G., Heo, J., & Abidi, B. (2005). Recent advances in visual and infrared face recognition -- A review. *Computer Vision and Image Understanding*, *97*(1), 103–135. doi:10.1016/j.cviu.2004.04.001

Kong, S. G., Heo, J., Abidi, B. R., Paik, J., & Abidi, M. A. (2005). Recent advances in visual and infrared face recognition - a review. *Computer Vision and Image Understanding*, *97*, 103–135. .doi:10.1016/j.cviu.2004.04.001

Kononenko, I. (1994). Estimating attributes: Analysis and extensions of relief. In *Proceedings of European Conference on Machine Learning* (pp. 171–182).

Kopriva, I., & Nuzillard, D. (2006). Non-negative matrix factorization approach to blind image deconvolution. *Lecture Notes in Computer Science, 3889*, 966–973.

Kotsia, I., Zafeiriou, S., & Pitas, I. (2007). A novel discirminant non-negative matrix factorization algorithm with applications to facial image characterization problems. *IEEE Transactions on Information Sorensics and Security, 2*(3), 588–595.

Kramer, M. A. (1991). Nonlinear principal components analysis using auto-associative neural networks. *AIChE Journal. American Institute of Chemical Engineers, 32*(2), 233–243. doi:10.1002/aic.690370209

Kreyszig, E. (1978). *Introductory functional analysis with applications*. New York: Wiley.

Kruger, U., Zhang, J. P., & Xie, L. (2008). Developments and applications of nonlinear principal component analysis - A review. *Lecture Notes in Computational Science and Engineering, 58*, 1–43. doi:10.1007/978-3-540-73750-6_1

Kuncheva, L., Bezdek, J., & Duin, R. (2001). Decision templates for multiple classifier fusion: An experimental comparison. *Pattern Recognition, 34*(2). doi:10.1016/S0031-3203(99)00223-X

Kuncheva, L. I., & Whitaker, C. J. (2003). Measures of diversity in classifier ensembles. *Machine Learning, 51*(2), 181–207. doi:10.1023/A:1022859003006

Kurita, T., & Taguchi, T. (2005). A kernel-based Fisher discriminant analysis for face detection. *IEICE Transactions on Information and Systems, E88*(3), 628–635. doi:10.1093/ietisy/e88-d.3.628

Kurita, T., Pic, M., & Takahashi, T. (2003). Recognition and detection of occluded faces by a neural network classifier with recursive data reconstruction. In *IEEE Conf. on Advanced Video and Signal Based Surveillance*, July (pp. 53–58).

Kyperountas, M., Tefas, A., & Pitas, I. (2007). Weighted Piecewise LDA for solving the small sample size problem in face verification. *IEEE Transactions on Neural Networks, 18*(2), 506–519. doi:10.1109/TNN.2006.885038

Kyperountas, M., Tefas, A., & Pitas, I. (2008). Dynamic Training using Multistage Clustering for Face Recognition. *Pattern Recognition, Elsevier, 41*(3), 894–905. doi:10.1016/j.patcog.2007.06.017

Kyperountas, M., Tefas, A., & Pitas, I. (2010). Salient feature and reliable classifier selection for facial expression classification. *Pattern Recognition, 43*(3), 972–986. doi:10.1016/j.patcog.2009.07.007

La Cara, G. E., Ursino, M., & Bettini, M. (2003). Extraction of Salient Contours in Primary Visual Cortex: A Neural Network Model Based on Physiological Knowledge. In *Proceedings of the 25th Annual International Conference of the IEEE* (Vol. 3, pp. 2242 – 2245).

Lades, M., Vorbruggen, J. C., Buhmann, J., Lange, J., von der Malsburg, C., Wurtz, R. P., & Konen, M. (1993). Distortion invariant object recognition in the dynamic link architecture. *IEEE Transactions on Computers, 42*, 300–311. .doi:10.1109/12.210173

Lai, J., Yuen, P. C., Chen, W., Lao, S., & Kawade, M. (2001). Robust facial feature point detection under non-linear illuminations. In *2nd International Workshop on Recognition, Analysis and Tracking of Faces and Gestures in Real-Time Systems* (pp. 168-174).

Lam, K., & Yan, H. (1998). An analytic-to-holistic approach for face recognition based on a single frontal view. *IEEE Transactions on Pattern Analysis and Machine Intelligence, 20*(7), 673–686. doi:10.1109/34.689299

Land, E. H., & McCann, J. J. (1971). Lightness and Retinex Theory. *Journal of the Optical Society of America, 61*(1), 1–11. doi:10.1364/JOSA.61.000001

Lando, M., & Edelman, S. (1995). Generalization from a single view in face recognition. In *Proceedings of the International Workshop on Automatic Face and Gesture Recognition* (pp. 80-85). doi: 10.1.1.45.9570

Lanitis, A., Taylor, J. C., & Timothy, F. C. (2002). Toward automatic simulation of aging effects on face images. *IEEE Transactions on Pattern Analysis and Machine Intelligence, 24*(4), 442–455. doi:10.1109/34.993553

Lanitis, A. T., C.J., Cootes, T.F. (1997). Automatic interpretation and coding of face images using flexible models. *Pattern Analysis and Machine Intelligence, IEEE Transactions on, 19*(7), 743-756.

Lawrence, S., Giles, C. L., Tsoi, A. C., & Back, A. D. (1997). Face recognition: a convolutional neural network approach. *IEEE Transactions on Neural Networks, 8*, 89–113. doi:10.1109/72.554195

Lê Cao, K. A., Gonçalves, O., Besse, P., & Gadat, S. (2007). Selection of biologically relevant genes with a wrapper stochastic algorithm. *Statistical Applications in Genetics and Molecular Biology, 6*(1). doi:10.2202/1544-6115.1312

Leder, H., & Bruce, V. (2000). When inverted faces are recognized: The role of configural information in face recognition. *Quarterly Journal of Experimental Psychology, 53A*, 513–536. doi:10.1080/027249800390583

Leder, H., & Carbon, C.-C. (2006). Face-specific configural processing of relational information. *The British Journal of Psychology, 97*, 19–29. doi:10.1348/000712605X54794

Lee, D. D., & Seung, H. S. (1999). Learning the parts of objects by non-negative matrix factorization. *Nature, 401*, 788–791. doi:10.1038/44565

Lee, D. D., & Seung, H. S. (1999). Learning the parts of objects by non-negative matrix factorization. *Nature, 401*(6755), 788–791.

Lee, K., Ho, J., Yang, M., & Kriegman, D. (2005). *Visual Tracking and Recognition using Probabilistic Appearance Manifolds*. CVIU.

Lee, K., & Kriegman, D. (2005). *Online Probabilistic Appearance Manifolds for Video-based Recognition and Tracking*. CVPR.

Lee, D. D., & Seung, H. S. (2001). Algorithms for non-negative matrix factorization. *Advances in Neural Information Processing Systems, 13*, 556–562.

Levner, I. (2005). Feature selection and nearest centroid classification for protein mass spectrometry. *BMC Bioinformatics, 6*, 68. doi:10.1186/1471-2105-6-68

Li, L., & Zhang, Y. J. (2009). FastNMF: Highly efficient monotonic fixed-point nonnegative matrix factorization algorithm with good applicability. *Journal of Electronic Imaging, 18*(3), 033004. doi:10.1117/1.3184771

Li, M., & Yuan, B. (2005). 2D-LDA: A novel statistical linear discriminant analysis for image matrix. *PRL, 26*(5), 527–532.

Li, S. Z., & Jain, A. K. (2004). *Handbook of Face Recognition*. New York: Springer.

Li, L., & Zhang, Y. J. (2007). Survey on algorithms of non-negative matrix factorization. *Acta Electronica Sinica, 36*(4), 737–743.

Li, S. Z., & Jain, A. K. (2005). *Handbook of Face Recognition*. Berlin: Springer.

Li, S. Z., & Jain, A. K. (Eds.). (2005). *Handbook of Face Recognition*. New York: Springer.

Li, F., Fergus, R., & Perona, P. (2004). Learning generative visual models from few training examples: an incremental Bayesian approach tested on 101 object categories. *Computer Vision and Pattern Recognition Workshop on Generative-Model Based Vision*. Retrieved from http://www.vision.caltech.edu/Image_Datasets/Caltech101/Caltech101.html

Li, L., & Zhang, Y. J. (2007). Non-negative matrix-set factorization. *Proc. ICIG*, 564-569.

Li, Q., Ye, J., & Kambhamettu, C. (2004). Linear projection methods in face recognition under unconstrained illuminations: A comparative study. In *IEEE Computer Society Conf. on Computer Vision and Pattern Recognition (CVPR04)*.

Liang, D., Yang, J., & Chang, Y. C. (2006). Relevance feedback based on non-negative matrix factorization for image retrieval. *IEE Proceedings. Vision Image and Signal Processing, 153*(4), 436–444.

Lien, J. J., Kanade, T., Cohn, J. F., & Li, C. (1998). Subtly different facial expression recognition and expression intensity estimation. In *Proceedings of IEEE Computer Vision and Pattern Recognition*, Santa Barbara, CA (pp. 853–859).

Lin, S.-H., Kung, S.-Y., & Lin, L.-J. (1997). Face recognition/detection by probabilistic decision-based neural network. *IEEE Transactions on Neural Networks, 8*(1), 114–132. doi:10.1109/72.554196

Littlewort, G., Bartlett, M. S., Fasel, I., Susskind, J., & Movellan, J. (2006). Dynamics of facial expression extracted automatically from video. *J. Image & Vision Computing, 24*(6), 615–625. doi:10.1016/j.imavis.2005.09.011

Littlewort, G. C., Bartlett, M. S., & Kang, L. (2007 November). Faces of Pain: Automated Measurement of Spontaneous Facial Expressions of Genuine and Posed Pain. In *Proc. ICMI*, Nagoya, Aichi, Japan

Liu, C. J., & Wechsler, H. (2000). Robust coding schemes for indexing and retrieval from large face databases. *IEEE Trans. IP, 9*(1), 132–137.

Liu, C. (2004). Gabor-based kernel PCA with fractional power polynomial models for face recognition. *IEEE Transactions on Pattern Analysis and Machine Intelligence, 26*(5), 572–581. doi:10.1109/TPAMI.2004.1273927

Liu, C. (2002). Gabor Feature Based Classification Using the Enhanced Fisher Linear Discriminant Model for Face Recognition. *IEEE Transactions on Image Processing*, 467–476.

Liu, C., & Wechsler, H. (2003). Independent Component Analysis of Gabor Features for Face Recognition. *IEEE Transactions on Neural Networks*, 919–928.

Liu, C. (2004). Gabor based kernel PCA with fractional power polynomial models for face recognition. *IEEE Transactions on Pattern Analysis and Machine Intelligence, 26*(5), 572–581. doi:10.1109/TPAMI.2004.1273927

Liu, C., & Wechsler, H. (2001). A shape and texture based enhanced Fisher classifier for face recognition. *IEEE Transactions on Image Processing, 10*(4), 598–607. doi:10.1109/83.913594

Liu, C., & Wechsler, H. (2002). Gabor feature based classification using the enhanced Fisher linear discriminant model for face recognition. *IEEE Transactions on Image Processing, 11*(4), 467–476. doi:10.1109/TIP.2002.999679

Liu, Q., Lu, H., & Ma, S. (2004). Improving kernel Fisher discriminant analysis for face recognition. *IEEE Transactions on Circuits and Systems for Video Technology, 14*(1), 42–49. doi:10.1109/TCSVT.2003.818352

Liu, W. X., & Zheng, N. N. (2004a). Learning sparse features for classification by mixture models. *Pattern Recognition Letters, 25*(2), 155–161.

Liu, W. X., Zheng, N. N., & Li, X. (2004b). Relative gradient speeding up additive updates for nonnegative matrix factorization. *Neurocomputing, 57*, 493–499.

Liu, W. X., Zheng, N. N., & You, Q. B. (2006). Nonnegative matrix factorization and its applications in pattern recognition. *Chinese Science Bulletin, 51*(1), 7–18.

Liu, L., Wang, Y., & Tan, T. (2007). *Online Appearance Model*. CVPR.

Liu, C. H., & Chaudhuri, A. (2003). What determines whether faces are special? *Visual Cognition, 10*, 385–408. doi:10.1080/13506280244000050

Liu, C. (2004). Gabor-Based Kernel PCA with Fractional Power Polynomial Models for Face Recognition. *IEEE Trans. PAMI*, 572-581.

Ljung, L. (1987). *System Identification: Theory for the User*. Upper Saddle River, NJ: Prentice Hall.

Logothetis, N. K., & Sheinberg, D. L. (1996). Visual object recognition. *Annual Review of Neuroscience*, *19*(1), 577–621.

Lowe, D. G. (2004). Distinctive Image Features from Scale-Invariant Keypoints. *International Journal of Computer Vision*, *60*, 91–110. doi:10.1023/B:VISI.0000029664.99615.94

Lowe, D. (1999). Object recognition from local scale-invariant features. In *Intl. Conf. on Computer Vision* (pp. 1150-1157).

Lu, J., Plataniotis, Kostantinos, N., & Venetsanopoulos, A. N. (2003). Face Recognition Using LDA-Based Algorithms. *IEEE Transactions on Neural Networks*, *14*(1), 195–200. doi:10.1109/TNN.2002.806647

Lu, J., Plataniotis, K. N., & Venetsanopoulos, A. N. (2003). Face recognition using LDA based algorithms. *IEEE Transactions on Neural Networks*, *14*(1), 195–200. doi:10.1109/TNN.2002.806647

Lu, J., Plataniotis, K. N., & Venetsanopoulos, A. N. (2003). Face recognition using kernel direct discriminant analysis algorithms. *IEEE Transactions on Neural Networks*, *14*(1), 117–126. doi:10.1109/TNN.2002.806629

Lu, J., Plataniotis, K. N., & Venetsanopoulos, A. N. (2005). Regularization studies of linear discriminant analysis in small sample size scenarios with application to face recognition. *Pattern Recognition Letters*, *26*(2), 181–191. doi:10.1016/j.patrec.2004.09.014

Lu, J., Yuan, X., & Yahagi, T. (2007). A method for face recognition based on fuzzy c-means clustering and associated sub-NNs. *IEEE Transactions on Neural Networks*, *18*(1), 150–160. doi:10.1109/TNN.2006.884678

Lucas, B. D., & Kanade, T. (1981). An iterative image registration technique with an application to stereo vision . In *Image Understanding Workshop* (pp. 121–130). US Defense Advanced Research Projects Agency.

Lucey, S., & Chen, T. (2006). Learning patch dependencies for improved pose mismatched face verification. In *IEEE Computer Society Conference on Computer Vision and Pattern Recognition* (pp. 17–22).

Lyons, M. J., & Akamatsu, S. (1998, 14-16 Apr 1998). Coding facial expressions with gabor wavelets. In *Proc. Third IEEE International Conference on Automatic Face and Gesture Recognition*, Nara, Japan (pp. 200–205).

Lyons, M. J., Budynek, J., & Akamatsu, S. (1999). Automatic Classification of Single Facial Images. *IEEE Trans. PAMI*, 1357-1362.

Lyons, M. J., Budynek, J., Plante, A., & Akamatsu, S. (2000). Classifying Facial Attributes Using a 2-D Gabor Wavelet Representation and Discriminant Analysis. *FG*, 202-207.

Macura, T. J. (2008). *Open Microscopy Environment Analysis System: end-to-end software for high content, high throughput imaging*. Cambridge, UK: Ph.D Dissretation, University of Cambridge.

Magli, E., Olmo, G., & Lo Presti, L. (1999). Pattern Recognition by means of the Radon transform and the continuous wavelet transform. *Signal Processing*, *73*, 277–289. doi:10.1016/S0165-1684(98)00198-4

Mahoor, M., & Abdel Mottaleb, M. (2006). Facial features extraction in color images using enhanced active shape model. In *International Conference on Automatic Face and Gesture Recognition* (pp. 144–148).

Malciu, M., & Preteux, F. (2001 May). Mpeg-4 compliant tracking of facial features in video sequences. In *Proc. of International Conference on Augmented, Virtual Environments and 3D Imaging*, Mykonos, Greece (pp. 108–111).

Mallat, S. G. (1989). A theory for multi-resolution signal decomposition, the wavelet representation. *IEEE Transactions on Pattern Analysis and Machine Intelligence*, *11*, 674–693. doi:10.1109/34.192463

Marcel, S., Rodriguez, Y., & Heusch, G. (2007). On the Recent Use of Local Binary Patterns for Face Authentication. *International Journal of Image and Video Processing*.

Marcelja, S. (1980). Mathematical Description of the Responses of Simple Cortical Cells. *Journal of the Optical Society of America*, 1297–1300. doi:10.1364/JOSA.70.001297

Martinez, A. M. (2002). Recognizing imprecisely localized, partially occluded, and expression variant faces from a single sample per class. *IEEE Transactions on Pattern Analysis and Machine Intelligence, 24*(6), 748–763. doi:10.1109/TPAMI.2002.1008382

Martinez, A. M., & Kak, A. C. (2001). PCA versus LDA. *IEEE Transactions on Pattern Analysis and Machine Intelligence, 23*(2), 228–233. doi:10.1109/34.908974

Martinez, A. M., & Benavente, R. (1998). *The AR Face Database. CVC Technical Report #24*. West Lafayette, Indiana, USA: Purdue University.

Martinez, A., & Benavente, R. (1998). *The AR Face Database*. CVC.

Martinez, A. M. (2002). Recognizing imprecisely localized, partially occluded, and expression variant faces from a single sample per class. *IEEE Transactions on Pattern Analysis and Machine Intelligence, 24*(6), 748–763. doi:10.1109/TPAMI.2002.1008382

Martinez, A. M., & Benavente, R. (1998). The AR face database (Tech. Rep. No. 24). *CVC*.

Mase, K., & Pentland, A. (1991). Recognition of facial expression from optical flow. *IEICE Trans., 74*(10), 3474–3483.

Matas, J., Chum, O., Urba, M., & Pajdla, T. (2002). Robust wide baseline stereo from maximally stable extremal regions. In *Proceedings of British Machine Vision Conference* (pp. 384-396).

Matas, J., Hamouz, M., Jonsson, K., Kittler, J., Li, Y., Kotropoulos, C., et al. (2000). Comparison of face verification results on the XM2VTS database. In *Proceedings of the 15th International Conference on Pattern Recognition* (Vol. 4, pp. 858–863).

Matsuno, K., Iee, C.-W., & Tsuji, S. (1994). *Recognition of Human Facial Expressions Without Feature Extraction*. Paper presented at the ECCV.

Maurer, D., Le Grand, R., & Mondloch, C. J. (2002). The many faces of configural processing. *Trends in Cognitive Sciences, 6*, 255–260. doi:10.1016/S1364-6613(02)01903-4

McKone, E., & Robbins, R. (2007). The evidence rejects the expertise hypothesis: Reply to Gauthier & Bukach. *Cognition, 103*, 331–336. doi:10.1016/j.cognition.2006.05.014

McKone, E., Crookes, K., & Kanwisher, N. (in press). The cognitive and neural development of face recognition in Humans . In Gazzaniga, M. (Ed.), *The cognitive Neurosciences*.

Mehrabian, A. (1968). Communication without words. *Psychology Today, 2*(4), 53–56.

Meng, J. E., Shiqian, W., Juwei, L., & Hock, L. T. (2002). Face recognition with radial basis function (RBF) neural networks. *IEEE Transactions on Neural Networks, 13*(3), 697–710. doi:10.1109/TNN.2002.1000134

Menser, B., & Muller, F. (1999). Face detection in color images using principal components analysis. In *7th International Conference on Image Processing and Its Applications* (Vol. 2, p. 620-624).

Messer, K., Matas, J., Kittler, J., Luettin, J., & Maitre, G. (1999). XM2VTSDB: The extended M2VTS database. In *2nd International Conference on Audio and Video-based Biometric Person Authentication* (pp. 72-77).

Micheli-Tzanakou, E., Uyeda, E., & Ray, R. (1995). Comparison of neural network algorithms for face recognition. *Simulation, 65*(1), 37–51. doi:10.1177/003754979506500105

Mika, G., Ratsch, J., Weston, B., et al. (1999). Fisher discriminant analysis with kernels. *Proc. IWNNSP IX*, 41-48.

Mikolajczyk, M., & Schmid, C. (2004). Scale & Affine Invariant Interest Point Detectors. *International Journal of Computer Vision, 60*, 63–86. doi:10.1023/B:VISI.0000027790.02288.f2

Moghaddam, B. (2002). Principal manifolds and probabilistic subspaces for visual recognition. *IEEE Trans. PAMI, 24*(6), 780–788.

Moghaddam, B., & Pentland, A. P. (1997). *Probabilistic Visual Learning for Object Representation*. IEEE Trans. on PAMI.

Moghaddam, B., Jebara, T., & Pentland, A. (2000). Bayesian face recognition. *PR, 33*(11), 1771-1782.

Moore, A., Allman, J., & Goodman, R. M. (1991). A Real Time Neural System for Color Consistency. *IEEE Transactions on Neural Networks, 2*, 237–247. doi:10.1109/72.80334

Moreels, P., & Perona, P. (2004). *Common-Frame Model for Object Recognition*. NIPS.

Moreels, P., & Perona, P. (2005). Evaluation of features detectors and descriptors based on 3D objects. In *IEEE International Conference on Computer Vision* (Vol. 1, pp. 800- 807).

Mtiller, K. R., Mika, S., Riitsch, G., Tsuda, K., & Scholopf, B. (2001). An introduction to kernel based learning algorithm. *IEEE Transactions on Neural Networks, 12*, 181–201. doi:10.1109/72.914517

Murase, H., & Nayar, S. (1995). Visual learning and recognition of 3D objects from appearance. *International Journal of Computer Vision, 14*, 5–24. .doi:10.1007/BF01421486

Nachson, I. (1995). On the modularity of face perception: The riddle of domain specificity. *Journal of Clinical and Experimental Neuropsychology, 9*, 353–383.

Nagesh, P., & Li, B. X. (2009). *A Compressive Sensing Approach for Expression-Invariant Face Recognition*. CVPR.

Naseem, I., Togneri, R., & Bennamoun, M. (2009). *Linear Regression for Face Recognition*. IEEE Trans. on Pattern Analysis and Machine Intelligence.

Nastar, C., & Ayach, N. (1996). Frequency-based non-rigid motion analysis. *IEEE Transactions on Pattern Analysis and Machine Intelligence, 18*(11), 1067–1079. doi:10.1109/34.544076

Nguyen, M. H., Perez, J., & de la Torre Frade, F. (2008). Facial feature detection with optimal pixel reduction SVMs. In *8th IEEE International Conference on Automatic Face and Gesture Recognition*.

Nikolaos, E., & Feng, D. (2008). Building highly realistic facial modeling and animation: A survey. *The Visual Computer, 24*(1), 13–30.

Nilsson, M., Nordberg, J., & Claesson, I. (2007). Face Detection using Local SMQT Features and Split up Snow Classifier. In *IEEE International Conference on Acoustics, Speech and Signal Processing* (Vol. 2, pp. 589-592).

North, B., Blake, A., Isard, M., & Rittscher, J. (2000). Learning and classification of complex dynamics. *IEEE Transactions on Pattern Analysis and Machine Intelligence, 22*(9), 1016–1034. doi:10.1109/34.877523

Nusseck, M., Cunningham, D. W., Wallraven, C., & Bülthoff, H. (2008). The contribution of different facial regions to the recognition of conversational expressions. *Journal of Vision (Charlottesville, Va.), 8*(8). doi:10.1167/8.8.1

Obdrzalek, S., & Matas, J. (2002). Object recognition using local affine frames on distinguished regions. In *Proceedings of British Machine Vision Conference*.

Ohmoto, Y., Ueda, K., & Ohno, T. (2008). Real-time system for measuring gaze direction and facial features: towards automatic discrimination of lies using diverse nonverbal information. *AI & Society, 23*(2), 187–200. doi:10.1007/s00146-007-0138-x

Oliver, N., Pentland, A., & Bérard, F. (2000). Lafter: a real-time face and tracker with facial expression recognition. *Pattern Recognition, 33*, 1369–1382. doi:10.1016/S0031-3203(99)00113-2

ORL face database. (n.d.). Retrieved from http://www.uk.research.att.com/facedatabase

Orlov, N., Shamir, L., Macura, T., Johnston, J., Eckley, D. M., & Goldberg, I. G. (2008). WND-CHARM: Multipurpose image classification using compound image transforms. *Pattern Recognition Letters, 29*, 1684–1693. .doi:10.1016/j.patrec.2008.04.013

Otsuka, T., & Ohya, J. (1998). *Spotting segments displaying facial expression from image sequences using HMM.* Paper presented at the IEEE Proceedings of the Second International Conference on Automatic Face and Gesture Recognition, Japan.

Ouhsain, M., & Hamza, A. B. (2009). Image watermarking scheme using nonnegative matrix factorization and wavelet transform. *International Journal on Expert Systems with Applications, 36*(2), 2123–2129.

Palmer, S. E. (1977). Hierarchical structure in perceptual representation. *Cognitive Psychology, 9*(3), 441–474.

Pan, Z., Healey, G., & Prasad, M. (2003). Face recognition in hyperspectral images. *IEEE Trans. PAMI, 25*, 1552–1560.

Pan, Z., Healey, G., Prasad, M., & Tromberg, B. (2003). Face recognition in hyperspectral images. *IEEE Transactions on Pattern Analysis and Machine Intelligence, 25*(12), 1552–1560. doi:10.1109/TPAMI.2003.1251148

Pang, S., Kim, S., & Bang, S. Y. (2005). Face membership authentication using SVM classification tree generated by membership-based LLE data partition. *IEEE Transactions on Neural Networks, 16*(2), 436–446. doi:10.1109/TNN.2004.841776

Pang, Y., Tao, D., Yuan, Y., & Li, X. (2008). Binary Two-Dimensional PCA. *IEEE Trans. on Systems, Man, and Cybernetics, Part B*, 1176-1180.

Pantic, M., & Patras, I. (2006). Dynamics of facial expression: Recognition of facial actions and their temporal segments from face profile image sequences. *IEEE Transactions on System Systems, Man, and Cybernetics . Part B: Cybernetics, 36*, 433–449. doi:10.1109/TSMCB.2005.859075

Pantic, M., & Rothkrantz, L. J. M. (2000). Automatic analysis of facial expressions: the state of the art. *Pattern Analysis and Machine Intelligence . IEEE Transactions on, 22*(12), 1424–1445.

Pantic, M., & Bartlett, M. S. (2007). Machine analysis of facial expressions . In Delac, K., & Grgic, M. (Eds.), *Face recognition* (pp. 377–416). Vienna, Austria: I-Tech Education and Publishing.

Pantic, M. (2005). Affective computing . In Pagani, M. (Eds.), *Encyclopedia of Multimedia Technology and Networking* (*Vol. 1*, pp. 8–14). Hershey, PA: Idea Group Publishing.

Papatheodorou, T., & Rueckert, D. (2004). Evaluation of automatic 4D face recognition using surface and texture registration. In *IEEE Internat. Conf. on Automatic Face and Gesture Recognition* Seoul . *Korea & World Affairs*, (May): 321–326.

Pardas, M., & Bonafonte, A. (2002). Facial animation parameters extraction and expression detection using hmm. *Signal Processing Image Communication, 17*, 675–688. doi:10.1016/S0923-5965(02)00078-4

Pardas, M., & Sayrol, E. (2001, November). Motion estimation based tracking of active contours. *Pattern Recognition Letters, 22*(13), 1447–1456. doi:10.1016/S0167-8655(01)00084-8

Pardas, M. (2000, Jun 2000). Extraction and tracking of the eyelids. In *Proc. International Conference on Acoustics, Speech and Signal Processing*, Istambul, Turkey (Vol. 4, pp. 2357–2360).

Pardas, M. B. A., Landabaso, J.L. (2002). *Emotion recognition based on mpeg4 facial animation parameters.* Paper presented at the IEEE International Conference on Acoustics, Speech, and Signal Processing.

Park, S. W., & Savvides, M. (2007). Individual kernel tensor-subspaces for robust face recognition: A computationally efficient tensor framework without requiring mode factorization. *IEEE Trans. SMC-B, 37*(5), 1156–1166.

Park, S., & Kim, D. (2009). Subtle facial expression recognition using motion magnification. *Pattern Recognition Letters*, *30*(7), 708–716. doi:10.1016/j.patrec.2009.02.005

Park, Y. K., Park, S. L., & Kim, J. K. (2008). Retinex Method Based on Adaptive smoothing for Illumination Invariant Face Recognition. *Signal Processing*, *88*(8), 1929–1945. doi:10.1016/j.sigpro.2008.01.028

Park, C. H., & Park, H. (2008). A comparison of generalized linear discriminant analysis algorithms. *PR, 41*(3), 1083-1097.

Pascual-Montano, A., Carzzo, J. M., & Lochi, K. (2006). Non-smooth nonnegative matrix factorization (nsNMF). *IEEE Transactions on Pattern Analysis and Machine Intelligence*, *28*(3), 403–415.

Penev, P. S., Ayache, M., & Fruchter, J. (2004). Independent manifold analysis for sub-pixel tracking of local features and face recognition in video sequences. *SPIE*, *5404*, 523–533.

Penev, P. S., & Atick, J. J. (1996). Local feature analysis: a general statistical theory for object representation. *Network: Computation in Neural Systems, 7*, 477–500. doi: 10.1.1.105.4097

Perlibakas, V. (2003). Automatical detection of face features and exact face contour. *Pattern Recognition Letters*, *24*(16), 2977–2985. doi:10.1016/S0167-8655(03)00158-2

Peterson, M. A., & Rhodes, G. (2003). Introduction: analytic and holistic processing – the view through different lenses . In Peterson, M. A., & Rhodes, G. (Eds.), *Perception of faces, objects, and scenes: Analytic and holistic processes*. Oxford, UK: Oxford University Press.

Phillips, J. P., Moon, H., Rizvi, A. S., & Rauss, P. J. (2000). The FERET evaluation methodology for face-recognition algorithms. *IEEE Transactions on Pattern Analysis and Machine Intelligence*, *22*(10), 1090–1104. doi:10.1109/34.879790

Phillips, P., Wechsler, H., Huang, J., & Rauss, P. (1998). The FERET database and evaluation procedure for face-recognition algorithms. *Image and Vision Computing*, *16*(5), 295–306. doi:10.1016/S0262-8856(97)00070-X

Phillips, P. J., Flynn, P. J., Scruggs, T., Bowyer, K. W., Chang, J., & Hoffman, K. (2005). Overview of the face recognition grand challenge . In *IEEE Computer Vision and Pattern Recognition conference* (*Vol. 1*, pp. 947–954). CVPR.

Phillips, P. J., Scruggs, W. T., O'Toole, A. J., Flynn, P. J., Bowyer, K. W., Schott, C. L., & Sharpe, M. (2007, March). FRVT 2006 and ICE 2006 Large-Scale Results. *NISTIR 7408*.

Picard, R. (1997). *Affective computing*. Cambridge, MA: MIT Press.

Picard, R. W., Vyzas, E., & Healy, J. (2001). Toward machine emotional intelligence: Analysis of affective physiological state. *IEEE Transactions on Pattern Analysis and Machine Intelligence*, *23*(10), 1175–1191. doi:10.1109/34.954607

Pinto, N., DiCarlo, J. J., & Cox, D. D. (2009). How far can you get with a modern face recognition test set using only simple features? *CVPR*, 2591-2598.

Price, J. R., & Gee, T. F. (2005). Face recognition using direct, weighted linear discriminant analysis and modular subspaces. *PR, 38*(2), 209-219.

Prince, S. J. D., Elder, J. H., Warrell, J., & Felisberti, F. M. (2008). Tied factor analysis for face recognition across large pose differences. *IEEE Transactions on Pattern Analysis and Machine Intelligence*, *30*(6), 970–984. doi:10.1109/TPAMI.2008.48

Prince, S. J. D., & Elder, J. H. (2007). Probabilistic linear discriminant analysis for inferences about identity. In *IEEE International Conference on Computer Vision* (pp. 1–8).

Pujol, A., Vitria, J., & Lumbreras, F. (2001). Topological principal component analysis for face encoding and recognition. *PRL*, *22*(6-7), 769–776.

Qing Shan, L., Rui, H., Han Qing, L., & Song De, M. (2003). Kernel-based nonlinear discriminant analysis for face recognition. *Journal of Computer Science and Technology*, *18*(6), 788–795. doi:10.1007/BF02945468

Quinlan, J. R. (1993). *C4.5: Program for Machine Learning*. San Francisco: Morgan Kaufmann.

Rakover, S. S. (1990). *Metapsychology: missing links in behavior, mind and science*. New York: Solomon/Paragon.

Rakover, S. S. (2002). Featural vs. configurational information in faces: A conceptual and empirical analysis. *The British Journal of Psychology, 93*, 1–30. doi:10.1348/000712602162427

Rakover, S. S. (2008). Is facial beauty an innate response to the Leonardian Proportion? *Empirical Studies of the Arts, 26*, 155–179. doi:10.2190/EM.26.2.b

Rakover, S. S., & Cahlon, B. (2001). *Face recognition: Cognitive and computational processes*. Philadelphia, PA: John Benjamins.

Rakover, S. S., & Teucher, B. (1997). Facial inversion effects: part and whole relationship. *Perception & Psychophysics, 59*, 752–761.

Ramasubramanian, D., & Venkatesh, Y. V. (2000). Encoding and recognition of faces based on the human visual model and DCT. *Pattern Recognition, 34*, 2447–2458. doi:10.1016/S0031-3203(00)00172-2

Reilly, J., Ghent, J., & McDonald, J. (2006, November 6-8). Investigating the dynamics of facial expression. In G. Bebis et al. (Eds.), *Advances in Visual Computing: Proc. of the Second International Symposium on Visual Computing (ISVC 2006)*, Lake Tahoe, Nevada, USA (LNCS 4292, pp, 334-343).

Reinders, M. J. T., Koch, R. W. C., & Gerbrands, J. J. (1996). Locating facial features in image sequences using neural networks. In *2nd International Conference on Automatic Face and Gesture Recognition* (pp. 230-235).

Reyment, R. A., & Jvreskog, K. G. (1996). *Applied Factor Analysis in the Natural Sciences* (2nd ed.). Cambridge, UK: Cambridge University Press.

Rhodes, G., Brake, K., & Atkinson, A. (1993). What's lost in inverted faces? *Cognition, 47*, 25–57. doi:10.1016/0010-0277(93)90061-Y

Riaz, Z., Gilgiti, A., & Mirza, S. M. (2004). Face recognition: a review and comparison of HMM, PCA, ICA and neural networks. *E-Tech*, 41-46.

Riccio, D., & Nappi, M. (2003 September). Defering range/domain comparisons in fractal image compression. In *Internat. Conf. on Image Analysis and Processing* (Vol. 1, pp. 412–417).

Riesenhuber, M., Jarudi, I., Gilad, S., & Sinha, P. (2004). Face processing in humans is compatible with a simple shape-based model of vision. *Proceedings. Biological Sciences, 271*(Suppl.), S448–S450. doi:10.1098/rsbl.2004.0216

Rish I. (2001). *An empirical study of the naïve Bayes classifier*. Technical Report RC 22230.

Rissanen, J. (1983). A universal prior for integers and estimation by minimum description length. *Annals of Statistics, 11*(2), 416–431. doi:10.1214/aos/1176346150

Robbins, R., & McKone, E. (2007). No face-like processing for objects-of-expertise in three behavioral tasks. *Cognition, 103*, 34–79. doi:10.1016/j.cognition.2006.02.008

Robinson, J. O. (1998). *The psychology of visual illusion*. New York: Dover Publications.

Rodenacker, K., & Bengtsson, E. (2003). A feature set for cytometry on digitized microscopic images. *Annals of Cellular Pathology, 25*, 1–36. doi: 10.1.1.33.9697

Romdhani, S., Psarrou, A., & Gong, S. (2000). On utilizing templates and feature-based correspondence in multi-view appearance models. In *Proceedings of the 6th European Conference on Computer Vision* (Vol. 1, pp. 799-813). doi: 10.1.1.63.6036

Rosenblum, M., Yacoob, Y., & Davis, L. S. (1996). Human expression recognition from motion using a radial basis function network architecture. *IEEE Transactions on Neural Networks, 7*, 1121–1137. doi:10.1109/72.536309

Rosenblum, M., Yacoob, Y., & Davis, L. S. (1996). Human Expression Recognition from Motion Using a Radial Basis Function Network Architecture. *IEEE Transactions on Neural Networks*, *7*(5), 1121–1138. doi:10.1109/72.536309

Rossion, B. (2008). Picture-plane inversion leads to qualitative changes of face perception. *Acta Psychologica*, *128*, 274–289. doi:10.1016/j.actpsy.2008.02.003

Rossion, B., & Gauthier, I. (2002). How does the brain process upright and inverted faces? *Behavioral and Cognitive Neuroscience Reviews*, *1*, 63–75. doi:10.1177/1534582302001001004

Rubin, D., & Thayer, D. (1982). EM algorithms for ML factor analysis. *Psychometrika*, *47*(1), 69–76. doi:10.1007/BF02293851

Samal, A., & Iyengar, P. (1992). Automatic recognition and analysis of human faces and facial expressions: A survey. *Pattern Recognition*, 65–77. doi:10.1016/0031-3203(92)90007-6

Samal, A., & Iyengar, P. A. (1992). Automatic recognition and analysis of human faces and facial expressions: A survey. *PR, 25*, 65-77.

Samaria, F., & Fallside, F. (1993). Face identification and feature extraction using Hidden Markov Models . In Vernazza, G. (Ed.), *Image Processing: Theory and Application*. Amsterdam: Elsevier.

Samaria, F., & Harter, A. C. (1994). Parameterization of a stochastic model for human face identification. In *Proceedings of the Second IEEE Workshop Applications of Computer Vision*. doi: 10.1109/ACV.1994.341300

Sanderson, C. (2008). *Biometric Person Recognition: Face*. Speech and Fusion.

Sanderson, C., & Paliwal, K. K. (2004). Identity Verification Using Speech and Face Information. *Digital Signal Processing*, 449–480. doi:10.1016/j.dsp.2004.05.001

Savvides, M., Vijaya Kumar, B. V. K., & Khosla, P. (2002). Face verification using correlation filters. In *Proceedings of the 3rd IEEE Conference on Automatic Identification Advanced Technologies* (pp. 56–61). doi: 10.1109/ICISIP.2004.1287684

Schaffalitzky, F., & Zisserman, A. (2002). Automated scene matching in movies. In *Proceedings of the International Conference on Image and Video Retrieval* (pp. 186-197).

Schmid, C., & Moger, R. (1997). Local Grayvalue Invariants for Image Retrieval. *IEEE Transactions on Pattern Analysis and Machine Intelligence*, *19*, 530–535. doi:10.1109/34.589215

Scholof, B., Smola, A., & Muller, K. R. (1998). Nonlinear component analysis as a kernel eigenvalue problem. *Neural Computation*, *10*(5), 1299–1319. doi:10.1162/089976698300017467

Schwaninger, A., Ryf, S., & Hofer, F. (2003). Configural information is processed differently in perception and recognition of faces. *Vision Research*, *43*, 1501–1505. doi:10.1016/S0042-6989(03)00171-8

Schwaninger, A., Carbon, C.-C., & Leder, H. (2003). Expert face processing: Specialization and constraints . In Schwarzer, G., & Leder, H. (Eds.), *Development of face processing*. Göttingen, Germany: Hogrefe.

Searcy, J. H., & Bartlett, J. C. (1996). Inversion and processing of component and spatial-relational information in faces. *Journal of Experimental Psychology. Human Perception and Performance*, *22*, 904–915. doi:10.1037/0096-1523.22.4.904

Sekuler, A. B., Gaspar, C. M., Gold, J. M., & Bennett, P. J. (2004). Inversion leads to quantitative, not qualitative, changes in face processing. *Current Biology*, *14*, 391–396. doi:10.1016/j.cub.2004.02.028

Shahnaz, F., Berry, M. W., & Pauca, V. P., & PLemmons, R. J. (2006). Document clustering using nonnegative matrix factorization. *Journal of Information Processing and Management*, *42*(3), 373–386.

Shakhnarovich, G., & Moghaddam, B. (2004). Face Recognition in Subspaces. In *Handbook of Face Recognition*. Berlin: Springer-Verlag.

Shamir, L., Ling, S., Rahimi, S., Ferrucci, L., & Goldberg, I. (2009b). Biometric identification using knee X-rays. *International Journal of Biometrics*, *1*, 365–370. .doi:10.1504/IJBM.2009.024279

Shamir, L., Orlov, N., Eckley, D. M., Macura, T., & Goldberg, I. (2008a). IICBU-2008 - A proposed benchmark suite for biological image analysis. *Medical & Biological Engineering & Computing*, *46*, 943–947. .doi:10.1007/s11517-008-0380-5

Shamir, L., Orlov, N., Eckley, D. M., Macura, T., Johnston, J., & Goldberg, I. (2008b). Wndchrm - An open source utility for biological image analysis. *BMC - . Source Code for Biology and Medicine*, *3*, 13. .doi:10.1186/1751-0473-3-13

Shamir, L., Orlov, N., & Goldberg, I. (2009a). Evaluation of the informativeness of multi-order image transforms. In *International Conference on Image Processing Computer Vision and Pattern Recognition (IPCV'09)* (pp. 37-41).

Shan, C., Gong, S., & McOwan, P. W. (2006, September 4-7). Dynamic facial expression recognition using a bayesian temporal manifold model. In *Proceedings of British Machine Vision Conference (BMVC 2006)*, Edinburgh, United Kingdom (Vol. 1, pp. 297–306). New York: BMVA Press.

Shan, S., Cao, B., Su, Y., Qing, L., Chen, X., & Gao, W. (2008). Unified principal component analysis with generalized covariance matrix for face recognition. In *IEEE Computer Society Conference on Computer Vision and Pattern Recognition* (pp. 1–7).

Shan, S., et al. (2008). Unified principal component analysis with generalized covariance matrix for face recognition. *Proc. CVPR*, 1-7.

Shan, S., Gao W., & Zhao, D. (2003). Face Identification Based On Face-Specific Subspace. *International Journal of Image and System Technology*, 23-32.

Shan, S., Zhang, W., Su, Y., Chen, X., & Gao, W. (2006). Ensemble of piecewise FDA based on spatial histograms of local (Gabor) binary patterns for face recognition. In *International Conference on Pattern Recognition* (pp. 606–609).

Shawe-Taylor, J., & Cristianini, N. (2000). *Support Vector Machines and Other Kernel-based Learning Methods*. Cambridge, UK: Cambridge University Press.

Sherrah, J. (2004 May). False alarm rate: A critical performance measure for face recognition. In *Sixth IEEE Internat. Conf. on Automatic Face and Gesture Recognition*, (pp. 189–194).

Shih, F. Y., & Chuang, C.-F. (2004). Automatic extraction of head and face boundaries and facial features. *Information Sciences Informatics and Computer Science: An International Journal*, *158*(1), 117–130.

Shin, Y., Lee, S. S., Chung, C., & Lee, Y. (2000, 21-25 Aug 2000). *Facial expression recognition based on two-dimensional structure of emotion*. Paper presented at the International Conference on Signal Processing Proceedings.

Short, J., Kittler, J., & Messer, K. (2004). A Comparison of Photometric Normalization Algorithms for Face Verification. In *Proc. of AFGR'04* (pp. 254- 259).

Short, J., Kittler, J., & Messer, K. (2004). Comparison of photometric normalisation algorithms for face verification. *Proc. ICAFGR*, 254-259.

Sim, T., Baker, S., & Bsat, M. (2003). The CMU pose, illumination, and expression database. *IEEE Transactions on Pattern Analysis and Machine Intelligence*, *25*(12), 1615–1618. doi:10.1109/TPAMI.2003.1251154

Singh, R., Vasta, M., & Noore, A. (2005). Textural feature based face recognition for single training images. *Electronics Letters*, *41*, 640–641. .doi:10.1049/el:20050352

Sivic, J. (2006). *Efficient visual search of images and videos*. Ph.D. Thesis, University of Oxford, Oxford, UK.

Sivic, J., & Zisserman, A. (2003). Video Google: A Text Retrieval Approach to Object Matching in Videos. In *Proceedings of the International Conference on Computer Vision*.

Sivic, J., Everingham, M., & Zisserman, A. (2005). Person spotting: video shot retrieval for face sets. In *International Conference on Image and Video Retrieval*.

Sivic, J., Schaffalitzky, F., & Zisserman, A. (2004). Efficient Object Retrieval from Videos. In *Proceedings of the 12th European Signal Processing Conference*.

Smets, P. (1998). The transferable belief model for quantified belief representation . In *Handbook of defeasible reasoning and uncertainty management system* (*Vol. 1*, pp. 267–301). Dordrecht: Kluwer Academic.

Smets, P. (2005). Decision making in the TBM: the necessity of the pignistic transformation. *International Journal of Approximate Reasoning*, *38*, 133–147. doi:10.1016/j.ijar.2004.05.003

Smets, P. (2000 July). Data fusion in the transferable belief model. In *Proc. of International Conference on Information Fusion*, Paris, France (pp. 21–33).

Smeulders, M., Santini, S., Gupta, A., & Jain, R. (2000). Content-based image retrieval at the end of early years. *IEEE Transactions on Pattern Analysis and Machine Intelligence*, *22*, 1349–1380. doi:10.1109/34.895972

Smith, P., Shah, M., & da Vitoria Lobo, N. (2003). Determining driver visual attention with one camera. *IEEE Transactions on Intelligent Transportation Systems*, *4*(4), 205–218. doi:10.1109/TITS.2003.821342

Smith, M., Cottrell, G., Gosselin, F., & Schyns, P. G. (2005). Transmitting and decoding facial expressions of emotions. *Psychological Science*, *16*, 184–189. doi:10.1111/j.0956-7976.2005.00801.x

Socolinsky, D. A., & Selinger, A. (2004). Thermal face recognition over time. In *Internat. Conf. on Pattern Recognition (ICPR04)*.

Solso, R. L., & McCarthy, J. E. (1981). Prototype formation of faces: A case of pseudo-memory. *The British Journal of Psychology*, *72*, 499–503.

Song, M., Wang, H., Bu, J., Chen, C., & Liu, Z. (2006, October 8-11). Subtle facial expression modelling with vector field decomposition. In *Proceedings of IEEE International Conference on Image Processing (ICIP 2006)*, Atlanta, Georgia, USA (Vol. 1, pp. 2101-2104). Washington, DC: IEEE Press

Spacek, L. (2002). *University of Essex Face Database*. Retrieved from http://www.essex.ac.ukmvallfacesindex.html

Specht, D. F. (1990). Probabilistic Neural Networks. *Neural Networks*, 109–118. doi:10.1016/0893-6080(90)90049-Q

Stone, M. (1974). Cross-validatory choice and assessment of statistical predictions. *Journal of the Royal Statistical Society. Series B. Methodological*, *36*, 111–147.

Stouten, V., Demuynck, K., & Hamme, H. V. (2008). Discovering phone patterns in spoken utterances by non-negative matrix factorization. *IEEE Signal Processing Letters*, *15*(1), 131–134.

Strang, G., & Nguyen, T. (1996). *Wavelets and Filter Banks*. Wellesley, MA: Wellesley-Cambridge Press.

Štruc, V., & Pavešić, N. (2009). Gabor-Based Kernel Partial-Least-Squares Discrimination Features for Face Recognition. *Informatica*, *20*(1), 115–138.

Štruc, V., Žibert, J., & Pavešić, N. (2009). Histogram Remapping as a Preprocessing Step for Robust Face Recognition. *WSEAS Transactions on Information Science and Applications*, *6*(3), 520–529.

Su, Y. (2003). RankGene: identification of diagnostic genes based on expression data. *Bioinformatics (Oxford, England)*, *19*, 1578–1579. doi:10.1093/bioinformatics/btg179

Sun, Y. (2007). Iterative relief for feature weighting: Algorithms, theories, and applications. *IEEE Transactions on Pattern Analysis and Machine Intelligence*, *29*, 1035–1051. doi:10.1109/TPAMI.2007.1093

Sun, Y., & Lijun, Y. (2007). A genetic algorithm based feature selection approach for 3d face recognition. *Biometrics Symposium in 3D Imaging for Safety and Security, Springer - Computational Imaging and Vision, 35*, 95–118.

Sundaresan, A., & Chellappa, R. (2008). Model driven segmentation of articulating humans in Laplacian Eigenspace. *IEEE Trans. PAMI, 30*(10), 1771–1785.

Sung, J., Lee, S., & Kim, D. (2006, August 20-24). A real-time facial expression recognition using the staam. In *Proceedings of IEEE International Conference on Pattern Recognition (ICPR 2006)*, Hong Kong, PR China (Vol. 1, pp. 275–278). Washington, DC: IEEE Press

Swedlow, J. R., Goldberg, I., Brauner, E., & Peter, K. S. (2003). Informatics and quantitative analysis in biological Imaging. *Science, 300*, 100–102. .doi:10.1126/science.1082602

Swets, D. L., & Weng, J. (1999). Hierarchical discriminant analysis for image retrieval. *IEEE Transactions on Pattern Analysis and Machine Intelligence, 21*(5), 386–401. doi:10.1109/34.765652

Tan, T., & Yan, H. (1999). Face recognition by fractal transformations. In *IEEE Internat. Conf. on Acoustics, Speech, and Signal Processing (ICASSP '99)* (pp. 3537–3540).

Tanaka, J. W., & Farah, M. J. (1993). Parts and their configuration in face recognition. *Quarterly Journal of Experimental Psychology, 46A*, 225–245.

Tanaka, J. W., & Farah, M. J. (2003). The holistic representation of faces . In Peterson, M. A., & Rhodes, G. (Eds.), *Perception of faces, objects, and scenes: Analytic and holistic processes*. Oxford, UK: Oxford University Press.

Tanaka, H. T., Ikeda, M., & Chiaki, H. (1998). Curvature-based face surface recognition using spherical correlation principal directions for curved object recognition. In *3rd IEEE International Conference on Automatic Face and Gesture Recognition* (pp. 372-377).

Tarr, M. J., & Cheng, Y. D. (2003). Learning to see faces and objects. *Trends in Cognitive Sciences, 7*, 23–30. doi:10.1016/S1364-6613(02)00010-4

Tarr, M. J. (2003). Visual object recognition: Can a single mechanism suffice? In Peterson, M. A., & Rhodes, G. (Eds.), *Perception of faces, objects, and scenes: Analytic and holistic processes*. Oxford, UK: Oxford University Press.

Tefas, A., Kotropoulos, C., & Pitas, I. (2001). Using Support vector machines to enhance the performance of elastic graph matching for frontal face authentication. *IEEE Transactions on Pattern Analysis and Machine Intelligence, 23*(7), 735–746. doi:10.1109/34.935847

Tefas, A., Kotropoulos, C., & Pitas, I. (2002). Face verification using elastic graph matching based on morphological signal decomposition. *Signal Processing, 82*(6), 833–851. doi:10.1016/S0165-1684(02)00157-3

Tekalp, M. (1999). *Face and 2d mesh animation in mpeg-4. Tutorial Issue on the MPEG-4 Standard.* Image Communication Journal.

The BioID face database. (n.d.). Retrieved from http://www.bioid.com/downloads/facedb /facedatabase.html

The JAFFE database. (n.d.). Retrieved from http://www.mis.atr.co.jp/ mlyons/jaffe.html

Tian, Y., Kanade, T., & Cohn, J. F. (2001). Recognizing action units for facial expression analysis. *IEEE Transactions on Pattern Analysis and Machine Intelligence, 23*, 97–115. doi:10.1109/34.908962

Tian, Y. L., Kanade, T., & Cohn, J. F. (2005). Facial expression analysis . In Li, S. Z., & Jain, A. K. (Eds.), *Handbook of face recognition* (pp. 247–276). New York: Springer. doi:10.1007/0-387-27257-7_12

Tian, Y., Kanade, T., & Cohn, J. (2000 March). Dual state parametric eye tracking. In *Proc. 4th IEEE International Conference on Automatic Face and Gesture Recognition*, Grenoble (pp. 110–115).

Tibshirani, R. (1996). Regression shrinkage and selection via the lasso. *Journal of the Royal Statistical Society. Series B. Methodological, 58*, 267–288.

Tipping, M. E., & Bishop, C. M. (1999). Probabilistic principal component analysis. *Journal of the Royal Statistical Society. Series B. Methodological*, *61*, 611–622. doi:10.1111/1467-9868.00196

Tong, Y., Liao, W., & Ji, Q. (2006). Inferring facial action units with causal relations. In *Proc. IEEE Computer Vision and Pattern Recognition* (pp. 1623–1630).

Tsalakanidou, F., Tzovaras, D., & Strintzis, M. G. (2003). Use of depth and colour Eigenfaces for face recognition. *Pattern Recognition Letters*, *24*(9-10), 1427–1435. doi:10.1016/S0167-8655(02)00383-5

Tsapatsoulis, N., Karpouzis, K., Stamou, G., Piat, F., & Kollias, S. (2000 September). A fuzzy system for emotion classification based on the mpeg-4 facial definition parameter set. In *Proceedings of the 10th European Signal Processing Conference*, Tampere, Finland.

Tsekeridou, S., & Pitas, I. (1998 September). Facial feature extraction in frontal views using biometric analogies. In *Proc. 9th European Signal Processing Conference*, Island of Rhodes, Greece (Vol. 1, pp. 315–318).

Turk, M., & Pentland, A. (1991). Eigenfaces for Recognition. *Journal of Cognitive Neuroscience*, 71–86. doi:10.1162/jocn.1991.3.1.71

Turk, M., & Pentland, A. (1991). Eigenfaces for recognition. *Journal of Cognitive Neuroscience*, *13*(1), 71–86. doi:10.1162/jocn.1991.3.1.71

Turk, M., & Pentland, A. (1991). Eigenfaces for recognition. *Journal of Cognitive Neuroscience*, *3*, 71–86. doi:10.1162/jocn.1991.3.1.71

Turk, M., & Pentland, A. (1991). Face recognition using eigenfaces. In *IEEE Computer Society Conference on Computer Vision and Pattern Recognition* (pp. 586–591).

Valentine, T. (1988). Upside-down faces: A review of the effect of inversion on face recognition. *The British Journal of Psychology*, *79*, 471–491.

Valentine, T. (1991). A unified account of the effects of distinctiveness, inversion and race in face recognition. *Quarterly Journal of Experimental Psychology*, *43A*, 161–204.

Valstar, M. F., Gunes, H., & Pantic, M. (2007 November). How to Distinguish Posed from Spontaneous Smiles using Geometric Features. In *Proc. ACM Int'l Conf on Multimodal Interfaces*, Nagoya, Japan (pp. 38-45).

Valstar, M. F., Pantic, M., Ambadar, Z., & Cohn, J. F. (2006). Spontaneous vs. posed facial behavior: automatic analysis of brow actions. In *Proc. ACM Intl. Conference on Multimodal Interfaces* (pp. 162–170).

van Dijck, G., van Hulle, M., & Wevers, M. (2004). Genetic algorithm for feature subset selection with exploitation of feature correlations from continuous wavelet transform: a real-case application. *International Journal of Computational Intelligence*, *1*, 1–12.

Vapnik, V. (1998). *Statistical learning theory. Adaptive and Learning Systems for Signal Processing, Communications, and Control*. New York: John Wiley & Sons Inc.

Vapnik, V. N. (1995). *The Nature of Statistical Learning Theory*. New York: Springer-Verlag.

Vasilescu, M. A. O., & Terzopoulos, D. (2002). Multilinear Analysis of Image Ensembles: TensorFace. *ECCV*, 447-46.

Vetter, T., & Poggio, T. (1997). Linear object classes and image synthesis from a single example image. *IEEE Transactions on Pattern Analysis and Machine Intelligence*, *19*, 733–741. .doi:10.1109/34.598230

Vijaya, K., Bhagavatula, V. K., & Savvides, M. (2006). Correlation pattern recognition for face recognition. *Proceedings of the IEEE*, *94*(11), 1963–1975. doi:10.1109/JPROC.2006.884094

Viola, P., & Jones, M. (2001). Rapid object detection using a boosted cascade of simple features . In *IEEE Computer Vision and Pattern Recognition* (*Vol. 1*, pp. 511–518). CVPR.

Viola, P., & Jones, M. (2004). Robust Real-time Face Detection. *International Journal of Computer Vision*, 137–154. doi:10.1023/B:VISI.0000013087.49260.fb

Vukadinovec, D., & Pantic, M. (2005). Fully automatic facial feature point detection using Gabor feature based boosted classifiers. In *International Conference on Systems Man and Cybernetics*.

Wachsmuth, E., Oram, M. W., & Perrett, D. I. (1994). Recognition of objects and their component parts: responses of single units in the temporal cortex of the macaque. *Cerebral Cortex*, *4*(5), 509–522.

Wallraven, C., Breidt, M., Cunningham, D. W., & Bülthoff, H. (2008). Evaluating the perceptual realism of animated facial expressions. *TAP*, *4*(4).

Wang, X., Xiao, B., Ma, J. F., & Bi, X.-L. (2007). Scaling and rotation invariant approach to object recognition based on Radon and Fourier-Mellin transforms. *Pattern Recognition*, *40*, 3503–3508. doi:10.1016/j.patcog.2007.04.020

Wang, G. L., Kossenkov, A. V., & Ochs, M. F. (2006b). LS-NMF: a modified non-negative matrix factorization algorithm utilizing uncertainty estimates. *BMC Bioinformatics*, *7*, 175.

Wang, X., & Tang, X. (2006). Random sampling for subspace face recognition. *International Journal of Computer Vision*, *70*(1), 91–1042. doi:10.1007/s11263-006-8098-z

Wang, J. G., Sung, E., & Venkateswarlu, R. (2005). Estimating the eye gaze from one eye. *Computer Vision and Image Understanding*, *98*, 83–103. doi:10.1016/j.cviu.2004.07.008

Wang, L., & Fu, X. (2005). *Data Mining with Computational Intelligence*. Berlin: Springer.

Wang, F. (2006a). *Research of Face Detection Technology Based on Skin Color and Non-negative Matrix Factorization*. Master dissertation, Huaqiao University, China.

Wang, H. X., Zheng, W. M., & Hu, Z. L. (2007). Local and weighted maximum margin discriminant analysis. *Proc. CVPR*, *1*, 1-8.

Wang, H., Li, S. Z., Wang, Y., & Zhang, J. (2004). Self Quotient Image for Face Recognition. In *Proc. of the ICPR'04* (pp. 1397- 1400).

Wang, H., Yan, S., Huang, T., Liu, J., & Tang, X. (2008). Misalignment-robust face recognition. In *IEEE Computer Society Conference on Computer Vision and Pattern Recognition* (pp. 1–6).

Wang, X., & Tang, X. (2004). Dual-space linear discriminant analysis for face recognition. In *IEEE Computer Society Conference on Computer Vision and Pattern Recognition* (Vol. 2, pp. 564–569).

Wayman, J. L. (2002). Digital signal processing in biometric identification: A review. *Proc. ICIP, 1*, 37-40.

Wehrle, T., Kaiser, S., Schmidt, S., & Scherer, K. R. (2000). Studying the dynamics of emotional expression using synthesized facial muscle movements. *Journal of Personality and Social Psychology*, *78*(1), 105–119. doi:10.1037/0022-3514.78.1.105

Wen, Z., & Huang, T. S. (2004). *3D Face Processing: Modeling, Analysis and Synthesis*. Amsterdam: Kluwer Academic Publishers.

Weng, J., & Hwang, W.-S. (2007). Incremental Hierarchical Discriminant Regression. *IEEE Transactions on Neural Networks*, *18*(2), 397–415. doi:10.1109/TNN.2006.889942

Weschler, H. (2007). *Reliable Face Recognition Methods: System Design, Implementation and Evaluation*. New York: Springer.

Weyers, P., Mühlberger, A., Hefele, C., & Pauli, P. (2006). Electromyografic responses to static and dynamic avatar emotional facial expressions. *Psychophysiology*, *43*, 450–453. doi:10.1111/j.1469-8986.2006.00451.x

Whitehill, J., & Omlin, C. 2006). Haar Features for FACS AU Recognition. In *Proc. IEEE Int'l Conf. Face and Gesture Recognition* (pp. 5).

Widanagamaachchi, W. N., & Dharmaratne, A. T. (2008). 3D face reconstruction from 2D images: A survey. *Proc. Digital Image Computing: Techniques and Applications*, 365-371.

Wild, S., Curry, J., & Dougherty, A. (2004). Improving non-negative matrix factorizations through structured initialization. *Pattern Recognition*, *37*(11), 2217–2232.

Wiskott, L., Fellous, J. M., Kruger, N., & von der Malsburg, C. (1997). Face recognition by elastic bunch graph matching. *IEEE Transactions on Pattern Analysis and Machine Intelligence, 19*(July), 775–779. doi:10.1109/34.598235

Wolfrum, P., Wolff, C., Lucke, J., & von der Malsburg, C. (2008). A recurrent dynamic model for correspondence-based face recognition. *Journal of Vision (Charlottesville, Va.), 8*(7), 1–18. doi:10.1167/8.7.34

Wong, J.-J., & Cho, S.-Y. (2006). *Facial emotion recognition by adaptive processing of tree structures.* Paper presented at the Proceedings the 2006 ACM symposium on Applied computing, Dijon, France.

Wright, J., Yang, A. Y., Ganesh, A., Sastry, S. S., & Ma, Y. (2009). Robust Face Recognition via Sparse Representation. *IEEE Transactions on Pattern Analysis and Machine Intelligence, 2*(31), 210–227. doi:10.1109/TPAMI.2008.79

Wu, J., & Zhou, Z.-H. (2003). Efficient face candidates selector for face detection. *Pattern Recognition, 36*(5), 1175–1186. doi:10.1016/S0031-3203(02)00165-6

Wu, B. (2003). Comparison of statistical methods for classification of ovarian cancer using mass spectrometry data. *Bioinformatics (Oxford, England), 19*, 1636–1643. doi:10.1093/bioinformatics/btg210

Wu, Y., Liu, H., & Zha, H. (2005). *Modeling facial expression space for recognition.* Paper presented at the IEEE/RSJ International Conference on Intelligent Robots and Systems.

Xiang, T., Leung, M. K. H., & Cho, S. Y. (2007). Expression recognition using fuzzy spatio-temporal modeling. *Pattern Recognition, 41*(1), 204–216. doi:10.1016/j.patcog.2007.04.021

Xiao, R., Li, W., Tian, Y., & Tang, X. (2006). Joint boosting feature selection for robust face recognition. In *Proceedings of the IEEE Conference on Computer Vision and Pattern Recognition (CVPR 06)* (pp. 1415–1422).

Xiaogang, W., & Xiaoou, T. (2004). A unified framework for subspace face recognition. *IEEE Transactions on Pattern Analysis and Machine Intelligence, 26*(9), 1222–1228. doi:10.1109/TPAMI.2004.57

Xie, X., Sudhakar, R., & Zhuang, H. (1993). Corner detection by a cost minimization approach. *Pattern Recognition, 26*, 1235–1243. doi:10.1016/0031-3203(93)90208-E

Xie, X., & Lam, K.-M. (2006). Gabor based kernel PCA with doubly nonlinear mapping for face recognition with a single face image. *IEEE Transactions on Image Processing, 15*(9), 2481–2492. doi:10.1109/TIP.2006.877435

Xiujuan, C., Shiguang, S., Xilin, C., & Wen, G. (2007). Locally Linear Regression for Pose-Invariant Face Recognition. *IEEE Transactions on Image Processing, 7*(16), 1716–1725. doi:10.1109/TIP.2007.899195

Xu, C., Tan, T., Wang, Y., & Quan, L. (2006). Combining local features for robust nose location in 3D facial data. *Pattern Recognition Letters, 27*(13), 1487–1494. doi:10.1016/j.patrec.2006.02.015

Xu, D., Tao, D., Li, X., & Yan, S. (2007). Face Recognition - a Generalized Marginal Fisher Analysis Approach. *International Journal of Image and Graphics*, 583–591. doi:10.1142/S0219467807002817

Xudong, J., Mandal, B., & Kot, A. (2008). Eigenfeature regularization and extraction in face recognition. *IEEE Transactions on Pattern Analysis and Machine Intelligence, 30*(3), 383–394. doi:10.1109/TPAMI.2007.70708

Yacoob, Y., & Davis, L. S. (1996). Recognizing human facial expressions from long image sequences using optical flow. *IEEE Transactions on Pattern Analysis and Machine Intelligence, 18*, 636–642. doi:10.1109/34.506414

Yacoob, Y., & Davis, L. S. (1996). Recognizing Human Facial Expressions from Long Image Sequences using Optical Flow. *IEEE Transactions on Pattern Analysis and Machine Intelligence, 18*(6), 636–642. doi:10.1109/34.506414

Yale face database. (n.d.). Retrieved from http://cvc.yale.edu./projects/yalefaces/yalefaces.html

Yan, Y., & Zhang, Y. J. (2008b). Tensor correlation filter based class-dependence feature analysis for face recognition. *Neurocomputing, 71*(16-18), 3534–3543. doi:10.1016/j.neucom.2007.09.013

Yan, S., Hu, Y., Niyogi, P., He, X., Cai, D., & Zhang, H.-J. (2005). Face recognition using laplacianfaces. *IEEE Transactions on Pattern Analysis and Machine Intelligence, 27,* 328–340. doi:10.1109/TPAMI.2005.55

Yan, Y., & Zhang, Y.-J. (2008a). Tensor Correlation Filter Based Class-dependence Feature Analysis for Face Recognition. *Neurocomputing,* 3434–3438. doi:10.1016/j.neucom.2007.11.006

Yan, Y., & Zhang, Y.-J. (2008b). 1D Correlation Filter Based Class-Dependence Feature Analysis for Face Recognition. *Pattern Recognition,* 3834–3841. doi:10.1016/j.patcog.2008.05.028

Yang, J., & Yang, J. Y. (2001). An optimal FLD algorithm for facial feature extraction. *SPIE, 4572,* 438–444.

Yang, M. H., Kriegman, D. J., & Ahuja, N. (2002). Detecting faces in images: A survey. *IEEE Trans. PAMI, 24*(1), 34–58.

Yang, J., & Li, Y. (2006). Orthogonal relief algorithm for feature selection. *Lecture Notes in Computer Science, 4113,* 227–234. doi:10.1007/11816157_22

Yang, J., Frangi, A. F., & Yang, J. yu, & Jin, Z. (2005). KPCA plus LDA: A complete kernel fisher discriminant framework for feature extraction and recognition. *IEEE Transactions on Pattern Analysis and Machine Intelligence, 27*(2), 230–244. doi:10.1109/TPAMI.2005.33

Yang, J., Zhang, D., Frangi, A. F., & Yang, J.-Y. (2004). Two-dimensional PCA: a new approach to appearance-based face representation and recognition. *IEEE Transactions on Pattern Analysis and Machine Intelligence, 26*(1), 131–137. doi:10.1109/TPAMI.2004.1261097

Yang, M. H., Kriegman, D. J., & Ahuja, N. (2002). Detecting faces in images: A survey. *IEEE Transactions on Pattern Analysis and Machine Intelligence, 24*(1), 34–58. doi:10.1109/34.982883

Yang, J., Zhang, D., Frangi, A. F., et al. (2004). Two-dimensional PCA: A new approach to appearance-based face representation and recognition. *IEEE Trans. PAMI, 26*(1):), 131-137.

Yang, M. H. (2002). Kernel eigenfaces vs. kernel fisherfaces: face recognition using kernel methods. In *Proc. IEEE 5th Int. Conf. on Automatic Face and Gesture Recognition* (pp. 215-220).

Yang, P., Liu, Q., & Metaxas, D. N. (2007, July 2-5). Facial expression recognition using encoded dynamic features. In *Proceedings of IEEE International Conference on Multimedia and Expo (ICME 2007)*, Beijing, PR China (Vol. 1, pp. 1107-1110). Washington, DC: IEEE Press.

Yeasin, M., Bullot, B., & Sharma, R. (2006). Recognition of facial expressions and measurement of levels of interest from video. *IEEE Transactions on Multimedia, 8*(3), 500–508. doi:10.1109/TMM.2006.870737

Yilmaz, A., & Shah, M. A. (2002). Automatic feature detection and pose recovery for faces. *In Asian Conference on Computer Vision* (pp. 23-25).

Yin, R. K. (1969). Looking at upside-down faces. *Journal of Experimental Psychology, 81,* 141–145. doi:10.1037/h0027474

Yin, L., Chen, X., Sun, Y., Worm, T., & Reale, M. (2008, September 17-19). A high-resolution 3D dynamic facial expression database. In *Proceedings of IEEE International Conference on Automatic Face and Gesture Recognition (AFGR 2008)*, Amsterdam, The Netherlands. Washington, DC: IEEE Press

Young, A. W., Rowland, D., Calder, A. J., Etcoff, N. L., Seth, A., & Perrett, D. I. (1997). Facial expression megamix: Tests of dimensional and category accounts of emotion recognition. *Cognition, 63,* 271–313. doi:10.1016/S0010-0277(97)00003-6

Yovel, G., & Kanwisher, N. (2004). Face perception: Domain specific not process specific. *Neuron, 44,* 889–898.

Yovel, G., & Kanwisher, N. (2008). The representations of spacing and part-based information are associated for upright faces but dissociated for objects: Evidence from individual differences. *Psychonomic Bulletin & Review*, *15*, 933–939. doi:10.3758/PBR.15.5.933

Yu, W. W., Teng, X. L., & Liu, C. Q. (2006). Face recognition using discriminant locality preserving projections. *Image and Vision Computing*, *24*(3), 239–248. doi:10.1016/j.imavis.2005.11.006

Yu, H., & Yang, J. (2001, October). A direct LDA algorithm for high-dimensional data with application to face recognition. *Pattern Recognition*, *34*, 2067–2070. doi:10.1016/S0031-3203(00)00162-X

Yu, H., & Bennamoun, M. (2006). Complete invariants for robust face recognition. *Pattern Recognition*, *40*, 1579–1591. doi:10.1016/j.patcog.2006.08.010

Yu, H., & Yang, J. (2001). A direct LDA algorithm for high-dimensional data with application to face recognition. *Pattern Recognition, Elsevier*, *34*(12), 2067–2070. doi:10.1016/S0031-3203(00)00162-X

Yu, H., & Yang, J. (2001). A direct LDA algorithm for high-dimensional data with application to face recognition. *Pattern Recognition*, *34*, 2067–2070. .doi:10.1016/S0031-3203(00)00162-X

Yu, H., & Yang, J. (2001). A direct LDA algorithm for high-dimensional data with application to face recognition. *PR, 34*(10), 2067-2070.

Yuen, P. C., & Lai, J. H. (2002). *Face Representation using Independent Component Analysis*. Pattern Recognition.

Yuille, A., Hallinan, P., & Cohen, D. (1992, August). Feature extraction from faces using deformable templates. *International Journal of Computer Vision*, *8*(2), 99–111. doi:10.1007/BF00127169

Zafeiriou, S., Tefas, A., Buciu, I., & Pitas, I. (2006). Exploiting discriminant information in nonnegative matrix factorization with application to frontal face verification. *IEEE Transactions on Neural Networks*, *17*(3), 683–695.

Zdunek, R., & Cichocki, A. (2006). Non-negative matrix factorization with quasi-newton optimization. *Lecture Notes in Artificial Intelligence*, *4029*, 870–879.

Zeng, Z., Pantic, M., Roisman, G. I., & Huang, T. S. (2009). A Survey of Affect Recognition Methods: Audio, Visual, and Spontaneous Expressions. *IEEE Transactions on Pattern Analysis and Machine Intelligence*, *31*(1), 39–58. doi:10.1109/TPAMI.2008.52

Zeng, Z., Fu, Y., Roisman, G. I., Wen, Z., Hu, Y., & Huang, T. S. (2006). *One-class classification for spontaneous facial expression analysis*. Paper presented at the International Conference on Automatic Face and Gesture Recognition.

Zhang, X., Gao, Y., & Leung, M. K. H. (2008). Recognizing Rotated Faces From Frontal and Side Views: An Approach Toward Effective Use of Mugshot Databases. *IEEE Transactions on Information Forensics and Security*, *3*(4), 1966–1979. doi:10.1109/TIFS.2008.2004286

Zhang, B., Shan, S., Chen, X., & Gao, W. (2006). Histogram of Gabor Phase Patterns (HGPP), A Novel Object Representation Approach for Face Recognition. *IEEE Transactions on Image Processing*, 57–68.

Zhang, G., Huang, X., Li, S., Wang, Y., & Wu, X. (2004). Boosting local binary pattern (lbp)-based face recognition . In *SINOBIOMETRICS*. Berlin: Springer Verlag.

Zhang, B. L., Zhang, H., & Ge, S. S. (2004). Face recognition by applying wavelet subband representation and kernel associative memory. *IEEE Transactions on Neural Networks*, *15*(1), 166–177. doi:10.1109/TNN.2003.820673

Zhang, Y., & Martinez, A. (2006). A weighted probabilistic approach to face recognition from multiple images and video sequences. *Image and Vision Computing*, *24*(6), 626–638. doi:10.1016/j.imavis.2005.08.004

Zhang, B., Zhang, H., & Ge, S. (2004). Face recognition by applying wavelet subband representation and Kernel Associative Memories. *IEEE Transactions on Neural Networks*, *15*(1), 166–177. doi:10.1109/TNN.2003.820673

Zhang, Y., & Qiang, J. (2005). Active and dynamic information fusion for facial expression understanding from image sequences. *IEEE Transactions on Pattern Analysis and Machine Intelligence, 27*, 699–714. doi:10.1109/TPAMI.2005.93

Zhang, Y., & Ji, Q. (2005). Active and dynamic information fusion for facial expression understanding from image sequences. *IEEE Transactions on Pattern Analysis and Machine Intelligence, 27*(5), 699–714. doi:10.1109/TPAMI.2005.93

Zhang, T., Fang, B., Yuan, Y., Tang, Y. Y., Shang, Z., Li, D., & Lang, F. (2009). Multiscale Facial Structure Representation for Face Recognition Under Varying Illumination. *Pattern Recognition, 42*(2), 252–258. doi:10.1016/j.patcog.2008.03.017

Zhao, W., Chellappa, R., & Rosenfeld, A. (2003). Face recognition: A literature survey. *ACM Computing Surveys, 35*, 399–458. doi:10.1145/954339.954342

Zhao, W., Chellappa, R., & Phillips, P. J. (1999). *Subspace linear discriminant analysis for face recognition. Technical report, CAR-TR-914.* MD: Center for Automation Research, University of Maryland.

Zhao, W., Chellappa, R., Phillips, P. J., & Rosenfeld, A. (2003). Face Recognition: A Literature Survey. *ACM Computing Surveys*, 399–458. doi:10.1145/954339.954342

Zhao, H., & Pong, C., Y. (2008). Incremental Linear Discriminant Analysis for Face Recognition, *IEEE Transactions on Systems, Man and Cybernetics – Part B, 38*(1), 210-221.

Zhao, W., Chellappa, R., & Krishnaswamy, A. (1998). Discriminant analysis of principal components for face recognition. *FG, 336*–341.

Zhou, Z. H., & Geng, X. (2004). Projection functions for eye detection. *Pattern Recognition, 37*(5), 1049–1056. doi:10.1016/j.patcog.2003.09.006

Zhou, D., Yang, X., Peng, N., & Wang, Y. (2005). Improved LDA based face recognition using both global and local information. *Pattern Recognition Letters, 27*, 536–543. doi:10.1016/j.patrec.2005.09.015

Zhou, S., & Chellappa, R. (2004). Probabilistic identity characterization for face recognition. In *IEEE Computer Society Conference on Computer Vision and Pattern Recognition* (pp. 805–812).

Zhou, X. J., & Dillion, T. S. (1988). A Heuristic - Statistical Feature Selection Criterion For Inductive Machine Learning In The Real World. In *Proceedings of the 1988 IEEE International Conference on Systems, Man, and Cybernetics* (Vol. 1, pp. 548–552).

Zhu, M., & Martinez, A. (2006). Subclass discriminant analysis. *IEEE Transactions on Pattern Analysis and Machine Intelligence, 28*(8), 1274–1286. doi:10.1109/TPAMI.2006.172

Zhu, Y. F., Torre, F., Cohn, J. F., et al. (2009). Dynamic cascades with bidirectional bootstrapping for spontaneous facial action unit detection. *Proc. the Third International Conference on Affective Computing and Intelligent Interaction and Workshops*, 1-8.

Zou, H., Hastie, T., & Tibshirani, R. (2006). Sparse principal component analysis. *Journal of Computational and Graphical Statistics, 15*, 262–286. doi:10.1198/106186006X113430

Zou, J., Ji, Q., & Nagy, G. A. (2007). A comparative study of local matching approach for face recognition. *IEEE Transactions on Image Processing, 16*, 2617–2628. .doi:10.1109/TIP.2007.904421

Zou, X., Kittler, J., & Messer, K. (2007). Illumination Invariant Face Recognition: A Survey. In *Proc. of BTAS '07* (pp. 1-8).

Zou, X., Kittler, J., & Messer, K. (2007). Illumination invariant face recognition: A survey. *Proc. International Conference on Biometrics: Theory, Applications, and Systems*, 1-8.

Zuo, W., Zhang, D., & Wang, K. (2006). Bidirectional PCA with assembled matrix distance metric for image recognition. *IEEE Trans. SMC-B, 36*, 863–872.

About the Contributors

Yu-Jin Zhang, (zhang-yj@tsinghua.edu.cn) PhD, State University of Liège, Belgium, is Professor of Image Engineering at Tsinghua University, Beijing, China. Previously, he was with the Delft University of Technology, the Netherlands. In 2003, he spent the sabbatical year as visiting professor at National Technological University, Singapore. His research interests are mainly in the area of image engineering, including image processing, image analysis and image understanding, as well as their applications. He has published nearly 400 research papers and more than 20 books, including three monographs: *Image Segmentation* (Science Press, 2001), *Content-based Visual Information Retrieval* (Science Press, 2003) and *Subspace-based Face Recognition* (Tsinghua University Press, 2009), as well as two edited collections: *Advances in Image and Video Segmentation* (IRM Press, 2006) and *Semantic-based Visual Information Retrieval* (IRM Press, 2007). He is vice president of China Society of Image and Graphics and the director of the academic committee of the society. He is deputy editor-in-chief of *Journal of Image and Graphics* and at the editorial board of several international journals. He was the program co-chair of The First, Second, Fourth, and Fifth International Conference on Image and Graphics (ICIG'2000, ICIG'2002, ICIG'2007, and ICIG'2009). He is a senior member of IEEE.

* * *

M. Ashraful Amin (aminmdashraful@yahoo.com) received his B.Sc. degree in Computer Science from North South University of Bangladesh in 2002, the M.Sc. degree in Computer Science from Asian Institute of Technology, Thailand in 2005, and he completed doctoral studies in the department of Electrical Engineering at City University of Hong Kong in August 2009. His research interests include Facial Recognition, Pattern Recognition, and Biometrics.

Stylianos Asteriadis (stiast@image.ntua.gr) graduated from the School of Electrical and Computer Engineering of Aristotle University of Thessaloniki, Greece, in 2004. In 2006, he received his MSc degree on Digital Media from the Department of Informatics of the same University. He is currently with the Image, Video and Multimedia Systems Laboratory of the School of Electrical and Computer Engineering of National Technical University of Athens, where he is pursuing his PhD degree. His research interests include Image and Video Analysis, Stereovision, Pattern analysis and Human-Computer interaction.

Mohammed Bennamoun (bennamou@csse.uwa.edu.au) received his M.Sc. from Queen's University, Kingston, Canada in the area of Control Theory, and his PhD from Queen's /Q.U.T in Brisbane, Australia in the area of Computer Vision. He lectured Robotics at Queen's, and then joined QUT in

1993 as an Associate Lecturer. He then became a Lecturer in 1996 and a Senior Lecturer in 1998 at QUT. He was also the Director of a research Centre from 1998-2002. In Jan. 2003, he joined the Department of Computer Science and Software Engineering at The University of Western Australia (UWA) as an Associate Professor and was promoted to Professor in 2007. He has been the Head of the School of Computer Science and Software Engineering at UWA since February 2007. He was an Erasmus Mundus Scholar and Visiting Professor in 2006 at the University of Edinburgh. He was also Visiting Professor at CNRS (Centre National de la Recherche Scientifique) and Telecom Lille1, France in 2009, the Helsinki University of Technology in 2006, and the University of Bourgogne and Paris 13 in France in 2002-2003. He is the co-author of the book "Object Recognition: Fundamentals and Case Studies", Springer-Verlag, 2001. He won the "Best Supervisor of the Year" Award at QUT. He also received an award for research supervision at UWA in 2008. He published over 120 journal and conference publications. He served as a guest editor for a couple of special issues in International journals, such as the International Journal of Pattern Recognition and Artificial Intelligence (IJPRAI). He was selected to give conference tutorials at the European Conference on Computer Vision (ECCV) and the International Conference on Acoustics Speech and Signal Processing (IEEE ICASSP). He organized several special sessions for conferences; including a special session for the IEEE International Conference in Image Processing (IEEE ICIP). He was on the program committee of many conferences e.g. 3D Digital Imaging and Modeling (3DIM) and the International Conference on Computer Vision. He also contributed in the organization of many local and international conferences. His areas of interest include control theory, robotics, obstacle avoidance, object recognition, artificial neural networks, signal/image processing and computer vision (particularly 3D).

Siu-Yeung Cho (davidcho@pmail.ntu.edu.sg) is an Assistant Professor in School of Computer Engineering at Nanyang Technological University (NTU). Concurrently, he is the Director of Forensics and Security Laboratory (ForSe Lab) in the same school. Before joining NTU in 2003, he was a Research Fellow for The Hong Kong Polytechnic University and City University of Hong Kong between 2000-03, where he worked some projects for neural networks and adaptive image processing. He also leaded a project of content-based image analysis by novel machine learning model, which is one of the projects attached in the Centre for Multimedia Signal Processing at PolyU HK. Dr. Cho received his PhD and BEng(Hons) from the City University of Hong Kong and University of Brighton, UK, respectively, all in electronic and computer engineering. His research interests include neural networks and its applications, image analysis and 3D computer vision. He is also the co-inventor of Efficient Adaptive Processing of Data Structures, a novel machine-learning model to generalize objects in structural representation. Dr. Cho has published one monograph book, three book chapters, and over 50 technical papers in which more than 15 papers are in the top-notch international journals and conferences.

Maria De Marsico (demarsico@di.uniroma1.it) was born in Salerno, Italy, in 1963. She received the Laurea degree (cum laude) in Computer Science from the University of Salerno, Italy, in 1988. She is currently an Assistant Professor of Computer Science at Sapienza University of Rome. Her main research interests include Image processing, Multibiometric systems, Human-Computer Interaction. Maria De Marsico is a member of IEEE, ACM and IAPR.

Fadi Dornaika (fadi_dornaika@ehu.es) received the B.S. degree in electrical engineering from the Lebanese University, Tripoli, Lebanon, in 1990 and the M.S. and Ph.D. degrees in signal, image, and speech processing from the Institut National Polytechnique de Grenoble, France, in 1992 and 1995, respectively. He has worked at several research institutes including INRIA Rhône-Alpes, France, the Chinese University of Hong Kong, Linkoping University, Sweden, and the Computer Vision Center, Spain. He has published more than 100 papers in the field of computer vision. His research concerns geometrical and statistical modeling with focus on 3D object pose, real-time visual serving, calibration of visual sensors, cooperative stereo-motion, image registration, facial gesture tracking, and facial expression recognition.

Yuanjia Du (yuanjia.du@nxp.com) received the B.Eng. degree in Electronic Engineering from the Zhejiang University, China and the M.Sc. degree in Electronic Engineering from the Eindhoven University of Technology under the supervision of Prof. Gerard de Haan. Mr. Yuanjia Du is currently a Research Scientist in Trident Microsystems Europe B.V., Eindhoven, The Netherlands. Before joined Trident Microsystems, he was a research scientist in NXP Semiconductors Research Laboratories. Before that, he worked for 1 year as student intern in the Video Processing and Analysis Group, Philips Research Laboratories, Eindhoven, The Netherlands. His research interests include Multimedia Signal Post-Processing, Video Data Mining, Human Action/Activity Recognition, etc.

Sebastien Gadat (sebastien.gadat@math.univ-toulouse.fr) was born in 1978 in France. He is graduated from the "Centre de Mathématiques et de Leurs applications" (CMLA) from the ENS Cachan – FRANCE in 2004. He defended his thesis on the subject of feature extraction in signal processing and has published several papers in international journal on this topic. He is now "Maître de Conférences" in the Probability and Statistic Team of University Paul Sabatier in Toulouse. His actual research focuses on several fields of image processing. Among them: machine learning, statistical applications to signal processing, stochastic algorithms and statistical planning.

Zakia Hammal (zakia_hammal@yahoo.fr) graduated in Computer Science Engineering from the Institut National d'Informatique d'Alger (Algeria) in 2000. She obtained a master degree in Artificial Intelligence and Algorithmic from the Université de Caen (France) in 2002. She received her PhD degree in Cognitive Science from the Université Joseph Fourier at Grenoble (France) in 2006. Currently she is completing a post-doctoral position at the Université de Montréal at the Brain Music and Sound laboratory. Her main research topics include segmentation and analysis of facial features, affective computing, multimodal Human-Machine Interaction and visual perception.

Raghunath S. Holambe (rsholambe@sggs.ac.in) received the Ph.D. degree from Indian Institute of Technology, Kharagpur in India and he is presently a professor in Instrumentation Engineering in SGGS Institute of Engineering and Technology, Nanded (India). He has published several papers in international journals, and conferences. The areas of his research interest are Digital Signal Processing, Image Processing, Applications of Wavelet Transform, Biometrics, and real time signal processing using DSP Processors.

Dattatray V. Jadhav (dvjadhao@yahoo.com) received the B.E. degree in Electronics engineering from Marathwada University in 1991 and M. Tech. degree in 1997 from Dr. B. A. Marathwada University, India. He has received Ph. D. degree from S. G. G. S. Institute of Engineering and Technology, Nanded, India. Presently he is a professor in Electronics Engineering Department of Vishwakarma Institute of

Technology, Pune. He has published several papers in international journals, and conferences. He is the recipient of ISTE National award 2008 for outstanding research work in Pattern Recognition. His areas of interests include computer vision, biometrics and image processing.

Marios Kyperountas (marioskyperountas@yahoo.com) received the B.Sc. in Electrical Engineering in 2002 and the M.Sc. in Electrical Engineering in 2003, both from Florida Atlantic University in Boca Raton, Florida, where he graduated Summa Cum Laude. He was a research assistant at the FAU Imaging Technology Center from 2000 until 2003 where he worked on several high-resolution imaging R&D projects funded by NASA, DARPA and the US NAVY. From 2003 until 2005, he was a researcher at the Artificial Intelligence and Information Analysis lab of Aristotle University of Thessaloniki, in Greece. Currently, he is a PhD candidate of the Department of Informatics at AUTh and works as an Image Processing Engineer in Santa Barbara, California. His research interests include real-time video processing, pattern recognition, ultrasonic imaging, DSP algorithms, and medical imaging. Mr. Kyperountas is a member of the Golden Key Honor Society, Phi-Kappa-Phi Honor Society and Tau-Beta-Pi Engineering Honor Society.

Le Li (lile05@mails.tsinghua.edu.cn) received the Ph.D. degree in Electric Engineering from Tsinghua University, Beijing, 2009. His research interests are mainly in matrix factorization and image engineering. His current research interests are focused on non-negative matrix factorization and its applications to image engineering.

Peng Li (P.Li@cs.ucl.ac.uk) received the B. Eng and M. Eng. from North China Electric Power University, and the PhD degree in Electrical and Electronic Engineering from the Nanyang Technological University, Singapore, in 2006. He was a lecturer in North China Electric Power University from 1998 to 2002. From 2005 to 2007, he was a computer vision engineer in Stratech Systems Ltd. Singapore. He was a research associate in University of Bristol in 2007. He is now a research fellow in the Department of Computer Science, University College London, United Kingdom. His research interests include computer vision and machine learning, particularly in face recognition and kernel methods, etc. He is a member of IEEE.

Michele Nappi (mnappi@unisa.it) was born in Naples, Italy, in 1965. He received the laurea degree (cum laude) in computer science from the University of Salerno, Salerno, Italy, in 1991, the M.Sc. degree in information and communication technology from I.I.A.S.S. 'E.R. Caianiello,' Vietri sul Mare, Salerno, and the Ph.D. degree in applied mathematics and computer science from the University of Padova, Padova, Italy. He is currently an Associate Professor of computer science at the University of Salerno. His research interests include pattern recognition, image processing, compression and indexing, multimedia databases and visual languages. Dr. Nappi is a member of IAPR.

Imran Naseem (imran.naseem@ee.uwa.edu.au) is a PhD candidate with the School of EEC Engineering, UWA. His research areas are related to biometric recognition systems with an emphasis on face technology. In particular, he has proposed novel face recognition algorithms based on regression methods to demonstrate improvement over the benchmark systems. In his research, he has used robust estimation to address several robustness issues in the paradigm of face recognition. From his current research, he has already registered fifteen international papers in the most prestigious journals and conferences in pattern recognition and image processing including IEEE TPAMI and ICIP.

Yok-Yen Nguwi (yokyen@gmail.com) is currently a Ph.D. Candidate at Nanyang Technological University, Singapore. She is doing research at the Centre for Computational Intelligence with Dr. Cho Siu-Yeung, David. She received her BEng degree (Class I hons) in Computer Engineering from The University of Newcastle, Australia. Her research interest includes neuroscience, neural networks, and computer vision.

Nikos Nikolaidis (nikolaid@aiia.csd.auth.gr) received the Diploma of Electrical Engineering in 1991 and the PhD degree in Electrical Engineering in 1997, both from the Aristotle University of Thessaloniki, Greece. From 1998 to 2002 he was postdoctoral researcher and teaching assistant at the Department of Informatics, Aristotle University of Thessaloniki. He is currently an Assistant Professor in the same Department. Dr. Nikolaidis is the co-author of the book "3-D Image Processing Algorithms:" (Wiley, 2000). He has co-authored 13 book chapters, 34 journal papers and 97 conference papers. His research interests include computer graphics, image and video processing and analysis, copyright protection of multimedia, computer vision and 3-D image processing. Dr. Nikolaidis is a Senior Member of IEEE and is currently serving as associate editor for the EURASIP Journal on Image and Video Processing, the International Journal of Innovative Computing, Information and Control the Innovative Computing, Information and Control Express Letters and the Journal of Information Hiding and Multimedia Signal Processing.

Nikola Pavešić (nikola.pavesic@fe.uni-lj.si) received his B.Sc. degree in electronics, M.Sc. degree in automatics, and Ph.D. degree in electrical engineering from the University of Ljubljana, Slovenia, in 1970, 1973 and 1976, respectively. Since 1970, he has been a staff member at the Faculty of Electrical Engineering in Ljubljana, where he is currently head of the Laboratory of Artificial Perception, Systems and Cybernetics. His research interests include pattern recognition, neural networks, image processing, speech processing, and information theory. He is the author and co-author of more than 200 papers and 3 books addressing several aspects of the above areas. Professor Nikola Pavešić is a member of IEEE, the Slovenian Association of Electrical Engineers and Technicians (Meritorious Member), the Slovenian Pattern Recognition Society, and the Slovenian Society for Medical and Biological Engineers.

Ioannis Pitas (pitas@aiia.csd.auth.gr) received the Diploma of Electrical Engineering in 1980 and the PhD degree in Electrical Engineering in 1985 both from the Aristotle University of Thessaloniki, Greece. Since 1994, he has been a Professor at the Department of Informatics, Aristotle University of Thessaloniki. From 1980 to 1993 he served as Scientific Assistant, Lecturer, Assistant Professor, and Associate Professor in the Department of Electrical and Computer Engineering at the same University. He served as a Visiting Research Associate or Visiting Assistant Professor at several Universities. He has published 194 journal papers, 443 conference papers and contributed in 31 books in his areas of interest and edited or co-authored another 7. He has also been an invited speaker and/or member of the program committee of several scientific conferences and workshops. In the past he served as Associate Editor or co-Editor of four international journals and General or Technical Chair of three international conferences. His current interests are in the areas of digital image and video processing and analysis, medical image analysis, multidimensional signal processing, copyright protection of multimedia and computer vision. Prof. Pitas is an IEEE Fellow and member of the National Research Council of Greece.

Simon J. D. Prince (S.Prince@cs.ucl.ac.uk) received his Ph.D. in 1999 from the University of Oxford for work concerning the study of human stereo vision. He has a diverse background in biological and computing sciences and has published papers across the fields of biometrics, psychology, physiology, medical imaging, computer vision, computer graphics and human computer interaction. He previously worked as a postdoctoral research scientist in Oxford, Singapore and Toronto. Dr. Prince is currently a senior lecturer in the Department of Computer Science at University College London. He is a member of the IEEE and ACM Computing Society.

Bogdan Raducanu (bogdan@cvc.uab.es) received the B.Sc, in computer science from the University "Politehnica" of Bucharest (PUB), Romania, in 1995 and the Ph.D. *'cum laude'*, also in computer science, from the University of The Basque Country (UPV/EHU), Spain in 2001. Currently, he is a senior researcher at the Computer Vision Center in Barcelona, Spain. His research interests include computer vision, pattern recognition, artificial intelligence and social robotics.

Sam S. Rakover: (rakover@psy.haifa.ac.il) Areas of interest are fear and avoidance learning in animals (in the past), philosophy of science and mind, and face perception and recognition. His list of publications includes about eighty professional papers and four books: *Metapsychology: Missing links in behavior, mind and science* (1990); *Face recognition: cognitive and computational processes* (Rakover & Cahlon, 2001); *Explanation: theoretical approaches and applications* (Hon & Rakover, Eds., 2001); *To understand a cat: methodology and philosophy* (2007). Rakover has also published six novels and many short stories (in Hebrew).

Daniel Riccio (driccio@unisa.it) was born in Cambridge, United Kingdom, in 1978. He received the laurea degree (cum laude) and the Ph.D. in computer science from the University of Salerno in 2002 and 2006. He is currently an Assistant Professor at the University of Salerno. His research interests include biometrics, fractal image compression and indexing. He is a member of GIRPR since 2004.

Lior Shamir (shamirl@mail.nih.gov) received the Bachelor's degree in Computer Science from Tel Aviv University, Tel Aviv, Israel, and the Ph.D. degree from Michigan Tech. He is a Research Fellow in Laboratory of Genetics, National Institute on Aging, National Institutes of Health, Baltimore, MD.

Ling Shao (ling.shao at sheffield.ac.uk) received the B.Eng. degree in Electronic Engineering from the University of Science and Technology of China (USTC), the M.Sc. degree in Medical Image Analysis and the Ph.D. (D.Phil.) degree in Computer Vision at the Robotics Research Group from the University of Oxford. Dr. Shao is currently a Senior Lecturer (Associate Professor) in the Department of Electronic and Electrical Engineering at the University of Sheffield. Before joining Sheffield University, he worked for 4 years as a Senior Research Scientist in the Video Processing and Analysis Group, Philips Research Laboratories, The Netherlands. His research interests include Multimedia Signal Processing, Video Search and Mining, Human Action/Activity Recognition, Content Based Multimedia Retrieval, Human-Computer Interaction, etc. Dr. Shao has published over 50 academic papers in refereed journals and conference proceedings and has filed 9 patent applications. He is an associate editor of the International Journal of Image and Graphics and the EURASIP Journal on Advances in Signal Processing, a guest editor of IEEE Journal of Selected Topics in Signal Processing and EURASIP Journal on Image and Video Processing, and serves on the editorial boards of several other journals.

Vitomir Štruc (vitomir.struc@fe.uni-lj.si) received his B.Sc. degree in electrical engineering from the University of Ljubljana in 2005. In 2007, he became a staff member at the Laboratory of Artificial Perception, Systems and Cybernetics of the Faculty of Electrical Engineering, where he is currently working as a researcher. His research interests include pattern recognition, machine learning, image processing, face and palm-print recognition as well as biometrics in general. He has authored and co-authored more than 20 papers and 2 books addressing different aspects of the above areas. He participates in research projects related to biometric security systems, human-machine interaction, secure communications and others. Vitomir Štruc is also a member of the Slovenian Pattern Recognition Society.

Anastasios Tefas (tefas@aiia.csd.auth.gr) received the B.Sc. in informatics in 1997 and the Ph.D. degree in informatics in 2002, both from the Aristotle University of Thessaloniki, Greece. Since 2008, he has been a Lecturer at the Department of Informatics, Aristotle University of Thessaloniki. From 2006 to 2008, he was an Assistant Professor at the Department of Information Management, Technological Institute of Kavala. From 2003 to 2004, he was a temporary lecturer in the Department of Informatics, University of Thessaloniki. From 1997 to 2002, he was a researcher and teaching assistant in the same department. He has co-authored over 70 journal and conference papers and contributed 2 chapters in edited books, with over 400 third researcher citations. His current research interests include computational intelligence, pattern recognition, statistical machine learning, digital signal and image processing and computer vision. Dr. Tefas participated in 10 research projects financed by national and European funds.

Teik-Toe Teoh (TEOH0065@ntu.edu.sg) is currently a PHD candidate at Nanyang Technological University, Singapore. He received his Master of Science in Computer Engineering from University of Southern California and Bachelor of Science in Electrical Engineering (Hons) from same school. His current research is on Computational modeling of human emotion using machine learning.

Roberto Togneri (roberto@ee.uwa.edu.au) received the B.E. degree in 1985 and the Ph.D. degree in 1989 both from the University of Western Australia. He joined the School of Electrical, Electronic and Computer Engineering at The University of Western Australia in 1998 as a Senior Tutor, appointed to Lecturer in 1992 and then Senior Lecturer in 1997. His research activities include signal processing and robust feature extraction of speech signals, statistical and neural network models for speech and speaker recognition, and related aspects of communications, information retrieval, and pattern recognition. He has published over 70 refereed journal and conference papers in the areas of spoken language and information systems and was co-author of the book "Fundamentals of Information Theory and Coding Design", Chapman & Hall/CRC, 2003. Dr. Togneri is currently a member of the Signals and Systems Engineering Research Group and heads the Signal and Information Processing Lab. He is a senior member of IEEE.

Sergio Vitulano (vitulano@vaxca1.unica.it) was born in Milan in 1940. He graduated in nuclear physics at the University of Naples "Federico II" in 1974 and received the Ph.D. in Cybernetics from the University of Salerno in 1976, where he taught image processing until 1992. Presently, he is Associate

Professor of Computer Science at the University of Cagliari, he is interested in image processing, pattern recognition and medical imaging. He is a member of IAPR and IASTED.

Hong Yan (h.yan@cityu.edu.hk) received his Ph.D. degree from Yale University. He was a professor in electrical and information engineering at the University of Sydney and is currently a professor in electronic engineering at City University of Hong Kong. His research interests include image processing, pattern recognition and bioinformatics and he has over 300 journal and conference publications in these areas. Professor Yan is a fellow of the Institute of Electrical and Electronics Engineers (IEEE), the International Association of Patten Recognition (IAPR) and the Institution of Engineers, Australia (IEAust).

Index